From the publi

Nursing™

THE SERIES FOR CLINICAL EXCELLENCE

Perfecting Clinical Procedures

Wolters Kluwer Health | Lippincott Williams & Wilkins

Philadelphia • Baltimore • New York • London
Buenos Aires • Hong Kong • Sydney • Tokyo

Staff

Executive Publisher
Judith A. Schilling McCann, RN, MSN

Editorial Director
H. Nancy Holmes

Clinical Director
Joan M. Robinson, RN, MSN

Art Director
Elaine Kasmer

Editorial Project Manager
Jennifer Santambrosio Kowalak

Clinical Project Manager
Jennifer Meyering, RN, BSN, MS, CCRN

Editor
Julie Munden

Copy Editors
Kimberly Bilotta (supervisor), Scotti Cohn, Heather Ditch, Jen Fielding, Elizabeth Mooney, Dona Perkins, Dorothy P. Terry, Pamela Wingrod

Designers
Joseph John Clark (project manager and cover design), Lynn Foulk (book design)

Digital Composition Services
Diane Paluba (manager), Joyce Rossi Biletz, Donna S. Morris

Manufacturing
Beth J. Welsh

Editorial Assistants
Megan L. Aldinger, Karen J. Kirk, Linda K. Ruhf

Design Assistant
Georg W. Purvis IV

Indexer
Barbara Hodgson

NSPCP010407

Library of Congress Cataloging-in-Publication Data

Nursing. Perfecting clinical procedures.
p. ; cm.
Includes bibliographical references and index.
1. Nursing—Handbooks, manuals, etc. I. Lippincott Williams & Wilkins.
[DNLM: 1. Nursing Care—Handbooks. WY 49 N9749 2007]
RT41.N866 2007
610.73--dc22 2007000194
ISBN-13: 978-1-58255-664-2 (alk. paper)
ISBN-10: 1-58255-664-4 (alk. paper)

Contents

Contributors and consultants

Katrina D. Allen, RN, MSN, CCRN
Nursing Faculty
Faulkner State Community College
Bay Minette, Ala.

Helen C. Ballestas, RN, MSN, CRRN, PhD(C)
Nurse Educator
New York Institute of Technology
Old Westbury

Rita Bates, RN, MSN
Assistant Professor
College of Health Sciences
University of Arkansas
Fort Smith

JoAnn C. Green, RN, MSN, CCRN, CNS
Clinical Nurse Specialist, Cardiac Services
Lakeland (Fla.) Regional Medical Center

Patrick Kenny, RN, EdD, ACRN, CAN, BC, C
Director of Nursing Education & Research
Penn Presbyterian Medical Center
Philadelphia

Emily Karwacki Sheff, RN, MS, APRN,BC
Registered Nurse
Massachusetts General Hospital
Lecturer
Massachusetts General Hospital/Institute of Health Professions
Clinical Instructor
Boston College

A

Admixture of drugs in a syringe

Combining two drugs into one syringe avoids the discomfort of two injections. Typically, drugs can be mixed in a syringe in one of four ways: from two multidose vials (for example, regular and long-acting insulin), from one multidose vial and one ampule, from two ampules, or from a cartridge-injection system combined with either a multidose vial or an ampule.

Drug combinations are contraindicated when the drugs aren't compatible and when the combined doses exceed the amount of solution that can be absorbed from a single injection site.

Equipment

Prescribed medications ♦ patient's medication record and chart ♦ alcohol pads, syringe, and needle ♦ optional: cartridge-injection system and filter needle

The type and size of the syringe and needle depend on the prescribed medications, patient's body build, and route of administration. Medications that come in prefilled cartridges require a cartridge-injection system. (See *Cartridge-injection system.*)

Key steps

- Verify that the drugs to be administered agree with the patient's medication record and the prescriber's orders.
- Calculate the dose to be given.
- Wash your hands.

Cartridge-injection system

A cartridge-injection system, such as Tubex or Carpuject, is a convenient, easy-to-use method of injection that facilitates accuracy and sterility. The device consists of a plastic cartridge-holder syringe and a prefilled medication cartridge with a needle attached.

The medication in the cartridge is premixed and premeasured, saving time and helping to ensure an exact dose. The medication remains sealed in the cartridge and sterile until the injection is administered to the patient.

The disadvantage of this system is that not all drugs are available in cartridge form. However, compatible drugs can be added to partially filled cartridges.

Mixing drugs from two multidose vials

- Using an alcohol pad, wipe the rubber stopper on the first vial. This decreases the risk of contaminating the medication as you insert the needle into the vial.
- Pull back the syringe plunger until the volume of air drawn into the syringe equals the volume to be withdrawn from the drug vial.
- Without inverting the vial, insert the needle into the top of the vial, making sure that the needle's bevel tip doesn't touch the solution. Inject the air into the vial and withdraw the needle. This replaces air in

the vial, thus preventing creation of a partial vacuum on withdrawal of the drug.
- Repeat the steps above for the second vial. Then, after injecting the air into the second vial, invert the vial, withdraw the prescribed dose, and then withdraw the needle.
- Wipe the rubber stopper of the first vial again and insert the needle, taking care not to depress the plunger. Invert the vial, withdraw the prescribed dose, and then withdraw the needle.

Mixing drugs from a multidose vial and an ampule

- Using an alcohol pad, clean the vial's rubber stopper.
- Pull back on the syringe plunger until the volume of air drawn into the syringe equals the volume to be withdrawn from the drug vial.
- Insert the needle into the top of the vial and inject the air. Then invert the vial and keep the needle's bevel tip below the level of the solution as you withdraw the prescribed dose. Put the sterile needle cover over the needle.
- Wrap a sterile gauze pad or an alcohol pad around the ampule's neck to protect yourself from injury in case the glass splinters. Break open the ampule, directing the force away from you.
- If desired, switch to the filter needle at this point to filter out any glass splinters.
- Insert the needle into the ampule. Be careful not to touch the outside of the ampule with the needle. Draw the correct dose into the syringe.
- If you switched to the filter needle, change back to a regular needle to administer the injection.

Mixing drugs from two ampules

- An opened ampule doesn't contain a vacuum. To mix drugs from two ampules in a syringe, calculate the prescribed doses and open both ampules, using sterile technique. If desired, use a filter needle to draw up the drugs. Then change to a regular needle to administer them.

Special considerations

- Insert the needle through the vial's rubber stopper at a slight angle, bevel up, and exert slight lateral pressure. This way you won't cut a piece of rubber out of the stopper, which can then be pushed into the vial.
- When mixing drugs from multidose vials, be careful not to contaminate one drug with the other. Ideally, the needle should be changed after drawing the first medication into the syringe. This isn't always possible because many disposable syringes don't have removable needles.

DO'S & DON'TS

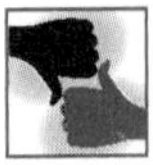

Never combine drugs if you're unsure of their compatibility, and never combine more than two drugs. Although drug incompatibility usually causes a visible reaction, such as clouding, bubbling, or precipitation, some incompatible combinations produce no visible reaction even though they alter the chemical nature and action of the drugs. Check appropriate references and consult a pharmacist when you're unsure about specific compatibility. When in doubt, administer two separate injections.

- Some medications are compatible for only a brief time after being combined and should be administered within 10 minutes after mixing. After this time, environmental factors, such as temperature, exposure to light, and humidity, may alter compatibility.
- To reduce the risk of contamination, most health care facilities dispense parenteral medications in single-dose vials. Insulin is one of the few drugs still packaged in multidose vials. Be careful when mixing regular and long-acting insulin. Draw up the regular insulin first to avoid contamination by the long-acting suspension. (If a minute amount of the regular insulin is accidentally mixed with the long-acting insulin, it won't appreciably change the effect of the long-acting insulin.) Check your facility's policy before mixing insulins.
- When you combine a cartridge-injection system and a multidose vial, use a separate

Diseases requiring airborne precautions

Disease	Precautionary period
Chickenpox (varicella)	Until lesions are crusted and no new lesions appear
Herpes zoster (disseminated)	Duration of illness
Herpes zoster (localized in immunocompromised patient)	Duration of illness
Measles (rubeola)	Duration of illness
Tuberculosis (TB)—pulmonary or laryngeal, confirmed or suspected	Depends on clinical response; patient must be on effective therapy, be improving clinically (decreased cough and fever and improved findings on chest X-ray), and have three consecutive negative sputum smears collected on different days, or TB must be ruled out

needle and syringe to inject air into the multidose vial. This prevents contamination of the multidose vial by the cartridge-injection system.

Complications

None

Documentation

Record the drugs administered, injection site, and time of administration. Document adverse drug effects or other pertinent information.

Airborne precautions

Airborne precautions, used in addition to standard precautions, prevent the spread of infectious diseases transmitted by droplet nuclei 5 µm or smaller that are breathed, sneezed, or coughed into the environment. (See *Diseases requiring airborne precautions.*)

To effectively guard against the spread of infection from an airborne transmitted infection, an isolation patient requires a monitored negative-pressure room with the door kept closed to maintain the proper air pressure balance in the isolation room, the anteroom, and the adjoining hallway or corridor. The air should be appropriately discharged directly to the outside of the building or filtered through high-efficiency particulate air (HEPA) filtration before it's circulated to other areas of the health care facility. If for some reason a private room isn't available, patients infected with the same disease can share a room, but consultation with infection control professionals is advised before patient placement.

Everyone who enters the patient's room must wear respiratory protection. Regardless of the type of respirator used, the health care worker must make sure that the respirator properly fits his face, covering the mouth and nose, each time he wears it. If the patient must leave the room for an essential procedure, he should wear a surgical mask to cover his nose and mouth while out of the room. Personnel in the area where the patient is going should be notified and instructed to take airborne precautions.

Equipment

Respirators (either disposable N95 or HEPA respirators or reusable HEPA respirators or powered air purifying respirators) ♦ surgical masks ♦ isolation door card ♦

other personal protective equipment as needed for standard precautions

Gather additional supplies needed for routine patient care, such as a thermometer, stethoscope, and blood pressure cuff.

Preparation

- Keep airborne precaution supplies outside the patient's room in a cart or anteroom.

Key steps

- Situate the patient in a negative-pressure room with the door closed. If possible, the room should have an anteroom, and it should be possible to monitor the negative pressure. If necessary, two patients with the same infection may share a room. Explain isolation precautions to the patient and his family.
- Keep the patient's door (and the anteroom door) closed at all times to maintain the negative pressure and contain the airborne pathogens. Put an airborne precautions sign on the door to notify anyone entering the room.
- Put your respirator on according to the manufacturer's directions. Adjust the straps for a firm but comfortable fit. Check the fit.
- Instruct the patient to cover his nose and mouth with a facial tissue while coughing or sneezing.
- Tape an impervious bag to the patient's bedside so the patient can dispose of facial tissues correctly.
- Make sure that visitors wear respiratory protection while in the patient's room.
- Limit the patient's movement from the room. If he must leave the room for essential procedures, make sure he wears a surgical mask over his nose and mouth. Notify the receiving department or area of the patient's isolation precautions so that the precautions will be maintained and the patient can be returned to his room promptly.
- All negative-pressure rooms require constant monitoring usually via electronic devices. When the monitor's alarm sounds, it indicates a problem with negative pressure.

Special considerations

- Before leaving the room, remove gloves (if worn), and wash your hands. Remove your respirator outside the patient's room after closing the door.
- Depending on the type of respirator and recommendations from the manufacturer, follow your facility's policy and either discard your respirator or store it until the next use. If your respirator is to be stored until the next use, store it in a dry, well-ventilated place (not a plastic bag) to prevent microbial growth. Nondisposable respirators must be cleaned according to the manufacturer's recommendations.

Complications

None

Patient teaching

- Explain isolation precautions to the patient and his family.
- Tell the patient that visitors shouldn't be immunocompromised.
- Instruct the patient to cover his nose and mouth with a facial tissue when coughing or sneezing.

Documentation

Record the need for airborne precautions on the nursing care plan and as otherwise indicated by your facility. Document initiation and maintenance of the precautions, the patient's tolerance of the procedure, and any patient or family teaching. Also document the date airborne precautions were discontinued.

Antiembolism stocking application

The use of elastic antiembolism stockings helps to prevent deep vein thrombosis (DVT) and pulmonary embolism by compressing the patient's superficial leg veins. This compression increases venous return by forcing blood into the deep venous system rather than allowing it to pool in the legs and form clots.

Applying antiembolism stockings helps to provide equal pressure over the patient's entire leg or a graded pressure that's greatest at the ankle and decreases over the length of the leg. Usually indicated for the postoperative, bedridden, elderly, or other patient at risk for DVT, these stockings shouldn't be used on the patient with dermatoses or open skin lesions, gangrene, severe arteriosclerosis or other ischemic vascular diseases, pulmonary or any massive edema, recent vein ligation, or vascular or skin grafts. For the patient with chronic venous problems, intermittent pneumatic compression stockings may be worn during surgery and postoperatively.

Equipment

Tape measure ♦ antiembolism stockings of correct size and length ♦ talcum powder

Preparation

- Obtain the correct size stocking according to the manufacturer's specifications.
- If the patient's measurements are outside the range indicated by the manufacturer or if his legs are deformed or edematous, ask the practitioner if he wants to order custom-made stockings.

Before applying a knee-length stocking

Measure the circumference of the patient's calf at its widest point and leg length from the bottom of the heel to the back of the knee. (See *Measuring for antiembolism stockings*, page 6.)

Before applying a thigh-length stocking

Measure the circumference of the calf and thigh at their widest points and the leg length from the bottom of the heel to the gluteal fold.

Before applying a waist-length stocking

Measure the circumference of the calf and thigh at their widest points and the leg length from the bottom of the heel along the side to the waist.

Key steps

- Check the practitioner's order, and assess the patient's condition. If his legs are cold or cyanotic, notify the practitioner before proceeding.
- Explain the procedure to the patient, provide privacy, and wash your hands thoroughly.
- Have the patient lie down. Then dust his ankle with talcum powder to ease application.

Applying a knee-length stocking

- Insert your hand into the stocking from the top, and grasp the heel pocket from the inside. Holding the heel, turn the stocking inside out so that the foot is inside the stocking leg. This method allows easier application than gathering the entire stocking and working it up over the foot and ankle.
- With the heel pocket down, hook the index and middle fingers of both your hands into the foot section. Facing the patient, ease the stocking over the toes, stretching it sideways as you move it up the foot.
- Support the patient's ankle with one hand, and use the other hand to pull the heel pocket under the heel. Then center the heel in the pocket.
- Gather the loose portion of the stocking at the toe, and pull only this section over the heel. Gather the loose material at the ankle, and slide the rest of the stocking up over the heel with short pulls, alternating front and back.
- Insert your index and middle fingers into the gathered stocking at the ankle, and ease the fabric up the leg to the knee.
- Supporting the patient's ankle with one hand, use your other hand to stretch the stocking toward the knee, front and back, to distribute the material evenly. The stocking top should be 1″ to 2″ (2.5 to 5 cm) below the bottom of the patella.
- Gently snap the fabric around the ankle to ensure a tight fit and eliminate gaps that could reduce pressure.
- Adjust the foot section for fabric smoothness and toe comfort by tugging on the toe section. Properly position the toe window, if any.
- Repeat the procedure for the second stocking, if ordered.

Measuring for antiembolism stockings

Measure the patient carefully to ensure that his antiembolism stockings provide enough compression for adequate venous return.

To choose the correct *knee-length* stocking, measure the circumference of the calf at its widest point (top left) and the leg length from the bottom of the heel to the back of the knee (bottom left).

To choose a *thigh-length* stocking, measure the calf as for a knee-length stocking and the thigh at its widest point (top right). Then measure leg length from the bottom of the heel to the gluteal fold (bottom right).

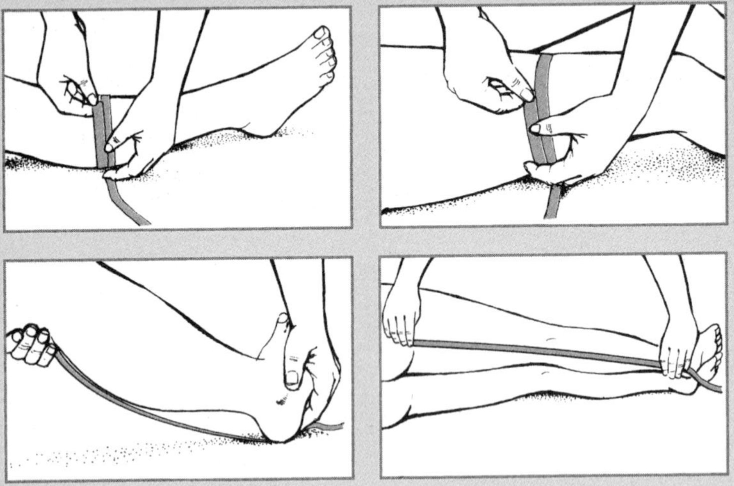

Applying a thigh-length stocking

- Follow the procedure for applying a knee-length stocking, taking care to distribute the fabric evenly below the knee before continuing the procedure.
- With the patient's leg extended, stretch the rest of the stocking over the knee.
- Flex the patient's knee, and pull the stocking over the thigh until the top is 1″ to 3″ (2.5 to 7.5 cm) below the gluteal fold.
- Stretch the stocking from the top, front and back, to distribute the fabric evenly over the thigh.
- Gently snap the fabric behind the knee to eliminate gaps that could reduce pressure.

Applying a waist-length stocking

- Follow the procedure for applying knee-length and thigh-length stockings, and extend the stocking top to the gluteal fold.
- Fit the patient with the adjustable belt that accompanies the stockings. Make sure the waistband and the fabric don't interfere with any incision, drainage tube, catheter, or other device.

Special considerations

- Apply the stockings in the morning, if possible, before edema develops. If the patient has been ambulating, ask him to lie down and elevate his legs for 15 to 30 minutes before applying the stockings to facilitate venous return.

Do's & don'ts

Don't allow the stockings to roll or turn down at the top or toe because the excess pressure could cause venous strangulation.

- Have the patient wear the stockings in bed and during ambulation to provide continuous protection against thrombosis.
- Check the patient's toes at least once every 4 hours—more often in the patient with a faint pulse or edema. Note skin color and temperature, sensation, swelling, and ability to move. If complications occur, remove the stockings and notify the practitioner immediately.
- Be alert for an allergic reaction because some patients can't tolerate the sizing in new stockings. Laundering the stockings before applying them reduces the risk of an allergic reaction to sizing. Remove the stockings at least once daily to bathe the skin and observe for irritation and breakdown.
- Using warm water and mild soap, wash the stockings when soiled. Keep a second pair handy for the patient to wear while the other pair is being laundered.

Complications

- Arterial blood flow obstruction (characterized by cold and bluish toes, dusky toenail beds, decreased or absent pedal pulses, and leg pain or cramps)
- Allergic reaction and skin irritation

Patient teaching

- If the patient will require antiembolism stockings after discharge, teach him or a family member how to apply them correctly and explain why he needs to wear them.
- Instruct the patient or family member to care for the stockings properly and to replace them when they lose elasticity.

Documentation

Record the date and time of stocking application and removal, stocking length and size, condition of the leg before and after treatment, condition of the toes during treatment, any complications, and the patient's tolerance of the treatment.

Arterial pressure monitoring

Direct arterial pressure monitoring permits continuous measurement of the patient's systolic, diastolic, and mean blood pressures and allows arterial blood sampling. Because direct measurement reflects systemic vascular resistance as well as blood flow, it's generally more accurate than indirect methods (such as palpation and auscultation of Korotkoff, or audible pulse, sounds), which are based on blood flow.

Direct monitoring is indicated when highly accurate or frequent blood pressure measurements are required—for example, in patients with low cardiac output and high systemic vascular resistance. It may also be used for hospitalized patients who are obese or have severe edema, if these conditions make indirect measurement difficult to perform. In addition, it may be used for patients who are receiving titrated doses of vasoactive drugs or who need frequent blood sampling.

Indirect monitoring, which carries few associated risks, is commonly performed by applying pressure to an artery (such as by inflating a blood pressure cuff around the arm) to decrease blood flow. As pressure is released, flow resumes and can be palpated or auscultated.

Equipment

Arterial catheter insertion

Gloves ♦ gown ♦ mask ♦ protective eyewear ♦ sterile gloves ♦ sterile gown ♦ 16G to 20G catheter (type and length depend on the insertion site, patient's size, and other anticipated uses of the line) ♦ preassembled preparation kit (if available) ♦ povidone-iodine ♦ sterile drapes ♦ sheet protector ♦ sterile towels ♦ prepared pressure transducer system ♦ ordered local anesthetic ♦ sutures ♦ syringe and needle (21G to 25G, 1″) ♦ I.V. pole ♦ tubing and medication labels ♦ site care kit (containing sterile dressing, antimicrobial ointment, and hypoallergenic tape) ♦ arm board and soft wrist restraint (for a femoral site, an ankle restraint) ♦ optional: clippers (for femoral artery insertion)

Blood sample collection: Open system

Gloves ♦ gown ♦ mask ♦ sterile 4″ × 4″ gauze pads ♦ protective eyewear ♦ sheet protector ♦ 5- or 10-ml syringe for discard sample ♦ syringes of appropriate size and number for ordered laboratory tests, laboratory request forms and labels, 16G or 18G needles (depending on your facility's policy) ♦ vacutainers

Blood sample collection: Closed system

Gloves ♦ gown ♦ mask ♦ protective eyewear ♦ syringes of appropriate size and number for ordered laboratory tests, laboratory request forms and labels ♦ alcohol swab ♦ blood transfer unit ♦ vacutainers

Arterial line tubing changes

Gloves ♦ gown ♦ mask ♦ protective eyewear ♦ sheet protector ♦ preassembled arterial pressure tubing with flush device and disposable pressure transducer ♦ sterile gloves ♦ 500-ml bag of I.V. flush solution (usually normal saline solution) ♦ 500 or 1,000 units of heparin ♦ syringe and needle (21G to 25G, 1″) ♦ alcohol swabs ♦ medication label ♦ pressure bag ♦ site care kit ♦ tubing labels

Arterial catheter removal

Gloves ♦ mask ♦ gown ♦ protective eyewear ♦ two sterile 4″ × 4″ gauze pads ♦ sheet protector ♦ sterile suture removal set ♦ dressing ♦ alcohol swabs ♦ hypoallergenic tape

Femoral line removal

Additional sterile 4″ × 4″ gauze pads ♦ small sandbag (which you may wrap in a towel or place in a pillowcase) ♦ adhesive bandage ♦ optional: your facility may use a compression device

Catheter-tip culture

Sterile scissors ♦ sterile container

Preparation

- Before setting up and priming the monitoring system, wash your hands thoroughly.
- Maintain asepsis by wearing personal protective equipment throughout preparation. (For instructions on setting up and priming the monitoring system, see "Transducer system setup," page 544.)
- Label all medications, medication containers, and other solutions on and off the sterile field.
- When you've completed equipment preparation, set the alarms on the bedside monitor according to your facility's policy.

Key steps

- Confirm the patient's identity using two patient identifiers according to your facility's policy.
- Explain the procedure to the patient and his family, including the purpose of arterial pressure monitoring and the anticipated duration of catheter placement. Make sure the patient signs a consent form. If he can't sign, ask a responsible family member to give written consent.
- Check the patient's history for an allergy or a hypersensitivity to iodine, heparin, or the ordered local anesthetic.
- Maintain asepsis by wearing personal protective equipment throughout all procedures described below.
- Position the patient for easy access to the catheter insertion site. Place a sheet protector under the site.
- If the catheter will be inserted into the radial artery, perform Allen's test to assess collateral circulation in the hand.

Inserting an arterial catheter

- Using a preassembled preparation kit, the practitioner prepares and anesthetizes the insertion site. He covers the surrounding area with either sterile drapes or towels and cleans the area with povidone-iodine. The catheter is then inserted into the artery and attached to the fluid-filled pressure tubing.
- While the practitioner holds the catheter in place, activate the fast-flush release to flush blood from the catheter. After each fast-flush operation, observe the drip

chamber to verify that the continuous flush rate is as desired. A waveform should appear on the bedside monitor.

- The practitioner may suture the catheter in place, or you may secure it with hypoallergenic tape. Apply antimicrobial ointment and cover the insertion site with a dressing, as specified by your facility's policy.
- Immobilize the insertion site. With a radial or brachial site, use an arm board and soft wrist restraint (if the patient's condition so requires). With a femoral site, assess the need for an ankle restraint; maintain the patient on bed rest, with the head of the bed raised no more than 15 to 30 degrees, to prevent the catheter from kinking. Level the zeroing stopcock of the transducer with the phlebostatic axis. Then zero the system to atmospheric pressure.
- Activate monitor alarms, as appropriate.

Obtaining a blood sample from an open system

- Assemble the equipment, taking care not to contaminate the dead-end cap, stopcock, and syringes. Turn off or temporarily silence the monitor alarms, depending on your facility's policy. (However, some facilities require that alarms be left on.)
- Locate the stopcock nearest the patient. Open a sterile 4″ × 4″ gauze pad. Remove the dead-end cap from the stopcock, and place it on the gauze pad.
- Insert the syringe for the discard sample into the stopcock. (This sample is discarded because it's diluted with flush solution.) Follow your facility's policy on how much discard blood to collect. In most cases, you'll withdraw 5 to 10 ml into a 5- or 10-ml syringe.
- Next, turn the stopcock off to the flush solution. Slowly retract the syringe to withdraw the discard sample. If you feel resistance, reposition the affected extremity and check the insertion site for obvious problems (such as catheter kinking). After correcting the problem, resume blood withdrawal. Then turn the stopcock halfway back to the open position to close the system in all directions.
- Remove the discard syringe, and dispose of the blood in the syringe, observing standard precautions.
- Place the syringe for the laboratory sample in the stopcock, turn the stopcock off to the flush solution, and slowly withdraw the required amount of blood. For each additional sample required, repeat this procedure. If the practitioner has ordered coagulation tests, obtain blood for this sample from the final syringe to prevent dilution from the flush device.
- After you've obtained blood for the final sample, turn the stopcock off to the syringe and remove the syringe. Activate the fast-flush release to clear the tubing. Then turn off the stopcock to the patient, and repeat the fast flush to clear the stopcock port.
- Turn the stopcock off to the stopcock port, and replace the dead-end cap. Reactivate the monitor alarms. Attach needles to the filled syringes, and transfer the blood samples to the appropriate Vacutainers, labeling them according to facility policy. Send all samples to the laboratory with appropriate documentation.
- Check the monitor for return of the arterial waveform and pressure reading. (See *Understanding the arterial waveform,* page 10.)

Obtaining a blood sample from a closed system

- Assemble the equipment, maintaining sterile technique. Locate the closed-system reservoir and blood sampling site. Deactivate or temporarily silence monitor alarms. (However, some facilities require that alarms be left on.)
- Clean the sampling site with an alcohol swab.
- Holding the reservoir upright, grasp the flexures and slowly fill the reservoir with blood over a 3- to 5-second period. (This blood serves as discard blood.) If you feel resistance, reposition the affected extremity, and check the catheter site for obvious problems (such as kinking). Then resume blood withdrawal.
- Turn the one-way valve off to the reservoir by turning the handle perpendicular to the tubing. Using a syringe with at-

Understanding the arterial waveform

Normal arterial blood pressure produces a characteristic waveform, representing ventricular systole and diastole. The waveform has five distinct components: the anacrotic limb, systolic peak, dicrotic limb, dicrotic notch, and end diastole.

The *anacrotic limb* marks the waveform's initial upstroke, which results as blood is rapidly ejected from the ventricle through the open aortic valve into the aorta. The rapid ejection causes a sharp rise in arterial pressure, which appears as the waveform's highest point. This is called the *systolic peak.*

As blood continues into the peripheral vessels, arterial pressure falls, and the waveform begins a downward trend. This part is called the *dicrotic limb.* Arterial pressure usually will continue to fall until pressure in the ventricle is less than pressure in the aortic root. When this occurs, the aortic valve closes. This event appears as a small notch (the *dicrotic notch*) on the waveform's downside. When the aortic valve closes, diastole begins, progressing until the aortic root pressure gradually descends to its lowest point. On the waveform, this is known as *end diastole.*

Normal arterial waveform

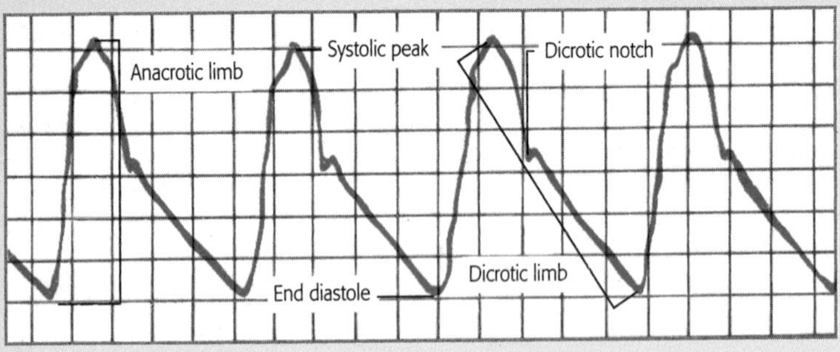

tached cannula, insert the cannula into the sampling site. (Make sure the plunger is depressed to the bottom of the syringe barrel.) Slowly fill the syringe. Then grasp the cannula near the sampling site, and remove the syringe and cannula as one unit. Repeat the procedure as needed to fill the required number of syringes. If the practitioner has ordered coagulation tests, obtain blood for those tests from the final syringe to prevent dilution from the flush solution.

- After filling the syringes, turn the one-way valve to its original position, parallel to the tubing. Now smoothly and evenly push down on the plunger until the flexures lock in place in the fully closed position and all fluid has been reinfused. The fluid should be reinfused over a 3- to 5-second period. Then activate the fast-flush release to clear blood from the tubing and reservoir.
- Clean the sampling site with an alcohol swab. Reactivate the monitor alarms. Using the blood transfer unit, transfer blood samples to the appropriate Vacutainers, labeling them according to your facility's policy. Send all samples to the laboratory with appropriate documentation.

Changing arterial line tubing

- Wash your hands and follow standard precautions. Assemble the new pressure monitoring system.
- Consult your facility's policy and procedure manual to determine how much tubing length to change.
- Inflate the pressure bag to 300 mm Hg, and check it for air leaks. Then release the pressure.
- Prepare the I.V. flush solution, and prime the pressure tubing and transducer system. At this time, add both medication and tub-

ing labels. Place the I.V. solution into the pressure bag and apply 300 mm Hg of pressure to the system. Then hang the I.V. bag on a pole.

- Place the sheet protector under the affected extremity. Remove the dressing from the catheter insertion site, taking care not to dislodge the catheter or cause vessel trauma. Turn off or temporarily silence the monitor alarms. (However, some facilities require that alarms be left on.)
- Turn off the flow clamp of the tubing segment that you'll change. Disconnect the tubing from the catheter hub, taking care not to dislodge the catheter. Immediately insert new tubing into the catheter hub. Secure the tubing and then activate the fast-flush release to clear it.
- Reactivate the monitor alarms. Apply an appropriate dressing.
- Level the zeroing stopcock of the transducer with the phlebostatic axis, and zero the system to atmospheric pressure.

Removing an arterial catheter

- Consult your facility's policy to determine whether you're permitted to perform this procedure.
- Explain the procedure to the patient.
- Assemble all equipment. Wash your hands. Observe standard precautions, including wearing personal protective equipment, for this procedure.
- Record the patient's systolic, diastolic, and mean blood pressures. If a manual, indirect blood pressure hasn't been assessed recently, obtain one now to establish a new baseline.
- Turn off the monitor alarms. Then turn off the flow clamp to the flush solution.
- Carefully remove the dressing over the insertion site. Remove any sutures, using the suture removal kit, and then carefully check that all sutures have been removed.
- Withdraw the catheter using a gentle, steady motion. Keep the catheter parallel to the artery during withdrawal to reduce the risk of traumatic injury.
- Immediately after withdrawing the catheter, apply pressure to the site with a sterile 4″ × 4″ gauze pad. Maintain pressure for at least 10 minutes (longer if bleeding or oozing persists). Apply additional pressure to a femoral site or if the patient has coagulopathy or is receiving anticoagulants. In some facilities, a compression device may be used to apply pressure to the femoral site.
- Cover the site with an appropriate dressing and secure the dressing with tape. If stipulated by your facility's policy, make a pressure dressing for a femoral site by folding in half four sterile 4″ × 4″ gauze pads, and apply the dressing. Cover the dressing with a tight adhesive bandage; then cover the bandage with a sandbag. Maintain the patient on bed rest for 6 hours with the sandbag in place.
- If the practitioner has ordered a culture of the catheter tip (to diagnose a suspected infection), gently place the catheter tip on a 4″ × 4″ sterile gauze pad. When the bleeding is under control, hold the catheter over the sterile container. Using sterile scissors, cut the tip so it falls into the sterile container. Label the specimen and send it to the laboratory.
- Observe the site for bleeding. Assess circulation in the extremity distal to the site by evaluating color, pulses, and sensation. Repeat this assessment every 15 minutes for the first 4 hours, every 30 minutes for the next 2 hours, then hourly for the next 6 hours.

Special considerations

- Observing the pressure waveform on the monitor can enhance assessment of arterial pressure. An abnormal waveform may reflect an arrhythmia (such as atrial fibrillation) or other cardiovascular problems, such as aortic stenosis, aortic insufficiency, pulsus alternans, or pulsus paradoxus. (See *Recognizing abnormal waveforms,* page 12.)
- Change the pressure tubing every 2 to 3 days, according to your facility's policy. Change the dressing at the catheter site at intervals specified by your facility's policy. Regularly assess the site for signs of infection, such as redness and swelling. Notify the practitioner immediately if you note any such signs.
- Be aware that erroneous pressure readings may result from a catheter that's clotted or positional, loose connections, addi-

Recognizing abnormal waveforms

Understanding a normal arterial waveform is relatively straightforward. An abnormal waveform, however, is more difficult to decipher. Abnormal patterns and markings may provide important diagnostic clues to the patient's cardiovascular status, or they may simply signal trouble in the monitor. Use this chart to help you recognize and resolve waveform abnormalities.

Abnormality	Possible causes	Nursing interventions
Alternating high and low waves in a regular pattern 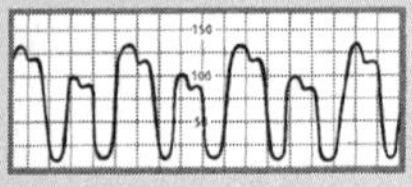	Ventricular bigeminy	▪ Check the patient's electrocardiogram to confirm ventricular bigeminy. The tracing should reflect premature ventricular contractions every second beat.
Flattened waveform 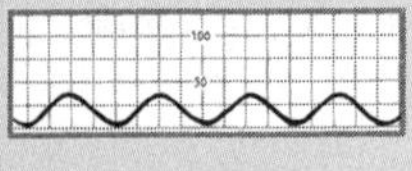	Overdamped waveform or hypotensive patient	▪ Check the patient's blood pressure with a sphygmomanometer. If you obtain a reading, suspect overdamping. Correct the problem by checking the pressure on the pressure infusion bag and increasing, if necessary, or by trying to aspirate the arterial line. If you succeed, flush the line. If the reading is very low or absent, suspect hypotension.
Slightly rounded waveform with consistent variations in systolic height 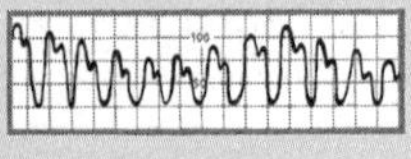	Patient on ventilator with positive end-expiratory pressure	▪ Check the patient's systolic blood pressure regularly. The difference between the highest and lowest systolic pressure reading should be less than 10 mm Hg. If the difference exceeds that amount, suspect pulsus paradoxus, possibly from cardiac tamponade.
Slow upstroke 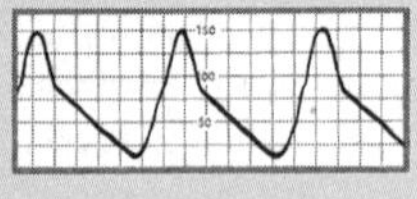	Aortic stenosis	▪ Check the patient's heart sounds for signs of aortic stenosis. Also notify the practitioner
Diminished amplitude on inspiration 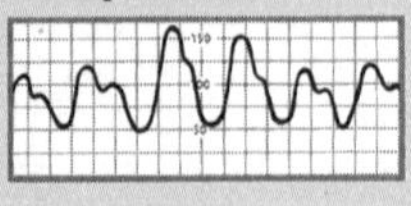	Pulsus paradoxus, possibly from cardiac tamponade, constrictive pericarditis, or lung disease	▪ Note systolic pressure during inspiration and expiration. If inspiratory pressure is at least 10 mm Hg less than expiratory pressure, call the practitioner. ▪ If you're also monitoring pulmonary artery pressure, observe for a diastolic plateau. This occurs when the mean central venous pressure , mean pulmonary artery pressure, and mean pulmonary artery wedge pressure are within 5 mm Hg of one another.

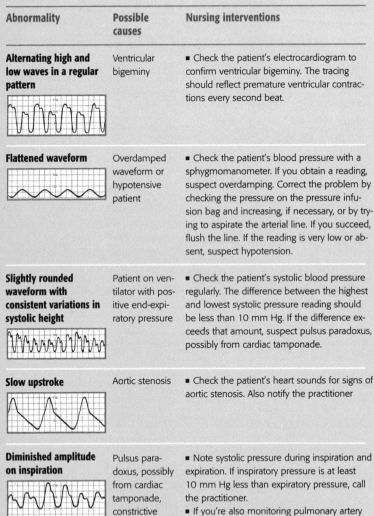

tion of extra stopcocks or extension tubing, inadvertent entry of air into the system, or improper calibrating, leveling, or zeroing of the monitoring system. If the catheter lumen clots, the flush system may be improperly pressurized. Regularly assess the amount of flush solution in the I.V. bag, and maintain 300 mm Hg of pressure in the pressure bag.

Complications

- Arterial bleeding
- Infection
- Air embolism
- Arterial spasm
- Thrombosis
- Vessel trauma

Documentation

Document the date of system setup so that all caregivers will know when to change the components. Document systolic, diastolic, and mean pressure readings as well. Record circulation in the extremity distal to the site by assessing color, pulses, and sensation. Carefully document the amount of flush solution infused to avoid hypervolemia and volume overload, and to ensure accurate assessment of the patient's fluid status.

Make sure the patient's position is documented when each blood pressure reading is obtained. This is important for determining trends.

Arterial puncture for blood gas analysis

Obtaining an arterial blood sample requires percutaneous puncture of the brachial, radial, or femoral artery or withdrawal of a sample from an arterial line. Once collected, the sample can be analyzed to determine the patient's arterial blood gas (ABG) values.

ABG analysis evaluates ventilation by measuring blood pH and the partial pressure of arterial oxygen ($Pa{O_2}$) and partial pressure of arterial carbon dioxide ($Pa{CO_2}$). Blood pH measurement reveals the blood's acid-base balance, the $Pa{O_2}$ indicates the amount of oxygen that the lungs deliver to the blood, and the $Pa{CO_2}$ indicates the lungs' capacity to eliminate carbon dioxide. ABG samples also can be analyzed for oxygen content and saturation and for bicarbonate values.

Typically, ABG analysis is ordered for patients who have chronic obstructive pulmonary disease, pulmonary edema, acute respiratory distress syndrome, myocardial infarction, or pneumonia. It's also performed during episodes of shock and after coronary artery bypass surgery, resuscitation from cardiac arrest, changes in respiratory therapy or status, and prolonged anesthesia.

A specially trained nurse can draw most ABG samples. Only nurses who have had additional specialized training should use the femoral artery. This artery is best used in an emergency, such as cardiac arrest or hypovolemic shock, when pulses are difficult to palpate. Before attempting a radial puncture, Allen's test should be performed.

Equipment

Plastic luer-lock syringe specially made for drawing blood for ABG analysis ♦ 1 ml ampule of aqueous heparin (1:1,000) ♦ 20G 1¼" needle ♦ 22G 1" needle ♦ gloves ♦ alcohol pad ♦ two 2" × 2" gauze pads ♦ rubber cap for syringe hub or rubber stopper for needle ♦ ice-filled plastic bag ♦ label ♦ laboratory request form ♦ adhesive bandage ♦ optional: 1% lidocaine solution

Many health care facilities use a commercial ABG kit that contains all the equipment listed above except the adhesive bandage and ice. If your facility doesn't use such a kit, obtain a sterile syringe specially made for drawing ABG samples, and use a clean emesis basin filled with ice instead of the plastic bag to transport the sample to the laboratory.

Preparation

- Prepare the collection equipment before entering the patient's room.
- Wash your hands thoroughly, then open the ABG kit and remove the sample label and the plastic bag.

- Record on the label the patient's name and room number, date and collection time, and the practitioner's name.
- Fill the plastic bag with ice and set it aside. If the syringe isn't heparinized, you'll have to do so.
- Attach the 20G needle to the syringe, and then open the ampule of heparin.
- Draw all the heparin into the syringe to prevent the sample from clotting. Hold the syringe upright, and pull the plunger back slowly to about the 7-ml mark. Rotate the barrel while pulling the plunger back to allow the heparin to coat the inside surface of the syringe. Then slowly force the heparin toward the hub of the syringe, and expel all but about 0.1 ml of heparin.
- To heparinize the needle, first replace the 20G needle with the 22G needle. Then hold the syringe upright, tilt it slightly, and eject the remaining heparin. Excess heparin in the syringe alters blood pH and $Pa{O_2}$ values.

Key steps

- Confirm the patient's identity using two patient identifiers according to your facility's policy.
- Tell the patient that you need to collect an arterial blood sample, and explain the procedure to help ease anxiety and promote cooperation. Tell him that the needle insertion will cause some discomfort but that he must remain still during the procedure.
- Wash your hands and put on gloves.
- Place a rolled towel under the patient's wrist for support. Locate the artery and palpate it for a strong pulse.
- Clean the puncture site with an alcohol pad, starting in the center of the site and spiraling outward in a circular motion with friction for 30 seconds or until the final pad comes away clean. Allow the skin to dry.
- Palpate the artery with the index and middle fingers of one hand while holding the syringe over the puncture site with the other hand. The puncture site should be between your index and middle fingers as they palpate the pulse.
- Puncture the skin and the arterial wall in one motion, following the path of the artery. When puncturing the radial artery, hold the needle bevel up at a 30- to 45-degree angle. When puncturing the brachial artery, hold the needle at a 60-degree angle. (See *Arterial puncture technique.*)
- Watch for blood backflow in the syringe. Don't pull back on the plunger because arterial blood should enter the syringe automatically. Fill the syringe to the 5-ml mark.
- After collecting the sample, press a gauze pad firmly over the puncture site until the bleeding stops—at least 5 minutes. If the patient is receiving anticoagulant therapy or has a blood dyscrasia, apply pressure for 10 to 15 minutes; if necessary, ask a coworker to hold the gauze pad in place while you prepare the sample for transport to the laboratory. Don't ask the patient to hold the pad. If he fails to apply sufficient pressure, a large, painful hematoma may form, hindering future arterial punctures at that site.
- Check the syringe for air bubbles. If any appear, remove them by holding the syringe upright and slowly ejecting some of the blood onto a 2″ × 2″ gauze pad.
- Insert the needle into a rubber stopper, or remove the needle and place a rubber cap directly on the needle hub. This prevents the sample from leaking and keeps air out of the syringe.
- Put the labeled sample in the ice-filled plastic bag or emesis basin. Attach a properly completed laboratory request form, and send the sample to the laboratory immediately.
- When bleeding stops, apply a small adhesive bandage to the site.
- Monitor the patient's vital signs, and observe for signs of circulatory impairment, such as swelling, discoloration, pain, numbness, or tingling in the arm or leg. Watch for bleeding at the puncture site.

Special considerations

- If the patient is receiving oxygen, make sure that his therapy has been underway for at least 15 minutes before collecting an arterial blood sample.

Do's & don'ts

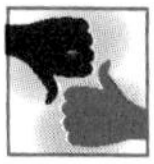

Unless ordered, don't turn off existing oxygen therapy before collecting arterial blood samples. Be sure to indicate on the laboratory request slip the amount and type of oxygen therapy the patient is receiving.

- If the patient isn't receiving oxygen, indicate that he's breathing room air. If the patient has received a nebulizer treatment, wait about 20 minutes before collecting the sample.
- If necessary, anesthetize the puncture site with 1% lidocaine solution or normal saline with 0.9% benzyl alcohol. Consider such use of lidocaine carefully because it delays the procedure, the patient may be allergic to the drug, or the resulting vasoconstriction may prevent successful puncture.
- When filling out a laboratory request form for ABG analysis, be sure to include the following information to help the laboratory staff calibrate the equipment and evaluate results correctly: the patient's current temperature, most recent hemoglobin level, current respiratory rate and, if the patient is on a ventilator, fraction of inspired oxygen and tidal volume.
- If you use too much force when attempting to puncture the artery, the needle may touch the periosteum of the bone, causing the patient considerable pain, or you may advance the needle through the opposite wall of the artery. If this happens, slowly pull the needle back a short distance and check to see if you obtain a blood return. If blood still doesn't enter the syringe, withdraw the needle completely and start with a fresh heparinized needle. Don't make more than two attempts to withdraw blood from the same site. Probing the artery may injure it and the radial nerve. Also, hemolysis will alter test results.
- If arterial spasm occurs, blood won't flow into the syringe and you won't be able to collect the sample. If this happens, replace the needle with a smaller one and try the puncture again. A smaller-bore needle is less likely to cause arterial spasm.

Arterial puncture technique

The angle of needle penetration in arterial blood gas sampling depends on which artery will be sampled. For the radial artery, which is used most commonly, the needle should enter bevel-up at a 30- to 45-degree angle over the radial artery.

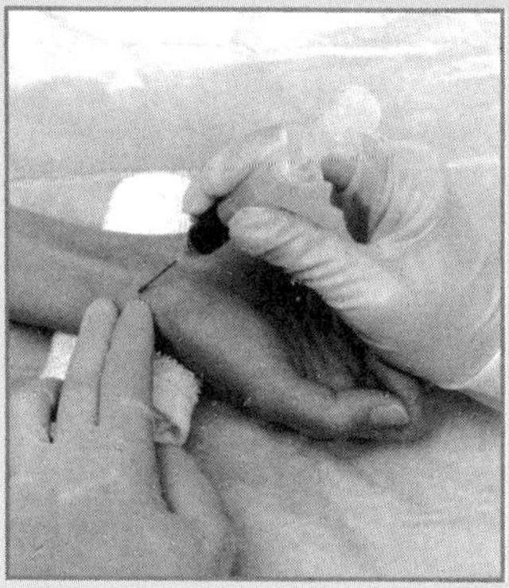

Complications

- Hematoma

Documentation

Record the results of Allen's test, the time the sample was drawn, the patient's temperature, site of the arterial puncture, how long pressure was applied to the site to control bleeding, and the type and amount of oxygen therapy the patient was receiving.

Arteriovenous fistula care

An arteriovenous (AV) fistula consists of two segments of tubing joined (in a U-shape) to divert blood from an artery to a vein. Created surgically, usually in a forearm or upper arm, the AV fistula provides access to the circulatory system for hemodialysis. (See *An inside look at an AV fistula,* page 16.) After insertion, you should regularly assess the fistula for patency and

An inside look at an AV fistula

The illustration below shows how an arteriovenous (AV) fistula is created in the forearm by connecting the vein to the arterial wall.

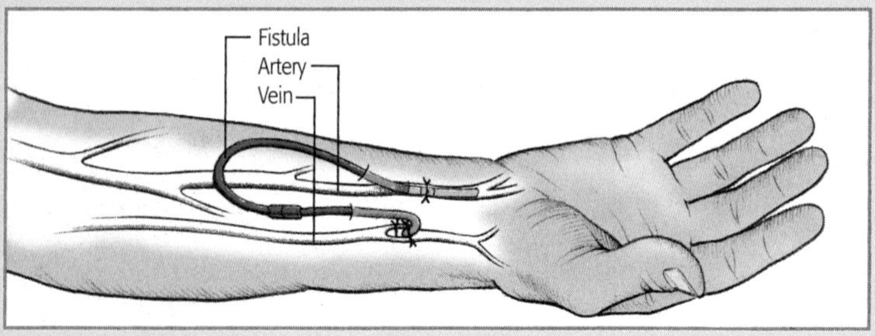

examine the surrounding skin for signs of infection.

AV fistula care also includes aseptically cleaning the arterial and venous exit sites, applying antiseptic ointment, and dressing the sites with sterile bandages. When done just before hemodialysis, this procedure prolongs the life of the fistula, helps prevent infection, and allows for the early detection of clotting. Care is required more often if the dressing becomes wet or nonocclusive.

Equipment

Drape ♦ stethoscope ♦ sterile gloves ♦ sterile 4″ × 4″ gauze pads ♦ sterile cotton-tipped applicators ♦ antiseptic ♦ bulldog clamps ♦ plasticized or hypoallergenic tape ♦ optional: swab specimen kit, prescribed antimicrobial ointment (povidone-iodine), sterile elastic gauze bandage, 2″ × 2″ gauze pads, hydrogen peroxide

Kits containing the necessary equipment can be prepackaged and stored for use.

Key steps

- Explain the procedure to the patient. Provide privacy and wash your hands.
- Place the drape on a stable surface, such as a bedside table, to reduce the risk of traumatic injury to the fistula or graft site. Place the patient's arm on the draped surface.
- Remove the two bulldog clamps from the elastic gauze bandage, and unwrap the bandage from the fistula or graft area.
- Carefully remove the gauze dressing covering the shunt and the 4″ × 4″ gauze pad under the fistula or graft.
- Assess the arterial and venous exit sites for signs and symptoms of infection, such as erythema, swelling, excessive tenderness, or drainage. Obtain a swab specimen of any purulent drainage, and notify the practitioner immediately of any signs of infection.
- Check blood flow through the fistula by inspecting the color of the blood and comparing the warmth of the fistula with that of the surrounding skin. The blood should be bright red; the fistula should feel as warm as the skin.

ACTION STAT!

If the blood is dark purple or black and the temperature of the fistula or graft is lower than the surrounding skin, clotting has occurred. Notify the practitioner immediately.

- Use the stethoscope to auscultate the fistula between the arterial and venous exit sites. A bruit confirms normal blood flow. Palpate the fistula for a thrill (by lightly placing your fingertips over the access site and feeling for vibration), which also indicates normal blood flow.

Caring for an AV fistula at home

Before the patient leaves the health care facility, teach him how to care for his arteriovenous (AV) fistula. Be sure to cover:

- keeping the incision clean and dry to prevent infection
- cleaning the site daily until it heals completely and the sutures are removed (usually 10 to 14 days after surgery)
- notifying the practitioner about pain, swelling, redness, or drainage at the site
- how to palpate a thrill
- using the arm freely after the site heals
- not allowing treatments or procedures on the arm with the AV fistula, including blood pressure monitoring or needle punctures
- avoiding excessive pressure on the arm
- avoiding lifting heavy objects, sleeping on the arm with the AV fistula, or wearing tight-sleeved shirts
- the need to avoid getting the hemodialysis access site wet for several hours after dialysis
- exercises for the affected arm to promote vascular dilation and blood flow, starting by squeezing a small rubber ball or other soft object for 15 minutes, when advised by the practitioner.

- Open a few packages of 4″ × 4″ gauze pads and cotton-tipped applicators, and soak them with the antiseptic. Put on the sterile gloves.
- Using a soaked 4″ × 4″ gauze pad, start cleaning the skin at one of the exit sites. Wipe away from the site to remove bacteria and reduce the chance of contaminating the fistula.
- Use the soaked cotton-tipped applicators to remove crusted material from the exit site because the encrustations provide a medium for bacterial growth.
- Clean the other exit site, using fresh, soaked 4″ × 4″ gauze pads and cotton-tipped applicators.
- Clean the rest of the skin that was covered by the gauze dressing with fresh, soaked 4″ × 4″ gauze pads.
- If ordered, apply antimicrobial ointment to the exit sites to help prevent infection.
- Cover the exit sites with a dry, sterile 4″ × 4″ gauze pad, and tape it securely to keep the exit sites clean and protected.
- For routine daily care, wrap the fistula or graft lightly with an elastic gauze bandage.

Special considerations

- Blood pressure measurement and venipuncture should be avoided in the affected arm to prevent fistula or graft occlusion.
- Always handle the arm with the fistula or graft and dressings carefully. Don't use scissors or other sharp instruments to remove the dressing because you may accidentally cut into the fistula.
- When cleaning the fistula exit sites, use each 4″ × 4″ gauze pad only once and avoid wiping the area more than once to minimize the risk of contamination. When redressing the site, make sure that the tape doesn't kink or occlude the fistula. If the exit sites are heavily encrusted, place a 2″ × 2″ hydrogen peroxide-soaked gauze pad on the area for about 1 hour to loosen the crust. Make sure that the patient isn't allergic to iodine before using povidone-iodine.

Complications

- Clotting
- Hemorrhage
- Infection

Patient teaching

- Teach the patient how to care for the fistula for proper home care. (See *Caring for an AV fistula at home*.)

Documentation

Record that graft or fistula care was administered, the condition of the graft or fistula and surrounding skin, any ointment used, and any instructions given to the patient.

Arthroplasty care

Care of the patient after arthroplasty—surgical replacement of all or part of a joint—helps restore mobility and normal use of the affected extremity; it also helps prevent such complications as infection, phlebitis, and respiratory problems. Arthroplasty care includes maintaining alignment of the affected joint, assisting with exercises, and providing routine postoperative care. An equally important nursing responsibility is teaching home care and exercises that may continue for several years, depending on the type of arthroplasty performed and the patient's condition.

The two most common arthroplastic procedures are cup arthroplasty and total joint replacement. In cup arthroplasty, the surgeon inserts a moveable cup between the hip joint surfaces. The prosthesis has a porous coating that promotes bone ingrowth. This procedure is usually indicated for a young patient who has rheumatoid arthritis, degenerative joint disease from traumatic injury, or an acetabulum fracture.

Total joint replacement (usually of the hip or knee) is commonly performed in patients over age 50. Total hip replacement may be used to treat osteoarthritis and severe crippling rheumatoid arthritis; total knee replacement is commonly used to treat severe joint pain, joint contractures, and deterioration of joint surfaces, conditions that prohibit full extension or flexion. (See *Total hip replacement*.)

Nursing care after these operations—as well as care after less common surgical procedures (such as shoulder, elbow, wrist, ankle, or finger joint replacement)—requires similar skills.

Equipment

Traction frame with trapeze ♦ comfort device (such as static air mattress overlay, low-air-loss bed, or sheepskin) ♦ bedsheets ♦ incentive spirometer ♦ continuous passive motion (CPM) machine (for total knee or shoulder replacement) ♦ compression stocking ♦ sterile dressings ♦ hypoallergenic tape ♦ iuce bag ♦ skin lotion ♦ warm water ♦ crutches or walker ♦ pain medications ♦ closed-wound drainage system ♦ I.V. antibiotics, as ordered ♦ pillow ♦ abduction splint ♦ anticoagulants ♦ optional: closed drainage system, slings

After total knee or shoulder replacement, an immobilizer may be applied in the operating room, or the extremity may be placed in CPM.

Preparation

- After the patient goes to the operating room, make a Balkan frame with a trapeze on his bed frame. This will allow him some mobility after the operation.
- Make the bed, using a comfort device and clean sheets.
- Have the bed taken to the operating room. This enables immediate placement of the patient on his hospital bed after surgery and eliminates the need for an additional move from his bed on the postanesthesia care unit.

Key steps

- Check the patient's vital signs every 15 minutes twice, every 30 minutes until they stabilize, and then every 2 to 4 hours and routinely thereafter, according to your facility's protocol. Report changes in his vital signs because they may indicate infection, hemorrhage, or postoperative complications.
- Encourage the patient to perform deep-breathing and coughing exercises. Assist with incentive spirometry as ordered to prevent respiratory complications.
- Assess the patient's neurovascular status every 2 hours for the first 48 hours and then every 4 hours for signs of complications. Check the affected leg for color, temperature, toe movement, sensation, edema, capillary refill, and pedal pulse. Investigate complaints of pain, burning, numbness, or tingling.
- Apply the compression stocking to the unaffected leg, as ordered, to promote venous return and prevent phlebitis and pulmonary emboli. Once every 8 hours, remove it, inspect the leg—especially the heel—for pressure ulcers, and reapply it.
- Administer pain medication, as ordered.

- For 24 hours after surgery, administer I.V. antibiotics, as ordered, to minimize the risk of wound infection.
- Administer anticoagulant therapy, as ordered, to minimize the risk of thrombophlebitis and embolus formation. Observe for bleeding. Observe the leg for signs and symptoms of phlebitis, such as warmth, swelling, tenderness, redness, and a positive Homans' sign.
- Check dressings for excessive bleeding. Circle any drainage on the dressing and mark it with your initials, the date, and the time. As needed, apply more sterile dressings, using hypoallergenic tape. Report excessive bleeding to the practitioner.
- Observe the closed-wound drainage system for discharge color and amount. Proper drainage prevents hematoma. Purulent discharge and fever may indicate infection. Empty and measure drainage as ordered, using clean technique.
- Monitor fluid intake and output every shift; include wound drainage in the output measurement.
- Apply an ice bag, as ordered, to the affected site for the first 48 hours to reduce swelling, relieve pain, and control bleeding.
- Reposition the patient every 2 hours. These position changes enhance comfort, prevent pressure ulcers, and help prevent respiratory complications.
- Help the patient use the trapeze to reposition himself every 2 hours. Provide skin care for the back and buttocks, using warm water and lotion, as indicated.
- Instruct the patient to perform muscle-strengthening exercises for affected and unaffected extremities, as ordered, to help maintain muscle strength and range of motion (ROM) and to help prevent phlebitis.
- Before ambulation, give an analgesic, as ordered, 30 minutes before activity because movement is very painful. Encourage the patient during exercise.
- Help the patient with progressive ambulation, using adjustable crutches or a walker when needed.

After hip arthroplasty

- Keep the affected leg in abduction and in the neutral position to stabilize the hip and keep the cup and femur head in the acetabulum. Place a pillow between the patient's legs to maintain hip abduction.
- Positioning of the patient after hip surgery varies, based on the surgical approach used and the surgeon's preference.

For anterior approach:
- No adduction past midline
- No flexion greater than 90 degrees
- No external rotation past midline

For posterior approach:
- No adduction past midline
- No flexion greater than 60 to 90 degrees
- No internal rotation past midline
- No extension past neutral

- Keep the patient in the supine position, with the affected hip in full extension, for 1 hour three times per day and at night. This will help prevent hip flexion contracture.
- On the day after surgery, have the patient begin plantar flexion and dorsiflexion exercises of the foot on the affected leg.

Total hip replacement

To form a totally artificial hip, the surgeon cements a femoral head prosthesis in place to articulate with a cup, which he then cements into the deepened acetabulum. He may avoid using cement by implanting a prosthesis with a porous coating that promotes bony ingrowth.

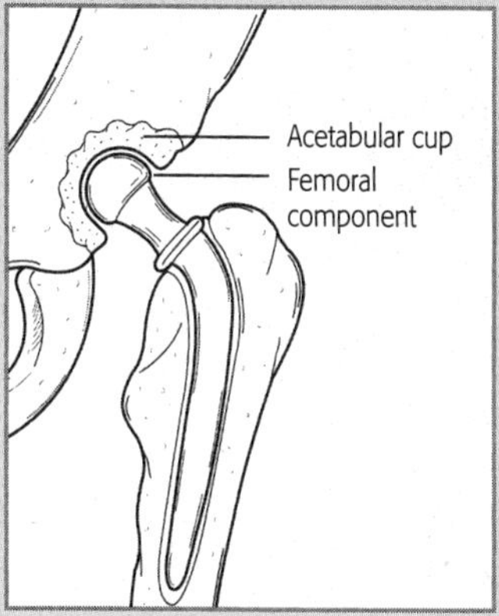

When ordered, instruct him to begin quadriceps exercises. Progressive ambulation protocols vary. In most cases, the patient is permitted to begin transfer and progressive ambulation with assistive devices on the first postoperative day.

After total knee replacement

- Elevate the affected leg, as ordered, to reduce swelling.
- Instruct the patient to begin quadriceps exercises and straight leg-raising, when ordered (usually on the first postoperative day). Encourage flexion-extension exercises, when ordered (usually after the first dressing change).
- If the practitioner orders use of the CPM machine, he'll adjust the machine daily to gradually increase the degree of flexion of the affected leg. Typically, the patient can dangle his feet on the first postoperative day and begin ambulation with partial weight bearing as tolerated (cemented knee) or toe-touch ambulation only (uncemented knee) by the second day. The patient may need to wear a knee immobilizer for support when walking; otherwise, he should be in CPM for most of the day and night or during waking hours only. Check your facility's protocol.
- The degree of flexion, extension, and weight bearing status will depend on the practitioner's specific orders, surgical approach used, and the surgeon's preference.

Special considerations

- Before surgery, explain the procedure to the patient. Emphasize that frequent assessment—including monitoring his vital signs, neurovascular integrity, and wound drainage—is normal after the operation.
- Inform the patient that he'll receive I.V. antibiotics for about 2 days. Make sure that he understands that he'll receive medication around the clock for pain control.
- Explain the need for immobilizing the affected leg and exercising the unaffected one.

Complications

- Pulmonary embolism
- Pneumonia
- Phlebitis
- Paralytic ileus
- Urine retention
- Bowel impaction

ALERT

A deep wound or infection at the prosthesis site is a serious complication that may force the removal of the prosthesis.

DEVICE SAFETY

Dislocation of a total hip prosthesis may occur after violent hip flexion or adduction or during internal rotation. Signs and symptoms of dislocation include the inability to rotate the hip or bear weight, shortening of the leg, and increased pain.

ALERT

Fat embolism, a potentially fatal complication resulting from the release of fat molecules in response to increased intermedullary canal pressure from the prosthesis, may develop within 72 hours after surgery.

Patient teaching

- Teach the patient to perform muscle-strengthening exercises for affected and unaffected extremities to maintain muscle strength and ROM to prevent phlebitis.
- Before discharge, instruct the patient about home care and exercises.
- Advise the patient he may return to work in 3 to 6 months, or as instructed by the practitioner.
- Tell the patient not to drive a car until after the 2-month follow-up.
- Tell the patient to keep wearing elastic stockings until the 2-month follow-up.

Documentation

Record the patient's neurovascular status. Describe his position (especially the position of the affected leg), skin care and condition, respiratory care and condition, and the use of compression stockings. Document all exercises performed and their effect, and record ambulatory efforts and the type of support used.

On the appropriate flowchart, record the patient's vital signs and fluid intake and output. Record discharge instructions and how well the patient seems to understand them.

Automated external defibrillation

Automated external defibrillators (AEDs) are commonly used to meet the need for early defibrillation, which is currently considered the most effective treatment for ventricular fibrillation. Some health care facilities now require an AED on every noncritical care unit. Their use is also becoming common in such public places as shopping malls, sports stadiums, and airplanes. Instruction in using the AED is required as part of basic life support (BLS) and advanced cardiac life support (ACLS) training.

AEDs are used to provide early defibrillation—even when no health care provider is present. The AED interprets the victim's cardiac rhythm and gives the operator step-by-step directions on how to proceed if defibrillation is indicated. Most AEDs have a "quick-look" feature that allows visualization of the rhythm with the paddles before electrodes are connected.

The AED is equipped with a microcomputer that senses and analyzes a patient's heart rhythm at the push of a button. Then it audibly or visually prompts you to deliver a shock. AED models all have the same basic function but offer different operating options. For example, all AEDs communicate directions via messages on a display screen, give voice commands, or both. Some AEDs simultaneously display a patient's heart rhythm.

All devices record your interactions with the patient during defibrillation, either on a cassette tape or in a solid-state memory module. Some AEDs have an integral printer for immediate event documentation. Your facility's policy determines who's responsible for reviewing all AED interactions; the patient's physician always has that option. Local and state regulations govern who's responsible for collecting AED case data for reporting purposes.

Equipment

AED ♦ two prepackaged electrodes

Key steps

- After discovering that your patient is unresponsive to your questions, pulseless, and apneic, follow BLS and ACLS protocols. Then ask a colleague to bring the AED into the patient's room and set it up before the code team arrives.
- Open the foil packets containing the two electrode pads. Attach the white electrode cable connector to one pad and the red electrode cable connector to the other. The electrode pads aren't site-specific.
- Expose the patient's chest. Remove the plastic backing film from the electrode pads, and place the electrode pad attached to the white cable connector on the right upper portion of the patient's chest, just beneath his clavicle.
- Place the pad attached to the red cable connector to the left of the heart's apex. To help remember where to place the pads, think "white—right, red—ribs." (Placement for both electrode pads is the same as for manual defibrillation or cardioversion.)
- Firmly press the device's ON button, and wait while the machine performs a brief self-test. Most AEDs signal their readiness by a computerized voice that says "Stand clear" or by emitting a series of loud beeps. (If the AED isn't functioning properly, it will convey the message "Don't use the AED. Remove and continue CPR.") Remember to report any AED malfunctions in accordance with your facility's procedure.
- Now the machine is ready to analyze the patient's heart rhythm. Ask everyone to stand clear, and press the ANALYZE button when the machine prompts you to. Be careful not to touch or move the patient while the AED is in analysis mode. (If you get the message "Check electrodes," make sure the electrodes are correctly placed and the patient cable is securely attached; then press the analyze button again.)

- In 15 to 30 seconds, the AED will analyze the patient's rhythm. When the patient needs a shock, the AED will display a "Stand clear" message and emit a beep that changes into a steady tone as it's charging.
- When the AED is fully charged and ready to deliver a shock, it will prompt you to press the SHOCK button. (Some fully automatic AED models automatically deliver a shock within 15 seconds after analyzing the patient's rhythm. If a shock isn't needed, the AED will display "No shock indicated" and prompt you to "Check patient.")
- Make sure no one is touching the patient or his bed, and call out "Stand clear." Then press the shock button on the AED. Most AEDs are ready to deliver a shock within 15 seconds.
- After the first shock, continue CPR, beginning with chest compressions until 5 cycles or about 2 minutes of CPR have been provided. Don't delay compressions to recheck rhythm or pulse. After 5 cycles of CPR, the AED should analyze the rhythm and deliver another shock, if indicated.
- If a nonshockable rhythm is detected, the AED should instruct you to resume CPR. Then continue the algorithm sequence until the code team leader arrives.
- After the code, remove and transcribe the AED's computer memory module or tape, or prompt the AED to print a rhythm strip with code data. Follow your facility's policy for analyzing and storing code data.

Special considerations

DEVICE SAFETY

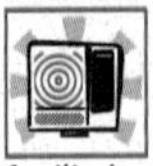

Defibrillators vary from one manufacturer to the next, so be sure to familiarize yourself with your facility's equipment.

- Defibrillator operation should be checked at least every 8 hours and after each use.

Complications

- Defibrillation causing accidental electric shock to those providing care
- Skin burns

Documentation

After using an AED, give a synopsis to the code team leader. Remember to report:

- the patient's name, age, medical history, and chief complaint
- the time you found the patient in cardiac arrest
- when you started CPR
- when you applied the AED
- how many shocks the patient received
- when the patient regained a pulse at any point
- what postarrest care was given, if any
- physical assessment findings.

Later, be sure to document the code on the appropriate form.

B

Balloon valvuloplasty

Although the treatment of choice for valvular heart disease is surgery, balloon valvuloplasty is an alternative to valve replacement in patients with critical stenoses. This technique enlarges the orifice of a heart valve that has been narrowed by a congenital defect, calcification, rheumatic fever, or aging. It evolved from percutaneous transluminal coronary angioplasty and uses the same balloon-tipped catheters for dilatation.

Balloon valvuloplasty was first performed successfully on pediatric patients, then on elderly patients who had stenotic valves complicated by other medical problems, such as chronic obstructive pulmonary disease. It's indicated for patients who face a high risk from surgery and for those who refuse surgery. Balloon valvuloplasty has proved to be more tolerable than surgery for elderly patients, especially those older than age 80.

This procedure is performed in the cardiac catheterization laboratory under local anesthesia. The physician inserts a balloon-tipped catheter through the patient's femoral vein or artery, threads it into the heart, and repeatedly inflates it against the leaflets of the diseased valve. This increases the size of the orifice, improving valvular function and helping prevent complications from decreased cardiac output. (See *How balloon valvuloplasty works,* page 24.)

Your role includes teaching the patient and his family about valvuloplasty and monitoring the patient for potential complications.

Equipment

Povidone-iodine solution ♦ local anesthetic ♦ valvuloplasty or balloon-tipped catheter ♦ I.V. solution and tubing ♦ electrocardiogram (ECG) monitor and electrodes ♦ pulmonary artery (PA) catheter ♦ contrast medium ♦ oxygen and nasal cannula ♦ sedative ♦ emergency medications ♦ clippers ♦ heparin for injection ♦ introducer kit for balloon catheter ♦ sterile gown, gloves, mask, cap, and drapes ♦ 5-lb (2.3-kg) sandbag ♦ optional: nitroglycerin (Nitro-Bid)

Key steps

Before balloon valvuloplasty

- Reinforce the physician's explanation of balloon valvuloplasty, including its risks and alternatives, to the patient and his family.
- Reassure the patient that although he'll be awake during the procedure, he'll receive a sedative and a local anesthetic beforehand.
- Teach the patient what to expect. For example, inform him that his groin hair will be clipped and the area cleaned with an antiseptic; he'll feel a brief, stinging sensation when the local anesthetic is injected; and he may feel pressure as the catheter moves along the vessel. Describe the warm, flushed feeling he's likely to experience from injection of the contrast medium.
- Tell him that the procedure may last up to 4 hours and that he may feel discomfort from lying on a hard table for that long.

How balloon valvuloplasty works

In balloon valvuloplasty, the physician inserts a balloontipped catheter through the femoral vein or artery and threads it into the heart. After locating the stenotic valve, he inflates the balloon, increasing the size of the valve opening.

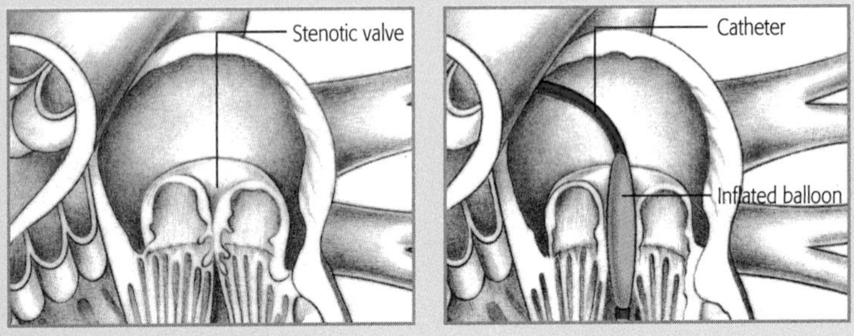

ALERT

Make sure the patient has no allergies to shellfish, iodine, or contrast media.

- Make sure that the patient or a responsible family member has signed a consent form.
- Withhold food and fluids (except for medications) for at least 6 hours before balloon valvuloplasty or as ordered (usually after midnight the night before the procedure).
- Make sure that the results of routine laboratory studies and blood typing and crossmatching are available.
- Insert an I.V. line to provide access for medications.
- Take baseline peripheral pulses in all extremities.
- Shave the insertion sites; then clean the sites with povidone-iodine solution.
- Give the patient a sedative as ordered.
- Have the patient void.
- When the patient arrives at the cardiac catheterization laboratory, apply ECG electrodes and ensure I.V. line patency.

During balloon valvuloplasty

- Administer oxygen by nasal cannula.
- The physician will put on a sterile gown, gloves, mask, and cap, and open the sterile supplies. A member of the team labels all medications, medication containers, and other solutions on and off the sterile field.
- The physician prepares and anesthetizes the catheter insertion site (usually at the femoral artery). He may insert a PA catheter if one isn't in place.
- He then inserts a large guide catheter into the site and threads a valvuloplasty or balloon-tipped catheter up into the heart.
- The physician injects a contrast medium to visualize the heart valves and assess the stenosis. He also injects heparin to prevent the catheter from clotting.
- Using low pressure, he inflates the balloon on the valvuloplasty catheter for a short time, usually 12 to 30 seconds, gradually increasing the time and pressure. If the stenosis isn't reduced, a larger balloon may be used.
- After completion of valvuloplasty, a series of angiograms is taken to evaluate the effectiveness of the treatment.
- The physician then sutures the guide catheter in place. He'll remove it after the effects of the heparin have worn off.

After balloon valvuloplasty

- When the patient returns to the unit, he may be receiving I.V. heparin or nitroglycerin. He may also have a sandbag over the insertion site to prevent formation of a hematoma.
- Monitor ECG rhythm and arterial pressures.

ACTION STAT!

Monitor the insertion site frequently for signs of hemorrhage because exsanguination can occur rapidly.

- To prevent excessive hip flexion and migration of the catheter, keep the affected leg straight and elevate the head of the bed no more than 15 degrees. If necessary, use a soft restraint.
- Monitor vital signs every 15 minutes for the first hour, every 30 minutes for the next 2 hours, and then hourly for the next 5 hours. If vital signs are unstable, notify the practitioner and continue to check them every 5 minutes.
- When you take vital signs, assess peripheral pulses distal to the catheter insertion site as well as the color, sensation, temperature, and capillary refill time of the affected extremity.
- Assess the catheter site for hematoma, ecchymosis, and hemorrhage. If the hematoma expands, mark the site and alert the practitioner.
- Auscultate regularly for murmurs, which may indicate worsening valvular insufficiency. Notify the practitioner if you detect a new or worsening murmur.
- To help the kidneys excrete the contrast medium, provide I.V. fluids at a rate of at least 100 ml/hour, as ordered. Assess the patient for signs of fluid overload: distended neck veins, atrial and ventricular gallops, dyspnea, pulmonary congestion, tachycardia, hypertension, and hypoxemia. Monitor intake and output closely.
- Encourage the patient to perform deep-breathing exercises to prevent atelectasis. This is especially important in elderly patients.
- After the guide catheter is removed (usually 6 to 12 hours after valvuloplasty), apply direct pressure for at least 10 minutes and monitor the site frequently. Alternatively, a compression device may be used as appropriate.
- Note the patient's tolerance of the procedure and his condition afterward.

Special considerations

- Assess the patient's vital signs constantly during the procedure, especially if it's an aortic valvuloplasty. During balloon inflation, the aortic outflow tract is completely obstructed, causing blood pressure to fall dangerously low. Ventricular ectopy is also common during balloon positioning and inflation. Start treatment for ectopy when signs or symptoms develop or when ventricular tachycardia is sustained. Carefully assess the patient's respiratory status; changes in rate and pattern can be the first sign of a complication, such as embolism.
- Assess pedal pulses with a Doppler stethoscope. They'll be difficult to detect, especially if the catheter sheath remains in place. Also assess for complications: embolism, hemorrhage, chest pain, and cardiac tamponade. Using heparin and a large-bore catheter can lead to arterial hemorrhage. This complication can be reversed with protamine sulfate when the sheath is removed, or the sheath can be left in place and removed 6 to 8 hours after the heparin is discontinued. Chest pain can result from obstruction of blood flow during aortic valvuloplasty, so assess for signs and symptoms of myocardial ischemia.

ACTION STAT!

Be alert for signs or symptoms of cardiac tamponade (decreased or absent peripheral pulses, pale or cyanotic skin, hypotension, and paradoxical pulse), which requires emergency surgery.

Complications

- Myocardial infarction or calcium emboli (embolization of debris released from the calcified valve) (rare)
- Bleeding or hematoma at the insertion site, arrhythmias, circulatory disorders distal to the insertion site, guide wire perforation of the ventricle leading to tamponade, disruption of the valve ring, restenosis of the valve, and valvular insufficiency, which can contribute to heart failure and reduced cardiac output

■ Infection and allergic reaction to contrast medium

Patient teaching

■ Stress the need for prophylactic antibiotics during dental surgery or other invasive procedures.
■ Explain the importance of regular follow-up care.

Documentation

Document any complications and interventions. Note the patient's tolerance of the procedure and his condition afterward.

Bedside hemoglobin testing

Monitoring hemoglobin levels at the patient's bedside provides fast, accurate results allowing for immediate intervention, if necessary. In contrast, traditional monitoring methods require blood samples to be sent to the laboratory for interpretation. Numerous testing systems are available for bedside monitoring. Bedside systems are also convenient for the patient's home use.

One system that's available is the HemoCue, which gives accurate results without having to pipette, dispense, or mix blood and reagents to obtain readings. This system eliminates the risk of leakage, broken tubes, and splattered blood. A plastic, disposable microcuvette functions as a combination pipette, test tube, and measuring vessel. It contains a reagent that produces a precise chemical reaction as soon as it contacts blood. The photometer is powered by a battery or an AC adapter. Another type of system is calibrated at the manufacturer and seldom needs to be recalibrated, returning to zero between tests. Use the control cuvette included with each system to test photometer function. (See *Using a bedside hemoglobin monitor.*)

Normal hemoglobin values range from 12.5 to 15 g/dl. A below-normal hemoglobin value may indicate anemia, recent hemorrhage, or fluid retention, causing hemodilution. An elevated hemoglobin value suggests hemoconcentration from polycythemia or dehydration.

Equipment

Lancet ♦ microcuvette ♦ photometer ♦ gloves ♦ alcohol pads ♦ gauze pads

Key steps

■ Confirm the patient's identity using two patient identifiers according to your facility's policy.
■ Take the equipment to the patient's bedside, and explain the purpose of the test to him. Tell him that he'll feel a pinprick in his finger during blood sampling.
■ Plug the AC adapter into the photometer power inlet. Plug the other end of the adapter into the wall outlet.
■ Turn the photometer on. If it hasn't been used recently, insert the control cuvette to make sure that the photometer is working properly.
■ Wash your hands and put on gloves.
■ Select an appropriate puncture site. You'll usually use a fingertip for an adult. The middle and fourth fingers are the best choices. The second finger is usually the most sensitive, and the thumb may have thickened skin or calluses. Blood should circulate freely in the finger from which you're collecting blood, so avoid using a ring-bearing finger.
■ For an infant, use the heel or great toe.
■ Keep the patient's finger straight and ask him to relax it. Holding his finger between the thumb and index finger of your nondominant hand, gently rock the patient's finger as you move your fingers from his top knuckle to his fingertip. This causes blood to flow to the sampling point.
■ Use an alcohol pad to clean the puncture site, wiping in a circular motion from the center of the site outward. Dry the site thoroughly with a gauze pad.
■ Pierce the skin quickly and sharply with the lancet and apply the microcuvette, which automatically collects a precise amount of blood (about 5 µl).
■ Place the microcuvette into the photometer. Results will appear on the photometer screen within 40 seconds to 4 minutes.
■ Place a gauze pad over the puncture site until the bleeding stops.
■ Dispose of the lancet and microcuvette according to your facility's policy. Remove your gloves and wash your hands. Notify

DEVICE SAFETY

Using a bedside hemoglobin monitor

Monitoring blood glucose and hemoglobin levels at the patient's bedside is a straightforward procedure. A photometer, such as the HemoCue analyzer shown here, relies on capillary action to draw blood into a disposable microcuvette. This method of obtaining blood minimizes a health care worker's exposure to the patient's blood and decreases the risk of cross-contamination. Follow the three steps shown here when using the HemoCue system.

Pierce the skin; the microcuvette draws blood automatically.

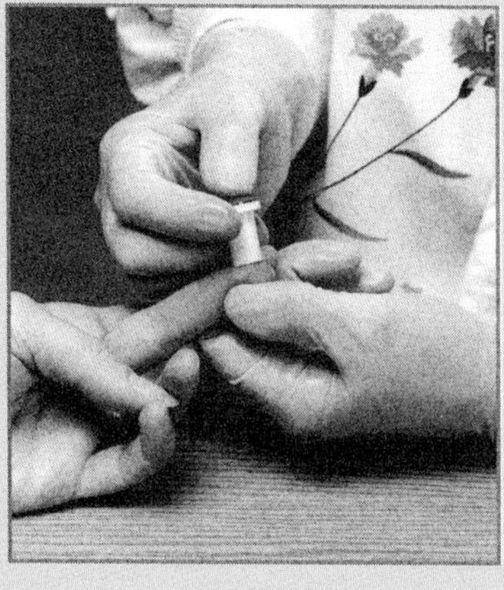

Place the microcuvette into the photometer.

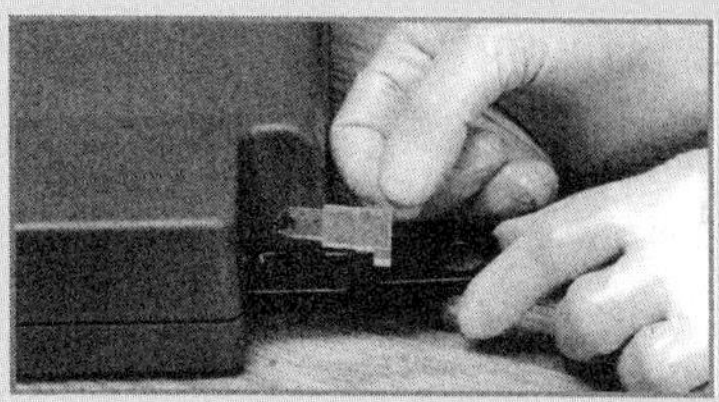

Read the blood glucose or hemoglobin levels from the photometer screen.

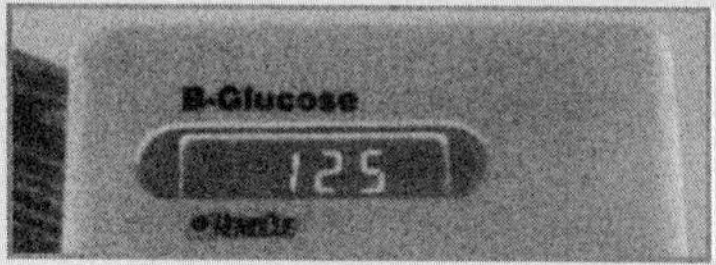

the practitioner if the test result is outside the expected parameters.

Special considerations

- Before using a microcuvette, note its expiration date. Microcuvettes can be stored for up to 2 years; however, after the microcuvette vial is opened, the shelf life is 90 days.
- Before collecting a blood sample, operate the photometer with the control cuvette to check for proper function. To ensure an adequate blood sample, don't use a cold, cyanotic, or swollen area as the puncture site.
- Follow your facility's policy and procedure for point-of-care testing when performing bedside hemoglobin testing.

Complications

None

Documentation

Document the values obtained from the photometer as well as the date and time of the test and any interventions performed.

Bispectral index monitoring

Bispectral index monitoring involves the use of an electronic device that converts EEG waves into a number. This number, statistically derived based on raw EEG data, indicates the depth or level of a patient's sedation and provides a direct measure of the effects of sedatives and anesthetics on the brain. Rather than relying on subjective assessments and vital signs, bispectral index monitoring provides objective, reliable data on which to base care, thus minimizing the risks of oversedation and undersedation.

Bispectral index monitoring equipment

Bispectral index monitoring consists of a monitor and cable connected to a sensor applied to the patient's forehead (as shown below).

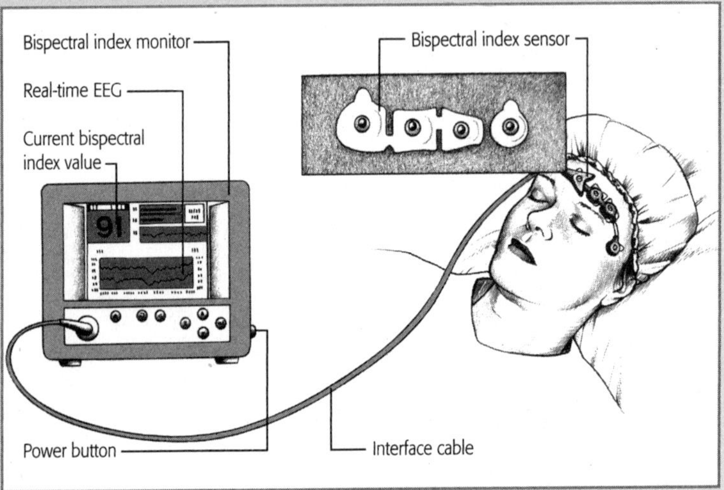

The bispectral index monitor is attached to a sensor that's applied to the patient's forehead. The sensor obtains information about the patient's electrical brain activity and translates this information into a number from 0 (indicating no brain activity) to 100 (indicating a patient who's awake and alert). On the intensive care unit, monitoring is used to assess sedation when the patient is receiving mechanical ventilation or neuromuscular blockers or during barbiturate coma or bedside procedures.

Equipment

Bispectral index monitor and cable ♦ bispectral index sensor ♦ alcohol swabs ♦ soap and water

Preparation

- Place the bispectral index monitor close to the patient's bed, and plug the power cord into the wall outlet.

Key steps

- Gather the necessary equipment and confirm the patient's identity using two patient identifiers according to your facility's policy. Explain the procedure and rationale to the patient and his family. (See *Bispectral index monitoring equipment*.)
- Provide privacy. Wash your hands and follow standard precautions.
- Clean the patient's forehead with soap and water and allow it to dry. If necessary, wipe the forehead with an alcohol swab to ensure that the skin is oil-free. Allow the alcohol to dry.
- Open the sensor package and apply the sensor to the patient's forehead. Position the circle labeled "1" midline—approximately 1½″ (about 4 cm) above the bridge of the nose.
- Position the circle labeled "3" on the right or left temple area, at the level of the outer canthus of the eye, between the corner of the eye and the patient's hairline.
- Ensure that the circle labeled "4" and the line below it are parallel to the eye on the appropriate side.

Sensor problems

When initiating bispectral index monitoring, be aware that the monitor may display messages that indicate a problem. This chart highlights these messages and offers possible solutions.

Message	Possible solutions
High impedance message	Check sensor adhesion; reapply firm pressure to each of the numbered circles on the sensor for 5 seconds each; if message continues, check the connection between the sensor and the monitor; if necessary, apply a new sensor.
Noise message	Remove possible pressure on the sensor; investigate possible electrical interference from equipment.
Lead-off message	Check sensor for electrode displacement or lifting; reapply with firm pressure or if necessary, apply a new sensor.

- Apply gentle, firm pressure around the edges of the sensor, including the areas in between the numbered circles, to ensure proper adhesion.
- Press firmly on each of the numbered circles for approximately 5 seconds to ensure that the electrodes adhere to the skin.
- Connect the sensor to the interface cable and monitor.
- Turn on the monitor.
- Watch the monitor for information related to impedance (electrical resistance) testing.

ALERT

Be aware that for the monitor to display a reading, impedance values must be below a specified threshold. If not, be prepared to troubleshoot sensor problems. (See *Sensor problems*.)

- Select a smoothing rate (the time during which data is analyzed for calculation of the bispectral index; usually 15 or 30 seconds) using the "advanced setup" button based on your facility's policy. Read and record the bispectral index value.

Special considerations

- Always evaluate the bispectral index value in light of other patient assessment findings—don't rely on the bispectral index value alone. (See *Interpreting bispectral index values*, page 30.)
- Keep in mind that movement may occur with low bispectral index values. Be alert for possible artifact that could falsely elevate bispectral index values.

ALERT

Bispectral index values may be elevated due to muscle shivering, tightening, or twitching, or the use of mechanical devices either with the patient or near the patient, bispectral index monitor, or sensor. Interpret the bispectral index value cautiously in these situations.

- Anticipate the need to adjust the dosage of sedation based on the patient's bispectral index value.

ALERT

Keep in mind that a decrease in stimulation, increased sedation, recent administration of a neuromuscular blocking agent or analgesia, or hypothermia may decrease bispectral index, thus indicating the need for a decrease in sedative agents. Pain may cause

Interpreting bispectral index values

Use the following guidelines to interpret your patient's bispectral index value.

Bispectral index	State	
100	Awake	
80	Light or moderate sedation	Light hypnotic state
70	Deep sedation (low probability of explicit recall)	Light hypnotic state
60	General anesthesia (low probability of consciousness)	Moderate hypnotic state
40	Deep hypnotic state	
0	Flat-line EEG	

an elevated bispectral index, indicating a need for an increase in sedation.

- Check the sensor site according to your facility's policy. Change the sensor every 24 hours.

Complications

None

Documentation

Document initiation of bispectral index monitoring, including baseline bispectral index value and location of the sensor. Record assessment findings in conjunction with the bispectral index value to provide a clear overall picture of the patient's condition.

Record any increases or decreases in bispectral index values, along with actions instituted based on values and any changes in sedative agents administered.

Bladder irrigation, continuous

Continuous bladder irrigation can help prevent urinary tract obstruction by flushing out small blood clots that form in the patient after prostate or bladder surgery. It may also be used to treat an irritated, inflamed, or infected bladder lining.

This procedure requires placement of a triple-lumen catheter: one lumen controls balloon inflation, one allows irrigant inflow, and one allows irrigant outflow. The continuous flow of irrigating solution through the bladder also creates a mild tamponade that may help prevent venous hemorrhage. Although the patient typically receives the catheter while he's in the operating room after prostate or bladder surgery, he may have it inserted at his bedside if he isn't a surgical patient.

Equipment

One 4,000-ml container or two 2,000-ml containers of irrigating solution (usually normal saline solution) or the prescribed amount of medicated solution ♦ Y-type tubing made specifically for bladder irrigation ♦ alcohol or a povidone-iodine pad ♦ I.V. pole or bedside pole attachment ♦ drainage bag and tubing

Preparation

- Before starting continuous bladder irrigation, double-check the irrigating solution against the practitioner's order.

Setup for continuous bladder irrigation

In continuous bladder irrigation, a triple-lumen catheter allows irrigating solution to flow into the bladder through one lumen and flow out through another, as shown in the inset. The third lumen is used to inflate the balloon that holds the catheter in place.

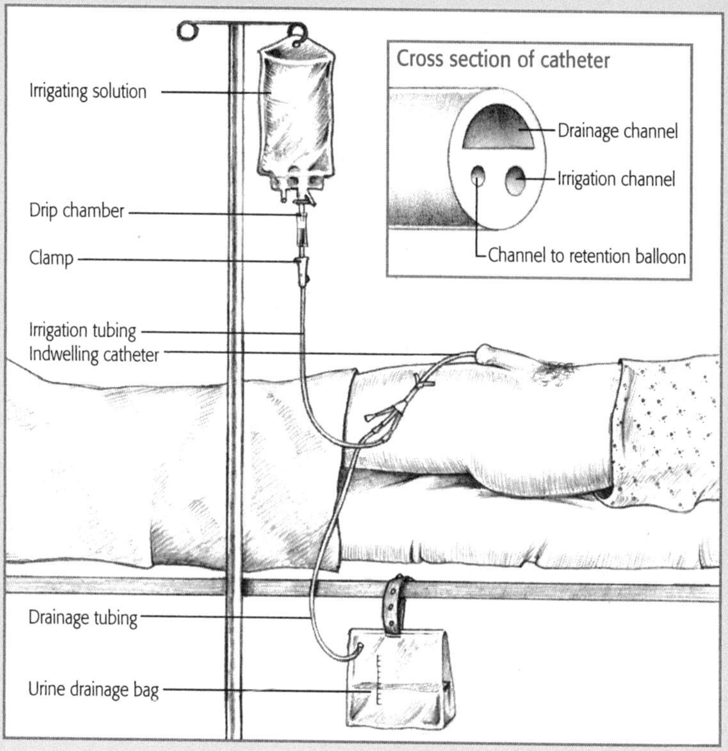

- If the solution contains an antibiotic, check the patient's chart to make sure that he isn't allergic to the drug.
- Unless otherwise specified, the patient should remain on bed rest throughout continuous bladder irrigation.

Key steps

- Confirm the patient's identity using two patient identifiers according to your facility's policy.
- Wash your hands. Assemble all equipment at the patient's bedside. Explain the procedure to the patient and provide privacy.
- Insert the spike of the Y-type tubing into the container of irrigating solution. (If you have a two-container system, insert one spike into each container.) (See *Setup for continuous bladder irrigation.*)
- Squeeze the drip chamber on the spike of the tubing.
- Open the flow clamp and flush the tubing to remove air, which could cause bladder distention. Then close the clamp.
- To begin, hang the irrigating solution on the I.V. pole.
- Clean the opening to the inflow lumen of the catheter with the alcohol or povidone-iodine pad.

- Insert the distal end of the Y-type tubing securely into the inflow lumen (third port) of the catheter.
- Make sure that the catheter's outflow lumen is securely attached to the drainage bag tubing.
- Open the flow clamp under the container of irrigating solution, and set the drip rate as ordered.
- To prevent air from entering the system, don't let the primary container empty completely before replacing it.
- If you have a two-container system, simultaneously close the flow clamp under the nearly empty container and open the flow clamp under the reserve container. This prevents reflux of irrigating solution from the reserve container into the nearly empty one. Hang a new reserve container on the I.V. pole and insert the tubing, maintaining asepsis.
- Empty the drainage bag about every 4 hours or as often as needed. Use sterile technique to avoid the risk of contamination.
- Monitor the patient's vital signs at least every 4 hours during irrigation; increase the frequency if his condition becomes unstable.

Special considerations

- Check the inflow and the outflow lines periodically for kinks to make sure that the solution is running freely. If the solution flows rapidly, check the lines frequently.
- Measure the outflow volume accurately. It should—allowing for urine production—exceed inflow volume.

ACTION STAT!

If inflow volume exceeds outflow volume postoperatively, suspect bladder rupture at the suture lines or renal damage, and notify the practitioner immediately.

- Assess outflow for changes in appearance and for blood clots, especially if irrigation is being performed postoperatively to control bleeding. If drainage is bright red, irrigating solution is usually infused rapidly with the clamp wide open until drainage clears. Notify the practitioner at once if you suspect hemorrhage. If drainage is clear, the solution is usually given at a rate of 40 to 60 gtt/minute. The practitioner typically specifies the rate for antibiotic solutions.
- Encourage oral fluid intake of 2 to 3 qt/day (2 to 3 L/day), unless contraindicated by another medical condition.
- Watch for interruptions in the continuous irrigation system.

DO'S & DON'TS

Check frequently for an obstruction in the catheter's outflow lumen.

Complications

- Infection due to interruptions of the continuous irrigation system
- Bladder distention caused by obstruction in the catheter's outflow lumen

Documentation

Each time you finish a container of solution, record the date, time, and amount of fluid given on the intake and output record. Also, record the time and amount of fluid each time you empty the drainage bag. Note the appearance of the drainage and any complaints the patient has.

Blood cultures

Blood is normally bacteria-free but susceptible to infection through infusion lines as well as from thrombophlebitis, infected shunts, and bacterial endocarditis due to prosthetic heart valve replacements. Bacteria may also invade the vascular system from local tissue infections through the lymphatic system and the thoracic duct.

Blood cultures are performed to detect bacterial invasion (bacteremia) and the systemic spread of such an infection (septicemia) through the bloodstream. In this procedure, a venous blood sample is collected by venipuncture at the patient's bedside and then transferred into two bottles, one containing an anaerobic medium and the other, an aerobic medium. The bottles are incubated, encouraging any organisms that are present in the sample to grow in the media. Blood cultures allow identification of about 67% of pathogens within 24 hours and up to 90% within 72 hours.

Although the timing of culture collections is debatable and possibly irrelevant, drawing three blood samples at least 1 hour apart is suggested. The first of these should be collected at the earliest sign of suspected bacteremia or septicemia. To check for suspected bacterial endocarditis, three or four samples may be collected at 5- to 30-minute intervals before starting antibiotic therapy.

Equipment

Tourniquet ♦ gloves ♦ alcohol ♦ povidone-iodine pads ♦ 10-ml syringe for an adult; 6-ml syringe for a child ♦ three or four 20G 1″ needles ♦ two or three blood culture bottles (50-ml bottles for adults, 20-ml bottles for infants and children) with sodium polyethanol sulfonate added (one aerobic bottle containing a suitable medium, such as Trypticase soy broth with 10% carbon dioxide atmosphere; one anaerobic bottle with prereduced medium; and, possibly, one hyperosmotic bottle with 10% sucrose medium) ♦ laboratory request form and laboratory biohazard transport bags ♦ 2″ × 2″ gauze pads ♦ small adhesive bandages ♦ labels

Preparation

- Check the expiration dates on the culture bottles and replace outdated bottles.

Key steps

- Confirm the patient's identity using two patient identifiers according to your facility's policy. Tell the patient that you need to collect a series of blood samples to check for infection. Explain the procedure to ease his anxiety and promote cooperation. Explain that the procedure usually requires three blood samples collected at different times.
- Wash your hands and put on gloves.
- Tie a tourniquet 2″ (5.1 cm) proximal to the area chosen. (See "Venipuncture," page 596.)
- Clean the venipuncture site with an alcohol pad. Start at the site and work outward in a circular motion. Wait 30 to 60 seconds for the skin to dry.
- Clean the venipuncture site with a povidone-iodine pad. Start at the site and work outward in a circular motion. Wait for the povidone-iodine to dry completely before performing the venipuncture.

DO'S & DON'TS

Don't wipe off the povidone-iodine with alcohol.

- Perform a venipuncture, drawing 10 ml of blood from an adult and only 2 to 6 ml of blood from a child.
- Wipe the diaphragm tops of the culture bottles with a povidone-iodine pad, and change the needle on the syringe used to draw the blood.
- Inject 5 ml of blood into each 50-ml bottle or 2 ml into each 20-ml pediatric culture bottle. (Bottle size may vary according to your facility's policy, but the sample dilution should always be 1:10.)
- Label the culture bottles with the patient's name and identification number, practitioner's name, and date and time of collection. Indicate the suspected diagnosis and the patient's temperature, and note on the laboratory request form any recent antibiotic therapy. Place the samples in the laboratory biohazard transport bag. Send the samples to the laboratory immediately.
- Discard syringes, needles, and gloves in the appropriate containers.

Special considerations

- Obtain each set of cultures from a different site.
- Avoid using existing blood lines for cultures unless the sample is drawn when the line is inserted or catheter sepsis is suspected.

Complications

- Hematoma

Documentation

Record the date and time of blood sample collection, name of the test, amount of blood collected, number of bottles used, patient's temperature, and adverse reactions to the procedure.

Blood glucose tests

Rapid, easy-to-perform reagent strip tests (such as Glucostix, Chemstrip bG, and Multistix) use a drop of capillary blood obtained by fingerstick, heelstick, or earlobe puncture as a sample. These tests can detect or monitor elevated blood glucose levels in patients with diabetes, screen for diabetes mellitus and neonatal hypoglycemia, and help distinguish diabetic coma from nondiabetic coma. They can be performed in the hospital, practitioner's office, or patient's home.

In blood glucose tests, a plastic strip that's inserted into a portable blood glucose meter (such as Glucometer, Accu-Chek, and OneTouch) provides quantitative measurements that compare in accuracy with other laboratory tests. Some meters store successive test results electronically to help determine glucose patterns.

Equipment

Reagent strips ♦ gloves ♦ portable blood glucose meter, if available ♦ alcohol pads ♦ gauze pads ♦ disposable lancets or mechanical blood-letting device ♦ small adhesive bandage ♦ watch or clock with a second hand

Key steps

- Confirm the patient's identity using two patient identifiers according to your facility's policy.
- Explain the procedure to the patient or child's parents.
- Next, select the puncture site—usually the fingertip or earlobe for an adult or a child. Use the heel or great toe for an infant.
- Wash your hands and put on gloves.
- If necessary, dilate the capillaries by applying warm, moist compresses to the area for about 10 minutes.
- Wipe the puncture site with an alcohol pad, and dry it thoroughly with a gauze pad.
- To collect a sample from the fingertip with a disposable lancet (smaller than 2 mm), position the lancet on the side of the patient's fingertip, perpendicular to the lines of the fingerprints. Pierce the skin sharply and quickly to minimize the patient's anxiety and pain and to increase blood flow. Alternatively, you can use a mechanical blood-letting device, such as an Autolet, which uses a spring-loaded lancet.
- After puncturing the fingertip, don't squeeze the puncture site to avoid diluting the sample with tissue fluid.
- Touch a drop of blood to the reagent patch on the strip; make sure you cover the entire patch.
- After collecting the blood sample, briefly apply pressure to the puncture site to prevent painful extravasation of blood into subcutaneous tissues. Ask the adult patient to hold a gauze pad firmly over the puncture site until bleeding stops.
- Make sure you leave the blood on the strip for exactly 60 seconds.
- Compare the color change on the strip with the standardized color chart on the product container. If you're using a blood glucose meter, follow the manufacturer's instructions. Meter designs vary, but they all analyze a drop of blood placed on a reagent strip that comes with the unit and provide a digital display of the resulting glucose level.
- After bleeding has stopped, you may apply a small adhesive bandage to the puncture site.

Special considerations

- Before using reagent strips, check the expiration date on the package and replace outdated strips. Check for special instructions related to the specific reagent. The reagent area of a fresh strip should match the color of the "0" block on the color chart. Protect the strips from light, heat, and moisture.
- Before using a blood glucose meter, calibrate it and run it with a control sample to ensure accurate test results. Follow the manufacturer's instructions for calibration.
- Follow your facility's policy for bedside point-of-care testing.

Oral and I.V. glucose tolerance tests

For monitoring trends in glucose metabolism, the two tests described here may offer benefits over blood testing with reagent strips.

Oral glucose tolerance test

The most sensitive test for detecting borderline diabetes mellitus, the oral glucose tolerance test (OGTT) measures carbohydrate metabolism after ingestion of a challenge dose of glucose. The body absorbs this dose rapidly, causing plasma glucose levels to rise and peak within 30 minutes to 1 hour. The pancreas responds by secreting insulin, causing glucose levels to return to normal within 2 to 3 hours. During this period, plasma and urine glucose levels are monitored to assess insulin secretion and the body's ability to metabolize glucose.

Although you may not collect the blood samples and urine specimens (usually five of each) required for this test, you're responsible for preparing the patient for the test and monitoring his physical condition during the test.

Begin by explaining the OGTT to the patient. Then tell him to maintain a high-carbohydrate diet for 3 days and to fast for 10 to 16 hours before the test, as ordered. The patient must not smoke, drink coffee or alcohol, or exercise strenuously for 8 hours before or during the test. Inform him that he'll then receive a challenge dose of 100 g of carbohydrate (usually a sweetened carbonated beverage or gelatin).

Tell the patient who will perform the venipunctures, when they'll be performed, and that he may feel slight discomfort from the needle punctures and the pressure of the tourniquet. Reassure him that collecting each blood sample usually takes less than 3 minutes. As ordered, withhold drugs that may affect test results. Remind him not to discard the first urine specimen voided after waking.

During the test period, watch for signs and symptoms of hypoglycemia—weakness, restlessness, nervousness, hunger, and sweating—and report them to the practitioner immediately. Encourage the patient to drink plenty of water to promote adequate urine excretion. Provide a bedpan, urinal, or specimen container when necessary.

A positive OGTT may indicate diabetes, but also may result from several metabolic diseases requiring further testing.

I.V. glucose tolerance test

The I.V. glucose tolerance test may be chosen for patients who can't absorb an oral dose of glucose; for example, those with malabsorption disorders and short-bowel syndrome or those who have had a gastrectomy. The test measures blood glucose after an I.V. infusion of 50% glucose over 3 to 4 minutes. Blood samples are then collected after 30 minutes, 1 hour, 2 hours, and 3 hours. After an immediate glucose peak of 300 to 400 mg/dl (accompanied by glycosuria), the normal glucose curve falls steadily, reaching fasting levels within 1 to 1¼ hours. Failure to achieve fasting glucose levels within 2 to 3 hours typically confirms diabetes.

- Avoid selecting cold, cyanotic, or swollen puncture sites to ensure an adequate blood sample. If you can't obtain a capillary sample, perform venipuncture and place a large drop of venous blood on the reagent strip. If you want to test blood from a refrigerated sample, allow the blood to return to room temperature before testing it.
- To help detect abnormal glucose metabolism and diagnose diabetes mellitus, the physician may order other blood glucose tests. (See *Oral and I.V. glucose tolerance tests.*)
- Newer blood glucose meters, such as the OneTouch Ultra, require smaller amounts

of blood; the puncture may be done on the patient's arm instead of his finger.

Complications

None

Patient teaching

- If the patient will be using the reagent strip system at home, teach him the proper use of the lancet or Autolet, reagent strips and color chart, and portable blood glucose meter, as necessary.
- Provide the patient with written guidelines.

Documentation

Record the reading from the reagent strip (using a portable blood glucose meter or a color chart) in your notes or on a special flowchart, if available. Also record the time and date of the test.

Blood pressure assessment

Blood pressure measures the pressure exerted by the blood as it flows through the arteries. Blood moves in waves as the heart contracts and relaxes. Systolic pressure occurs during left ventricular contraction at the height of the wave and reflects the integrity of the heart, arteries, and arterioles. Diastolic pressure occurs during left ventricular relaxation and directly indicates blood vessel resistance. Blood pressure is measured in millimeters of mercury (mm Hg) with a sphygmomanometer and a stethoscope, usually at the brachial artery (less commonly at the popliteal or radial artery).

Pulse pressure—the difference between systolic and diastolic pressures—varies inversely with arterial elasticity. Rigid vessels, incapable of distention and recoil, produce high systolic pressure and low diastolic pressure by about 40 mm Hg. Narrowed pulse pressure, a difference of less than 30 mm Hg, occurs when systolic pressure falls and diastolic pressure rises. These changes reflect reduced stroke column, increased peripheral resistance, or both. Widened pulse pressure, a difference of more than 50 mm Hg between systolic and diastolic pressures, occurs when systolic pressure rises and diastolic pressure remains constant, or when systolic pressure rises and diastolic pressure falls. These changes reflect increased stroke volume, decreased peripheral resistance, or both.

Equipment

Mercury or aneroid sphygmomanometer ♦ stethoscope ♦ automated vital signs monitor (if available)

The sphygmomanometer consists of an inflatable compression cuff linked to a manual air pump and a mercury manometer or an aneroid gauge. The mercury sphygmomanometer is more accurate and requires calibration less frequently than the aneroid model. However, a recently calibrated aneroid manometer may be used. To obtain an accurate reading from a mercury sphygmomanometer, you must rest its gauge on a level surface and view the meniscus at eye level; you can rest an aneroid gauge in any position, but you must view it directly from the front.

Cuffs come in sizes ranging from neonate to extra-large adult. Disposable cuffs and thigh cuffs are available. (See *Positioning the blood pressure cuff*.)

The automated vital signs monitor is a noninvasive device that measures the pulse rate, systolic and diastolic pressures, and mean arterial pressure at preset intervals. (See *Using an electronic vital signs monitor*, page 38.)

Preparation

- Carefully choose an appropriate-sized cuff for the patient; the bladder should encircle at least 80% at the upper arm. An excessively narrow cuff may cause a falsely high pressure reading; an excessively wide one, a falsely low reading.
- If you're using an automated vital signs monitor, collect the monitor, dual air hose, and pressure cuff. Then make sure that the monitor unit is firmly positioned near the patient's bed.

Key steps

- Tell the patient that you're going to take his blood pressure.

Positioning the blood pressure cuff

To properly position a blood pressure cuff, wrap the cuff snugly around the upper arm above the antecubital area (the inner aspect of the elbow). When measuring an adult's blood pressure, place the lower border of the cuff about 1" (2.5 cm) above the antecubital fossa. The center of the bladder should rest directly over the medial aspect of the arm; most cuffs have an arrow to be positioned over the brachial artery. Next, place the bell of the stethoscope on the brachial artery at the point where you hear the strongest beats.

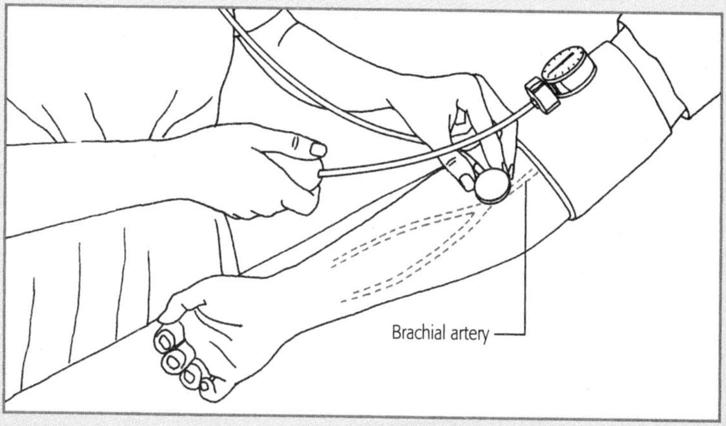

- Have the patient rest for at least 5 minutes before measuring his blood pressure. Make sure that he hasn't had caffeine or smoked for at least 30 minutes.
- The patient may lie supine or sit erect during blood pressure measurement. If the patient is sitting erect, make sure that he has both feet flat on the floor because crossing the legs may elevate blood pressure. His arm should be extended at heart level and be well supported. If the artery is below heart level, you may get a false-high reading. Make sure that the patient is relaxed and comfortable when you take his blood pressure so it stays at its normal level.
- To ensure proper cuff placement on the patient's arm, first palpate the brachial artery. Position the cuff 1" (2.5 cm) above the site of pulsation, center the bladder above the artery with the cuff fully deflated, and wrap the cuff evenly and snugly around the upper arm. If the arm is very large or misshapen and the conventional cuff won't fit properly, take leg or forearm measurements.
- To obtain a thigh blood pressure, apply the appropriate-sized cuff to the thigh, and auscultate the pulsations over the popliteal artery. To obtain a forearm blood pressure, apply the appropriate-sized cuff to the forearm 5" (12.7 cm) below the elbow.
- If necessary, connect the appropriate tube to the rubber bulb of the air pump and the other tube to the manometer. Then insert the stethoscope earpieces into your ears.
- To determine how high to pump the blood pressure cuff, first estimate the systolic blood pressure by palpation. As you feel the radial artery with the fingers of one hand, inflate the cuff with your other hand until the radial pulse disappears. Read this pressure on the manometer and add 30 mm Hg to it. Use this sum as the target inflation to prevent discomfort from overinflation. Deflate the cuff and wait at least 2 minutes.

Using an electronic vital signs monitor

An electronic vital signs monitor allows you to track a patient's vital signs continually, without having to reapply a blood pressure cuff each time. What's more, the patient won't need an invasive arterial line to gather similar data. The machine shown here is a Dinamap VS Monitor 8100, but these steps can be followed with most other monitors.

Some automated vital signs monitors are lightweight and battery-operated and can be attached to an I.V. pole for continual monitoring, even during patient transfers. Make sure you know the capacity of the monitor's battery, and plug the machine in whenever possible to keep it charged. Regularly calibrate the monitor to ensure accurate readings.

Before using any monitor, check its accuracy. Determine the patient's pulse rate and blood pressure manually, using the same arm you'll use for the monitor cuff. Compare your results when you get initial readings from the monitor. If the results differ, call your supply department or the manufacturer's representative.

Preparing the device

- Explain the procedure to the patient. Describe the alarm system so he won't be frightened if it's triggered.
- Make sure the power switch is off. Then plug the monitor into a properly grounded wall outlet.
- Make sure the air hose is secured to the monitor and the cuff. Keep the air hose away from the patient to avoid accidental dislodgment.
- Squeeze all air from the cuff, and wrap it loosely around the patient's arm about 1" (2.5 cm) above the antecubital fossa. If possible, avoid applying the cuff to a limb that has an I.V. line in place. Position the cuff's "artery" arrow over the palpated brachial artery. Then secure the cuff for a snug fit.

Selecting parameters

- When you turn on the monitor, it will default to a manual mode. (In this mode, you can obtain vital signs yourself before switching to the automatic mode.) Press the AUTO/MANUAL button to select the automatic mode. The monitor will give you baseline data for the pulse rate, systolic and diastolic pressures, and mean arterial pressure.
- Compare your previous manual results with these baseline data. If they match, you're ready to set the alarm parameters. Press the SELECT button to blank out all displays except systolic pressure.
- Use the HIGH and LOW limit buttons to set the specific parameters for systolic pressure. (These limits range from a high of 240 to a low of 0.) Repeat this three times for mean arterial pressure, pulse rate, and diastolic pressure. After setting the parameters for diastolic pressure, press the SELECT button again to display all current data. Even if you forget to do this last step, the monitor will automatically

- When you resume, locate the brachial artery by palpation. Center the bell of the stethoscope over the area of the artery where you detect the strongest beats, and hold it in place with one hand. The bell of the stethoscope transmits low-pitched arterial blood sounds more effectively than the diaphragm.
- Using the thumb and index finger of your other hand, turn the thumbscrew on the rubber bulb of the air pump clockwise to close the valve.
- Pump the cuff up to the predetermined level.
- Carefully open the valve of the air pump, and then slowly deflate the cuff—no faster than 2 to 3 mm Hg/second. While releasing air, watch the mercury column or aneroid gauge and auscultate for the sound over the artery.

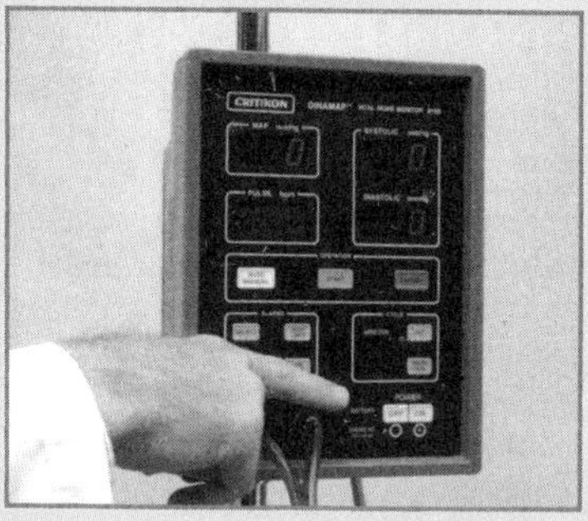

display current data 10 seconds after you set the last parameters.

Collecting data

- Program the monitor according to the desired frequency of assessments. Press the SET button until you reach the desired time interval in minutes. If you have chosen the automatic mode, the monitor will display a default cycle time of 3 minutes. You can override the default cycle time to set the interval you prefer.
- You can obtain a set of vital signs at any time by pressing the START button. Also, pressing the CANCEL button will stop the interval and deflate the cuff. You can retrieve stored data by pressing the PRIOR DATA button. The monitor will display the last data obtained along with the time elapsed since then. Scrolling backward, you can retrieve data from the previous 99 minutes. Make sure vital signs are documented frequently on a vital signs assessment sheet.

- When you hear the first beat or clear tapping sound, note the pressure on the column or gauge. This is the systolic pressure. (The beat or tapping sound is the first of five Korotkoff sounds. The second sound resembles a murmur or swish; the third sound, crisp tapping; the fourth sound, a soft, muffled tone; and the fifth, the last sound heard.)
- Continue to release air gradually while auscultating for the sound over the artery.
- Note the pressure where sound disappears. This is the diastolic pressure—the fifth Korotkoff sound.
- After you hear the last Korotkoff sound, deflate the cuff slowly for at least another 10 mm Hg to ensure that no further sounds are audible.
- Rapidly deflate the cuff. Record the pressure, wait 2 minutes, and then repeat the procedure. If the average of the readings is greater than 5 mm Hg, take the average of two more readings. After doing so, remove and fold the cuff, and return it to storage.
- Document the blood pressure results.

Special considerations

- If you can't auscultate blood pressure, you may estimate systolic pressure. To do this, first palpate the brachial or radial pulse. Then inflate the cuff until you no longer detect the pulse. Slowly deflate the cuff and, when you detect the pulse again, record the pressure as the palpated systolic pressure.
- Palpation of systolic blood pressure also may be important to avoid underestimating blood pressure in the patient with an auscultatory gap. This gap is a loss of sound between the first and second Korotkoff sounds; it may be as great as 40 mm Hg. You may find this in the patient with venous congestion or hypotension.
- When measuring blood pressure in the popliteal artery, position the patient on his abdomen, wrap a cuff around the middle of the thigh, and proceed with blood pressure measurement.
- If the patient is anxious or crying, delay blood pressure measurement, if possible, until he becomes calm to avoid falsely elevated readings.
- Occasionally, blood pressure must be measured in both arms or with the patient in two different positions (such as lying and standing or sitting and standing). In such cases, observe and record significant differences between the two readings, and record the blood pressure and the extremity and position used.
- Measure the blood pressure of the patient taking antihypertensive medications while he's in a sitting position to ensure accurate measurements.

DEVICE SAFETY

Remember that malfunction in an aneroid sphygmomanometer can be identified only by checking it against a mercury manometer of known accuracy. Be sure to check your aneroid manometer this way periodically. Malfunction in a mercury manometer is evident in abnormal behavior of the mercury column. Don't attempt to repair either type yourself; instead, send it to the appropriate service department.

Complications

- Inaccurate reading caused by impaired circulation

DO'S & DONT'S

Don't measure blood pressure on a patient's affected arm if the:

–shoulder, arm, or hand is injured or diseased.
–arm has a cast or bulky bandage.
–patient has had a mastectomy or removal of lymph nodes on that side.
–patient has an arteriovenous fistula in that limb.
–patient has a peripherally inserted central catheter on that side.

- Don't take blood pressure in the arm on the affected side of a mastectomy because it may decrease already compromised lymphatic circulation, worsen edema, and damage the arm.
- Likewise, don't take blood pressure on the same arm of an arteriovenous fistula or hemodialysis shunt because blood flow through the vascular device may be compromised.

Patient teaching

- Teach the patient about lifestyle modifications such as diet, exercise, and smoking cessation.
- Tell the patient about drug therapy such as antihypertensives.
- Make sure the patient understands the importance of follow-up care.

Documentation

In the patient's chart, record blood pressure as systolic over diastolic such as 120/78 mm Hg. Chart an auscultatory gap if present. If required by your facility, chart blood pressures on a graph, using dots or checkmarks. Also, document the limb used and the patient's position. Note the patient's response to patient teaching. Record the name of any practitioner notified of blood pressure results and any orders given.

Body mechanics

Many patient care activities require the nurse to push, pull, lift, and carry. By using proper body mechanics, the nurse can avoid musculoskeletal injury and fatigue and reduce the risk of injuring patients. Correct body mechanics can be summed up in three principles:

1. Keep a low center of gravity by flexing your hips and knees instead of bending at the waist. This position distributes weight evenly between the upper and lower body and helps maintain balance.
2. Create a wide base of support by spreading your feet apart. This tactic provides lateral stability and lowers the body's center of gravity.
3. Maintain proper body alignment and keep your body's center of gravity directly over the base of support by moving your feet rather than twisting and bending at your waist.

Equipment

No specified equipment

Key steps

- Follow the directions below to push, pull, stoop, lift, and carry correctly.

Pushing and pulling

- Stand close to the object and place one foot slightly ahead of the other, as in a walking position. Tighten the leg muscles and set the pelvis by simultaneously contracting the abdominal and gluteal muscles.
- To push, place your hands on the object and flex your elbows. Lean into the object

by shifting weight from the back leg to the front leg, and apply smooth, continuous pressure using leg muscles.

- To pull, grasp the object and flex your elbows. Lean away from the object by shifting weight from the front leg to the back leg. Pull smoothly, avoiding sudden, jerky movements.
- After you've started to move the object, keep it in motion; stopping and starting uses more energy.

Stooping

- Stand with your feet 10″ to 12″ (25.5 to 30.5 cm) apart and one foot slightly ahead of the other to widen the base of support.
- Lower yourself by flexing your knees, and place more weight on the front foot than on the back foot. Keep the upper body straight by not bending at the waist.
- To stand up again, straighten the knees and keep the back straight.

Lifting and carrying

- Assume the stooping position directly in front of the object to minimize back flexion and avoid spinal rotation when lifting.
- Grasp the object, and tighten your abdominal muscles.
- Stand up by straightening the knees, using the leg and hip muscles. Always keep your back straight to maintain a fixed center of gravity.
- Carry the object close to your body at waist height—near your center of gravity—to avoid straining the back muscles.

Special considerations

- Wear shoes with low heels, flexible nonslip soles, and closed backs to promote correct body alignment, facilitate proper body mechanics, and prevent accidents.
- When possible, pull rather than push an object because the elbow flexors are stronger than the extensors. Pulling an object allows the use of hip and leg muscles and avoids the use of lower back muscles.
- When doing heavy lifting or moving, remember to use assistive or mechanical devices, if available, or obtain assistance from coworkers. Know your limitations and use sound judgment.

DEVICE SAFETY

Mechanical and other assistive devices have been shown to significantly decrease incidences of low back injury in nursing personnel.

Complications

None

Documentation

- No specific documentation

Bone growth stimulation, electrical

Electrical bone growth stimulation—imitating the body's natural electrical forces—initiates or accelerates the healing process in a fractured bone that fails to heal. About 1 in 20 fractures may fail to heal properly, possibly as a result of infection, insufficient reduction or fixation, pseudoarthritis, or severe tissue trauma around the fracture.

Recent discoveries about the stimulating effects of electric currents on osteogenesis have led to using electrical bone stimulation to promote healing. The technique is also being investigated for treating spinal fractures.

Three basic electrical bone stimulation techniques are available: fully implantable direct current stimulation; semi-invasive percutaneous stimulation; and noninvasive electromagnetic coil stimulation. (See *Methods of electrical bone growth stimulation,* page 42.) The choice of the technique depends on the fracture type and location, the practitioner's preference, and the patient's ability and willingness to comply. The invasive device requires little or no patient involvement. With the other two methods, however, the patient must manage his own treatment schedule and maintain the equipment. Treatment time averages 3 to 6 months.

Equipment

Direct current stimulation

Small generator and leadwires connecting to a titanium cathode wire (surgically implanted into the nonunited bone site)

Methods of electrical bone growth stimulation

Electrical bone growth stimulation may be invasive or noninvasive.

Invasive system

An invasive system involves placing a spiral cathode inside the bone at the fracture site. A wire leads from the cathode to a battery-powered generator, also implanted in local tissues. The patient's body completes the circuit.

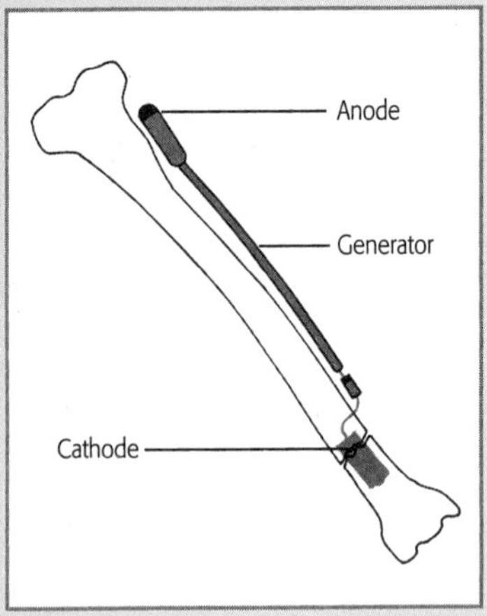

Noninvasive system

A noninvasive system may include a cuf-flike transducer or fitted ring that wraps around the patient's limb at the level of the injury. Electric current penetrates the limb.

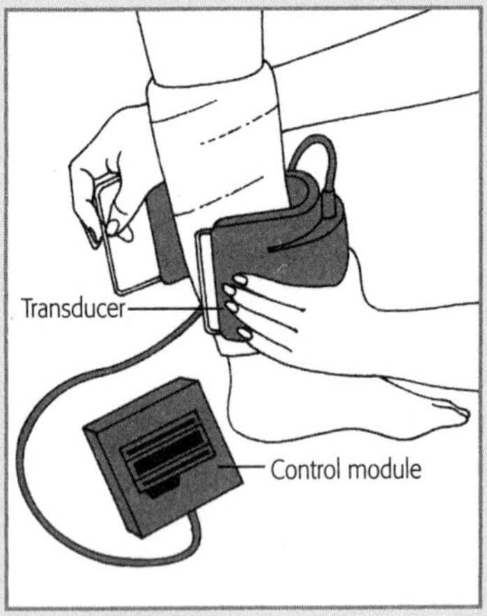

Percutaneous stimulation

External anode skin pad with a leadwire ♦ lithium battery pack ♦ one to four Teflon-coated stainless steel cathode wires (surgically implanted)

Electromagnetic stimulation

Generator that plugs into a standard 110-volt outlet ♦ two strong electromagnetic coils placed on either side of the injured area (The coils can be incorporated into a cast, cuff, or orthotic device.) (See *Using an external bone growth stimulator*.)

Preparation

- All equipment comes in sets with instructions provided by the manufacturer. Follow the instructions carefully.
- Make sure that all parts are included and are sterilized according to your facility's policy and procedure guidelines.

Key steps

- Confirm the patient's identity using two patient identifiers according to your facility's policy.
- Tell the patient whether he'll have an anesthetic and, if possible, which kind.

Direct current stimulation

- Implantation is performed with the patient under general anesthesia. Afterward, the practitioner may apply a cast or external fixator to immobilize the limb. The patient is usually hospitalized for 2 to 3 days after implantation. Weight bearing may be ordered as tolerated.
- After the bone fragments join, the generator and leadwire can be removed under local anesthesia. The titanium cathode remains implanted.

Using an external bone growth stimulator

An external bone growth stimulator (EBGS) is a noninvasive and painless alternative to surgical bone grafting. To use it, first gather the necessary equipment and familiarize your patient with the components of the EBGS system.

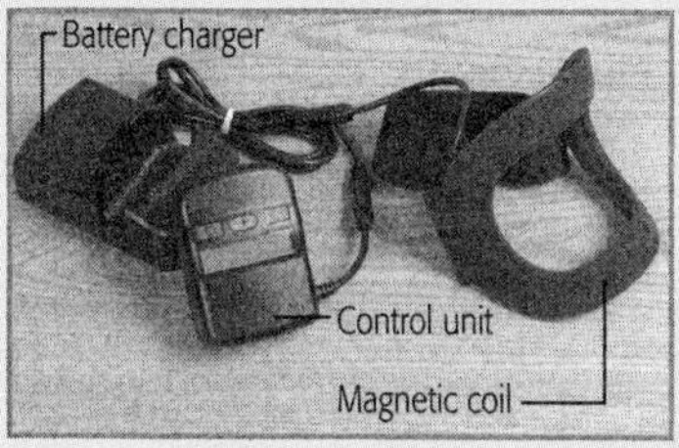

Teach the patient where and how to place the coil. Inform her that she may place the coil over her cast or against her skin. A layer of clothing between the coil and her skin will provide adequate protection against skin irritation. Show her how to secure the coil with the strap and connect the control unit to the coil.

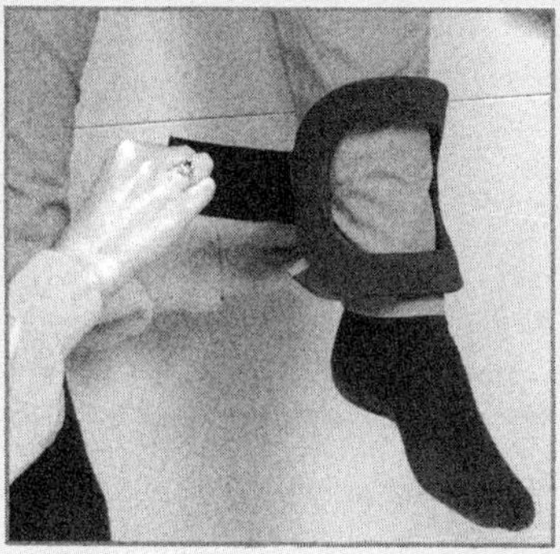

Pressing the button will start the unit, which will begin transmitting and recording. Be sure to show the patient when the battery needs changing. Depending on the type of unit, she may need to do this after each use or when the words "recharge battery" appear on the light-emitting diode (LED) screen. To charge the unit tell her to plug it into an outlet at home and leave it plugged in for at least 2 hours.

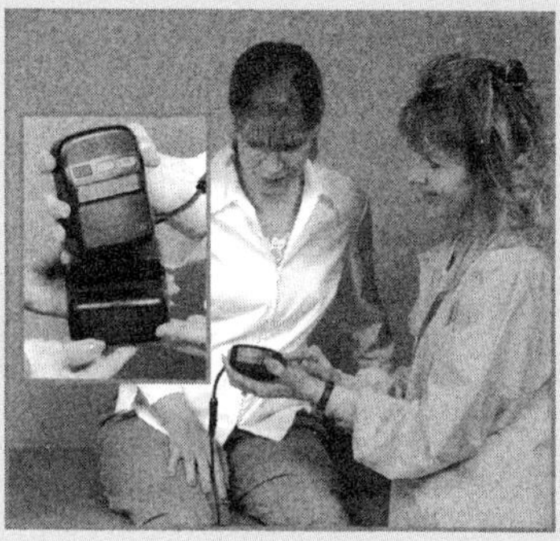

On the patient's return visits, turn on the control unit. The LED screen should display the hourly use per day and the number of days used and not used. Use this data to determine if she has used the EBGS according to her prescribed regimen. Be sure to document the usage times in her medical record.

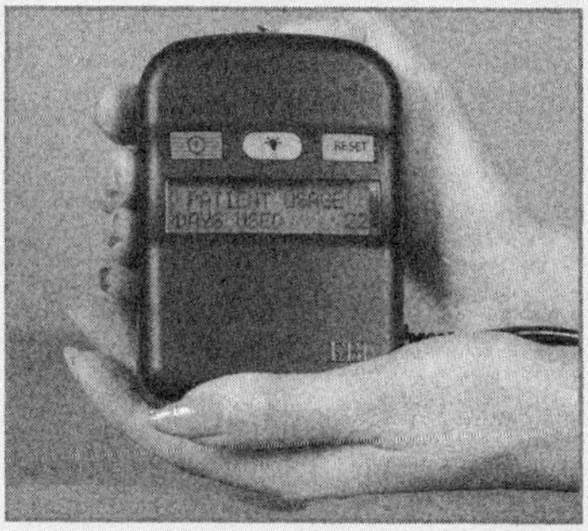

Adapted from Patterson, M. "What's the Buzz on External Bone Growth Stimulators?" *Nursing2000* 30(6):44-45, June 2000, with permission of the publisher.

Percutaneous stimulation

- Remove excessive body hair from the injured site before applying the anode pad. Avoid stressing or pulling on the anode wire. Instruct the patient to change the anode pad every 48 hours. Tell him to report local pain to his practitioner and not to bear weight for the duration of treatment.

Electromagnetic stimulation

- Show the patient where to place the coils, and tell him to apply them for 3 to 10 hours each day as ordered by his practitioner.
- Urge the patient not to interrupt the treatments for more than 10 minutes at a time.
- Teach the patient how to use and care for the generator.
- Relay the practitioner's instructions for weight bearing. Usually, the practitioner will advise against bearing weight until evidence of healing appears on X-rays.

Special considerations

- A patient with direct current electrical bone stimulation shouldn't undergo electrocauterization, diathermy, or magnetic resonance imaging (MRI). Electrocautery may "short" the system; diathermy may potentiate the electric current, possibly causing tissue damage; and the MRI will interfere with or stop the current.

ALERT

Percutaneous electrical bone stimulation is contraindicated if the patient has any kind of inflammatory process.

- Ask the patient if he's sensitive to nickel or chromium because both are present in the electrical bone stimulation system.
- Electromagnetic coils are contraindicated for a pregnant patient, a patient with a tumor, or a patient with an arm fracture or a pacemaker.

Complications

- Increased risk of infection occurring with direct current electrical bone stimulation equipment
- Local irritation or skin ulceration occurring around cathode pin sites with percutaneous devices

Patient teaching

- Teach the patient how to care for his cast or external fixation devices.
- Tell him how to care for the electrical generator.
- Urge him to follow treatment instructions faithfully.

Documentation

Record the type of electrical bone stimulation equipment provided, including the date, time, and location, as appropriate. Note the patient's skin condition and tolerance of the procedure. Record instructions given to the patient and his family as well as their ability to understand and act on those instructions.

Buccal, sublingual, and translingual drug administration

Certain drugs are given buccally, sublingually, or translingually to prevent their destruction or transformation in the stomach or small intestine. These drugs act quickly because the oral mucosa's thin epithelium and abundant vasculature allow direct absorption into the bloodstream.

Drugs given buccally include nitroglycerin (Nitro-Bid) and methyltestosterone; drugs given sublingually include ergotamine tartrate (Ergomar), isosorbide dinitrate (Isordil), and nitroglycerin. Translingual drugs, which are sprayed onto the tongue, include nitrate preparations for patients with chronic angina.

Equipment

Patient's medication record and chart ♦ prescribed medication ♦ medication cup

Key steps

- Verify the order on the patient's medication record by checking it against the prescriber's order on his chart.
- Wash your hands with warm water and soap. Explain the procedure to the patient if he's never taken a drug buccally, sublingually, or translingually before.
- Check the label on the medication before administering it to make sure you'll be giving the prescribed medication. Verify the expiration date of all medications, especially nitroglycerin.

- Confirm the patient's identity using two patient identifiers according to your facility's policy.
- If your facility utilizes a bar code scanning system, be sure to scan your ID badge, the patient's ID bracelet, and the medication's bar code.

Buccal and sublingual administration

- For buccal administration, place the tablet in the buccal pouch, between the cheek and gum. For sublingual administration, place the tablet under the patient's tongue.
- Tell the patient not to rinse his mouth until the tablet has been absorbed.
- Tell the patient with angina to wet the nitroglycerin tablet with saliva and to keep it under his tongue until it has been fully absorbed.
- Instruct the patient to keep the medication in place until it dissolves completely to ensure absorption.
- Caution him against chewing the tablet or touching it with his tongue to prevent accidental swallowing.
- Tell him not to smoke before the drug has dissolved because nicotine's vasoconstrictive effects slow absorption.

Translingual administration

- To administer a translingual drug, tell the patient to hold the medication canister vertically, with the valve head at the top and the spray orifice as close to his mouth as possible.
- Instruct him to spray the dose onto his tongue by pressing the button firmly.
- Remind the patient using a translingual aerosol form that he shouldn't inhale the spray but should release it under his tongue. Also tell him to wait 10 seconds or so before swallowing.

Special considerations

DO'S & DON'TS

Don't give liquids to a patient who's receiving buccal medication because some buccal tablets can take up to 1 hour to be absorbed.

Complications

- Mucosal irritation

DO'S & DONT'S

Alternate sides of the mouth for repeat doses to prevent continuous irritation of the same site.

- Tingling sensation under the tongue caused by sublingual medications such as nitroglycerin (If the patient finds this sensation annoying, try placing the drug in the buccal pouch instead.)

Patient teaching

- If the patient will be taking a buccal, sublingual, or translingual drug at home, make sure that he understands the proper administration.

Documentation

Record the medication administered, dose, date, and time, and patient's reaction, if any.

Burn care

The goals of burn care are to maintain the patient's physiologic stability, repair skin integrity, prevent infection, and promote maximal functioning and psychosocial health. Competent care immediately after a burn occurs can dramatically improve the success of overall treatment.

Burn severity is determined by the depth and extent of the burn and the presence of other factors, such as age, complications, and coexisting illnesses. (See *Estimating burn surfaces in adults and children*, page 46. See also *Evaluating burn severity*, page 47.)

To promote stability, you'll need to carefully monitor your patient's respiratory status, especially if he has suffered smoke inhalation. Be aware that a patient with burns involving more than 20% of his total body surface area usually needs fluid resuscitation, which aims to support the body's compensatory mechanisms without overwhelming them. Expect to give fluids (such as lactated Ringer's solution) to keep the patient's urine output at 30 to 50 ml/hour, and expect to monitor blood pres-

Estimating burn surfaces in adults and children

Different methods are required to assess body surface area (BSA) in adults and children because the proportion of BSA changes as the body grows.

Rule of Nines

The Rule of Nines quantifies BSA in percentages, either in fractions of nine or multiples of nine. To use this method, mentally assess the patient's burns by the body chart shown at right. Add the corresponding percentages for each body section burned. Use the total—a rough estimate of burn extent—to calculate initial fluid replacement needs.

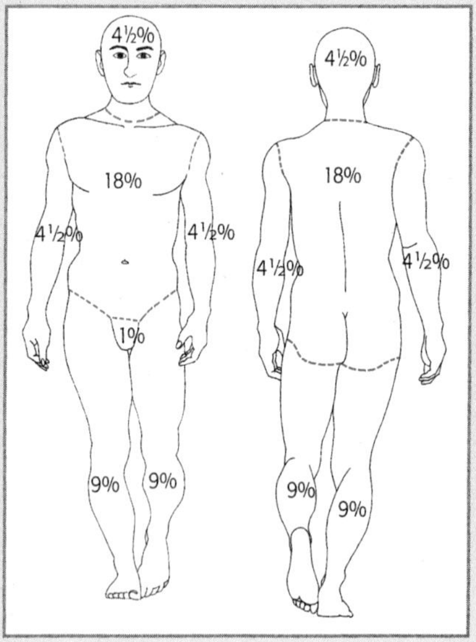

Lund-Browder chart

The Rule of Nines isn't accurate for infants and children because their body proportions differ from those of adults. An infant's head, for example, accounts for about 17% of his total BSA, whereas an adult's head comprises 7% of his BSA. The Lund-Browder chart, as shown here, is based on human anatomic studies relating the proportion of a specific body area to the body as a whole and can be used for infants, children, and adults.

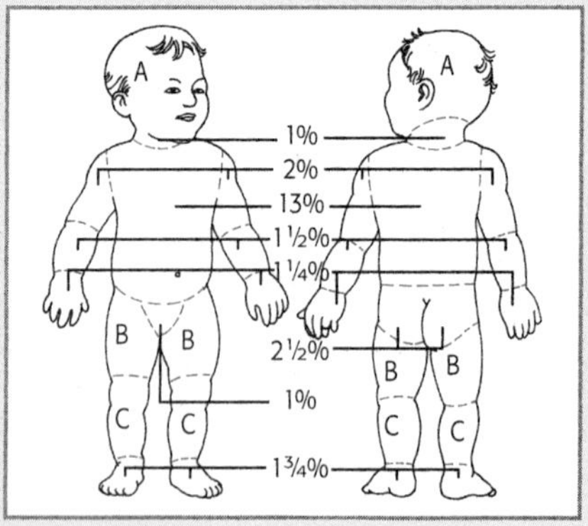

Percentage of burned body surface by age

At birth	0 to 1 year	1 to 4 years	5 to 9 years	10 to 15 years	Adult
A: Half of head					
9½%	8½%	6½%	5½%	4½%	3½%
B: Half of one thigh					
2¾%	3¼%	4%	4¼%	4½%	4¾%
C: Half of one leg					
2½%	2½%	2¾%	3%	3¼%	3½%

Evaluating burn severity

To judge a burn's severity, assess its depth and extent, color, and other factors, as shown below.

First-degree burn

Does the burned area appear pink or red with minimal edema? Is the area sensitive to touch and temperature changes? If so, the patient most likely has a first-degree burn affecting only the epidermal skin layer.

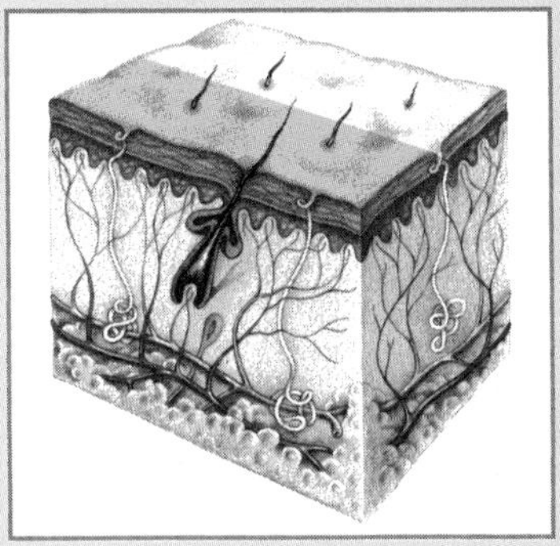

Second-degree deep partial-thickness burn

Does the burned area appear pink or red, with a mottled appearance? Do red areas blanch when you touch them? Does the skin have large, thick-walled blisters with subcutaneous edema? Does touching the burn cause severe pain? Is the hair still present? If so, the person most likely has a second-degree deep partial-thickness burn affecting the epidermal and dermal layers.

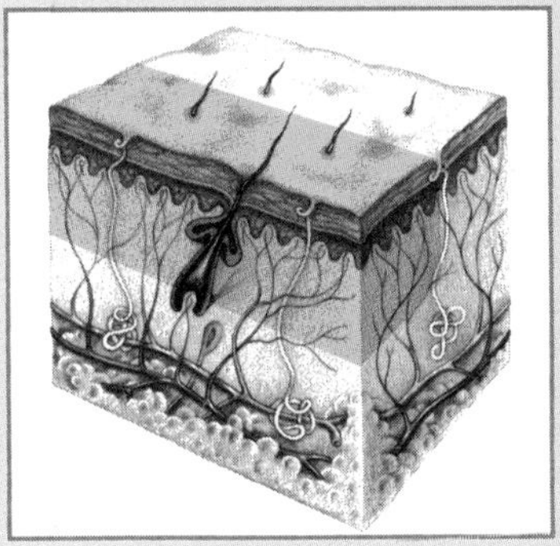

Third-degree burn

Does the burned area appear red, waxy white, brown, or black? Does red skin remain red with no blanching when you touch it? Is the skin leathery with extensive subcutaneous edema? Is the skin insensitive to touch? Does the hair fall out easily? If so, the patient most likely has a third-degree burn that affects all skin layers.

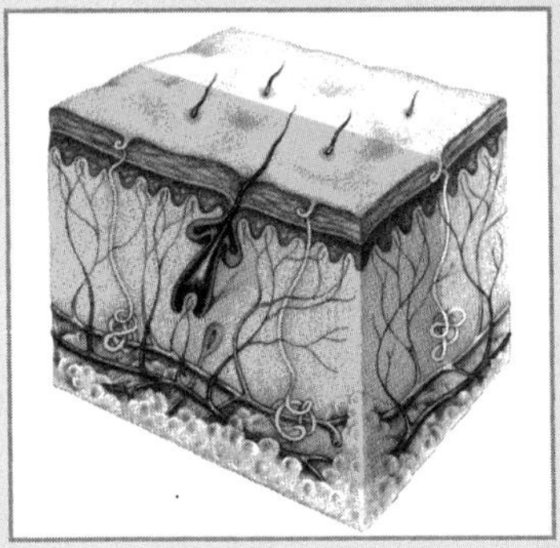

sure and heart rate. You'll also need to control body temperature because skin loss interferes with temperature regulation. Use warm fluids, heat lamps, and hyperthermia blankets, as appropriate, to keep the patient's temperature above 97° F (36.1° C) if possible. Additionally, you'll frequently review such laboratory values as serum electrolyte levels to detect early changes in the patient's condition.

Infection can increase wound depth, cause rejection of skin grafts, slow healing, worsen pain, prolong hospitalization, and even lead to death. To help prevent infection, use strict sterile technique during care, dress the burn site as ordered, monitor and rotate I.V. lines regularly, and carefully assess the burn's extent, body system function, and the patient's emotional status.

Other interventions, such as careful positioning and regular exercise for burned extremities, help maintain joint function, prevent contractures, and minimize deformity. (See *Positioning the burn patient to prevent deformity*.)

Skin integrity is repaired through aggressive wound debridement followed by maintenance of a clean wound bed until the wound heals or is covered with a skin graft. Third-degree burns and some second-degree deep partial-thickness burns must be debrided and grafted in the operating room. Surgery takes place as soon as possible after fluid resuscitation. Most wounds are managed with twice-daily dressing changes using topical antibiotics. Burn dressings encourage healing by barring germ entry and by removing exudate, eschar, and other debris that host infection. After thorough wound cleaning, topical antibacterial agents are applied and the wound is covered with absorptive, coarse-mesh gauze. Roller gauze typically tops the dressing and is secured with elastic netting or tape.

Equipment

Normal saline solution ♦ sterile bowl ♦ scissors ♦ tissue forceps ♦ ordered topical medication ♦ burn gauze ♦ roller gauze ♦ elastic netting or tape ♦ fine-mesh gauze ♦ elastic gauze ♦ cotton-tipped applicators ♦ ordered pain medication ♦ three pairs of sterile gloves ♦ sterile gown ♦ mask ♦ surgical cap ♦ heat lamps ♦ impervious plastic trash bag ♦ cotton bath blanket ♦ 4″ × 4″ gauze pads

A sterile field is required, and all equipment and supplies used in the dressing should be sterile.

Preparation

- Warm normal saline solution by immersing unopened bottles in warm water.
- Assemble equipment on the dressing table.
- Make sure the treatment area has adequate light to allow accurate wound assessment.
- Open equipment packages using sterile technique. Arrange supplies on a sterile field in order of use.
- To prevent cross-contamination, plan to dress the cleanest areas first and the dirtiest or most contaminated areas last.
- To help prevent excessive pain or cross-contamination, you may need to perform the dressing in stages to avoid exposing all wounds at the same time.

Key steps

- Administer the ordered pain medication about 20 minutes before beginning wound care to maximize patient comfort and cooperation.
- Explain the procedure to the patient and provide privacy.
- Turn on overhead heat lamps to keep the patient warm. Make sure they don't overheat the patient.
- Pour warmed normal saline solution into the sterile bowl in the sterile field.
- Wash your hands.

Removing a dressing without hydrotherapy

- Put on a gown, a mask, and sterile gloves.
- Remove dressing layers down to the innermost layer by cutting the outer dressings with sterile blunt scissors. Lay open these dressings.
- If the inner layer appears dry, soak it with warm normal saline solution to ease removal.
- Remove the inner dressing with sterile tissue forceps or your sterile gloved hand.
- Because soiled dressings harbor infectious microorganisms, dispose of the dressings carefully in the impervious plastic trash bag according to your facility's policy. Dispose of your gloves and wash your hands.

Positioning the burn patient to prevent deformity

For each of the potential deformities listed below, you can use the corresponding positioning and interventions to help prevent the deformity.

Burned area	Potential deformity	Preventive positioning	Nursing interventions
Neck	▪ Flexion contracture of neck ▪ Extensor contracture of neck	▪ Extension ▪ Prone with head slightly raised	▪ Remove pillow from bed. ▪ Place pillow or rolled towel under upper chest to flex cervical spine, or apply cervical collar.
Axilla	▪ Adduction and internal rotation ▪ Adduction and external rotation	▪ Shoulder joint in external rotation and 100- to 130-degree abduction ▪ Shoulder joint in forward flexion and 100- to 130-degree abduction	▪ Use an I.V. pole, bedside table, or sling to suspend arm. ▪ Use an I.V. pole, bedside table, or sling to suspend arm.
Pectoral region	▪ Shoulder protraction	▪ Shoulders abducted and externally rotated	▪ Remove pillow from bed.
Chest or abdomen	▪ Kyphosis	▪ Same as for pectoral region, with hips neutral (not flexed)	▪ Use no pillow under head or legs.
Lateral trunk	▪ Scoliosis	▪ Supine; affected arm abducted	▪ Put pillows or blanket rolls at sides.
Elbow	▪ Flexion and pronation	▪ Arm extended and supinated	▪Use an elbow splint, arm board, or bedside table.
Wrist	▪ Flexion ▪ Extension	▪ Splint in 15-degree extension ▪ Splint in 15-degree flexion	▪ Apply a hand splint. ▪ Apply a hand splint.
Fingers	▪ Adhesions of the extensor tendons; loss of palmar grasp	▪ Metacarpophalangeal joints in maximum flexion; interphalangeal joints in slight flexion; thumb in maximum abduction	▪ Apply a hand splint; wrap fingers separately.

(continued)

Positioning the burn patient to prevent deformity

(continued)

Burned area	Potential deformity	Preventive positioning	Nursing interventions
Hip	▪ Internal rotation, flexion, and adduction; possibly joint subluxation if contracture is severe	▪ Neutral rotation and abduction; maintain extension by prone position	▪ Put a pillow under buttocks (if supine) or use trochanter rolls or knee or long leg splints.
Knee	▪ Flexion	▪ Extension maintained	▪ Use a knee splint with no pillows under legs.
Ankle	▪ Plantar flexion if foot muscles are weak or their tendons are divided	▪ 90-degree dorsiflexion	▪ Use a footboard or ankle splint.

▪ Put on a new pair of sterile gloves. Using gauze pads moistened with normal saline solution, gently remove exudate and old topical medication.
▪ Carefully remove all loose eschar with sterile forceps and scissors, if ordered.
▪ Assess the wound's condition. It should appear clean, with no debris, loose tissue, purulence, inflammation, or darkened margins.
▪ Before applying a new dressing, remove your gown, gloves, and mask. Discard them properly, and put on a clean mask, a surgical cap, a gown, and sterile gloves.

Applying a wet dressing

▪ Soak fine-mesh gauze and the elastic gauze dressing in a large, sterile basin containing the ordered solution (for example, silver nitrate).
▪ Wring out the fine-mesh gauze until it's moist but not dripping, and apply it to the wound. Warn the patient that he may feel transient pain when you apply the dressing.
▪ Wring out the elastic gauze dressing, and position it to hold the fine-mesh gauze in place.
▪ Roll an elastic gauze dressing over the dressing to keep dressings intact.
▪ Cover the patient with a cotton bath blanket to prevent chills. Change the blanket if it becomes damp. Use an overhead heat lamp, if necessary.
▪ Change the dressings frequently, as ordered, to keep the wound moist, especially if you're using silver nitrate. Silver nitrate becomes ineffective and the silver ions may damage tissue if the dressing becomes dry. (To maintain moisture, some protocols call for irrigating the dressing with solution at least every 4 hours through small slits cut into the outer dressing.)

Applying a dry dressing with a topical medication

▪ Remove old dressings, and clean the wound (as described previously).
▪ Apply the ordered medication to the wound in a thin layer—about 2 to 4 mm thick—with your sterile gloved hand. Apply several layers of burn gauze over the wound to contain the medication but allow exudate to escape.
▪ Remember to cut the dressing to fit only the wound areas; don't cover unburned areas.

■ Cover the entire dressing with roller gauze, and secure it with elastic netting or tape.

Providing arm and leg care

■ Apply the dressings from the distal to the proximal area to stimulate circulation and prevent constriction. Wrap the burn gauze once around the arm or leg so the edges overlap slightly. Continue wrapping in this way until the gauze covers the wound.
■ Apply a dry roller gauze dressing to hold the bottom layers in place. Secure with elastic netting or tape.

Providing hand and foot care

■ Wrap each finger separately with a single layer of a 4″ × 4″ gauze pad to allow the patient to use his hands and to prevent webbing contractures.
■ Place the hand in a functional position, and secure this position using a dressing. Apply splints, if ordered.
■ Put gauze between each toe as appropriate, to prevent webbing contractures.

Providing chest, abdomen, and back care

■ Apply the ordered medication to the wound in a thin layer. Cover the entire burned area with sheets of burn gauze.
■ Wrap with roller gauze or apply a specialty vest dressing to hold the burn gauze in place.
■ Secure the dressing with elastic netting or tape. Make sure the dressing doesn't restrict respiratory motion, especially in very young or elderly patients or in those with circumferential injuries.

Providing scalp and facial care

■ If the patient has scalp burns, clip or shave the hair around the burn, as ordered. Clip other hair until it's about 2″ (5.1 cm) long to prevent contamination of burned scalp areas.
■ Shave facial hair if it comes in contact with burned areas.
■ Typically, facial burns are managed with milder topical agents (such as triple antibiotic ointment) and are left open to air. If dressings are required, make sure they don't cover the eyes, nostrils, or mouth.

Providing ear care

■ Clip or shave the hair around the affected ear.
■ Remove exudate and crusts with cotton-tipped applicators dipped in normal saline solution.
■ Place a layer of 4″ × 4″ gauze behind the auricle to prevent webbing.
■ Apply the ordered topical medication to 4″ × 4″ gauze pads, and place the pads over the burned area. Before securing the dressing with a roller bandage, position the patient's ears normally to avoid damaging the auricular cartilage.
■ Assess the patient's hearing ability.

Providing eye care

■ Clean the area around the eyes and eyelids with a cotton-tipped applicator and normal saline solution every 4 to 6 hours, or as needed, to remove crusts and drainage.
■ Administer ordered eye ointment or drops.
■ If the eyes can't be closed, apply lubricating ointment or drops, as ordered.
■ Be sure to close the patient's eyes before applying eye pads to prevent corneal abrasion. Don't apply topical ointment near the eyes without a practitioner's order.

Providing nasal care

■ Check the nostrils for inhalation injury, such as inflamed mucosa, singed vibrissae, and soot.
■ Clean the nostrils with cotton-tipped applicators dipped in normal saline solution. Remove crusts.
■ Apply the ordered ointment.
■ If the patient has a nasogastric tube, use tracheostomy ties to secure the tube. Be sure to check ties frequently for tightness resulting from facial tissue swelling. Clean the area around the tube every 4 to 6 hours.

Special considerations

■ Thorough assessment and documentation of the wound's appearance are essential to detect infection and other complications. A purulent wound or green-gray exudate indicates infection, an overly dry wound suggests dehydration, and a wound with a swollen, red edge suggests cellulitis. Suspect a fungal infection if the wound is white and powdery. Healthy granulation tissue appears clean, pinkish, faintly shiny, and free from exudate.

- Blisters protect underlying tissue, so leave them intact unless they impede joint motion, become infected, or cause patient discomfort.
- Keep in mind that the patient with healing burns has increased nutritional needs. He'll require extra protein and carbohydrates to accommodate an almost doubled basal metabolism.
- If you must manage a burn with topical medications, exposure to air, and no dressing, watch for such problems as wound adherence to bed linens, poor drainage control, and partial loss of topical medications.

Complications

- Infection
- Sepsis
- Allergic reaction to ointments or dressings
- Renal failure
- Multiple-organ-dysfunction syndrome
- Disfigurement, pain, and emotional issues

Patient teaching

- Begin discharge planning as soon as the patient enters the facility to help him (and his family) make a smooth transition from facility to home.
- To encourage therapeutic compliance, prepare him to expect scarring, teach him wound management and pain control, and urge him to follow the prescribed exercise regimen.
- Provide encouragement and emotional support, and urge the patient to join a burn survivor support group.
- Teach the family or caregivers how to encourage, support, and provide care for the patient.

Documentation

Record the date and time of all care provided. Describe the wound's condition, special dressing-change techniques, topical medications administered, positioning of the burned area, and the patient's tolerance of the procedure.

Burn dressings, biological

Biological dressings provide a temporary protective covering for burn wounds and clean granulation tissue. They also temporarily secure fresh skin grafts and protect graft donor sites. Three organic materials (pigskin, cadaver skin, and amniotic membrane) and one synthetic material (Biobrane) are commonly used. (See *Comparing biological dressings.*) Besides stimulating new skin growth, these dressings act like normal skin: They reduce heat loss, block infection, and minimize fluid, electrolyte, and protein losses.

Amniotic membrane or fresh cadaver skin is usually applied to the patient in the operating room, although it may be applied in a treatment room. Pigskin or Biobrane may be applied in either the operating room or a treatment room. Before applying a biological dressing, the nurse must clean and debride the wound. The frequency of dressing changes depends on the type of wound and the dressing's specific function.

Equipment

Ordered analgesic ♦ cap ♦ mask ♦ two pairs of sterile gloves ♦ sterile or clean gown ♦ shoe covers ♦ biological dressing ♦ sterile normal saline solution ♦ sterile basin ♦ xeroflo gauze ♦ elastic gauze dressing ♦ stockinette or elastic bandage ♦ sterile forceps ♦ sterile scissors ♦ sterile hemostat

Preparation

- Place the biological dressing in the sterile basin containing sterile normal saline solution (or open the Biobrane package).
- Using sterile technique, open the sterile dressing packages.
- Arrange the equipment on the dressing cart, and keep the cart readily accessible.
- Make sure the treatment area has adequate light to allow accurate wound assessment and dressing placement.

Comparing biological dressings

Different types of biological dressings are available and are used as appropriate for the type of graft required. Nursing considerations for each type are listed below.

Type	Description and uses	Nursing considerations
Amniotic membrane (homograft)	▪ Available from the obstetric department ▪ Must be sterile and come from an uncomplicated birth; serologic tests must be done ▪ Bacteriostatic condition doesn't require antimicrobials ▪ May be used to protect partial-thickness burns or (temporarily) granulation tissue before autografting ▪ Applied by the physician to clean wounds only	▪ Change the membrane every 48 hours. ▪ Cover the membrane with a gauze dressing or leave it exposed, as ordered. ▪ If you apply a gauze dressing, change it every 48 hours.
Biobrane (biosynthetic membrane)	▪ Comes in sterile, prepackaged sheets in various sizes and in glove form for hand burns ▪ Used to cover donor graft sites, superficial partial-thickness burns, debrided wounds awaiting autograft, and meshed autografts ▪ Provides significant pain relief ▪ Applied by the nurse	▪ Leave the membrane in place for 3 to 14 days, possibly longer. ▪ Don't use this dressing for preparing a granulation bed for subsequent autografting.
Cadaver (homograft)	▪ Obtained at autopsy up to 24 hours after death ▪ Applied in the operating room or at the bedside to debrided, untidy wounds ▪ Available as fresh cryopreserved homografts in tissue banks nationwide ▪ Provides protection, especially to granulation tissue after escharotomy ▪ May be used in some patients as a test graft for autografting ▪ Covers excised wounds immediately	▪ Observe for exudate. ▪ Watch for signs of rejection. ▪ Keep in mind that the gauze dressing may be removed every 8 hours to observe the graft.
Pigskin (heterograft or xenograft)	▪ Applied in the operating room or at the bedside ▪ Comes fresh or frozen in rolls or sheets ▪ Can cover and protect debrided, untidy wounds, mesh autografts, clean (eschar-free) partial-thickness burns, and exposed tendons	▪ Reconstitute frozen form with normal saline solution 30 minutes before use. ▪ Watch for signs of rejection. ▪ Cover with gauze dressing or leave exposed to air, as ordered.

Key steps

- If this is the patient's first treatment, explain the procedure to allay his fears and promote cooperation. Provide privacy.
- If ordered, administer an analgesic to the patient 20 minutes before beginning the procedure or give an analgesic I.V. immediately before the procedure to increase the patient's comfort and tolerance levels.
- Wash your hands and put on cap, mask, gown, shoe covers, and sterile gloves.
- Clean and debride the wound to reduce bacteria. Remove and dispose of gloves. Wash your hands and put on a fresh pair of sterile gloves.
- Place the dressing directly on the wound surface. Apply pigskin dermal with the shiny side down; apply Biobrane nylon-backed with the dull side down. Roll the dressing directly onto the skin if applicable. Place the dressing strips so that the edges touch but don't overlap. Use sterile forceps if necessary. Smooth the dressing. Eliminate folds and wrinkles by rolling out the dressing with the hemostat handle, the forceps handle, or your sterile-gloved hand to cover the wound completely and ensure adherence.
- Use the scissors to trim the dressing around the wound so that the dressing fits the wound without overlapping adjacent areas.
- Place Xeroflo gauze directly over an allograft, pigskin graft, or amniotic membrane. Place a few layers of gauze on top to absorb exudate, and wrap with a roller gauze dressing. Secure the dressing with tape or elastic netting. During daily dressing changes, the dressing will be removed down to the Xeroflo gauze, and the gauze will be replaced after the Xeroflo is inspected for drainage, adherence, and signs of infection.
- Place a nonadhesive dressing (such as Exu-Dry) over the Biobrane to absorb drainage and provide stability. Wrap the dressing with a roller gauze dressing, and secure it with tape or elastic netting. During daily dressing changes, the dressing will be removed down to the Biobrane and the site inspected for signs of infection. After the Biobrane adheres (usually in 2 to 3 days), it doesn't need to be covered with a dressing.
- Position the patient comfortably, elevating the area if possible. This reduces edema, which may prevent the biological dressing from adhering.

Special considerations

- Handle the biological dressing as little as possible.

Complications

- Infection
- Purulent wound drainage

Patient teaching

- Instruct the patient or caregiver to assess the site daily for signs of infection, swelling, blisters, drainage, and separation.
- Make sure the patient knows whom to contact if these complications develop.

Documentation

Record the time and date of dressing changes. Note areas of application, quality of adherence, and purulent drainage or other infection signs. Describe the patient's tolerance of the procedure.

C

Cardiac monitoring

Because it allows continuous observation of the heart's electrical activity, cardiac monitoring is used in patients with conduction disturbances and in those at risk for life-threatening arrhythmias. Like other forms of electrocardiography, cardiac monitoring uses electrodes placed on the patient's chest to transmit electrical signals that are converted into a tracing of cardiac rhythm on an oscilloscope.

Two types of monitoring may be performed: hardwire or telemetry. In hardwire monitoring, the patient is connected to a monitor at the bedside. The rhythm display appears at the bedside, but it may also be transmitted to a console at a remote location. Telemetry uses a small transmitter connected to the ambulatory patient to send electrical signals to another location, where they're displayed on a monitor screen. Battery powered and portable, telemetry frees the patient from cumbersome wires and cables and lets him be comfortably mobile and safely isolated from the electrical leakage and accidental shock occasionally associated with hardwire monitoring. Telemetry is especially useful for monitoring arrhythmias that occur during sleep, rest, exercise, or stressful situations. However, unlike hardwire monitoring, telemetry can monitor only cardiac rate and rhythm.

Regardless of the type, cardiac monitors can display the patient's heart rate and rhythm, produce a printed record of cardiac rhythm, and sound an alarm if the heart rate exceeds or falls below specified limits. Monitors also recognize and count abnormal heartbeats as well as changes. For example, ST-segment monitoring, helps detect myocardial ischemia, electrolyte imbalance, coronary artery spasm, and hypoxic events. The ST segment represents early ventricular repolarization, and any changes in this waveform component reflect alterations in myocardial oxygenation. Any monitoring lead that views an ischemic heart region will reveal ST-segment changes. The monitor's software establishes a template of the patient's normal QRST pattern from the selected leads; then the monitor displays ST-segment changes. Some monitors display such changes continuously, others only on command.

Equipment

Cardiac monitor ♦ leadwires ♦ patient cable ♦ disposable pregelled electrodes (number of electrodes varies from three to five, depending on patient's needs) ♦ alcohol pads ♦ 4″ × 4″ gauze pads ♦ optional: clippers, washcloth

Telemetry monitoring

Transmitter ♦ transmitter pouch ♦ telemetry battery pack ♦ leads ♦ electrodes

Preparation

- Plug the cardiac monitor into an electrical outlet and turn it on to warm up the unit while you prepare the equipment and the patient.

- Insert the cable into the appropriate socket in the monitor.
- Connect the leadwires to the cable. In some systems, the leadwires are permanently secured to the cable.
- Each leadwire should indicate the location for attachment to the patient: right arm (RA), left arm (LA), right leg (RL), left leg (LL), and chest (C). This should appear on the leadwire—if it's permanently connected—or at the connection of the leadwires and cable to the patient.
- Then connect an electrode to each of the leadwires, carefully checking that each leadwire is in its correct outlet.

Telemetry monitoring

- Insert a new battery into the transmitter.
- Be sure to match the poles on the battery with the polar markings on the transmitter case.
- By pressing the button at the top of the unit, test the battery's charge and test the unit to ensure that the battery is operational.
- If the leadwires aren't permanently affixed to the telemetry unit, attach them securely. If they must be attached individually, be sure to connect each one to the correct outlet.

Key steps

- Explain the procedure to the patient, provide privacy, and ask the patient to expose his chest. Wash your hands.
- Determine electrode positions on the patient's chest, based on which system and lead you're using. (See *Positioning monitoring leads*.)
- If the leadwires and patient cable aren't permanently attached, verify that the electrode placement corresponds to the label on the patient cable.
- If necessary, clip the hair from an area about 4" (10 cm) in diameter around each electrode site. Clean the area with an alcohol pad and dry it completely to remove skin secretions that may interfere with electrode function. Gently abrade the dried area by rubbing it briskly until it reddens to remove dead skin cells and to promote better electrical contact with living cells. (Some electrodes have a small, rough patch for abrading the skin; otherwise, use a dry washcloth or a dry gauze pad.)
- Remove the backing from the pregelled electrode. Check the gel for moistness. If the gel is dry, discard it and replace it with a fresh electrode.
- Apply the electrode to the site and press firmly to ensure a tight seal. Repeat with the remaining electrodes.
- When all the electrodes are in place, check for a tracing on the cardiac monitor. Assess the quality of the electrocardiogram (ECG). (See *Identifying cardiac monitor problems,* pages 59 and 60.)
- To verify that each beat is being detected by the monitor, compare the digital heart rate display with your count of the patient's heart rate.
- If necessary, use the gain control to adjust the size of the rhythm tracing, and use the position control to adjust the waveform position on the recording paper.
- Set the upper and lower limits of the heart rate alarm, based on unit policy. Turn the alarm on.

Telemetry monitoring

- Explain the procedure and how the machine works to the patient.
- If applicable, show him the button that will produce a recording of his ECG at the central station. Teach him how to push the button whenever he has symptoms. This causes the central console to print a rhythm strip.
- Wash your hands and provide privacy.
- Expose the patient's chest, and select the lead arrangement. Prepare the area for the electrode by clipping the hair and cleaning and abrading skin as described above. Remove the backing from one of the gelled electrodes. Check the gel for moistness. If it's dry, discard the electrode and obtain a new one.
- Apply the electrode to the appropriate site by pressing one side of the electrode against the patient's skin, pulling gently, and then pressing the other side against the skin. Press your fingers in a circular motion around the electrode to fix the gel and stabilize the electrode. Repeat for each electrode.

Positioning monitoring leads

This chart shows the correct electrode positions for some of the monitoring leads you'll use most often. For each lead, you'll see electrode placement for a five-leadwire system, a three-leadwire system, and a telemetry system.

In the two hardwire systems, the electrode positions for one lead may be identical to the electrode positions for another lead. In this case, you simply change the lead selector switch to the setting that corresponds to the lead you want. In some cases, you'll need to reposition the electrodes.

In the telemetry system, you can create the same lead with two electrodes that you do with three, simply by eliminating the ground electrode.

The illustrations below use these abbreviations: RA, right arm; LA, left arm; RL, right leg; LL, left leg; C, chest; and G, ground.

Five-leadwire system **Three-leadwire system** **Telemetry system**

Lead I

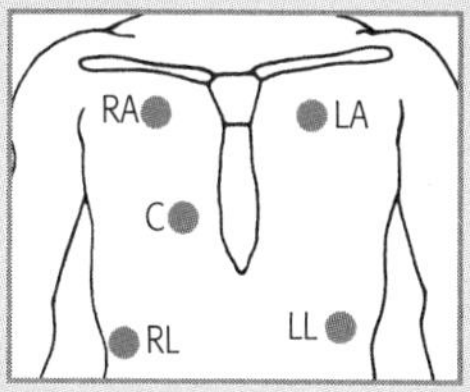

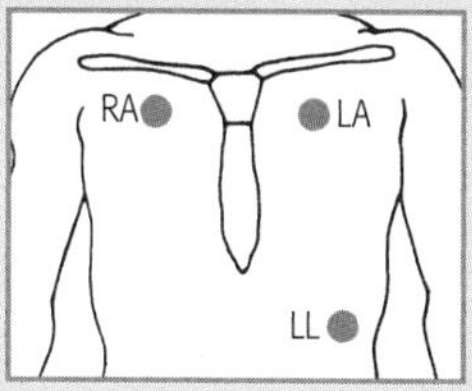

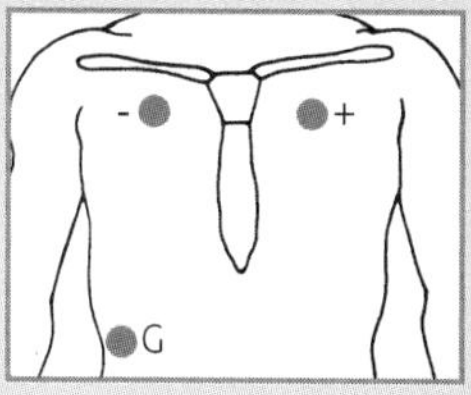

Lead II

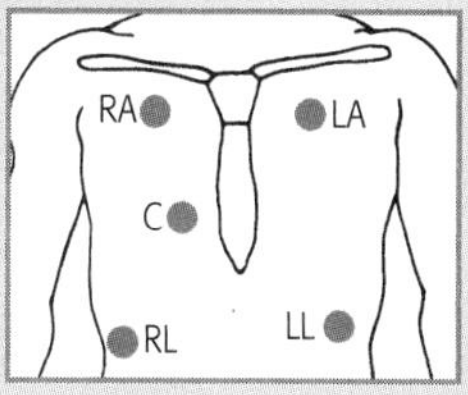

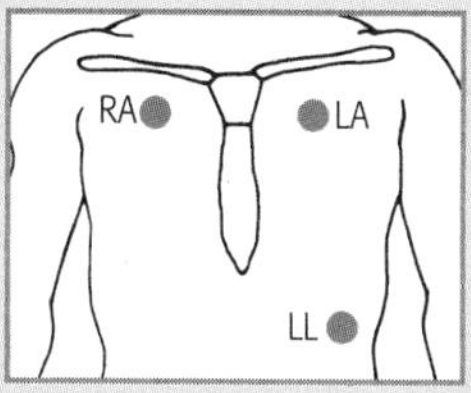

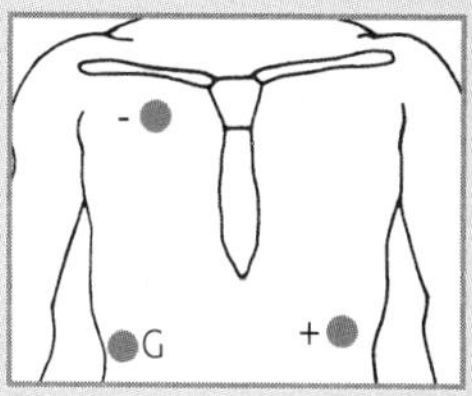

Lead II

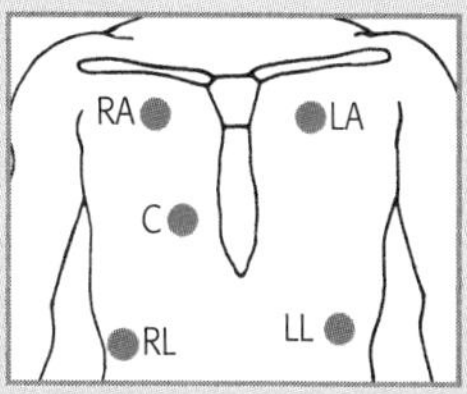

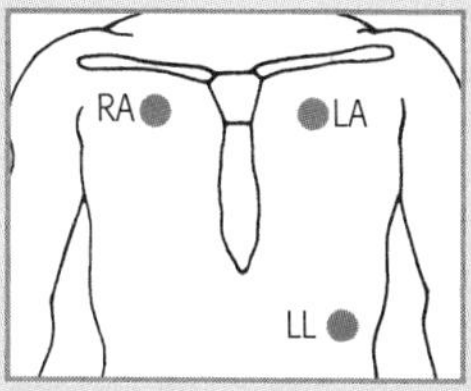

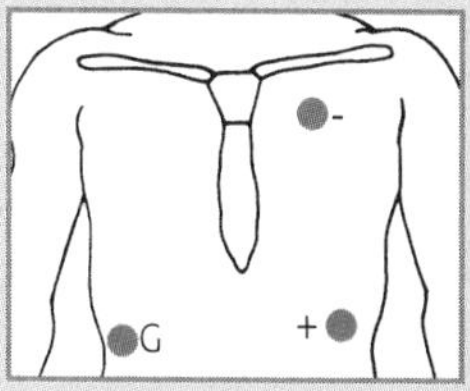

Lead MCL_1

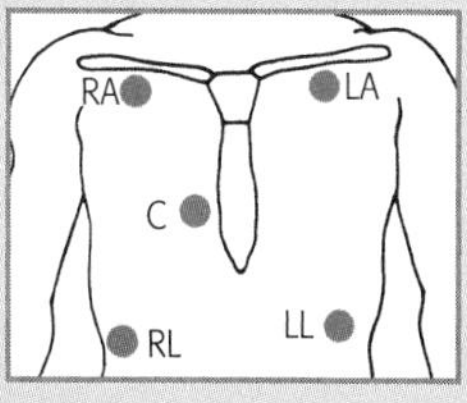

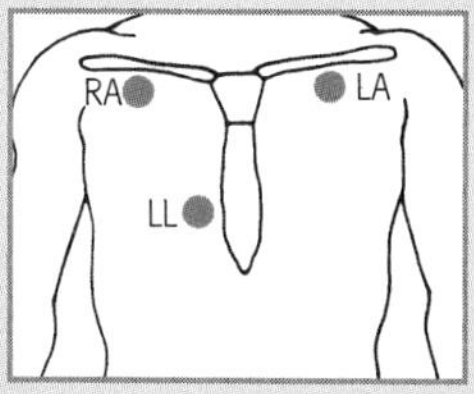

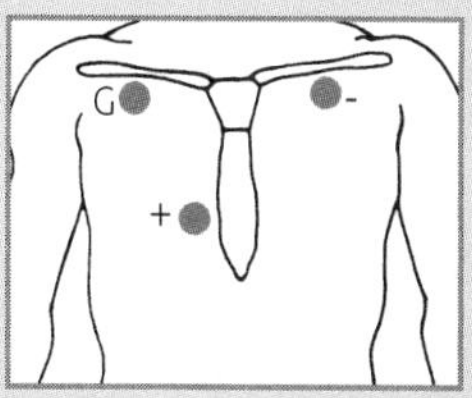

(continued)

Positioning monitoring leads *(continued)*

Five-leadwire system | **Three-leadwire system** | **Telemetry system**

Lead MCL_6

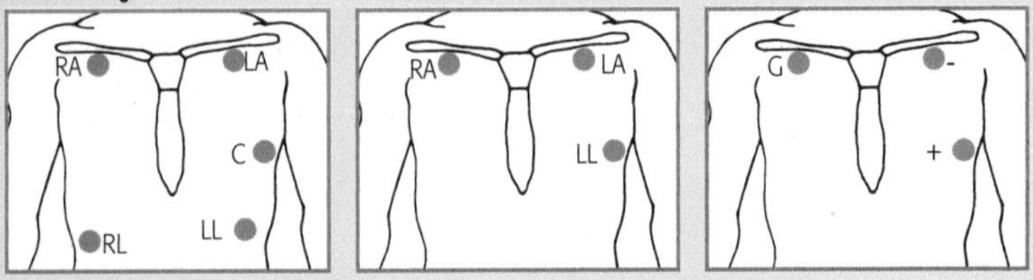

Sternal lead

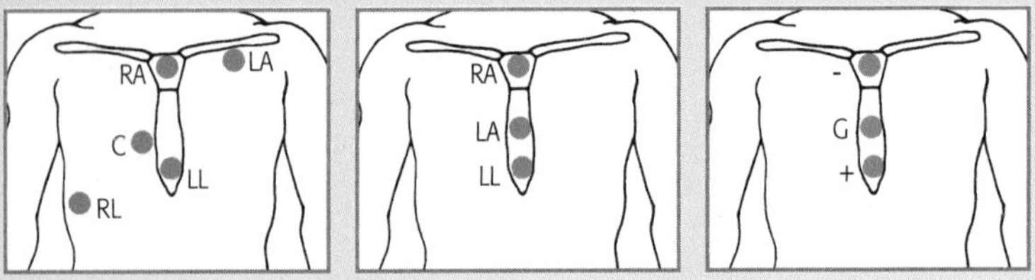

Lewis lead

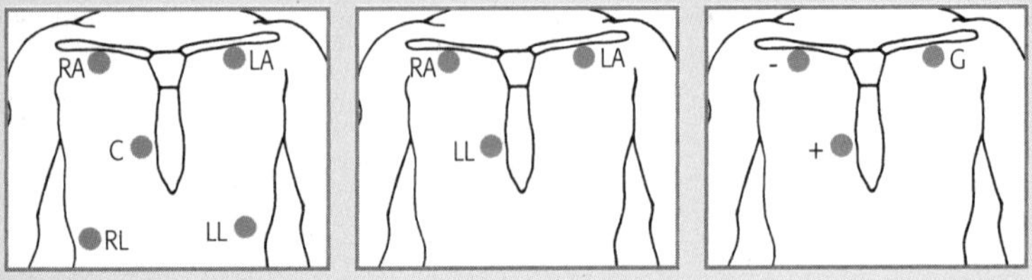

- Attach an electrode to the end of each leadwire.
- Place the transmitter in the pouch. Tie the pouch strings around the patient's neck and waist, making sure that the pouch fits snugly without causing him discomfort. If no pouch is available, place the transmitter in the patient's bathrobe pocket.
- Check the patient's waveform for clarity, position, and size. Adjust the gain and baseline as needed. (If necessary, ask the patient to remain resting or sitting in his room while you locate his telemetry monitor at the central station.)
- To obtain a rhythm strip, press the RECORD key at the central station. Label the strip with the patient's name and room number, date, and time. Also identify the rhythm. Place the rhythm strip in the appropriate location in the patient's chart.
- Tell the patient to remove the transmitter if he takes a shower or bath, but stress that he should let you know before he removes the unit.

Special considerations

DEVICE SAFETY

Make sure all electrical equipment and outlets are grounded to avoid electric shock and interference (artifacts). Also ensure that the patient is clean and dry to prevent electrical shock.

- Avoid opening the electrode packages until just before using to prevent the gel from drying out.

Identifying cardiac monitor problems

Problem	Possible causes	Solutions
False-high-rate alarm	▪ Monitor interpreting large T waves as QRS complexes, which doubles the rate	▪ Reposition electrodes to lead where QRS complexes are taller than T waves. Decrease gain if necessary.
	▪ Skeletal muscle activity	▪ Place electrodes away from major muscle masses.
False-low-rate alarm	▪ Shift in electrical axis from patient movement, making QRS complexes too small to register	▪ Reapply electrodes. Set gain so height of complex is greater than 1 mV.
	▪ Low amplitude of QRS	▪ Increase gain.
	▪ Poor contact between electrode and skin	▪ Reapply electrodes.
Low amplitude	▪ Gain dial set too low	▪ Increase gain.
	▪ Poor contact between skin and electrodes; dried gel; broken or loose leadwires; poor connection between patient and monitor; malfunctioning monitor; physiologic loss of QRS amplitude	▪ Check connections on all leadwires and monitoring cable. Replace electrodes as necessary.
Wandering baseline 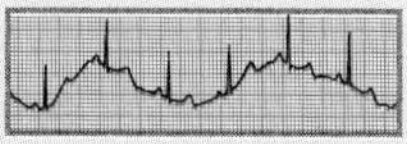	▪ Poor position or contact between electrodes and skin	▪ Reposition or replace electrodes.
	▪ Thoracic movement with respirations	▪ Reposition electrodes.
Artifact (waveform interference) 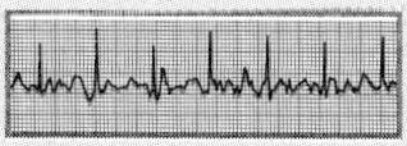	▪ Patient having seizures, chills, or anxiety	▪ Notify practitioner and treat patient as ordered. Keep patient warm and reassure him.
	▪ Patient movement	▪ Help patient relax.
	▪ Electrodes applied improperly	▪ Check electrodes and reapply, if necessary.
	▪ Static electricity	▪ Make sure cables don't have exposed connectors. ▪ Change patient's static-causing gown or pajamas.
	▪ Electrical short circuit in leadwires or cable	▪ Replace broken equipment. Use stress loops when applying leadwires.

(continued)

Identifying cardiac monitor problems *(continued)*

Problem	Possible causes	Solutions
Artifact (waveform interference) *(continued)*	■ Interference from decreased room humidity	■ Regulate humidity to 40%.
Broken leadwires or cable	■ Stress loops not used on leadwires ■ Cables and leadwires cleaned with alcohol or acetone, causing brittleness	■ Replace leadwires and retape them, using stress loops. ■ Clean cable and leadwires with soapy water. *Do not allow cable ends to become wet.* ■ Replace cable as necessary.
60-cycle interference (fuzzy baseline) 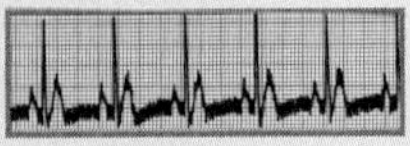	■ Electrical interference from other equipment in room ■ Patient's bed improperly grounded	■ Attach all electrical equipment to common ground. ■ Check plugs to make sure prongs aren't loose. ■ Attach bed ground to the room's common ground.
Skin excoriation under electrode	■ Patient allergic to electrode adhesive ■ Electrode on skin too long	■ Remove electrodes and apply nonallergenic electrodes and nonallergenic tape. ■ Remove electrode, clean site, and reapply electrode at new site.

■ Avoid placing the electrodes on bony prominences, hairy locations, areas where defibrillator pads will be placed, or areas for chest compression.
■ If the patient's skin is very oily, scaly, or diaphoretic, rub the electrode site with a dry 4″ × 4″ gauze pad before applying the electrode to help reduce interference in the tracing. Have the patient breathe normally during the procedure. If his respirations distort the recording, ask him to hold his breath briefly to reduce baseline wander in the tracing.
■ Assess skin integrity, and reposition the electrodes every 24 hours or as necessary.

Complications

■ None known

Documentation

Record the date and time that monitoring begins and the monitoring lead used. Document a rhythm strip at least every 8 hours and with any changes in the patient's condition (or as stated by your facility's policy). Label the rhythm strip with the patient's name and room number, the date, and the time.

Cardiac output measurement

Cardiac output—the amount of blood ejected by the heart—helps evaluate cardiac function. The most widely used method of calculating this measurement is the bolus thermodilution technique. Performed at the patient's bedside, the thermodilution technique is the most practical method of evaluating the cardiac status of critically ill patients and those suspected of having cardiac disease. Other methods in-

Cardiac output curves

These illustrations show cardiac output (CO) curves produced at the bedside using a pulmonary artery catheter (thermodilution method). Patients with a high CO have a curve with a small area beneath it, whereas patients with a low CO have a large area beneath the curve. Patients with uneven injection have an uneven upstroke on the curve. Presence of artifact commonly represents incorrect CO measurement.

Normal

High output

Low output

Uneven injection

Artifact

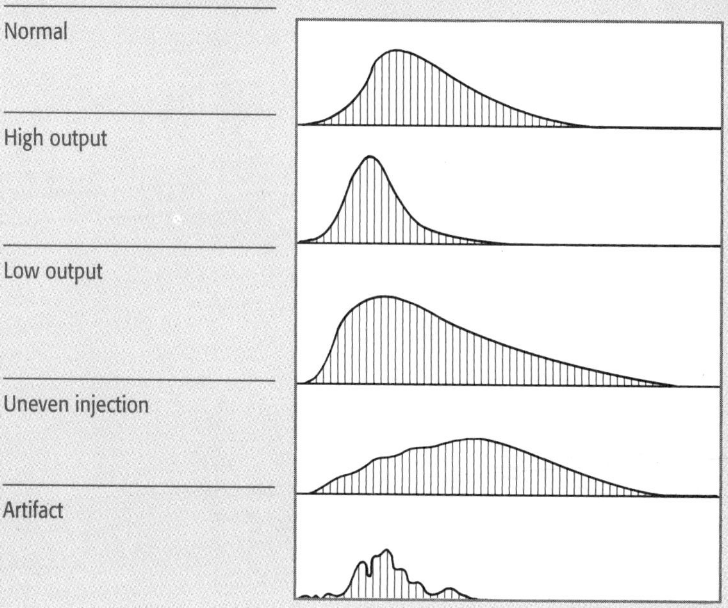

clude the Fick method and the dye dilution test.

To measure cardiac output, a quantity of solution colder than the patient's blood is injected into the right atrium via a port on a pulmonary artery (PA) catheter. This indicator solution mixes with the blood as it travels through the right ventricle into the pulmonary artery, and a thermistor on the catheter registers the change in temperature of the flowing blood. A computer then plots the temperature change over time as a curve, and calculates flow based on the area under the curve. (See *Cardiac output curves.*)

Iced or room-temperature injectant may be used. The choice should be based on your facility's policy as well as the patient's status. The accuracy of the bolus thermodilution technique depends on the computer being able to differentiate the temperature change caused by the injectate in the pulmonary artery and the temperature changes in the pulmonary artery. Because iced injectate is colder than room-temperature injectate, it provides a stronger signal to be detected.

Typically, however, room-temperature injectant is more convenient and provides equally accurate measurements. Iced injectant may be more accurate in patients with high or low cardiac outputs, hypothermic patients, or when smaller volumes of injectant must be used (3 to 5 ml), as in patients with volume restrictions or in children.

Equipment

Thermodilution PA catheter in position ◆ output computer and cables (or a module for the bedside cardiac monitor) ♦ closed injectant delivery system ♦ 10-ml syringe ♦ 500-ml bag of dextrose 5% in water or normal saline solution ♦ crushed ice and water (if iced injectant is used)

The newer bedside cardiac monitors measure cardiac output continuously, using either an invasive or a noninvasive method. If your bedside monitor doesn't have this capability, you'll need a freestanding cardiac output computer.

Preparation

- Wash your hands thoroughly, and assemble the equipment at the patient's bedside.
- Insert the closed injectant system tubing into the 500-ml bag of I.V. solution.
- Connect the 10-ml syringe to the system tubing, and prime the tubing with I.V. solution until it's free of air. Then clamp the tubing.

The steps that follow differ, depending on the temperature of the injectate.

Room-temperature injectate closed delivery system

- After clamping the tubing, connect the primed system to the stopcock of the proximal injectate lumen of the PA catheter.
- Next, connect the temperature probe from the cardiac output computer to the closed injectate system's flow-through housing device.
- Connect the cardiac output computer cable to the thermistor connector on the PA catheter and verify the blood temperature reading.
- Finally, turn on the cardiac output computer and enter the correct computation constant, as provided by the catheter's manufacturer. The constant is determined by the volume and temperature of the injectant as well as the size and type of catheter. For children, you'll need to adjust the computation constant to reflect a smaller volume and a smaller catheter size.

Iced injectate closed delivery system

- After clamping the tubing, place the coiled segment into the Styrofoam container and add crushed ice and water to cover the entire coil.
- Let the solution cool for 15 to 20 minutes.
- The rest of the steps are the same as those for the room-temperature injectate closed delivery system.

Key steps

- Make sure the patient is in a comfortable position. Tell him not to move during the procedure because movement can cause an error in measurement.
- Explain to the patient that the procedure will help determine how well his heart is pumping and that he'll feel no discomfort.

Room-temperature injectate closed delivery system

- Verify the presence of a PA waveform on the cardiac monitor.
- Unclamp the I.V. tubing and withdraw exactly 10 ml of solution. Reclamp the tubing.
- Turn the stopcock at the catheter injectate hub to open a fluid path between the injectate lumen of the PA catheter and the syringe.
- Press the START button on the cardiac output computer or wait for an INJECT message to flash.
- Inject the solution smoothly within 4 seconds, making sure it doesn't leak at the connectors.
- If available, analyze the contour of the thermodilution washout curve on a strip chart recorder for a rapid upstroke and a gradual, smooth return to the baseline.
- Repeat these steps until three values are within 10% to 15% of the median value. Compute the average, and record the patient's cardiac output.
- Return the stopcock to its original position, and make sure the injectate delivery system tubing is clamped.
- Verify the presence of a PA waveform on the cardiac monitor.
- Discontinue cardiac output measurements when the patient is hemodynamically stable and weaned from his vasoactive and inotropic medications. You can leave the PA catheter inserted for pressure measurements.

- Disconnect and discard the injectant delivery system and the I.V. bag. Cover any exposed stopcocks with air-occlusive caps.

Iced injectate closed delivery system

- Unclamp the I.V. tubing and withdraw 5 ml of solution into the syringe; with children, use 3 ml or less.
- Inject the solution to flow past the temperature sensor while observing the injectant temperature that registers on the computer. Verify that the injectate temperature is between 43° and 54° F (6.1° and 12.2° C).
- Verify the presence of a PA waveform on the cardiac monitor.
- Withdraw exactly 10 ml of cooled solution before reclamping the tubing.
- Turn the stopcock at the catheter injectant hub to open a fluid path between the injectate lumen of the PA catheter and syringe.
- Press the START button on the cardiac output computer, or wait for the INJECT message to flash.
- Inject the solution smoothly within 4 seconds, making sure it doesn't leak at the connectors.
- If available, analyze the contour of the thermodilution washout curve on a strip chart recorder for a rapid upstroke and a gradual, smooth return to baseline.
- Wait 1 minute between injections, and repeat the procedure until three values are within 10% to 15% of the median value. Compute the average, and record the patient's cardiac output.
- Return the stopcock to its original position, and make sure the injectant delivery system tubing is clamped.
- Verify the presence of a PA waveform on the cardiac monitor.
- Discontinue cardiac output measurements when the patient is hemodynamically stable and weaned from his vasoactive and inotropic medications. You can leave the PA catheter inserted for pressure measurements.
- Disconnect and discard the injectant delivery system and the I.V. bag. Cover any exposed stopcocks with air-occlusive caps.

Special considerations

ALERT

Monitor the patient for signs and symptoms of inadequate perfusion, including restlessness, fatigue, changes in level of consciousness, decreased capillary refill time, diminished peripheral pulses, oliguria, and pale, cool skin.

- The normal range for cardiac output is 4 to 8 L/minute. The adequacy of a patient's cardiac output is better assessed by calculating his cardiac index (CI), adjusted for his body size.
- To calculate the patient's CI, divide his cardiac output by his body surface area (BSA), a function of height and weight. For example, a cardiac output of 4 L/minute might be adequate for a 65″, 120-lb (165.1-cm, 54.4-kg) patient (normally a BSA of 1.59 and a CI of 2.5) but would be inadequate for a 74″, 230-lb (188-cm, 104.3-kg) patient (normally a BSA of 2.26 and a CI of 1.8). The normal CI for adults ranges from 2.5 to 4.2 L/minute/m^2; for pregnant women, 3.5 to 6.5 L/minute/m^2.
- Normal CI for infants and children is 3.5 to 4 L/minute/m^2.
- Normal CI for elderly adults is 2 to 2.5 L/minute/m^2.
- Add the fluid volume injected for cardiac output determinations to the patient's total intake. Injectate delivery of 30 ml/hour will contribute 720 ml to the patient's 24-hour intake.
- After cardiac output measurement, make sure the clamp on the injectate bag is secured to prevent inadvertent delivery of the injectate to the patient.

Complications

- None known

Documentation

Document your patient's cardiac output, CI, and other hemodynamic values and vital signs at the time of measurement. Note the patient's position during measurement and any other unusual occurrences, such as bradycardia or neurologic changes.

Cardiopulmonary resuscitation, adult

Cardiopulmonary resuscitation (CPR) seeks to restore and maintain the patient's respiration and circulation after his heartbeat and breathing have stopped. CPR is a basic life support (BLS) procedure that's performed on victims of cardiac arrest. Another BLS procedure is clearing the obstructed airway. (See "Foreign body airway obstruction," page 212.)

ALERT

For CPR purposes, the American Heart Association defines a patient by age. An infant is younger than age 1; a child is age 1 to age 8; and an adult is older than age 8.

Most adults who experience sudden cardiac arrest develop ventricular fibrillation and require defibrillation; CPR alone doesn't improve their chances of survival. Therefore, you must assess the victim and then contact emergency medical services (EMS) or call a code before starting CPR. Timing is critical. Early access to EMS, early CPR, and early defibrillation greatly improve a patient's chances of survival.

In most instances, you perform CPR to keep the patient alive until advanced cardiac life support (ACLS) can begin. Basic CPR procedure consists of assessing the victim, calling for help, and then following the ABC protocol: opening the Airway, restoring Breathing, then restoring Circulation. After the airway has been opened and breathing and circulation have been restored, drug therapy, diagnosis by electrocardiogram (ECG), or defibrillation may follow. CPR is contraindicated in "no code" patients.

Equipment

None needed

Key steps

- The following illustrated instructions provide a step-by-step guide for CPR as currently recommended by the American Heart Association (AHA):

One-person rescue

- If you're the sole rescuer, expect to determine unresponsiveness, call for help, open the patient's airway, check for breathing, assess for circulation, and begin compressions.

Opening the airway

- Assess the victim to determine if he's unconscious (as shown below). Gently shake his shoulders and shout, "Are you okay?" This helps ensure that you don't start CPR on a person who's conscious. Check whether he has an injury, particularly to the head or neck. If you suspect a head or neck injury, move him as little as possible to reduce the risk of paralysis.

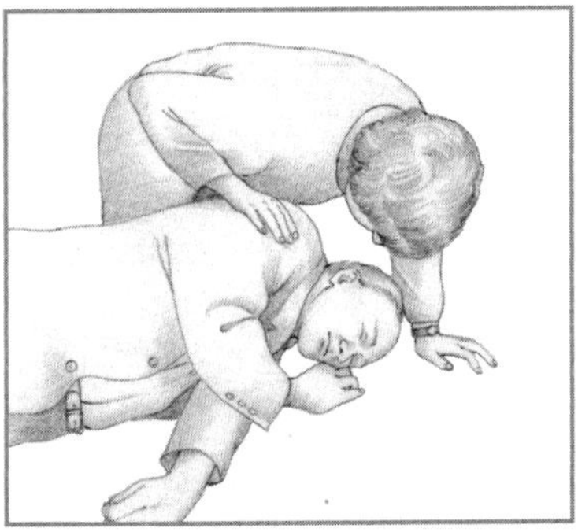

- Call out for help. Send someone to contact the EMS or call a code, and get the automated external defibrillator (AED). Place the victim in a supine position on a hard, flat surface. When moving him, roll his head and torso as a unit (as shown below). Avoid twisting or pulling his neck, shoulders, or hips.

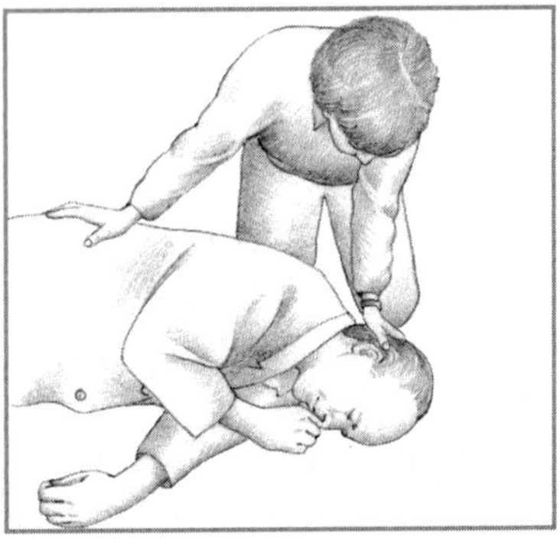

▪ Kneel near his shoulders (as shown below). This position will give you easy access to his head and chest.

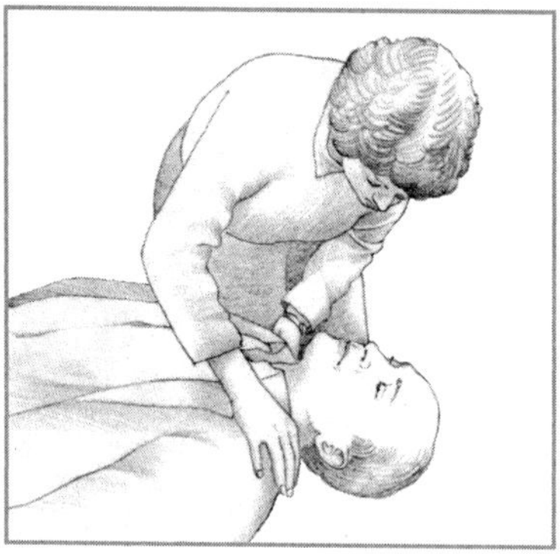

▪ In many cases, the muscles controlling the victim's tongue will be relaxed, causing the tongue to obstruct the airway. If the victim doesn't appear to have a neck injury, use the head-tilt, chin-lift maneuver to open his airway. To accomplish this, first place your hand that's closer to the victim's head on his forehead. Then apply firm pressure. The pressure should be firm enough to tilt the victim's head back. Next, place the fingertips of your other hand under the bony part of his lower jaw near the chin. Now lift the victim's chin (as shown below). At the same time, keep his mouth partially open.

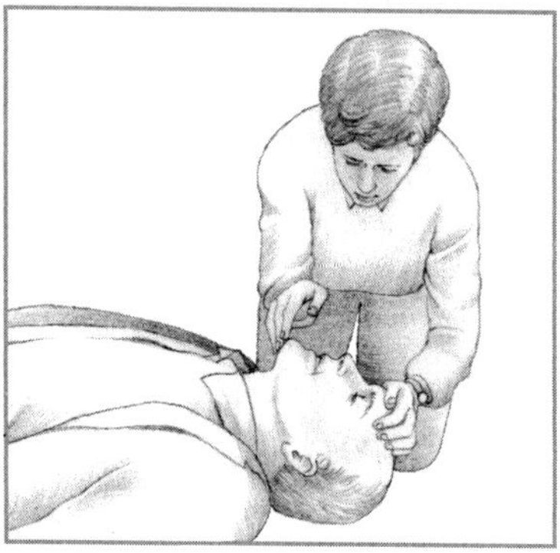

▪ Avoid placing your fingertips on the soft tissue under the victim's chin because this maneuver may inadvertently obstruct the airway you're trying to open.

▪ If you suspect a neck injury, use the jaw-thrust maneuver without head extension instead of the head-tilt, chin-lift maneuver. Kneel at the victim's head with your elbows on the ground. Rest your thumbs on his lower jaw near the corners of the mouth, pointing your thumbs toward his feet. Then place your fingertips around the lower jaw. To open the airway, lift the lower jaw with your fingertips (as shown below).

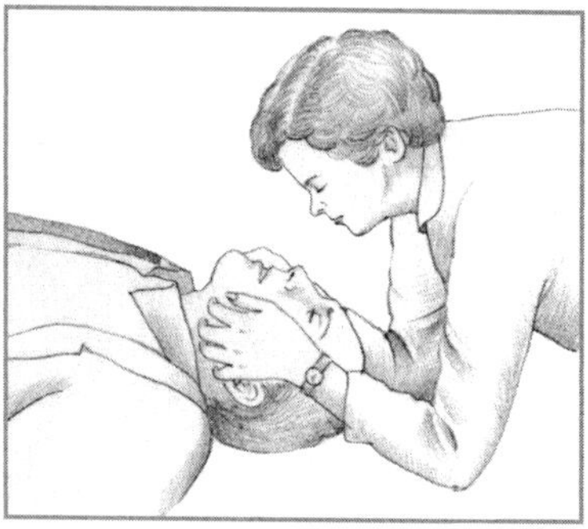

Checking for breathing

▪ While maintaining the open airway, look, listen and feel for breathing. Place your ear over the victim's mouth and nose (as shown below). Now, listen for the sound of air moving, and note whether his chest rises and falls. You may also feel airflow on your cheek. If he starts to breathe, keep the airway open and continue checking his breathing until help arrives.

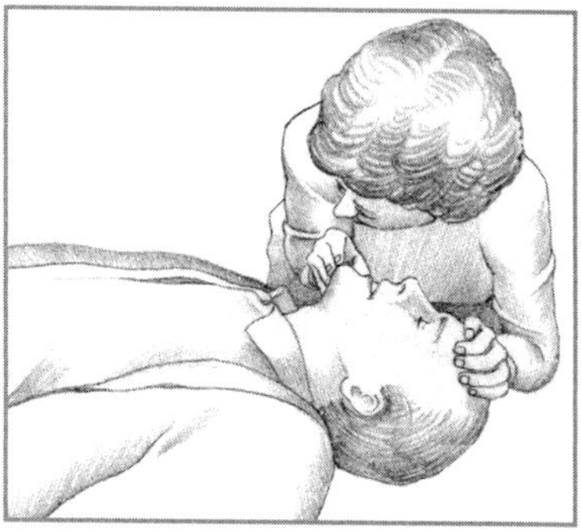

▪ If you don't detect adequate breathing within 10 seconds after opening his airway, begin rescue breathing. Pinch his nostrils shut with the thumb and index finger of the hand that you've had on his forehead (as shown below).

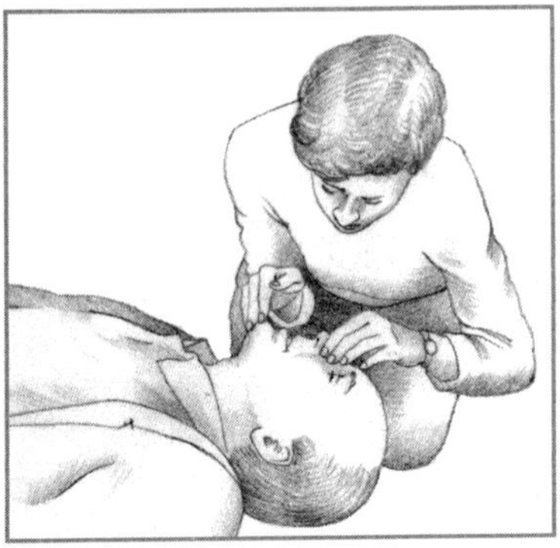

■ Take a regular (not deep) breath and place your mouth over the victim's mouth, creating a tight seal (as shown below). Give 2 breaths, each over 1 second. Each ventilation should have enough volume to produce a visible chest rise.

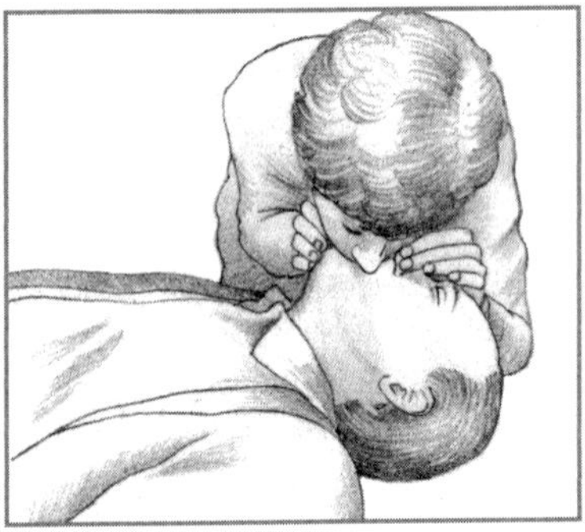

■ If the first ventilation isn't successful, reposition the victim's head and try again. If you still aren't successful, he may have a foreign-body airway obstruction. Check for loose dentures. If dentures or any other objects are blocking the airway, clear the airway.

Assessing circulation

■ Keep one hand on the victim's forehead so his airway remains open. With your other hand, palpate the carotid artery that's closer to you (as shown top of next column). To do this, place your index and middle fingers in the groove between the trachea and the sternocleidomastoid muscle. Palpate for 10 seconds.

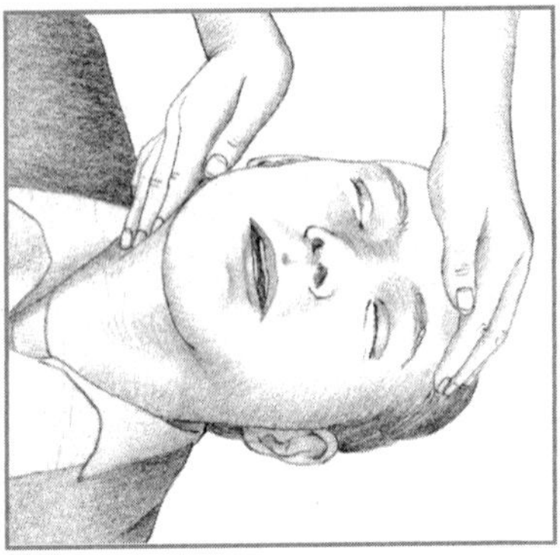

■ If you detect a pulse, don't begin chest compressions. Instead, perform rescue breathing by giving the victim 10 to 12 ventilations per minute (or one every 5 to 6 seconds). Each breath should be given over 1 second and cause a visible chest rise. After 2 minutes, recheck his pulse, but spend only 10 seconds doing so.

■ If there's no pulse, start giving chest compressions. Make sure the patient is lying on a hard surface. Make sure your knees are apart for a wide base of support. Using the hand closer to his feet, locate the lower margin of the rib cage (as shown below). Then move your fingertips along the margin to the notch where the ribs meet the sternum.

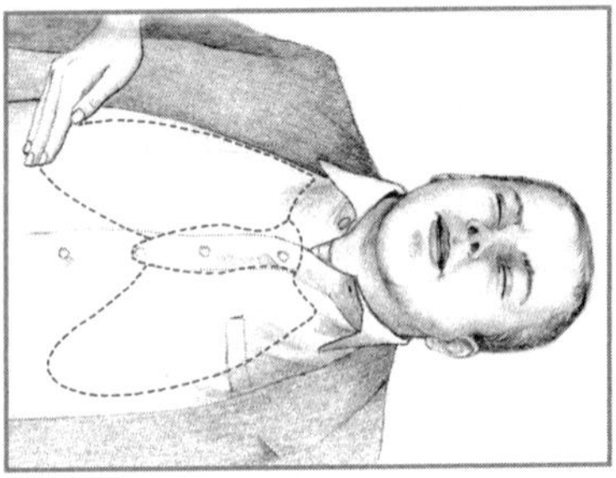

■ Place your middle finger on the notch and your index finger next to your middle finger. The long axis of the heel of your hand will be aligned with the long axis of the sternum in the center of the chest between the nipples (as shown top of next page).

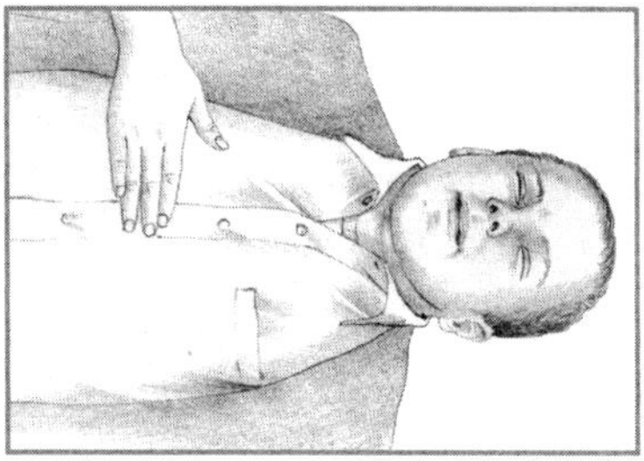

■ Put the heel of your other hand on the sternum, next to the index finger. The long axis of the heel of your hand will be aligned with the long axis of the sternum (as shown below).

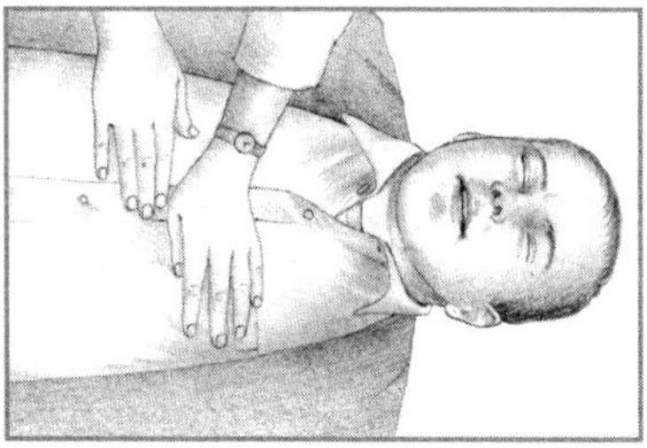

■ Take the first hand off the notch and put it on top of the hand on the sternum. Make sure you have one hand directly on top of the other and your fingers aren't on his chest (as shown below). This position will keep the force of the compression on the sternum and reduce the risk of a rib fracture, lung puncture, or liver laceration.

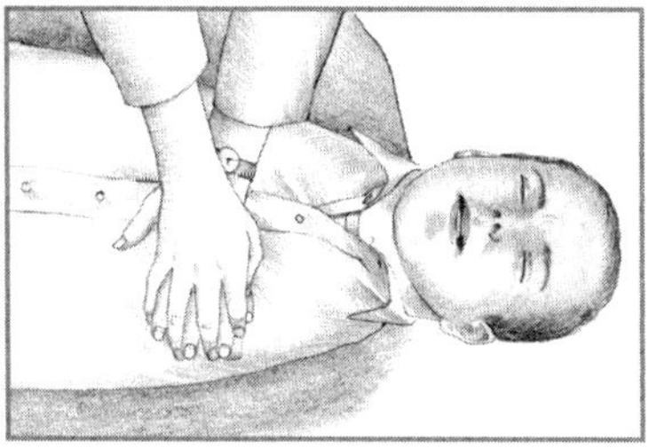

■ With your elbows locked, arms straight, and your shoulders directly over your hands (as shown top of next column), you're ready to give chest compressions. Using the weight of your upper body, compress the victim's sternum $1\frac{1}{2}''$ to 2″ (4 to 5 cm), delivering the pressure through the heels of your hands. After each compression, release the pressure and allow the chest to return to its normal position so that the heart can fill with blood. Don't change your hand position during compressions—you might injure the victim.

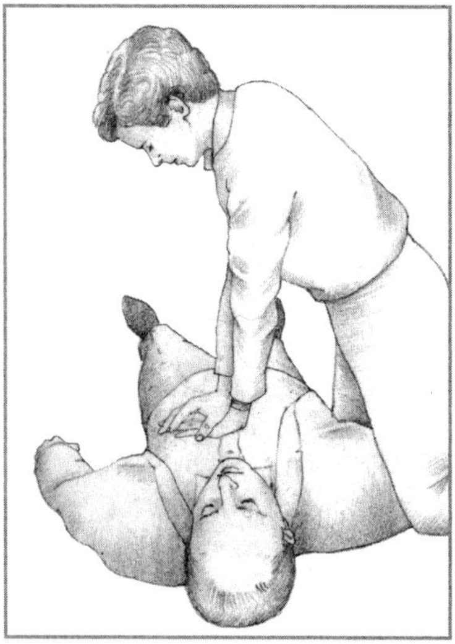

■ Give 30 chest compressions at a rate of approximately 100 per minute. Push hard and fast. Open the airway and give 2 ventilations. Then find the proper hand position again and deliver 30 more compressions. Continue chest compressions until EMS arrives or another rescuer arrives with the AED. Health care providers should interrupt chest compressions as infrequently as possible. Interruptions should last no longer than 10 seconds except for special interventions, such as the use of the AED or insertion of an airway.

Two-person rescue

If another rescuer arrives while you're giving CPR, follow these steps:

■ If the EMS team hasn't arrived, tell the second rescuer to repeat the call for help. If he isn't a health care professional, ask him to stand by (as shown top of next page). Then, after about 2 minutes or 5 cycles of compressions and ventilations, you should switch. The switch should occur in less than 5 seconds.

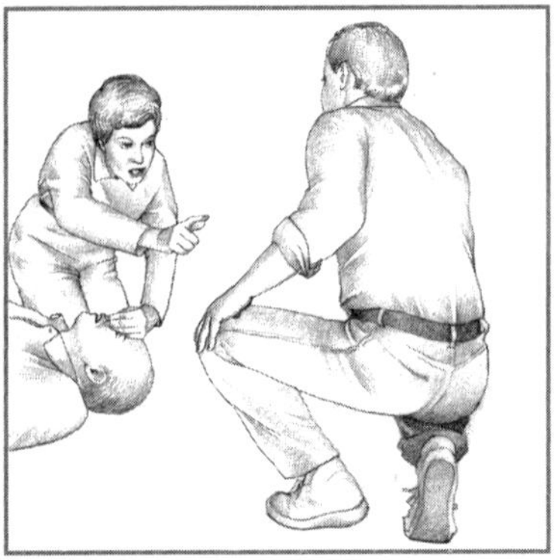

- If the rescuer is another health care professional, the two of you can perform two-person CPR. He should start assisting after you've finished 5 cycles of 30 compressions, 2 ventilations, and a pulse check.
- The second rescuer should get into place opposite you. While you're checking for a pulse, he should be finding the proper hand placement for delivering chest compressions (as shown below).

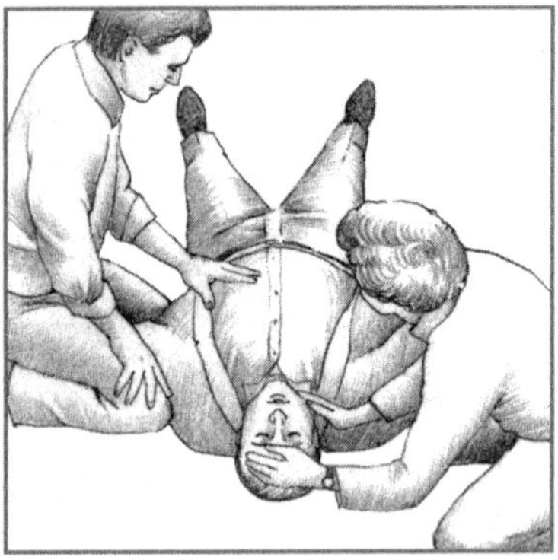

- If you don't detect a pulse, say, "No pulse, continue CPR." and give 2 ventilations. Then the second rescuer should begin delivering compressions at a rate of 100 per minute (as shown top of next column). Compressions and ventilations should be administered at a ratio of 30 compressions to 2 ventilations. The compressor (at this point, the second rescuer) should count out loud so the ventilator can anticipate when to give ventilations. To ensure that the ventilations are effective, they should cause a visible chest rise.

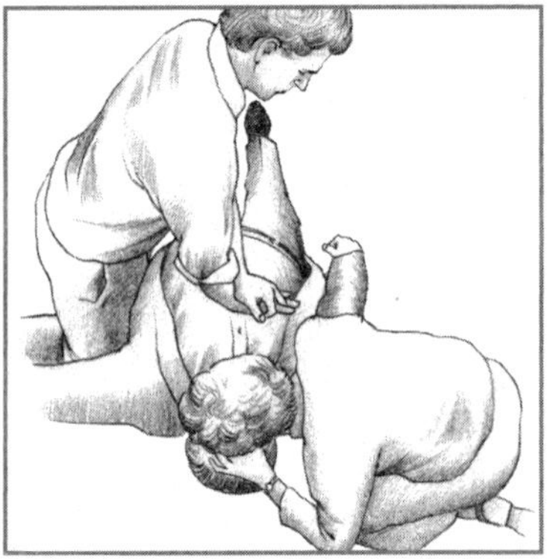

- The compressor role should switch after 5 cycles of compressions and ventilations. The switch should occur in less than 5 seconds.
- As shown below, both of you should continue giving CPR until an AED or defibrillator arrives, the ACLS providers take over, or the victim starts to move.

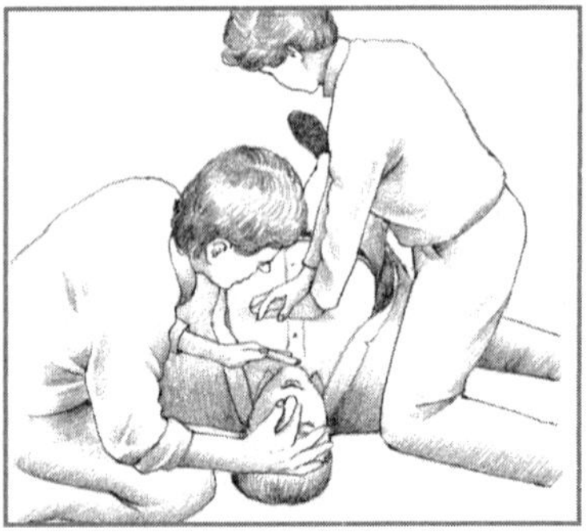

Special considerations

- Some health care professionals may hesitate to give mouth-to-mouth rescue breathing. For this reason, the AHA recommends that all health care professionals learn how to use disposable airway equipment.

Complications

- Fractured ribs, lacerated liver, and punctured lungs if the compressor doesn't place her hands properly on the sternum
- Gastric distention resulting from giving too much air during ventilation (see *Potential hazards of CPR*)

Potential hazards of CPR

Cardiopulmonary resuscitation (CPR) can cause various complications, including injury to bones and vital organs. This chart describes the causes of CPR hazards and lists preventive steps.

Hazard	Causes	Assessment findings	Preventive measures
Sternal and rib fractures	▪ Osteoporosis ▪ Malnutrition ▪ Improper hand placement	▪ Paradoxical chest movement ▪ Chest pain or tenderness that increases with inspiration ▪ Crepitus ▪ Palpation of movable bony fragments over the sternum ▪ On palpation, sternum feels unattached to surrounding ribs	**While performing CPR** ▪ Don't rest your hands or fingers on the patient's ribs. ▪ Interlock your fingers. ▪ Keep your bottom hand in contact with the chest, but release pressure after each compression. ▪ Compress the sternum at the recommended depth for the patient's age.
Pneumothorax, hemothorax, or both	▪ Lung puncture from fractured rib	▪ Chest pain and dyspnea ▪ Decreased or absent breath sounds over the affected lung ▪ Tracheal deviation from midline ▪ Hypotension ▪ Hyperresonance to percussion over the affected area along with shoulder pain	▪ Follow the measures listed for sternal and rib fractures.
Injury to the heart and great vessels (pericardial tamponade, atrial or ventricular rupture, vessel laceration, cardiac contusion, punctures of the heart chambers)	▪ Improperly performed chest compressions ▪ Transvenous or transthoracic pacing attempts ▪ Central line placement during resuscitation ▪ Intracardiac drug administration	▪ Jugular vein distention ▪ Muffled heart sounds ▪ Pulsus paradoxus ▪ Narrowed pulse pressure ▪ Electrical alternans (decreased electrical amplitude of every other QRS complex) ▪ Adventitious heart sounds ▪ Hypotension ▪ Electrocardiogram changes (arrhythmias, ST-segment elevation, T-wave inversion, and marked decrease in QRS voltage)	▪ Perform chest compressions properly.

(continued)

Potential hazards of CPR *(continued)*

Hazard	Causes	Assessment findings	Preventive measures
Organ laceration (primarily liver and spleen)	■ Forceful compression ■ Sharp edge of a fractured rib or xiphoid process	■ Persistent right upper quadrant tenderness (liver injury) ■ Persistent left upper quadrant tenderness (splenic injury) ■ Increasing abdominal girth	■ Follow the measures listed for sternal and rib fractures.
Aspiration of stomach contents	■ Gastric distention and an elevated diaphragm from high ventilatory pressures	■ Fever, hypoxia, and dyspnea ■ Auscultation of wheezes and crackles ■ Increased white blood cell count ■ Changes in color and odor of lung secretions	■ Intubate early. ■ Insert a nasogastric tube and apply suction, if gastric distention is marked.

Documentation

Whenever you perform CPR, document why you initiated it, whether the victim suffered from cardiac or respiratory arrest, when you found the victim and started CPR, and how long the victim received CPR. Note his response and any complications. Also include any interventions taken to correct complications.

If the victim also received ACLS, document which interventions were performed, who performed them, when they were performed, and what equipment was used.

Cardiopulmonary resuscitation, child (ages 1 to 8)

An adult who needs cardiopulmonary resuscitation (CPR) typically suffers from a primary cardiac disorder or an arrhythmia that has stopped the heart. An infant or a child who needs CPR typically suffers from hypoxia caused by respiratory difficulty or respiratory arrest.

Most pediatric crises requiring CPR are preventable. They include:
- motor vehicle accidents
- drowning
- burns
- smoke inhalation
- falls
- poisoning
- suffocation
- choking (usually from inhaling a plastic bag or small foreign bodies, such as toys and food).

Other causes of cardiopulmonary arrest in children include laryngospasm and edema from upper respiratory infections and sudden infant death syndrome.

Based on the same principle as CPR in adults, the procedure, when performed on children and infants, aims to restore cardiopulmonary function by pumping the victim's heart and ventilating the lungs until natural function resumes. However, CPR techniques differ depending on whether the patient is an adult, a child, or an infant.

ALERT

For CPR purposes, the American Heart Association defines a patient by age. An infant is under age 1; a child is age 1 to age 8; and an adult is over age 8.

Survival chances improve the sooner CPR begins and the faster advanced life-support systems are implemented. However speedily you undertake CPR for a child, though, first determine whether the patient's respiratory distress results from a mechanical obstruction or an infection, such as epiglottiditis or croup. Epiglottiditis or croup requires immediate medical attention, not CPR. CPR is appropriate only when the child isn't breathing.

Equipment

None needed

ALERT

A child-size bag-valve mask should be used if available.

Key steps

- Gently shake the apparently unconscious child's shoulder and shout at her to elicit a response.
- If the child is conscious but has difficulty breathing, help her into a position that best eases her breathing—if she hasn't naturally assumed this position.
- Call for help to alert others and to enlist emergency assistance. If you're alone and the child isn't breathing, perform CPR for five cycles (about 2 minutes), before calling for help. One cycle of CPR for the single rescuer is 30 compressions and two breaths.
- Position the child in a supine position on a firm, flat surface (usually the ground). The surface should provide the resistance needed for adequate chest compressions. If you must turn the child from a prone position, support her head and neck and turn her as a unit to avoid injuring her spine (as shown top of next column).

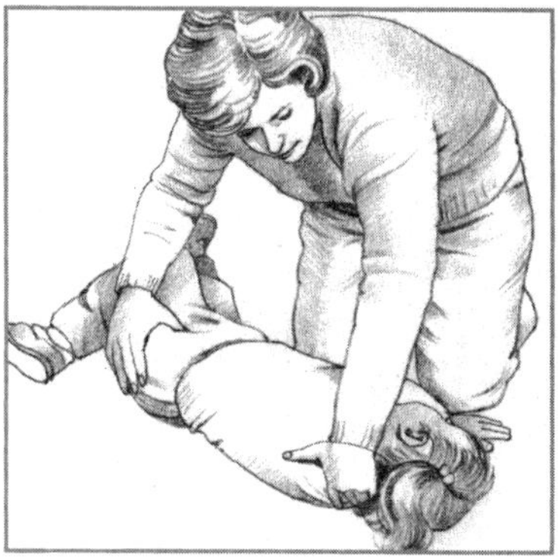

Establishing a patent airway

- Kneel beside the child's shoulder. Place one hand on the child's forehead and gently lift her chin with your other hand to open her airway (as shown below). Avoid fingering the soft neck tissue to avoid obstructing the airway. Never let the child's mouth close completely.

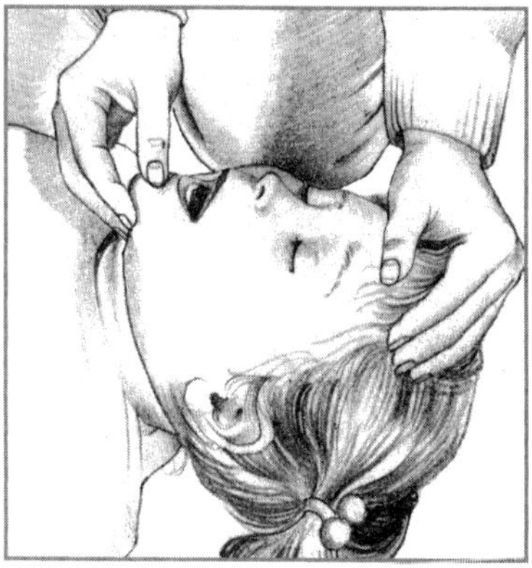

- If you suspect a neck injury, use the jaw-thrust maneuver to open the child's airway to keep from moving the child's neck. To do this, kneel beside the child's head. With your elbows on the ground, rest your thumbs at the corners of the child's mouth, and place two or three fingers of each hand under the lower jaw. Lift the jaw upward.
- While maintaining an open airway, place your ear near the child's mouth and nose to evaluate her breathing status. Look for chest movement, listen for exhaled air, and

feel for exhaled air on your cheek (as shown below).

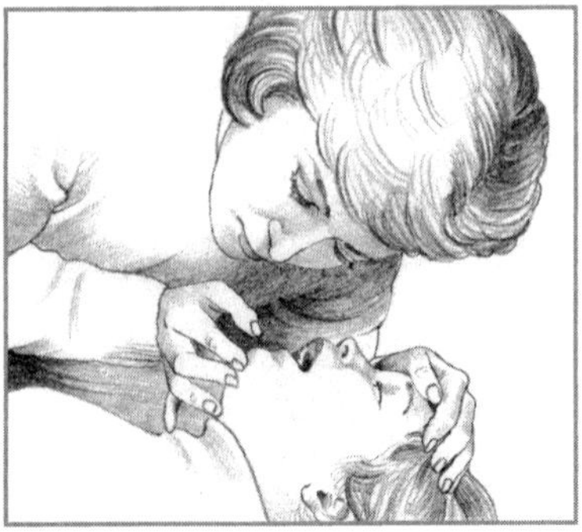

■ If the child is breathing, maintain an open airway and monitor respirations.

Restoring ventilation

■ If the child isn't breathing, maintain the open airway position, and take a breath. Then pinch the child's nostrils shut, and cover the child's mouth with your mouth (as shown below). Give two breaths that make the chest rise, pausing briefly after the first breath.

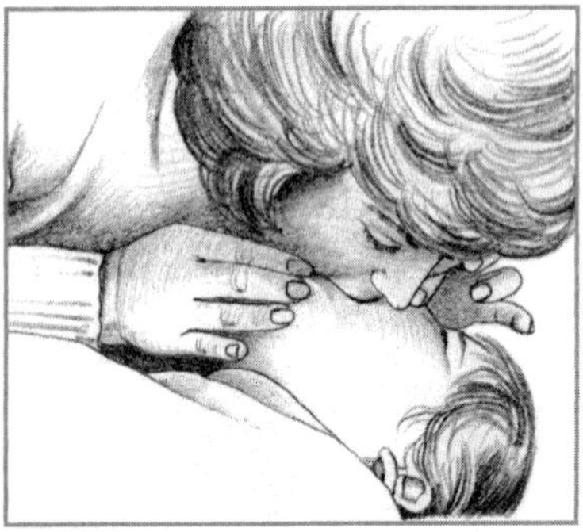

■ If your first attempt at ventilation fails to restore the child's breathing, reposition the child's head to open the airway and try again.

ALERT

If you're still unsuccessful, the airway may be obstructed by a foreign body.

■ Repeat the steps for establishing a patent airway.

■ After you free the obstruction, check for breathing and pulse.

■ If the child is breathing and there's no evidence of trauma, turn her on to her side or place her in the recovery position.

■ If breathing and pulse are absent, proceed with chest compressions.

Restoring heartbeat and circulation

■ Assess circulation by palpating the carotid artery for a pulse.

■ Locate the carotid artery with two or three fingers of one hand. (You'll need the other hand to maintain the head-tilt position that keeps the airway open.) Place your fingers in the center of the child's neck on the side closest to you, and slide your fingers into the groove formed by the trachea and the sternocleidomastoid muscle (as shown below). Palpate the artery for no more than 10 seconds to confirm the child's pulse status. The pulse should be greater than or equal to 60 beats/minute.

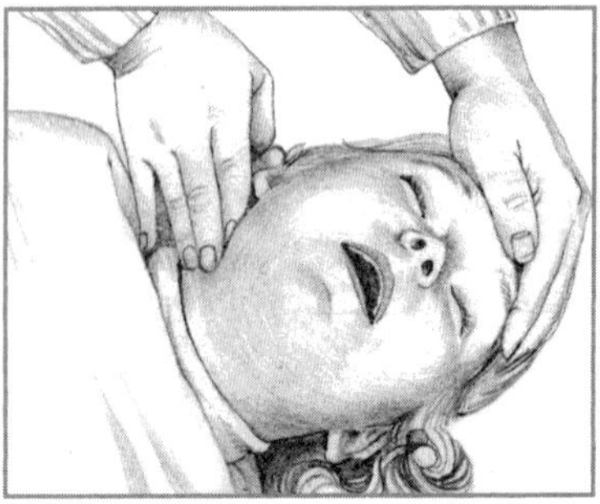

■ If you feel the child's pulse and it's greater than or equal to 60 beats/minute, continue rescue breathing, giving one breath every 3 seconds (20 breaths per minute) and recheck the pulse every 2 minutes.

■ If you can't feel a pulse or the pulse is less than 60 beats/minute with signs of poor perfusion, begin chest compressions.

■ Kneel next to the child's chest. Using the hand closest to her feet, locate the lower border of the rib cage on the side nearest you (as shown top of next page).

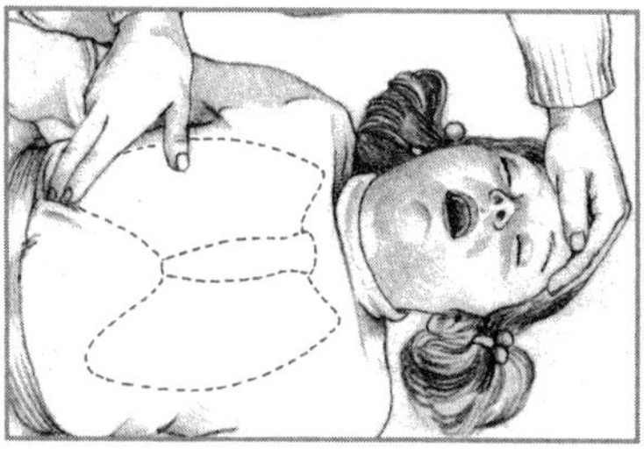

- Hold your middle and index fingers together, and move them up the rib cage to the notch where the ribs and sternum join. Put your middle finger on the notch and your index finger next to it (as shown below).

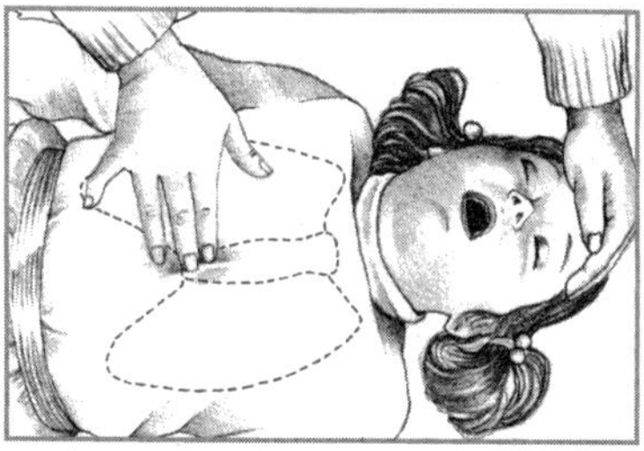

- Lift your hand and place the heel just above the spot where the index finger was (as shown below). The heel of your hand should be aligned with the long axis of the sternum.

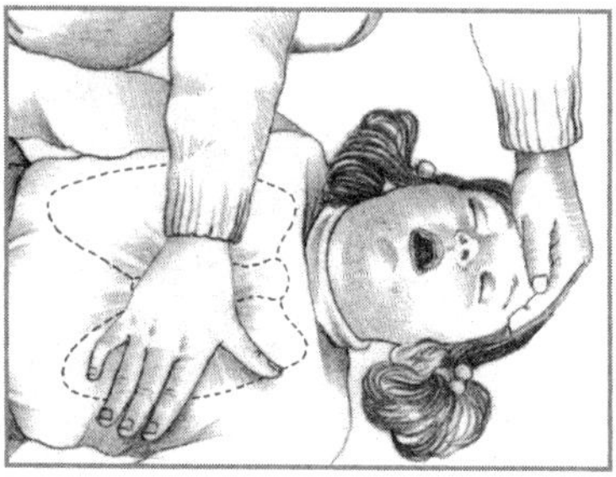

- Using the heel of one hand or with two hands, apply enough pressure to compress the child's chest downward approximately one-third to one-half the depth of the chest (as shown top of next column). Compressions should be hard and fast at a rate of 100 compressions/minute.

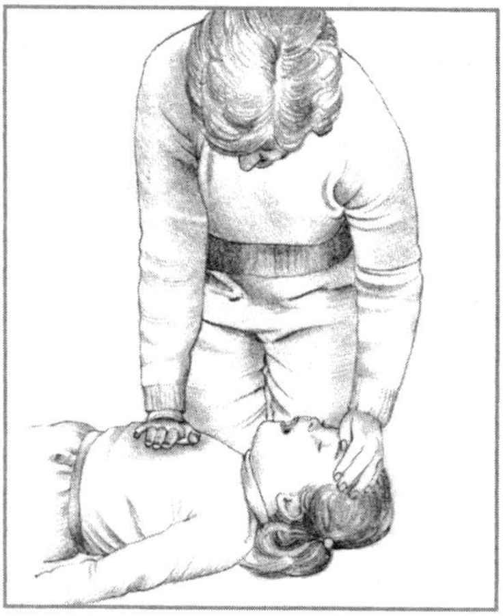

- After every thirty compressions, breathe two breaths into the child. Deliver two breaths for every fifteen compressions if you're working with a partner.
- If you can't detect a pulse, or if the pulse is less than 60 beats/minute and there are signs of poor perfusion, continue chest compression and rescue breathing. If you can detect a pulse, check for spontaneous respirations.
- If not already done, phone EMS or call a code and use an automated external defibrillator or defibrillator after 5 cycles of CPR.
- If the child begins breathing spontaneously, keep the airway open and place the child in a side-lying position to prevent aspiration.

Special considerations

- A child's tongue can easily block her small airway. If this occurs, simply opening the airway may eliminate the obstruction.
- When performing chest compressions, take care to ensure smooth motions. Keep your fingers off, and the heel of your hand on, the child's chest at all times. Also, time your motions so that the compression and relaxation phases are equal to promote effective compressions.
- If the child has breathing difficulty and a parent is present, find out whether the child recently had a fever or an upper respiratory tract infection. If so, suspect epiglottitis.

DO'S & DON'TS

Don't attempt to manipulate the airway because laryngospasm may occur and completely obstruct the airway. Allow the child to assume a comfortable position, and monitor her breathing until additional assistance arrives.

- Persist in attempts to remove an obstruction. As hypoxia develops, the child's muscles will relax, allowing you to remove the foreign object.
- During resuscitation efforts, make sure someone communicates support and information to the parents.
- If available, use a bag-valve mask over the child's nose and mouth when performing ventilations.

Complications

- Fractured ribs
- Lacerated liver
- Punctured lung
- Gastric distention

Documentation

Document all of the events of resuscitation and the names of the individuals who were present. Record whether the child suffered cardiac or respiratory arrest. Note where the arrest occurred, the time CPR began, how long the procedure continued, and the outcome. Document any complications—for example, a fractured rib, a bruised mouth, or gastric distention—as well as actions taken to correct them.

If the child received advanced cardiac life support, document which interventions were performed, who performed them, when they were performed, and what equipment was used.

Cardiopulmonary resuscitation, infant (younger than age 1)

The objective of cardiopulmonary resuscitation (CPR) in an infant is the same as in a child or adult, but the techniques for an infant vary.

Equipment

Infant-sized bag-valve mask, if available

Key steps

- Gently tap the foot of the apparently unconscious infant and call out his name.
- For a sudden witnessed collapse, call for help or call emergency medical services. If you didn't witness the collapse, perform resuscitation measures for 2 minutes; then call for help. You may move an uninjured infant close to a telephone, if necessary.
- Open the airway using the head-tilt, chin-lift maneuver, unless contraindicated by trauma; don't hyperextend the infant's neck.
- Place your ear near the infant's mouth and nose to evaluate his breathing status. Look for chest movement, listen for exhaled air, and feel for exhaled air on your cheek.
- If the infant is breathing, maintain an open airway and monitor respirations.

Restoring ventilation

- If the infant isn't breathing, take a breath and tightly seal your mouth over the infant's nose and mouth (as shown below). Give two breaths watching for the infant's chest to rise and fall.

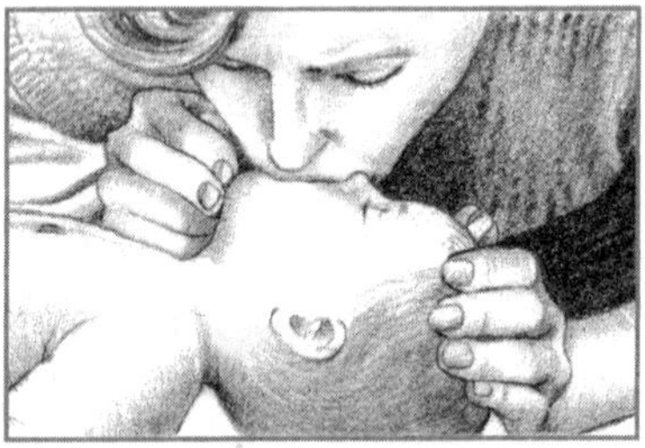

- Continue rescue breathing with one breath every 3 to 5 seconds (12 to 20 breaths per minute) if you can detect a pulse. Give each breath over 1 second.

Clearing the airway

- If you're unable to ventilate the infant, reposition the head and try again.
- To remove an airway obstruction, place the infant facedown on your forearm, with his head lower than his trunk. Support your forearm on your thigh.

■ Give five blows between the infant's should blades using the heel of your free hand.
■ If the airway remains obstructed, sandwich the infant between your hands and forearms and flip him over onto his back.

DO'S & DON'TS

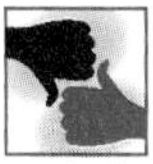

Don't do a blind finger sweep to find or remove an obstruction. In an infant, the maneuver may push the object back into the airway and cause further obstruction. Only place your fingers in the infant's mouth if you see an object to remove.

■ Keeping the infant's head lower than his trunk, give 5 midsternal chest thrusts, using your middle and ring fingers only, to raise the intrathoracic pressure enough to form a cough that will expel the obstruction (as shown below). Remember to hold the infant's head firmly to avoid injury.

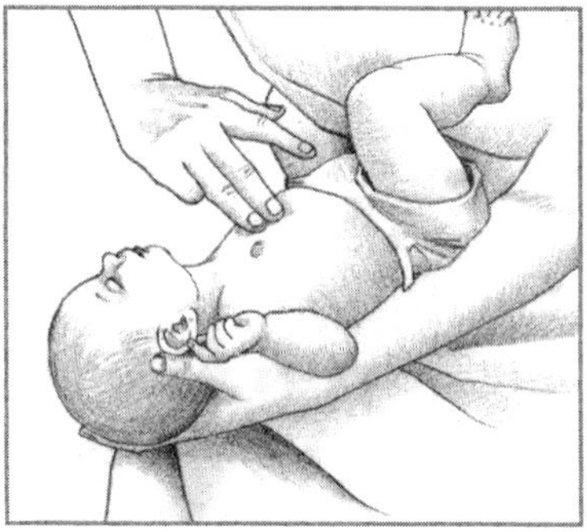

■ Repeat this sequence until the obstruction is dislodged or the infant loses consciousness. If the infant loses consciousness, start CPR. Every time you open the airway to deliver breaths, check the mouth and remove any object you see.

Restoring heartbeat and circulation

■ Assess the infant's pulse by palpating the brachial artery, located inside his upper arm between the elbow and the shoulder (as shown top of next column). Take no more than 10 seconds to assess the pulse.

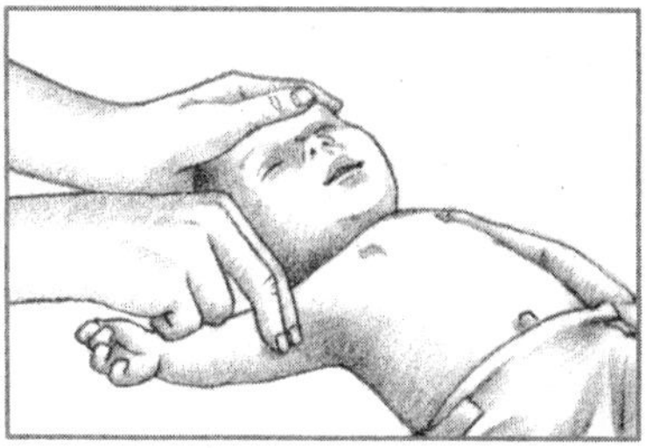

■ If you find a pulse, continue rescue breathing but don't initiate chest compressions.
■ Begin chest compressions if you find no pulse.
■ To locate the correct position on the infant's sternum for chest compression, draw an imaginary horizontal line between the infant's nipples.
■ Place two fingers on the sternum, directly below and perpendicular to, the nipple line. Use these two fingers to depress the sternum here 1/3″ to 1/2″ the depth of the chest at a rate of at least 100 compressions per minute (as shown below).

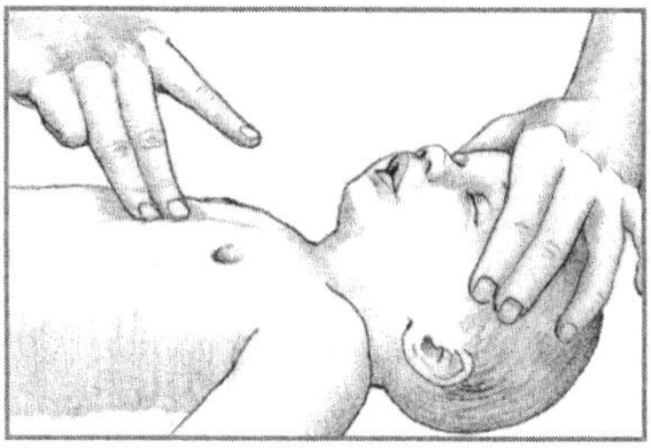

■ When two rescuers are present, use a 2-thumb encircling technique to provide chest compressions. Use both hands to encircle the infant's chest with both thumbs together over the lower half of the sternum. Forcefully compress the sternum with your thumbs as you squeeze the thorax with your fingers.
■ Supply two breaths after every 30 compressions or two ventilations for every 15 compressions if two rescuers are performing CPR. Maintain this ratio whether you're the helper or the lone rescuer. This ratio allows for about 100 compressions and 20 breaths/minute.

- If available, you should use a bag-valve mask over the infant's nose and mouth when performing ventilations.

Special considerations

- An infant's small airway can be easily blocked by his tongue. If this occurs, simply opening the airway may eliminate the obstruction.
- Take care to ensure smooth motions when performing cardiac compressions. Time your motions so that the compression and relaxation phases are equal to promote effective compressions.
- If the infant has breathing difficulty and a parent is present, find out whether the infant recently had a fever or an upper respiratory tract infection.
- If the infant recently had a fever or an upper respiratory tract infection, suspect epiglottiditis.

DO'S & DON'TS

Don't attempt to manipulate the airway because laryngospasm may occur and completely obstruct the airway. Place the infant in a comfortable position, and monitor his breathing until additional assistance arrives.

- Persist in attempts to remove an obstruction. As hypoxia develops, the infant's muscles will relax, allowing you to remove the foreign object.
- Make sure that someone communicates support and information to the parents during resuscitation efforts.

Complications

- Lacerated liver
- Punctured lungs
- Gastric distention

Documentation

Document all of the events of resuscitation and the names of the individuals who were present. Record whether the infant suffered cardiac or respiratory arrest. Note where the arrest occurred, the time CPR began, how long the procedure continued, and the outcome. Document any complications, such as a fractured rib, bruised mouth, or gastric distention, as well as actions taken to correct them.

If the infant received advanced cardiac life support, document which interventions were performed, who performed them, when they were perfumed, and what equipment was used.

Cardioversion, synchronized

Used to treat tachyarrhythmias, cardioversion delivers an electric charge to the myocardium at the peak of the R wave. This causes immediate depolarization, interrupting reentry circuits and allowing the sinoatrial node to resume control. Synchronizing the electrical charge with the R wave ensures that the current won't be delivered on the vulnerable T wave and thus disrupt repolarization.

Synchronized cardioversion is the treatment of choice for arrhythmias that don't respond to vagal massage or drug therapy, such as atrial tachycardia, atrial flutter, atrial fibrillation, and symptomatic ventricular tachycardia.

Cardioversion may be an elective or urgent procedure, depending on how well the patient tolerates the arrhythmia. For example, if the patient is hemodynamically unstable, he would require urgent cardioversion. Remember that, when preparing for cardioversion, the patient's condition can deteriorate quickly, necessitating immediate defibrillation.

Indications for cardioversion include stable paroxysmal atrial tachycardia, unstable paroxysmal supraventricular tachycardia, atrial fibrillation, atrial flutter, and ventricular tachycardia.

Equipment

Cardioverter-defibrillator ♦ conductive gel pads ♦ anterior, posterior, or transverse paddles ♦ electrocardiogram (ECG) monitor with recorder ♦ sedative ♦ oxygen therapy equipment ♦ airway ♦ handheld resuscitation bag ♦ emergency pacing equipment ♦ emergency cardiac medications ♦ automatic blood pressure cuff (if available) ♦ pulse oximeter (if available)

Key steps

- Explain the procedure to the patient, and make sure he has signed a consent form.
- Check the patient's recent serum potassium and magnesium levels and arterial blood gas results. Also check recent digoxin levels. Although digitalized patients may undergo cardioversion, they tend to require lower energy levels to convert. If the patient takes digoxin, withhold the dose on the day of the procedure.
- If possible, withhold all food and fluids for 6 to 12 hours before the procedure.
- Obtain a 12-lead ECG to serve as a baseline.
- Check to see if the practitioner has ordered administration of any cardiac drugs before the procedure. Also verify that the patient has a patent I.V. site in case drug administration becomes necessary.
- Connect the patient to a pulse oximeter and automatic blood pressure cuff, if available.
- Consider administering oxygen for 5 to 10 minutes before the cardioversion to promote myocardial oxygenation. If the patient wears dentures, evaluate whether they support his airway or might cause an airway obstruction. If they might cause an obstruction, remove them.
- Place the patient in the supine position and assess his vital signs, level of consciousness (LOC), cardiac rhythm, and peripheral pulses.
- Remove any oxygen delivery device just before cardioversion to avoid possible combustion.
- Have epinephrine, lidocaine, and atropine at the patient's bedside.
- Make sure that the resuscitation bag is at the patient's bedside.
- Administer a sedative, as ordered. The patient should be heavily sedated but still able to breathe adequately.
- Carefully monitor the patient's blood pressure and respiratory rate until he recovers.
- Press the POWER button to turn on the defibrillator. Next, push the SYNC button to synchronize the machine with the patient's QRS complexes. Make sure the SYNC button flashes with each of the patient's QRS complexes. You should also see a bright green flag flash on the monitor.
- Turn the ENERGY SELECT dial to the ordered amount of energy. Advanced cardiac life support protocols call for an initial shock of 50 to 100 joules for a patient with unstable supraventricular tachycardia, 100 to 200 joules for a patient with atrial fibrillation, 50 to 100 joules for a patient with atrial flutter, and 100 joules for a patient who has monomorphic ventricular tachycardia with a pulse. If there's no response with the first shock, the practitioner should increase the joules in a stepwise manner.
- Remove the paddles from the machine, and prepare them as you would if you were defibrillating the patient. Place the conductive gel pads or paddles in the same positions as you would to defibrillate.
- Make sure everyone stands away from the bed; then push the discharge buttons. Hold the paddles in place and wait for the energy to be discharged—the machine has to synchronize the discharge with the QRS complex.
- Check the waveform on the monitor. If the arrhythmia fails to convert, repeat the procedure two or three more times at 3-minute intervals. Gradually increase the energy level with each additional countershock.
- After the cardioversion, frequently assess the patient's LOC and respiratory status, including airway patency, respiratory rate and depth, and the need for supplemental oxygen. Because the patient will be heavily sedated, he may require airway support.
- Record a postcardioversion 12-lead ECG, and monitor the patient's ECG rhythm for 2 hours. Check the patient's chest for electrical burns.

Special considerations

DEVICE SAFETY

If the patient is attached to a bedside or telemetry monitor, disconnect the unit before cardioversion. The electric current it generates could damage the equipment.

- Be aware that improper synchronization may result if the patient's ECG tracing contains artifact-like spikes, such as peaked T waves or bundle-branch heart blocks when the R' wave may be taller than the R wave.

- Although the electric shock of cardioversion won't usually damage an implanted pacemaker, avoid placing the paddles directly over the pacemaker.
- Reset the synchronization mode after each cardioversion because many defibrillators automatically default back to the unsynchronized mode.

Complications

- Transient, harmless arrhythmias such as atrial, ventricular, and junctional premature beats
- Ventricular fibrillation (This type of arrhythmia is more likely to result from high amounts of electrical energy, digitalis toxicity, severe heart disease, electrolyte imbalance, or improper synchronization with the R wave.)

Patient teaching

- Review with the patient how to take his pulse and record it for the practitioner to review on follow-up visits.
- Review signs and symptoms to report, (recurrence of previous rhythm)

Documentation

Document the procedure, including the voltage delivered with each attempt, rhythm strips before and after the procedure, and how the patient tolerated the procedure.

Catheter (indwelling) care and removal

Intended to prevent infection and other complications by keeping the catheter site clean, routine catheter care is typically performed daily after the patient's morning bath and immediately after perineal care. (Bedtime catheter care may have to be performed before perineal care.)

Studies suggest that catheter care should include daily cleaning of the meatal-catheter area. The use of topical antibiotics is discouraged because it hasn't been proven to be effective in decreasing infection. The equipment and the patient's genitalia require inspection twice daily.

An indwelling urinary catheter should be removed when bladder decompression is no longer necessary, when the patient can resume voiding, or when the catheter is obstructed. Depending on the length of the catheterization, the practitioner may order bladder retraining before catheter removal.

Equipment

Catheter care

Soap and water ♦ sterile gloves ♦ eight sterile 4″ × 4″ gauze pads ♦ basin ♦ washcloth ♦ leg bag ♦ collection bag ♦ adhesive tape or leg band ♦ waste receptacle ♦ optional: safety pin, rubber band, gooseneck lamp or flashlight, adhesive remover, specimen container

Perineal cleaning

Washcloth ♦ additional basin ♦ gloves ♦ soap and water

Catheter removal

Gloves ♦ alcohol pad ♦ 10-ml syringe with a luer-lock ♦ bedpan ♦ linen-saver pad ♦ optional: clamp for bladder retraining

Key steps

- Confirm the patient's identity using two patient identifiers according to your facility's policy.
- Explain the procedure and its purpose to the patient.
- Provide the patient with the necessary equipment for self-cleaning, if possible.
- Provide privacy.

Catheter care

- Make sure that the lighting is adequate so you can see the perineum and catheter tubing clearly. Place a gooseneck lamp or flashlight at the bedside if needed.
- Inspect the catheter for problems and check the urine drainage for mucus, blood clots, sediment, and turbidity. Pinch the catheter between two fingers to determine if the lumen contains any material. If you notice any of these conditions (or if your

facility's policy requires it), obtain a urine specimen from the specimen collection port using a sterile needle and syringe. Collect at least 3 ml of urine, but don't fill the specimen cup more than halfway. Notify the practitioner about your findings.

ALERT

Be sure to clean the port with povidone-iodine solution before collecting the urine specimen.

- Inspect the outside of the catheter where it enters the urinary meatus for encrusted material and suppurative drainage. Inspect the tissue around the meatus for irritation or swelling.
- Remove the leg band, or if adhesive tape was used to secure the catheter, remove the adhesive tape. Inspect the area for signs and symptoms of adhesive burns—redness, tenderness, or blisters.
- Put on the gloves. Clean the outside of the catheter and the tissue around the meatus, using soap and water. To avoid contaminating the urinary tract, always clean by wiping away from—never toward—the urinary meatus. Use a dry gauze pad to remove encrusted material.

DO'S & DON'TS

Don't pull on the catheter while you're cleaning it. This can injure the urethra and the bladder wall. It can also expose a section of the catheter that was inside the urethra, so that when you release the catheter, the newly contaminated section will reenter the urethra, introducing potentially infectious organisms.

- Remove your gloves, reapply the leg band, and reattach the catheter to the leg band. If a leg band isn't available, tear a piece of adhesive tape from the roll.
- To prevent skin hypersensitivity or irritation, retape the catheter on the opposite side.

ALERT

Provide enough slack before securing the catheter to prevent tension on the tubing, which could injure the urethral lumen or bladder wall.

- Most drainage bags have a plastic clamp on the tubing to attach them to the sheet. If this isn't available, wrap a rubber band around the drainage tubing, insert the safety pin through a loop of the rubber band, and pin the tubing to the sheet below bladder level. Attach the collection bag, below bladder level, to the bed frame.
- If necessary, use an adhesive remover to clean residue from the previous tape site. Dispose of used supplies in the waste receptacle.

Catheter removal

- Wash your hands.
- Assemble the equipment at the patient's bedside. Explain the procedure and tell him that he may feel slight discomfort. Tell him that you'll check him periodically during the first 6 to 24 hours after catheter removal to make sure he resumes voiding.
- Put on gloves. Place a linen-saver pad under the patient's buttocks. Attach the syringe to the luer-lock mechanism on the catheter.
- Pull back on the plunger of the syringe. This deflates the balloon by aspirating the injected fluid. The amount of fluid injected is usually indicated on the tip of the catheter's balloon lumen and in the patient's chart.
- Because urine may leak as the catheter is removed, offer the patient a bedpan. Grasp the catheter, and pinch it firmly with your thumb and index finger to prevent urine from flowing back into the urethra. Gently pull the catheter from the urethra. If you meet resistance, don't apply force; instead, notify the practitioner. Remove the bedpan.
- Measure and record the amount of urine in the collection bag before discarding it. Remove and discard gloves, and wash your hands. For the first 24 hours after catheter removal, note the time and amount of each voiding.

Special considerations

- Your facility may require the use of specific cleaning agents for catheter care, so

Teaching about leg bags

A urine drainage bag attached to the leg provides the catheterized patient with greater mobility. Because the bag is hidden under clothing, it may also help him feel more comfortable about catheterization. Leg bags are usually worn during the day and are replaced at night with a standard collection device.

If your patient will be discharged with an indwelling catheter, teach him how to attach and remove a leg bag. To demonstrate, you'll need a bag with a short drainage tube, two straps, an alcohol pad, and adhesive tape.

Attaching the leg bag

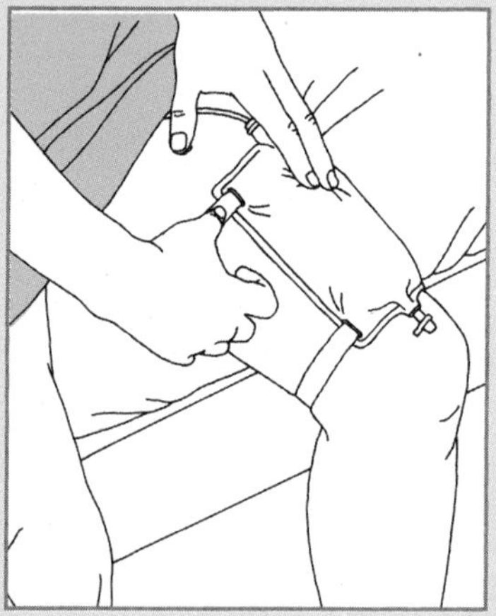

- Provide privacy, and explain the procedure. Describe the advantages of a leg bag, but caution the patient that a leg bag is smaller than a standard collection device and may have to be emptied more frequently.
- Remove the protective covering from the tip of the drainage tube. Then show the patient how to clean the tip with an alcohol pad, wiping away from the opening to avoid contaminating the tube. Show him how to attach the tube to the catheter.
- Place the drainage bag on the patient's calf or thigh. Have him fasten the straps securely (as shown), and then show him how to tape the catheter to his leg. Emphasize that he must leave slack in the catheter to minimize pressure on the bladder, urethra, and related structures. Excessive pressure or tension can lead to tissue breakdown.
- Also tell him not to fasten the straps too tightly to avoid interfering with his circulation.

Avoiding complications

- Although most leg bags have a valve in the drainage tube that prevents urine reflux into the bladder, urge the patient to keep the drainage bag lower than his bladder at all times because urine in the bag is a perfect growth medium for bacteria. Caution him not to go to bed or take long naps while wearing the drainage bag.
- To prevent a full leg bag from damaging the bladder wall and urethra, encourage the patient to empty the bag when it's only one-half full. He should also inspect the catheter and drainage tube periodically for compression or kinking, which could obstruct urine flow and result in bladder distention.
- Tell the patient to wash the leg bag with soap and water or a bacteriostatic solution before each use to prevent infection.

check the policy manual before beginning this procedure.

- Use a closed drainage system whenever possible to decrease the chance of the patient getting a urinary tract infection (UTI).
- Avoid raising the drainage bag above bladder level to prevent reflux of urine. To avoid damaging the urethral lumen or bladder wall, always disconnect the drainage bag and tubing from the bed linen and bed frame before helping the patient out of bed. Also, avoid contact with the floor.
- When possible, attach a leg bag to allow the patient greater mobility. If the patient will be discharged with an indwelling

catheter, teach him how to use a leg bag. (See *Teaching about leg bags*.)

- Encourage patients with unrestricted fluid intake to increase intake to at least 3 qt (3 L)/day. This helps flush the urinary system and reduces sediment formation. To prevent urinary sediment and calculi from obstructing the drainage tube, some patients are placed on an acid-ash diet to acidify urine.
- After catheter removal, assess the patient for incontinence, urgency, persistent dysuria or bladder spasms, fever, chills, or palpable bladder distention. The patient should void within 6 to 8 hours after catheter removal.
- When changing catheters after long-term use (usually 30 days), you may need a larger size catheter because the meatus enlarges, causing urine to leak around the catheter.

Complications

- Sediment buildup that can occur anywhere in a catheterization system, especially in a bedridden or dehydrated patient (To prevent this, keep the patient well hydrated if he isn't on fluid restriction.)
- Malfunction, obstruction, or contamination prompting change of the indwelling catheter as ordered
- Acute renal failure, resulting from a catheter obstructed by sediment (Stay alert for sharply reduced urine flow from the catheter. Assess for bladder discomfort or distention.)
- UTI that can result from catheter insertion or from intraluminal or extraluminal migration of bacteria up the catheter (Signs and symptoms may include cloudy urine, foul-smelling urine, hematuria, fever, malaise, tenderness over the bladder, and flank pain.)
- Failure of the balloon to deflate and rupture of the balloon from removing an indwelling catheter (If the balloon ruptures, cystoscopy is usually performed to ensure removal of balloon fragments.)

Patient teaching

- Instruct patients discharged with indwelling catheters to wash the urinary meatus and perineal area with soap and water twice daily, from front to back, and the anal area after each bowel movement.

Documentation

Record the care you performed, any modifications, patient complaints, and the condition of the perineum and urinary meatus. Note the character of the urine in the drainage bag, any sediment buildup, and whether a specimen was sent for laboratory analysis. Record fluid intake and output. An hourly record is usually necessary for critically ill patients and those with renal insufficiency who are hemodynamically unstable.

Catheter (indwelling) insertion

An indwelling urinary catheter (Foley catheter) remains in the bladder to provide continuous urine drainage. A balloon inflated at the catheter's distal end prevents it from slipping out of the bladder after insertion. Indwelling catheters are used most commonly to relieve bladder distention caused by urine retention and to allow continuous urine drainage when the urinary meatus is swollen from childbirth, surgery, or local trauma. Other indications for an indwelling catheter include urinary tract obstruction (by a tumor or enlarged prostate), urine retention or infection from neurogenic bladder paralysis caused by spinal cord injury or disease, and an illness in which the patient's urine output must be monitored.

An indwelling catheter is inserted using sterile technique and only when absolutely necessary. Insertion should be performed with extreme care to prevent injury and infection. To avoid trauma to the urethra and decrease the risk of infection, always use the smallest size catheter with the smallest balloon.

Equipment

Sterile indwelling catheter (latex or silicone #10 to #22 French [average adult sizes are # 14 to #16 French]) ♦ syringe filled with 10 ml of sterile water (normal saline solution is sometimes used) ♦

washcloth ♦ towel ♦ soap and water ♦ two linen-saver pads ♦ sterile gloves ♦ sterile drape ♦ sterile fenestrated drape ♦ sterile cotton-tipped applicators (or cotton balls and plastic forceps) ♦ antiseptic cleaning agent ♦ urine receptacle ♦ sterile water-soluble lubricant ♦ sterile drainage collection bag ♦ intake and output sheet ♦ adhesive tape ♦ optional: urine-specimen container and laboratory request form, leg band with Velcro closure, gooseneck lamp or flashlight, pillows or rolled blankets

Prepackaged sterile disposable kits that usually contain all the necessary equipment are available. The syringes in these kits are prefilled with 10 ml of normal saline solution.

Preparation

- Check the order on the patient's chart to determine if a catheter size or type has been specified.
- Wash your hands, select the appropriate equipment, and assemble it at the patient's bedside.

Key steps

- Confirm the patient's identity using two patient identifiers according to your facility's policy.
- Explain the procedure to the patient and provide privacy. Check his chart and ask when he voided last. Percuss and palpate the bladder to establish baseline data. Ask if he feels the urge to void.
- Have a coworker hold a flashlight or place a gooseneck lamp next to the patient's bed so that you can see the urinary meatus clearly.
- Place the female patient in the supine position, with her knees flexed and separated and her feet flat on the bed, about 2′ (61 cm) apart. If she finds this position uncomfortable, have her flex one knee and keep the other leg flat on the bed.
- Place the male patient in the supine position with his legs extended and flat on the bed. Ask the patient to hold the position to give you a clear view of the urinary meatus and to prevent contamination.
- If necessary, ask an assistant to help the patient stay in position or to direct the light. The elderly patient may need pillows or rolled towels or blankets to help with positioning.
- Wash your hands, and put on gloves. Use a washcloth to clean the patient's genital area and perineum thoroughly with soap and water. Dry the area with the towel.
- Place the linen-saver pads on the bed between the patient's legs and under the hips. To create the sterile field, open the prepackaged kit or equipment tray and place it between the female patient's legs or next to the male patient's hip. If the sterile gloves are the first item on the top of the tray, put them on. Place the sterile drape under the patient's hips. Drape the patient's lower abdomen with the sterile fenestrated drape so that only the genital area remains exposed. Take care not to contaminate your gloves.
- Open the rest of the kit or tray. Put on the sterile gloves if you haven't already done so.
- Make sure that the patient isn't allergic to iodine solution; if he's allergic, another antiseptic cleaning agent must be used.
- Tear open the packet of the antiseptic cleaning agent, and use it to saturate the sterile cotton balls or applicators. Be careful not to spill the solution on the equipment.
- Open the packet of water-soluble lubricant and apply it to the catheter tip; attach the drainage bag to the other end of the catheter. (If you're using a commercial kit, the drainage bag may be attached.) Make sure that all tubing ends remain sterile, and make sure that the clamp at the emptying port of the drainage bag is closed to prevent urine leakage from the bag. Some drainage systems have an air-lock chamber to prevent bacteria from traveling to the bladder from urine in the drainage bag. Note: Some urologists and nurses use a syringe prefilled with water-soluble lubricant and instill the lubricant directly into the male urethra, instead of on the catheter tip. This method helps prevent trauma to the urethral lining and, possibly, a urinary tract infection (UTI). Check your facility's policy.
- Before inserting the catheter, inflate the balloon with sterile water or normal saline

solution to inspect it for leaks. To do this, attach the prefilled syringe to the luer-lock, and then push the plunger and check for seepage as the balloon expands. Aspirate the solution to deflate the balloon. Inspect the catheter for resiliency. Rough, cracked catheters can injure the urethral mucosa during insertion, which can predispose the patient to infection.

- For the female patient, separate the labia majora and labia minora as widely as possible with the thumb, middle, and index fingers of your nondominant hand so you have a full view of the urinary meatus. Keep the labia well separated throughout the procedure (as shown below) so they don't obscure the urinary meatus or contaminate the area after it's cleaned.

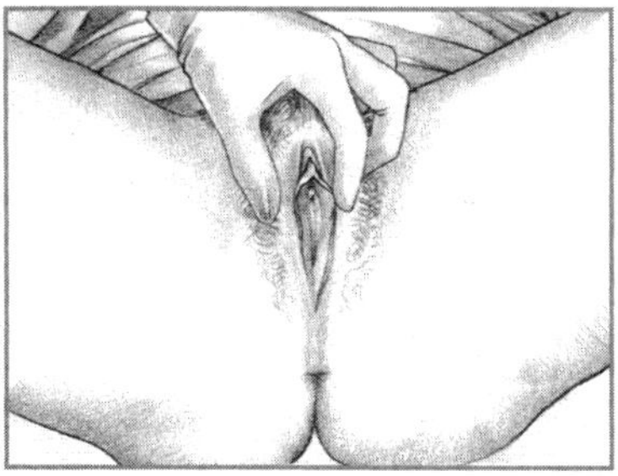

- With your dominant hand, use a sterile, cotton-tipped applicator (or pick up a sterile cotton ball with the plastic forceps) and wipe one side of the urinary meatus with a single downward motion (as shown below). Wipe the other side with another sterile applicator or cotton ball in the same way. Wipe directly over the meatus with still another sterile applicator or cotton ball. Take care not to contaminate your sterile glove.

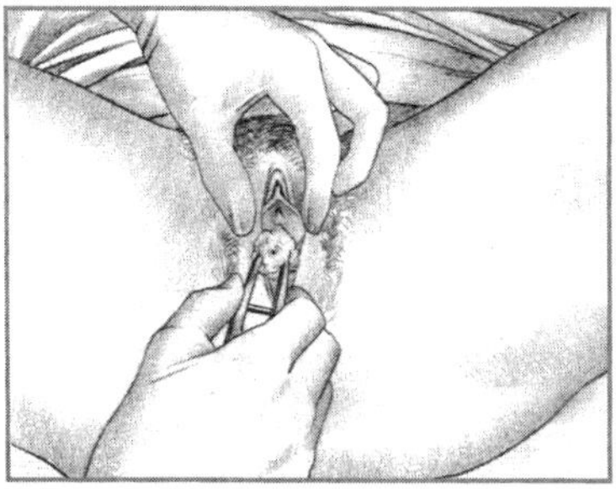

- For the male patient, hold the penis with your nondominant hand. If he's uncircumcised, retract the foreskin. Gently lift and stretch the penis to a 60- to 90-degree angle. Hold the penis this way throughout the procedure to straighten the urethra and maintain a sterile field (as shown below).

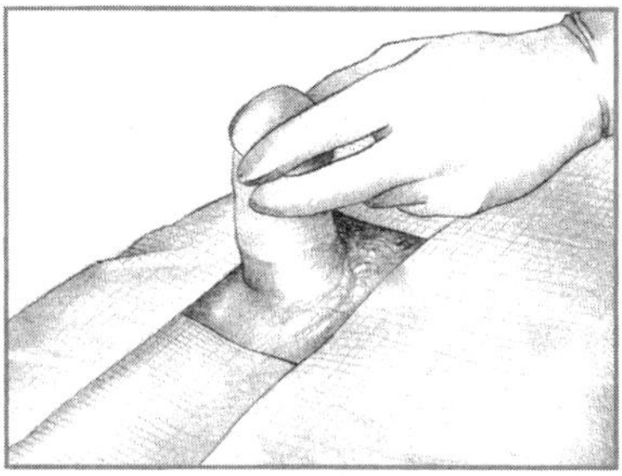

- Use your dominant hand to clean the glans with a sterile cotton-tipped applicator or a sterile cotton ball held in forceps. Clean in a circular motion, starting at the urinary meatus and working outward.
- Repeat the procedure using another sterile applicator or cotton ball and taking care not to contaminate your sterile glove.
- Pick up the catheter with your dominant hand and prepare to insert the lubricated tip into the urinary meatus. To facilitate insertion by relaxing the sphincter, ask the patient to cough as you insert the catheter. Tell the patient to breathe deeply and slowly to further relax the sphincter. Hold the catheter close to its tip to ease insertion and control its direction.

ALERT

Never force a catheter during insertion. Maneuver it gently as the patient bears down or coughs. If you still meet resistance, stop and notify the practitioner. Sphincter spasms, strictures, misplacement in the vagina (in females), or an enlarged prostate (in males) may cause resistance.

- For the female patient, advance the catheter about 2″ to 3″ (5 to 7.5 cm)—while continuing to hold the labia apart—until urine begins to flow (as shown top of next page). If the catheter is inadvertently inserted into the vagina, leave it there as a landmark. Begin the procedure over again using new supplies.

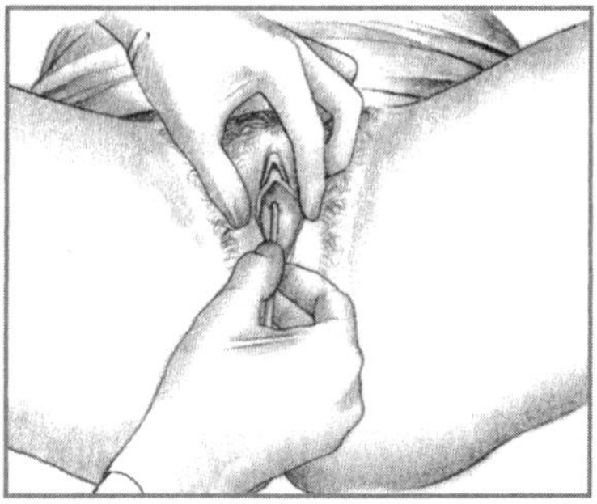

■ For the male patient, advance the catheter (to the bifurcation 5″ to $7^{1}/_{2}$″ [12.5 to 19 cm]) and check for urine flow (as shown below). If the foreskin was retracted, replace it to prevent compromised circulation and painful swelling.

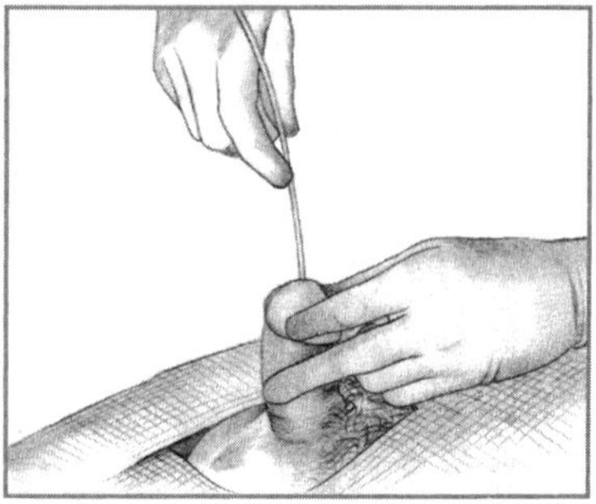

■ When urine stops flowing, attach the prefilled syringe to the luer-lock. Push the plunger and inflate the balloon to keep the catheter in place in the bladder (as shown below).

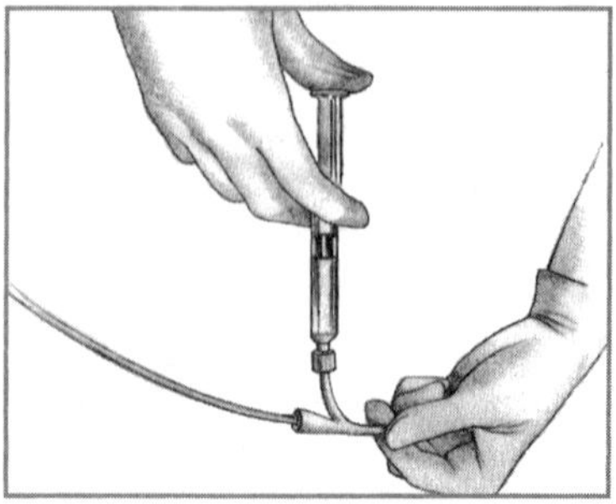

ALERT

Never inflate a balloon without first establishing urine flow, which assures you that the catheter is in the bladder.

■ Hang the collection bag below bladder level to prevent urine reflux into the bladder, which can cause infection, and to facilitate gravity drainage of the bladder. Make sure that the tubing doesn't get tangled in the bed's side rails.
■ Tape the catheter to the female patient's thigh (as shown below) to prevent possible tension on the urogenital trigone.

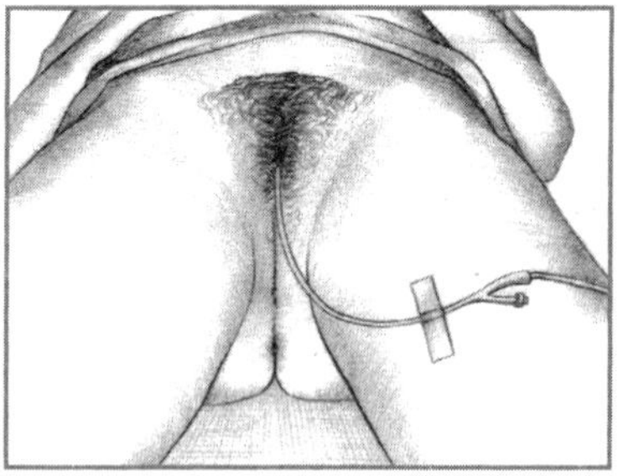

■ Tape the catheter to the male patient's abdomen (with penis directed toward chest) or anterior thigh to prevent pressure on the urethra at the penoscrotal junction, which can lead to the formation of urethrocutaneous fistulas. Taping also prevents traction on the bladder and alterations in the normal direction of urine flow in males.
■ As an alternative, secure the catheter to the patient's thigh using a leg band with a Velcro closure (as shown below). This decreases skin irritation, especially in patients with long-term indwelling catheters.

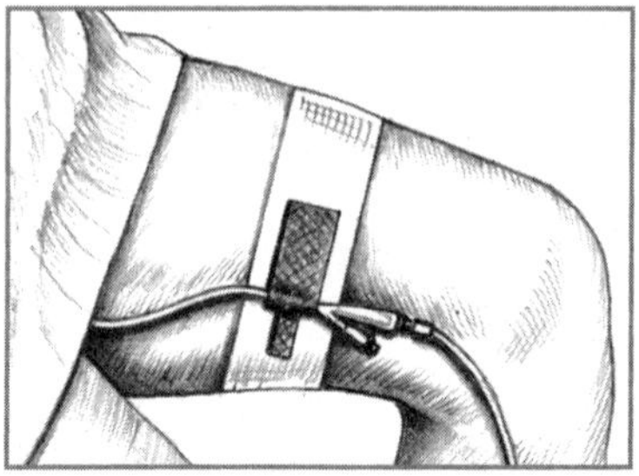

- Dispose of used supplies properly.

Special considerations

- Indwelling urinary catheters should be used only after all other means of management have been considered.
- The patient's need for a catheter should be reviewed regularly, and it should be removed as soon as possible.
- Several types of catheters are available with balloons of various sizes. Each type has its own method of inflation and closure. For example, in one type of catheter, sterile solution or air is injected through the inflation lumen, and then the end of the injection port is folded over itself and fastened with a clamp or rubber band. Note: Injecting a catheter with air makes identifying leaks difficult and doesn't guarantee deflation of the balloon for removal.
- A similar catheter is inflated when a seal in the end of the inflation lumen is penetrated with a needle or the tip of the solution-filled syringe. Another type of balloon catheter self-inflates when a prepositioned clamp is loosened. The balloon size determines the amount of solution needed for inflation, and the exact amount is usually printed on the distal extension of the catheter used for inflating the balloon.
- If necessary, ask the female patient to lie on her side with her knees drawn up to her chest during the catheterization procedure (as shown below). This position may be especially helpful for elderly or disabled patients such as those with severe contractures.

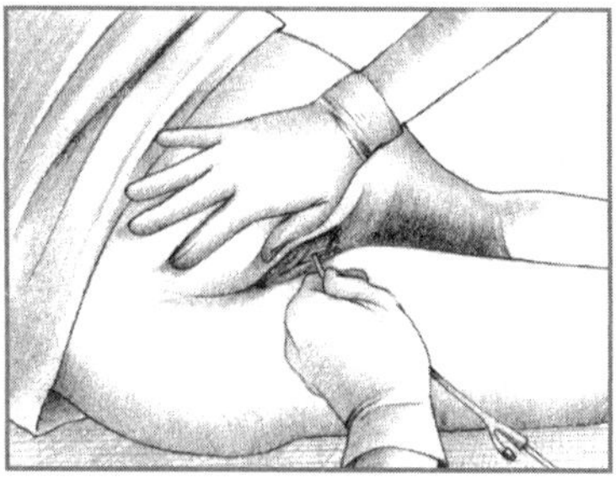

- If the practitioner orders a urine specimen for laboratory analysis, obtain it from the urine receptacle with a specimen collection container at the time of catheterization, and send it to the laboratory with the appropriate laboratory request form. Connect the drainage bag when urine stops flowing.
- Inspect the catheter and tubing periodically while they're in place to detect compression or kinking that could obstruct urine flow. Explain the basic principles of gravity drainage so the patient realizes the importance of keeping the drainage tubing and collection bag lower than his bladder at all times. If necessary, provide the patient with detailed instructions for performing clean intermittent self-catheterization. (See "Self-catheterization," page 451.)
- For monitoring purposes, empty the collection bag at least every 8 hours. Excessive fluid volume may require more frequent emptying to prevent traction on the catheter, which would cause the patient discomfort, and to prevent injury to the urethra and bladder wall. Some facilities encourage changing catheters at regular intervals, such as every 30 days, if the patient will have long-term continuous drainage.

ALERT

Observe the patient carefully for adverse reactions, such as hypovolemic shock, caused by removing excessive volumes of residual urine. Check your facility's policy beforehand to determine the maximum amount of urine that may be drained at one time (some facilities limit the amount to 700 to 1,000 ml). There's some controversy about whether to limit the amount of urine drained. Clamp the catheter at the first sign of an adverse reaction, and notify the practitioner.

Complications

- UTI resulting from the introduction of bacteria into the bladder
- Improper insertion causing traumatic injury to the urethral and bladder mucosa
- Bladder atony or spasms resulting from rapid decompression of a severely distended bladder

Patient teaching

- If the patient will be discharged with a long-term indwelling catheter, teach him and his family all aspects of daily catheter maintenance, including care of the skin and urinary meatus, signs and symptoms of a UTI or obstruction, how to irrigate the catheter (if appropriate), and the importance of adequate fluid intake to maintain patency.
- Explain that a home care nurse should visit every 4 to 6 weeks—or more often if needed—to change the catheter.

Documentation

Record the date, time, size, and type of indwelling catheter used. Describe the amount, color, and other characteristics of urine emptied from the bladder. Your facility may require only the intake and output sheet for fluid-balance data. If large volumes of urine have been emptied, describe the patient's tolerance for the procedure. Note whether a urine specimen was sent for laboratory analysis.

Central venous catheter therapy

A central venous (CV) catheter is a sterile catheter that's inserted through a large vein, such as the subclavian vein (or, less commonly, the internal jugular vein), and terminates in the superior vena cava. CV catheters allow long-term administration in situations requiring safe, repeated access to the venous system for administration of drugs, fluids and nutrition, and blood products. (See *Central venous catheter pathways.*)

By providing access to the central veins, CV therapy offers several benefits. It allows monitoring of CV pressure, which indicates blood volume or pump efficiency and permits aspiration of blood samples for diagnostic tests. It also allows administration of I.V. fluids in large amounts if necessary, in emergencies, or when decreased peripheral circulation makes peripheral vein access difficult; when prolonged I.V. therapy reduces the number of accessible peripheral veins; when solutions must be diluted (for large fluid volumes for irrigating of hypertonic fluids, such as total parenteral nutrition [TPN] solution); and when a patient requires long-term venous access. Because multiple blood samples can be drawn though it without repeated venipuncture, the CV line decreases the patient's anxiety and preserves peripheral veins.

CV therapy increases the risk of complications, such as pneumothorax, sepsis, thrombus formation, and vessel and adjacent organ perforation (all life-threatening conditions). Also, the CV catheter may decrease patient mobility, is difficult to insert, and costs more than a peripheral I.V. catheter.

Removal of a CV catheter, a sterile procedure, is usually performed by the practitioner at the end of therapy or the onset of complications. If the patient may have an infection, the removal procedure includes collection of the catheter tip as a specimen for culture by swabbing it over an agar plate, according to your facility's policy.

Equipment

Inserting a CV catheter

Electric clippers, if necessary ♦ sterile gloves and gowns ♦ blanket ♦ linen-saver pad ♦ sterile towel ♦ sterile drape ♦ masks ♦ antiseptic cleaning swabs ♦ normal saline solution ♦ 3-ml syringe with 25G 1″ needle ♦ 1% or 2% injectable lidocaine ♦ dextrose 5% in water (D_5W) ♦ syringes for blood sample collection ♦ suture material ♦ two 14G or 16G CV catheters ♦ I.V. solution with administration set prepared for use with an infusion pump or controller, as needed ♦ sterile 4″ × 4″ gauze pads ♦ 1″ adhesive tape ♦ sterile scissors ♦ heparin or normal saline flushes, as needed ♦ sterile marker ♦ sterile labels ♦ optional: transparent semipermeable dressing

Flushing a catheter

Normal saline solution or heparin flush solution ♦ alcohol pad

Changing an injection cap

Alcohol pad ♦ injection cap ♦ padded clamp

Central venous catheter pathways

The illustrations below show several common pathways for central venous (CV) catheter insertion. Typically, a CV catheter is inserted in the subclavian vein or the internal jugular vein. The catheter usually terminates in the superior vena cava. The CV catheter is tunneled when long-term placement is required.

Insertion: Subclavian vein
Termination: Superior vena cava

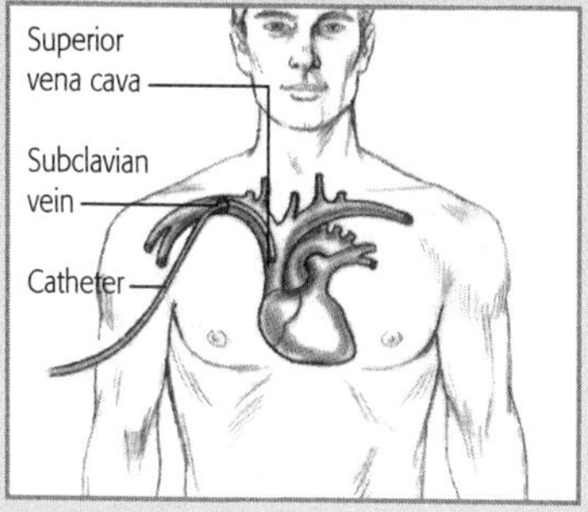

Insertion: Internal jugular vein
Termination: Superior vena cava

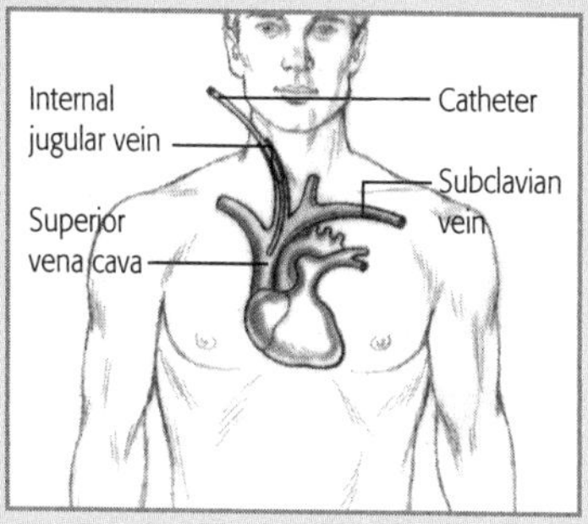

Insertion: Basilic vein (peripheral)
Termination: Superior vena cava

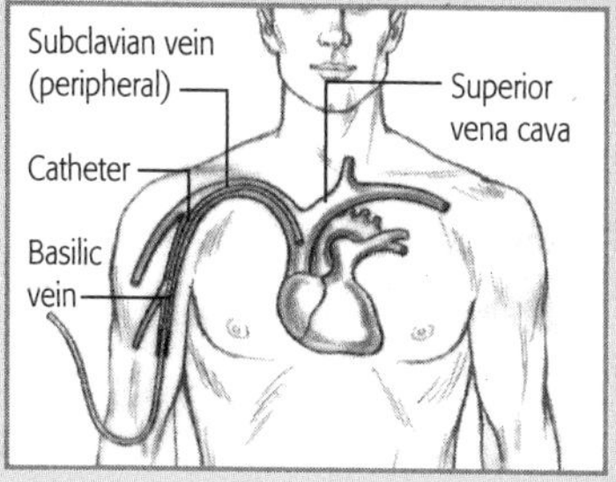

Insertion: Through a subcutaneous tunnel to the subclavian vein (Dacron cuff helps hold catheter in place)
Termination: Superior vena cava

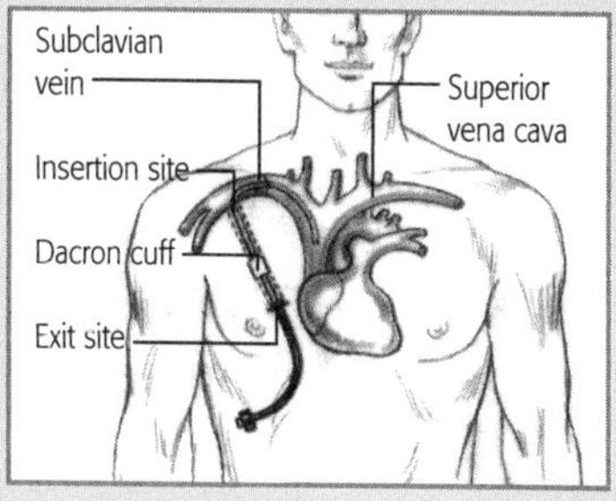

Removing a CV catheter

Clean gloves and sterile gloves ♦ sterile suture removal set ♦ antiseptic cleaning swabs ♦ alcohol pads ♦ sterile 4″ × 4″ gauze pads ♦ forceps ♦ tape ♦ sterile, plastic adhesive-backed dressing or transparent semipermeable dressing ♦ agar plate or culture tube, if necessary for culture

Some facilities have prepared trays containing most of the equipment for catheter insertion. The type of catheter selected depends on the type of therapy to be used. (See *Guide to central venous catheters,* pages 88 to 91.)

Preparation

- Before inserting a CV catheter, confirm catheter type and size with the practitioner; the most commonly used sizes are 14G and 16G.
- Set up the I.V. solution and prime the administration set using strict sterile technique.
- Attach the line to the infusion pump or controller, if ordered.
- Recheck all connections to make sure that they're tight.
- Label all medications, medication containers, and other solutions on and off the sterile field.

(Text continues on page 90.)

Guide to central venous catheters

Type	Description	Indications
Groshong catheter	■ Silicone rubber ■ About 35″ (89 cm) long ■ Closed end with pressure-sensitive three-way valve ■ Dacron cuff ■ Single or double lumen ■ Tunneled	■ Long-term central venous (CV) access ■ Patient with heparin allergy
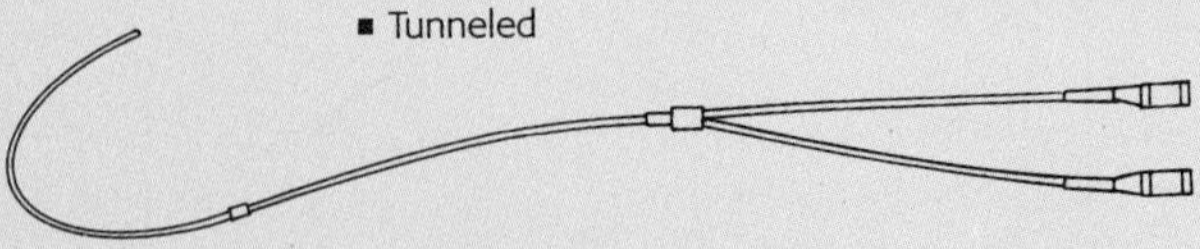		
Short-term single-lumen catheter	■ Polyurethane or silicone ruber (Silastic) ■ About 8″ (20.5 cm) long ■ Lumen gauge varies ■ Percutaneously placed	■ Short-term CV access ■ Emergency access ■ Patient who needs only one lumen
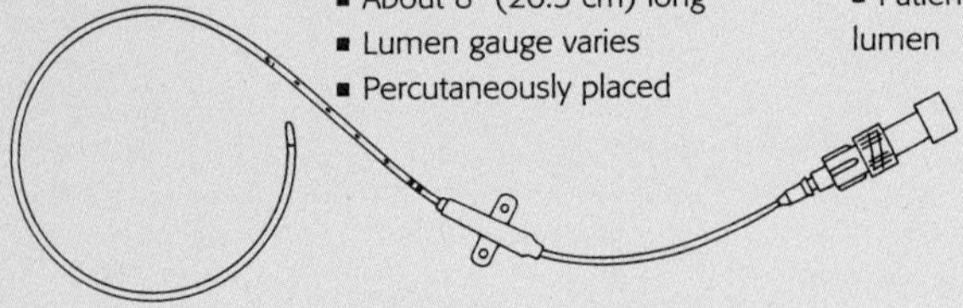		
Short-term multilumen catheter	■ Polyurethane or silicone rubber ■ Two, three, or four lumens exiting at ¾″ (2-cm) intervals ■ Lumen gauges vary ■ Percutaneously placed	■ Short-term CV access ■ Patient with limited insertion sites who requires multiple infusions
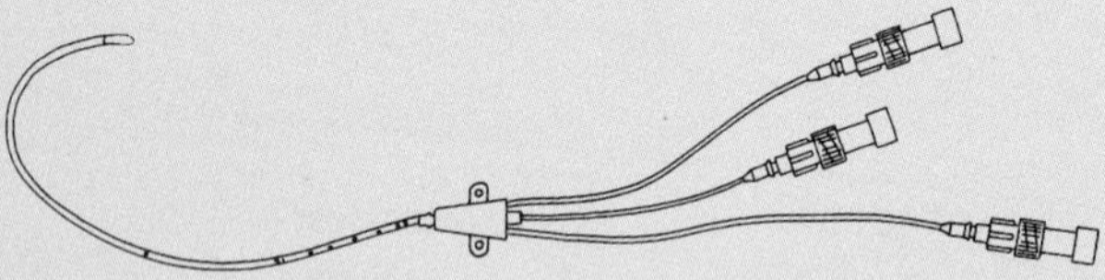		
Hickman catheter	■ Silicone rubber ■ About 35″ long ■ Open end with clamp ■ Dacron cuff 11¾″ (30 cm) from hub ■ Single lumen or multilumen ■ Tunneled	■ Long-term CV access ■ Home therapy
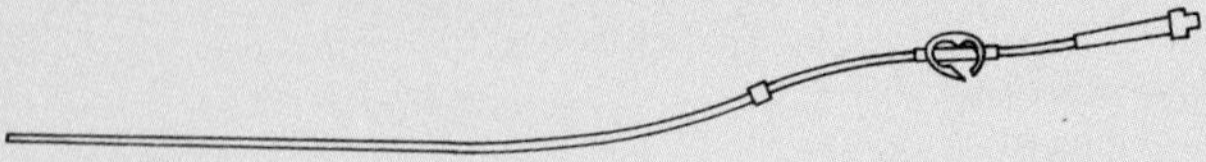		

Advantages and disadvantages	Nursing considerations
Advantages ▪ Less thrombogenic ▪ Pressure-sensitive three-way valve eliminates frequent heparin flushes ▪ Dacron cuff anchors catheter and prevents bacterial migration **Disadvantages** ▪ Requires surgical insertion ▪ Tears and kinks easily ▪ Blunt end makes it difficult to clear substances from its tip	▪ Two surgical sites require dressing after insertion. ▪ Handle catheter gently. ▪ Check the external portion frequently for kinks and leaks. ▪ Repair kit is available. ▪ Remember to flush with enough normal saline solution to clear the catheter, especially after drawing or administering blood. ▪ Change end caps weekly.
Advantages ▪ Easily inserted at bedside ▪ Easily removed ▪ Stiffness aids central venous pressure monitoring **Disadvantages** ▪ Limited functions ▪ Should be changed every 3 to 7 days (depending on your facility's policy)	▪ Assess frequently for signs of infection and clot formation.
Advantages ▪ Same as single-lumen catheter ▪ Allows infusion of multiple (even incompatible) solutions through the same catheter **Disadvantages** ▪ Same as single-lumen catheter	▪ Know gauge and purpose of each lumen. ▪ Use the same lumen for the same task (for example, to administer total parenteral nutrition [TPN] or collect a blood sample).
Advantages ▪ Dacron cuff prevents excess motion and migration of bacteria ▪ Clamps eliminate need for Valsalva's maneuver **Disadvantages** ▪ Requires surgical insertion ▪ Open end ▪ Requires physician for removal ▪ Tears and kinks easily	▪ Two surgical sites require dressing after insertion. ▪ Handle catheter gently. ▪ Observe frequently for kinks and tears. ▪ Repair kit is available. ▪ Clamp catheter with a nonserrated clamp any time it becomes disconnected or opens. ▪ Flush catheter daily when not in use with 3 to 5 ml of heparin (10 units/ml) and before and after each use, using SASH (S=saline, A=additive, S=saline, H=heparin) protocol.

(continued)

Guide to central venous catheters *(continued)*

Type	Description	Indications
Broviac catheter	■ Identical to Hickman except smaller inner lumen	■ Long-term CV access ■ Patient with small central vessels (pediatric or geriatric)
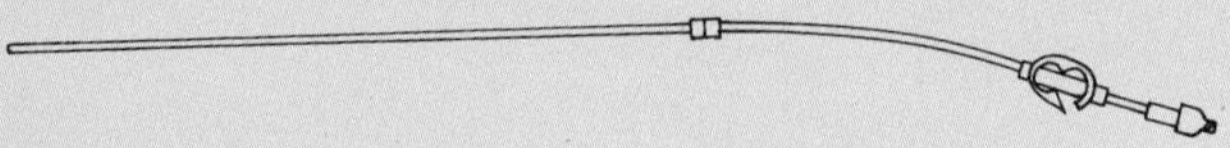		
Hickman/Broviac catheter	■ Hickman and Broviac catheters combined ■ Tunneled	■ Long-term CV access ■ Patient who needs multiple infusions
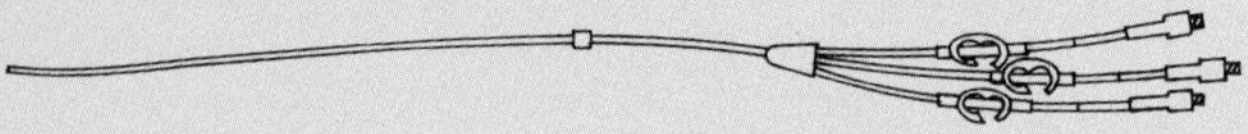		

■ As ordered, notify the radiology department that a chest X-ray machine will be needed.

Key steps
Inserting a CV catheter

■ Confirm the patient's identity using two patient identifiers according to your facility's policy.
■ Wash your hands thoroughly to prevent the spread of microorganisms.
■ Reinforce the practitioner's explanation of the procedure, and answer the patient's questions. Make sure that the patient has signed a consent form, if necessary, and check his history for hypersensitivity to iodine, latex, or the local anesthetic.
■ Place the patient in Trendelenburg's position to dilate the veins and reduce the risk of air embolism.
■ For subclavian vein insertion, place a rolled blanket lengthwise between the shoulders to increase venous distention. For jugular insertion, place a rolled blanket under the opposite shoulder to extend the neck, making anatomic landmarks more visible. Place a linen-saver pad under the patient to prevent soiling the bed.
■ Turn the patient's head away from the site to prevent possible contamination from airborne pathogens and to make the site more accessible. Place a mask on the patient if required by your facility's policy, unless doing so increases his anxiety or is contraindicated due to his respiratory status.
■ Prepare the insertion site. You may need to wash the skin with soap and water first. Make sure that the skin is free from hair because hair can harbor microorganisms. Infection-control practitioners recommend clipping the hair close to the skin rather than shaving, which may cause skin irritation and create multiple small open wounds, increasing the risk of infection. (If the practitioner orders that the area be shaved, try shaving it the evening before catheter insertion to allow partial healing of minor skin irritations.)
■ Establish a sterile field on a table, using a sterile towel or the wrapping from the instrument tray.
■ Put on a mask and sterile gloves and gown, and clean the area around the insertion site with an antiseptic cleaning swab using a vigorous back-and-forth motion. If

Advantages and disadvantages	Nursing considerations
Advantages ■ Smaller lumen for better comfort **Disadvantages** ■ Small lumen may limit uses ■ Single lumen may limit functions ■ In children, growth may cause catheter tip to move out of position	■ Check your facility's policy before drawing blood or administering blood or blood products. ■ Flush catheter daily when not in use with 3 to 5 ml of heparin (10 unites/ml) and before and after each use, using SASH protocol.
Advantages ■ Double-lumen Hickman catheter allows sampling and administration of blood ■ Broviac lumen delivers I.V. fluids, including TPN **Disadvantages** ■ Same as Hickman catheter	■ Know the purpose and function of each lumen. ■ Label lumens to prevent confusion. ■ Flush catheter daily when not in use with 3 to 5 ml of heparin (10 units/ml) and before and after each use, using SASH protocol.

the patient is sensitive to chlorhexidine, use an alcohol applicator.

■ After the practitioner puts on a sterile mask, a gown, and gloves and drapes the area to create a sterile field, open the packaging of the 3-ml syringe and 25G needle and hand it to him, using sterile technique.

■ Wipe the top of the lidocaine vial with an alcohol pad and invert it. The practitioner will then fill the 3-ml syringe and inject the anesthetic into the site.

■ Open the catheter package and give the catheter to the practitioner, using sterile technique. The practitioner should inspect the catheter for leaks before inserting the catheter.

■ Prepare the I.V. administration set for immediate attachment to the catheter hub. Ask the patient to perform Valsalva's maneuver while the practitioner attaches the I.V. line to the catheter hub. Valsalva's maneuver increases intrathoracic pressure, reducing the possibility of an air embolus.

■ After the practitioner attaches the I.V. line to the catheter hub, set the flow rate at a keep-vein-open rate to maintain venous access. (Alternatively, the catheter may be capped and flushed with heparin.) The practitioner then sutures the catheter in place.

■ After an X-ray confirms correct catheter placement in the midsuperior vena cava, set the flow rate as ordered.

■ Use normal saline solution to remove dried blood that could harbor microorganisms. Secure the catheter with adhesive tape, and apply a sterile 4″ × 4″ gauze pad. You may also use a transparent semipermeable dressing, either alone or placed over the gauze pad. Expect some serosanguineous drainage during the first 24 hours.

■ Place the patient in a comfortable position and reassess his status. Label the dressing with the time and date of catheter insertion and catheter length and gauge (if not imprinted on the catheter).

Flushing a catheter

■ To maintain patency, flush the catheter routinely according to your facility's policy. If the system is being maintained as a heparin lock and the infusions are intermittent, the flushing procedure will vary according to your facility's policy, the medication administration schedule, and the type of catheter used.

- All lumens of a multilumen catheter must be flushed regularly. Most facilities use a heparin flush solution available in premixed 10-ml multidose vials. Recommended concentrations vary from 10 to 100 units of heparin per milliliter. Use normal saline solution instead of heparin to maintain patency in two-way valved devices, such as the Groshong type, because research suggests that heparin isn't always needed to keep the line open.
- The recommended frequency for flushing CV catheters varies from once every 8 hours to once weekly.
- The recommended amount of flushing solution also varies. Some facilities recommend using twice the volume of the cannula and the add-on devices if this volume is known. If the volume is unknown, most facilities recommend 3 to 5 ml of solution to flush the catheter, although some call for as much as 10 ml of solution. Different catheters require different amounts of solution.
- To perform the flushing procedure, start by cleaning the cap with an alcohol pad. Allow the cap to dry. If using the needleless system, follow the manufacturer's guidelines.
- Access the cap and aspirate until blood appears to confirm the CV catheter patency.
- Inject the recommended type and amount of flush solution.
- After flushing the catheter, maintain positive pressure by keeping your thumb on the plunger of the syringe while withdrawing the needle. This prevents blood backflow and clotting in the line. If flushing a valved catheter, close the clamp just before the last of the flush solution leaves the syringe.

Changing an injection cap

- CV catheters used for intermittent infusions have needle-free injection caps (short luer-lock devices similar to the heparin lock adapters used for peripheral I.V. infusion therapy). These caps must be luer-lock types to prevent inadvertent disconnection and air embolism. Unlike heparin lock adapters, however, these caps contain a minimal amount of empty space, so you don't have to preflush the cap before connecting it.
- The frequency of cap changes varies according to your facility's policy and how often the cap is used; however, if the integrity of the product is compromised, it should be changed immediately. Use strict sterile technique when changing the cap.
- Clean the connection site with an alcohol pad or chlorhexidine.
- Instruct the patient to perform Valsalva's maneuver while you quickly disconnect the old cap and connect the new cap using sterile technique. If he can't perform this maneuver, use a padded clamp to prevent air from entering the catheter.

Removing a CV catheter

- If you're removing the CV catheter, first check the patient's record for the most recent placement (confirmed by an X-ray) to trace the catheter's path as it exits the body. Make sure that assistance is available if a complication, such as uncontrolled bleeding, occurs during catheter removal. (Some vessels, such as the subclavian vein, can be difficult to compress.)
- Confirm the patient's identity using two patient identifiers according to your facility's policy. Before you remove the catheter, explain the procedure to the patient.
- Place the patient in a supine position to prevent emboli.
- Wash your hands, and put on clean gloves and a mask.
- Turn off all infusions and prepare a sterile field, using a sterile drape.
- Remove and discard the old dressing, and change to sterile gloves.
- Clean the site with an alcohol pad or a gauze pad soaked in antiseptic cleaning solution. Inspect the site for signs of drainage or inflammation.
- Clip the sutures and, using forceps, remove the catheter in a slow, even motion. Have the patient perform Valsalva's maneuver as the catheter is withdrawn to prevent an air embolism.
- Apply pressure with a sterile gauze pad immediately after removing the catheter.
- Apply chlorhexidine to the insertion site to seal it. Cover the site with a gauze pad, and place a transparent semipermeable

dressing over the gauze. Label the dressing with the date and time of the removal and your initials. The site should be assessed every 24 hours until epithelialization occurs.

DEVICE SAFETY

Inspect the catheter tip and measure the length of the catheter to ensure that the catheter has been completely removed. If you suspect that the catheter hasn't been completely removed, notify the practitioner immediately and monitor the patient closely for signs of distress.

- If you suspect an infection, swab the catheter on a fresh agar plate, or clip the tip of the catheter, place it in a sterile container, and send it to the laboratory for culture.
- Dispose of the I.V. tubing and equipment properly.

Special considerations

- While you're awaiting chest X-ray confirmation of proper catheter placement, infuse an I.V. solution, such as D_5W or normal saline solution, at a keep-vein-open rate until correct placement is assured. Alternatively, use heparin to flush the line. Infusing an isotonic solution avoids the risk of vessel wall thrombosis.

ACTION STAT!

Stay alert for signs of air embolism, such as sudden onset of pallor, cyanosis, dyspnea, coughing, and tachycardia, progressing to syncope and shock. If any of these signs occur, place the patient on his left side in Trendelenburg's position and notify the practitioner.

- After insertion, watch for signs and symptoms of pneumothorax, such as shortness of breath, uneven chest movement, tachycardia, and chest pain. Notify the practitioner immediately if such signs and symptoms appear.
- Change the dressing every 48 hours if a gauze dressing is used or every 7 days if a transparent semipermeable dressing is used, according to your facility's policy, or whenever it becomes moist or soiled. While the CV catheter is in place, change the tubing every 72 hours and the solution every 24 hours or according to your facility's policy. Dressing, tubing, and solution changes for a CV catheter should be performed using sterile technique. (See *Changing a central venous catheter dressing,* page 94.) Assess the site for signs and symptoms of infection, such as discharge, inflammation, and tenderness.
- To prevent an air embolism, close the catheter clamp or have the patient perform Valsalva's maneuver each time the catheter hub is open to air. (A Groshong catheter doesn't require clamping because it has an internal valve.)

Complications

- Pneumothorax, typically occurring on catheter insertion but may not be noticed until after completion of procedure
- Sepsis, typically occurring later during infusion therapy
- Phlebitis (especially in peripheral CV therapy), thrombus formation, and air embolism

Patient teaching

- Care procedures used in the home are the same as those used in the health care facility, except that the home therapy patient uses clean instead of sterile technique. Teach the caregiver proper patient care technique.
- The overall goal of home therapy is patient safety, so your patient teaching must begin well before discharge.
- After discharge, a home therapy coordinator will provide follow-up care until the patient or someone close to him can independently provide catheter care and infusion therapy.
- Many home therapy patients learn to care for the catheter themselves and infuse their own medications and solution.

Documentation

Record the time and date of insertion, length and location of the catheter, solution infused, practitioner's name, and patient's response to the procedure. Docu-

Changing a central venous catheter dressing

Expect to change your patient's central venous (CV) catheter dressing every 3 to 7 days. Many facilities specify dressing changes whenever the dressing becomes soiled, moist, or loose. The illustrations here show the key steps you'll perform.

First, put on clean gloves, and remove the old dressing by pulling it toward the exit site of a long-term catheter or toward the insertion site of a short-term catheter. Remove and discard your gloves.

Next, put on sterile gloves, and clean the skin around the site three times, using a new alcohol pad each time. Start at the center and move outward, using a circular motion (as shown). Allow the skin to dry, and repeat the same cleaning procedure, using three applicators soaked in antiseptic cleaning solution.

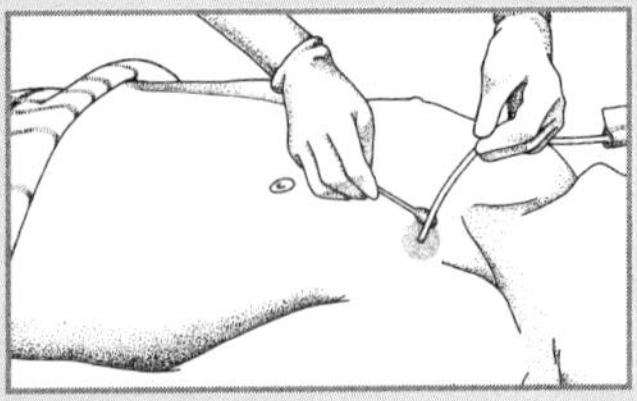

After the solution has dried, cover the site with a dressing, such as a gauze dressing or the transparent semipermeable dressing shown here. Write the time and date on the dressing.

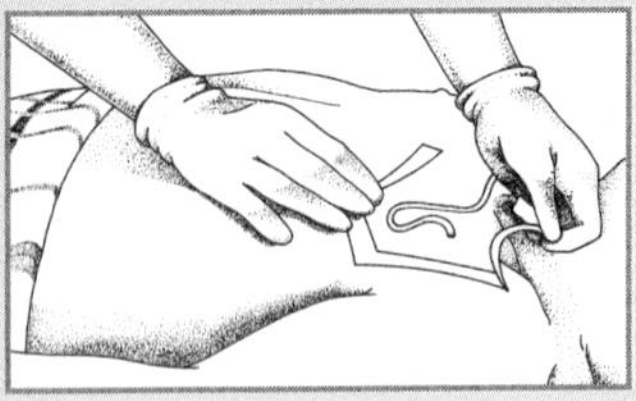

ment the time of the X-ray, its results, and your notification of the practitioner.

Record the time and date of removal and the type of antimicrobial ointment and dressing applied. Note the condition of the catheter insertion site and collection of a culture specimen.

Central venous pressure monitoring

In central venous pressure monitoring, the physician inserts a catheter through a vein and advances it until its tip lies in or near the right atrium. Because no major valves lie at the junction of the vena cava and right atrium, pressure at end diastole reflects back to the catheter. When connected to a manometer, the catheter measures central venous pressure (CVP), an index of right ventricular function.

CVP monitoring helps to assess cardiac function, to evaluate venous return to the heart, and to indirectly gauge how well the heart is pumping. The central venous (CV) line also provides access to a large vessel for rapid, high-volume fluid administration and allows frequent blood withdrawal for laboratory samples.

CVP monitoring can be done intermittently or continuously. The catheter is inserted percutaneously or using a cutdown method. Typically, a single lumen CVP line is used for intermittent pressure readings. To measure the patient's volume status, a disposable plastic water manometer is attached between the I.V. line and the central catheter with a three- or four-way stopcock. CVP is recorded in centimeters of water (cm H_2O) or millimeters of mercury (mm Hg) read from manometer markings.

Normal CVP ranges from 5 to 10 cm H_2O or 2 to 6 mm Hg. Any condition that alters venous return, circulating blood volume, or cardiac performance may affect CVP. If circulating volume increases (such as with enhanced venous return to the heart), CVP rises. If circulating volume decreases (such as with reduced venous return), CVP drops.

Equipment

Intermittent CVP monitoring

Disposable CVP manometer set ♦ leveling device (such as a rod from a reusable CVP pole holder or a carpenter's level or rule) ♦ additional stopcock (to attach the CVP manometer to the catheter) ♦ extension tubing (if needed) ♦ I.V. pole ♦ I.V. solution ♦ I.V. drip chamber and tubing ▪ dressing materials ♦ tape

Continuous CVP monitoring

Pressure monitoring kit with disposable pressure transducer ♦ leveling device ♦ bedside pressure module ♦ continuous I.V. flush solution ♦ pressure bag

Withdrawing blood samples through the CV line

Appropriate number of syringes for the ordered tests ♦ 5- or 10-ml syringe for the discard sample (syringe size depending on tests ordered)

Using an intermittent CV line

Syringe with normal saline solution ♦ syringe with heparin flush solution

Removing a CV catheter

Sterile gloves ♦ suture removal set ♦ sterile gauze pads ♦ antiseptic cleaning solution ♦ dressing ♦ tape

Key steps

- Confirm the patient's identity using two patient identifiers according to your facility's policy.
- Gather the necessary equipment. Explain the procedure to the patient to reduce his anxiety.
- Assist the physician as he inserts the CV catheter. (The procedure is similar to that used for pulmonary artery pressure monitoring, except that the catheter is advanced only as far as the superior vena cava.)

Obtaining continuous CVP readings with a pressure monitoring system

- Make sure the CV line or the proximal lumen of a pulmonary artery catheter is attached to the system. (If the patient has a CV line with multiple lumens, one lumen may be dedicated to continuous CVP monitoring and the other lumens used for fluid administration.)
- Set up a pressure transducer system. Connect pressure tubing from the CVP catheter hub to the transducer. Then connect the flush solution container to a flush device.
- To obtain values, position the patient flat. If he can't tolerate this position, use semi-Fowler's position. Locate the level of the right atrium by identifying the phlebostatic axis. Zero the transducer, leveling the transducer air-fluid interface stopcock with the right atrium. Read the CVP value from the digital display on the monitor, and note the waveform. Make sure the patient is still when the reading is taken to prevent artifact. Be sure to use this position for all subsequent readings.
- Perform and document the dynamic response or square wave test every 8 to 12 hours to verify the optimal waveform. (See *Square wave test,* page 96.)

Removing a CV line

- You may assist the physician in removing a CV line. (In some states, a nurse is permitted to remove the catheter with a physician's order or when acting under facility policy and protocol.)
- If the head of the bed is elevated, minimize the risk of air embolism during catheter removal—for example, by placing the patient in Trendelenburg's position if the line was inserted using a superior approach. If he can't tolerate this, position him flat.
- Turn the patient's head to the side opposite the catheter insertion site. Remove the dressing and exposes the insertion site. If sutures are in place, the physician removes them carefully.
- Turn the I.V. solution off.
- The physician pulls out the catheter out in a slow, smooth motion and then the nurse applies pressure to the insertion site.
- Clean the insertion site, apply an antiseptic cleaning solution, and cover it with a sterile gauze dressing as ordered. Remove gloves and wash your hands.

Square wave test

When using a pressure monitoring system, you must ensure and document the system's accuracy. Along with leveling and zeroing the system to atmospheric pressure at the phlebostatic axis and interpreting waveforms, you can ensure accuracy by performing the square wave test (or dynamic response test). To perform the test:

- Activate the fast-flush device for 1 second, and then release. Obtain a graphic printout.
- Observe for the desired response: the pressure wave rises rapidly, squares off, and is followed by a series of oscillations. (See illustration below.)

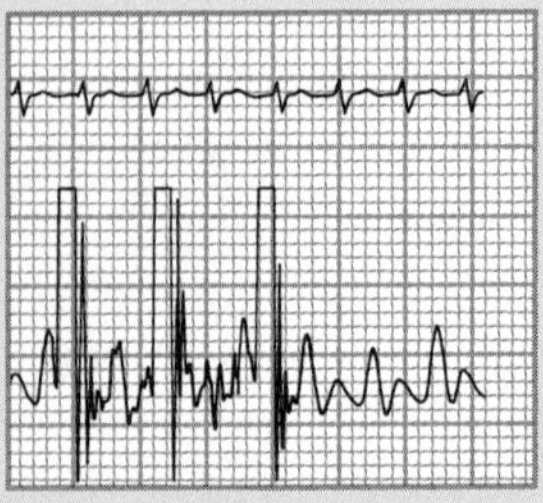

- Know that these oscillations should have an initial downstroke, which extends below the baseline and just 1 to 2 oscillations after the initial downstroke. Usually, but not always, the first upstroke is about one-third the height of the initial downstroke.
- Be aware that the intervals between oscillations should be no more than 0.04 to 0.08 second (1 to 2 small boxes).

Underdamped square wave

If you observe extra oscillations after the initial downstroke or more than 0.08 second between oscillations, the waveform is underdamped. (See illustration top of next column.) This can cause falsely high pressure readings and artifact in the waveforms. It can be corrected by:

- removing excess tubing or extra stopcocks from the system
- inserting a damping device (available from pressure tubing companies)
- dampening the wave by inserting a small air bubble at the transducer stopcock.

Repeat the square wave test, read the pressure waveform, and then remove the small air bubble.

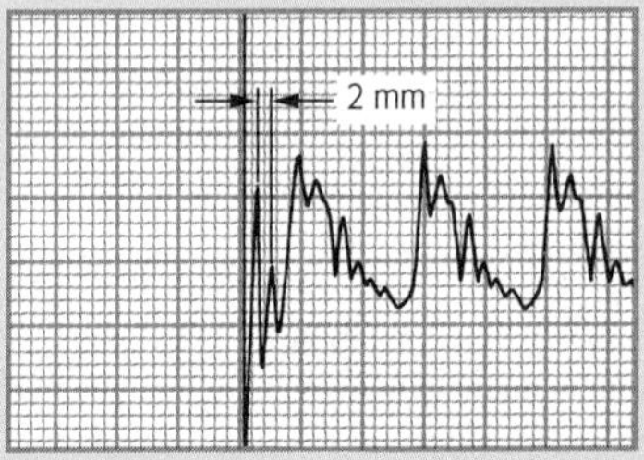

Overdamped square wave

If you observe a slurred upstroke at the beginning of the square wave and a loss of oscillations after the initial downstroke, the waveform is overdamped. (See illustration below.) This can cause falsely low pressure readings, and you can lose the sharpness of waveform peaks and the dicrotic notch. It can be corrected by:

- clearing the line of any blood or air
- checking to make sure there are no kinks or obstructions in the line
- ensuring that you're using short, low-compliance tubing.

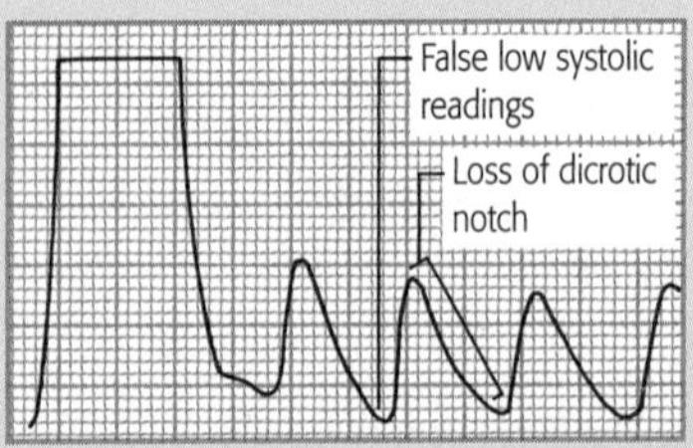

Adapted with permission from Quall, S.J. "Improving the Accuracy of Pulmonary Artery Catheter Measurements," *Journal of Cardiovascular Nursing* 15(2):71-82, January 2001. ©2001 Aspen Publishers.

- Assess the patient for signs of respiratory distress, which may indicate an air embolism.

Special considerations

- As ordered, arrange for daily chest X-rays to check catheter placement.
- Care for the insertion site according to your facility's policy. Typically, you'll change the dressing every 24 to 48 hours.
- Be sure to wash your hands before performing dressing changes and to use aseptic technique and sterile gloves when redressing the site. When removing the old dressing, observe for signs of infection such as redness, and note any patient complaints of tenderness. Apply ointment if directed by your facility's policy, and then cover the site with a sterile gauze dressing or a clear occlusive dressing.
- After the initial CVP reading, reevaluate readings frequently to establish a baseline for the patient. Authorities recommend obtaining readings at 15-, 30-, and 60-minute intervals to establish a baseline. If the patient's CVP fluctuates by more than 2 cm H_2O, suspect a change in his clinical status and report this finding to the practitioner.
- Change the I.V. solution every 24 hours and the I.V. tubing every 48 hours, according to your facility's policy. Expect the physician to change the catheter every 72 hours. Label the I.V. solution, tubing, and dressing with the date, time, and your initials.

Complications

- Pneumothorax (which typically occurs upon catheter insertion), sepsis, thrombus, vessel or adjacent organ puncture, and air embolism

Documentation

Document all dressing, tubing, and solution changes. Document the patient's tolerance of the procedure, the date and time of catheter removal, and the type of dressing applied. Note the condition of the catheter insertion site and whether a culture specimen was collected. Note any complications and actions taken.

Cerebral blood flow monitoring

Traditionally, caregivers have estimated cerebral blood flow (CBF) in neurologically compromised patients by calculating cerebral perfusion pressure. However, modern technology permits continuous regional blood flow monitoring at the bedside.

A sensor placed on the cerebral cortex calculates CBF in the capillary bed by thermal diffusion. Thermistors within the sensor detect the temperature differential between two metallic plates—one heated, one neutral. This differential is inversely proportional to CBF: As the differential decreases, CBF increases—and vice versa. This monitoring technique yields important information about the effects of interventions on CBF. It also yields continuous real-time values for CBF, which are essential in conditions in which compromised blood flow may put the patient at risk, such as ischemia and infarction.

CBF monitoring is indicated whenever CBF alterations are anticipated. It's used most commonly in patients with subarachnoid hemorrhage (in which a vasospasm may restrict blood flow), trauma associated with high intracranial pressure, or vascular tumors.

Equipment

CBF monitoring requires a special sensor that attaches to a computer data system or to a small analog monitor that operates on a battery for patient transport.

Caring for the site

Sterile 4″ × 4″ gauze pads ♦ clean gloves ♦ sterile gloves ♦ antiseptic cleaning solution

Removing the sensor

Sterile suture removal tray ♦ 1″ adhesive tape ♦ sterile 4″ × 4″ gauze pads ♦ clean gloves ♦ sterile gloves ♦ suture material

Preparation

- Make sure the patient or a family member is fully informed about the procedures involved in CBF monitoring, and obtain a signed consent form.

- If the patient will need CBF monitoring after surgery, advise him that a sensor will be in place for about 3 days.
- Tell the patient that the insertion site will be covered with a dry, sterile dressing. Mention that the sensor may be removed at the bedside.

Setting up the sensor monitor

- Depending on the type of system you're using, you may need to verify that a battery has been inserted in the monitor to allow CBF monitoring during patient transport to the intensive care unit.
- First, assemble the following equipment at the bedside: a monitor and a sensor cable with an attached sensor. Attach the distal end of the sensor cable (from the patient's head) to the SENSOR CONNECT port on the monitor. When the sensor cable is securely in place, press the ON key to activate the monitor.
- Next, calibrate the system by pressing the CAL key. You should see the red light appear on the CAL button. Ideally, you'll begin by calibrating the sensor to 00.0 by pressing the directional arrows. Readouts of plus or minus 0.1 are also acceptable.

Key steps

- The surgeon typically inserts the sensor in the operating room during or following a craniotomy. (Occasionally, he may insert it through a burr hole.) He implants the sensor far from major blood vessels and verifies that the metallic plates have good contact with the brain surface. (See *Inserting a CBF sensor*.)
- Press the RUN key to display the CBF reading. Observe the monitor's digital display, and document the baseline value.
- Record the CBF hourly. Be sure to watch for trends and correlate values with the patient's clinical status. Be aware that stimulation or activity may cause a 10% increase or decrease in CBF. If you detect a 20% increase or decrease, suspect poor contact between the sensor and the cerebral cortex.

Caring for the insertion site

- Wash your hands. Put on clean gloves, and remove the dressing from the sensor insertion site.
- Observe the site for cerebrospinal fluid (CSF) leakage, a potential complication. Then remove and discard your gloves.
- Next, put on sterile gloves. Using sterile technique, clean the insertion site with a gauze pad soaked in antiseptic cleaning solution. Clean the site, starting at the center and working outward in a circular pattern.
- Using a new gauze pad soaked with antiseptic cleaning solution, clean the exposed part of the sensor from the insertion site to the end of the sensor.
- Next, place sterile 4″ × 4″ gauze pads over the insertion site to completely cover it. Tape all edges securely to create an occlusive dressing.

Removing the sensor

- Usually, the CBF sensor remains in place for about 3 days when used for postoperative monitoring.
- Explain the procedure to the patient; then wash your hands. Put on clean gloves, remove the dressing, and dispose of the gloves and dressing properly.
- Open the suture removal tray and the package of suture material. The surgeon removes the anchoring sutures and then gently removes the sensor from the insertion site.
- After the surgeon closes the wound with stitches, put on sterile gloves, apply a folded gauze pad to the site, and tape it in place. Observe the condition of the site, including any leakage.

Special considerations

- CBF fluctuates with the brain's metabolic demands, ranging from 60 to 90 ml/100 g/minute normally. However, the patient's neurologic condition dictates the acceptable range. For example, in a patient in a coma, CBF may be one-half the normal value; in a patient in a barbiturate-induced coma with burst suppression on the EEG, CBF may be as low as 10 ml/100 g/minute. Vasospasm secondary to subarachnoid hemorrhage may result in CBF below 40 ml/100 g/minute. In an awake patient,

Inserting a CBF sensor

Typically, the surgeon inserts a cerebral blood flow (CBF) sensor during a craniotomy. He tunnels the sensor toward the craniotomy site and then carefully inserts the metallic plates of the thermistor to make sure they continuously contact the surface of the cerebral cortex. After closing the dura and replacing the bone flap, he closes the scalp.

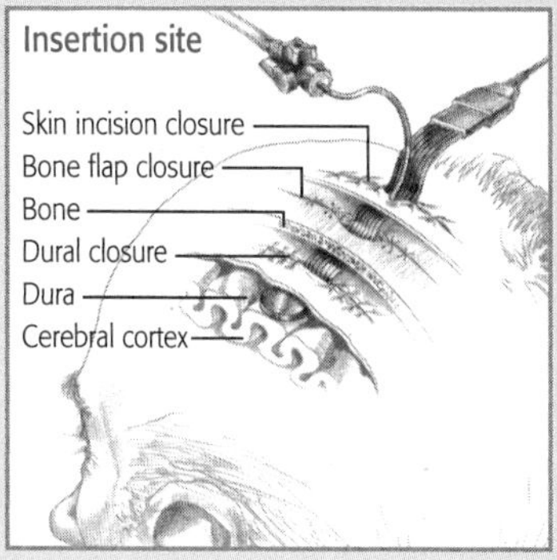

The sensor measures CBF by means of thermistors housed inside it. The thermistors consist of two metallic plates—one heated and one neutral. The sensor detects the temperature difference between the two plates. This difference is inversely proportional to CBF. As CBF increases, the temperature difference decreases—and vice versa.

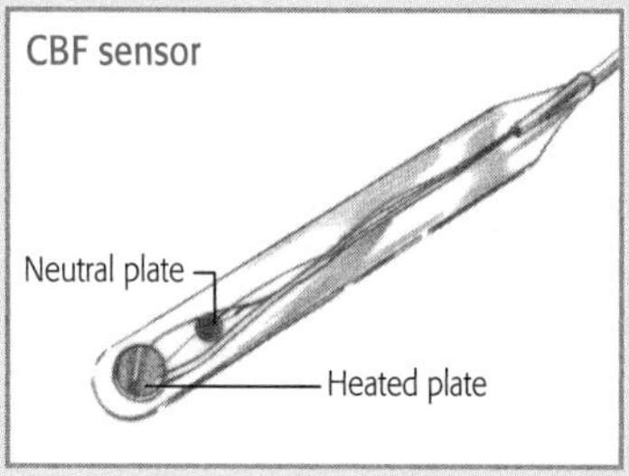

CBF above 90 ml/100 g/minute may indicate hyperemia.

- If you suspect poor contact between the sensor and the cerebral cortex, turn the patient toward the side of the sensor or gently wiggle the catheter back and forth (using a sterile-gloved hand). To determine whether these maneuvers have improved contact between the sensor and the cortex, observe the CBF value on the monitor as you perform them.
- If your patient has low CBF but no neurologic symptoms that indicate ischemia, suspect a fluid layer (a small hematoma) between the sensor and the cortex.
- As with intracranial pressure monitoring, CBF monitoring may lead to infection. Administer prophylactic antibiotics as ordered, and maintain a sterile dressing around the insertion site. CSF leakage, another potential complication, may occur at the sensor insertion site. To prevent leakage, the surgeon usually places an additional suture at the site.
- To reduce the risk of infection, change the dressing at the insertion site daily using sterile technique.

Complications

- CSF leakage at the sensor insertion site

Documentation

Document cleaning of the site, appearance of the site, and dressing changes. After sensor removal, document any leakage from the site.

Cerebrospinal fluid drains

Cerebrospinal fluid (CSF) drainage aims to reduce CSF pressure to the desired level and then to maintain it at that level. Fluid is withdrawn from the lateral ventricle

Methods of CSF drainage

Cerebrospinal fluid (CSF) drainage aims to control intracranial pressure (ICP) during treatment for traumatic injury or other conditions that cause a rise in ICP. Two procedures are commonly used, as detailed below.

Ventricular drain

For a ventricular drain, the physician makes a burr hole in the patient's skull and inserts the catheter into the ventricle. The distal end of the catheter is connected to a closed drainage system.

Lumbar drain

For a lumbar drain, the physician inserts a catheter beneath the dura into the L3-L4 interspace. The distal end of the catheter is connected to a sterile, closed drainage system affixed securely to the bed or to an I.V. pole. The drip chamber should be set at the level ordered by the physician.

Closed drainage system

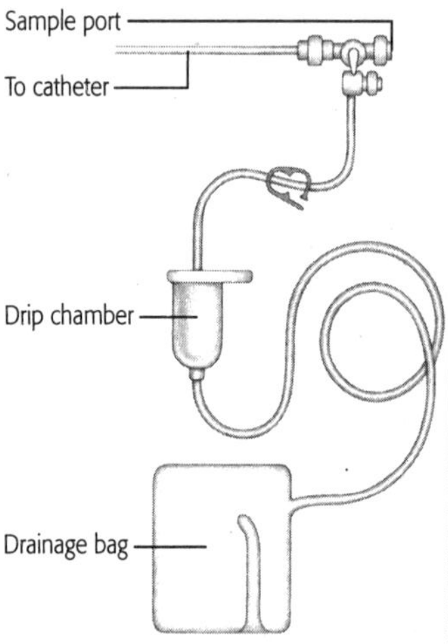

(ventriculostomy). Ventricular drainage is used to reduce increased intracranial pressure (ICP). External CSF drainage is used most commonly to manage increased ICP and to facilitate spinal or cerebral dural healing after traumatic injury or surgery. In either case, CSF is drained by a catheter or a ventriculostomy tube in a sterile, closed drainage collection system.

Other therapeutic uses include ICP monitoring via the ventriculostomy, direct instillation of medications, contrast media, or air for diagnostic radiology, and aspiration of CSF for laboratory analysis.

To place the ventricular drain, the physician inserts a ventricular catheter through a burr hole in the patient's skull. Usually, this is done in the operating room, with the patient receiving a general anesthetic. (See *Methods of CSF drainage*.)

Equipment

Overbed table ♦ sterile gloves ♦ sterile cotton-tipped applicators ♦ antiseptic cleaning solution ♦ alcohol pads ♦ sterile fenestrated drape ♦ 3-ml syringe for local anesthetic ♦ 25G ¾″ needle for injecting anesthetic ♦ local anesthetic (usually 1% lidocaine [Xylocaine]) ♦ 18G or 20G sterile spinal needle or Touhy needle ♦ #5 French whistle-tip catheter or ventriculostomy tube ♦ external drainage set (includes drainage tubing and sterile collection bag) ♦ suture material ♦ 4″ × 4″ dressings ♦ paper tape ♦ lamp or another light source ♦ I.V. pole ♦ ventriculostomy tray and twist drill ♦ sterile marker ♦ sterile labels ♦ optional: pain medication (such as an analgesic) and anti-infective agent (such as an antibiotic)

Preparation

- Open all equipment using sterile technique.
- Check all packaging for breaks in seals and for expiration dates.
- After the physician places the catheter, connect it to the external drainage system tubing. Secure connection points with tape or a connector.

- Place the collection system, including drip chamber and collection bag, on an I.V. pole.

Key steps

- Explain the procedure to the patient and his family. Consent should be obtained by the physician from the patient or a responsible family member and should be documented according to your facility's policy.
- Perform a baseline neurologic assessment, including vital signs, to help detect alterations or signs of deterioration.
- Wash your hands thoroughly.

Inserting a ventricular drain

- Place the patient in a supine position.
- Place the equipment tray on the overbed table, and unwrap the tray. Label all medications, medication containers, and other solutions on and off the sterile field.
- Adjust the height of the bed so that the physician can perform the procedure comfortably.
- Illuminate the area of the catheter insertion site.
- The physician will clean the insertion site and administer a local anesthetic. He'll put on sterile gloves and drape the insertion site.
- To insert the drain, the physician will request a ventriculostomy tray with a twist drill. After completing the ventriculostomy, he'll connect the drainage system and suture the ventriculostomy in place. He'll then cover the insertion site with a sterile dressing.

Monitoring CSF drainage

- Maintain a continuous hourly output of CSF. Ensure that the flow chamber of the ICP monitoring setup remains positioned as ordered.
- To drain CSF as ordered, put on sterile gloves, and then turn the main stopcock on to drainage. This allows CSF to collect in the graduated flow chamber. Document the time and the amount of CSF obtained. Turn the stopcock off to drainage. To drain the CSF from this chamber into the drainage bag, release the clamp below the flow chamber. Never empty the drainage bag. Instead, replace it when full using sterile technique.
- Check the dressing frequently for drainage, which could indicate CSF leakage.
- Check the tubing for patency by watching the CSF drops in the drip chamber.
- Observe CSF for color, clarity, amount, blood, and sediment. CSF specimens for laboratory analysis should be obtained from the collection port attached to the tubing, not from the collection bag.
- Change the collection bag when it's full or every 24 hours, according to your facility's policy.

Special considerations

- Maintenance of a continual hourly output of CSF is essential to prevent overdrainage or underdrainage. Underdrainage or lack of CSF may reflect kinked tubing, catheter displacement, or a drip chamber placed higher than the catheter insertion site. Overdrainage can occur if the drip chamber is placed too far below the catheter insertion site.
- Raising or lowering the head of the bed can affect the CSF flow rate. When changing the patient's position, reset the system to zero.
- If the patient is ambulatory or is allowed out of bed, advise him that he must call for assistance before getting out of bed. The drain must be closed before getting the patient out of bed.
- The patient may experience chronic headache during continuous CSF drainage. Reassure him that this isn't unusual; administer analgesics as appropriate.

DEVICE SAFETY

For ventricular drains, make sure ICP waveforms are being monitored at all times.

Complications

- Headache, tachycardia, diaphoresis, and nausea resulting from excessive CSF drainage
- Collapsed ventricles, tonsillar herniation, and medullary compression resulting from acute overdrainage

ACTION STAT!

If drainage accumulates too rapidly, clamp the system and immediately notify the practitioner because this constitutes a potential neurosurgical emergency.

- Clot formation due to cessation of drainage (If you can't quickly identify the cause of the obstruction, notify the practitioner. If drainage is blocked, the patient may develop signs of increased ICP.)
- Meningitis caused by infection (To prevent this, administer antibiotics as ordered.)

Documentation

Record the time and date of the insertion procedure and the patient's response. Record routine vital signs and neurologic assessment findings at least every 4 hours.

Document the color, clarity, and amount of CSF at least every 8 hours. Record hourly and 24-hour CSF output, and describe the condition of the dressing.

Chemotherapeutic drug administration

Administration of chemotherapeutic drugs requires specific skills in addition to those used when giving other drugs. For example, some drugs require special equipment or must be given through an unusual route. Others become unstable after a while, and still others must be protected from light. Finally, the drug dosage must be exact to avoid possible fatal complication. For these reasons, only specially trained nurses and practitioners should give chemotherapeutic drugs.

Chemotherapeutic drugs may be administered through various routes. Although the I.V. route (using peripheral or central veins) is used most commonly, these drugs may also be given orally, subcutaneously, I.M., intra-arterially, into a body cavity, through a central venous (CV) catheter, through an Ommaya reservoir into the spinal canal, or through a device implanted in a vein or subcutaneously such as through a patient-controlled analgesia device. They may also be administered into an artery, the peritoneal cavity, or the pleural space. (See *Intraperitoneal chemotherapy: An alternative approach.*)

Before administering chemotherapy, laboratory data (electrolyte levels and white blood cell count) should be reviewed, the patient should be assessed for the appropriateness of the prescribed therapy, and the drug order should be validated by two clinicians with special attention to medication concentration and the infusion rate.

The administration route depends on the drug's pharmacodynamics and the tumor's characteristics. For example, if a malignant tumor is confined to one area, the drug may be administered through a localized, or regional, method. Regional administration allows delivery of a high drug dose directly to the tumor. This is particularly advantageous because many solid tumors don't respond to drug levels that are safe for systemic administration.

If the drug to be administered is a vesicant, there are several factors for the nurse to remember: a low-pressure infusion device should be the instrument of choice; a positive blood return should be confirmed before administration; a new access site should be started before peripheral administration; and a peripheral access device shouldn't be used for a continuous infusion.

Chemotherapy may be administered to a patient whose cancer is believed to have been eradicated through surgery or radiation therapy. This treatment, called adjuvant chemotherapy, helps to ensure that no undetectable metastasis exists. A patient may also receive chemotherapy, or neoadjuvant or synchronous chemotherapy, before surgery or radiation therapy. Induction chemotherapy helps improve survival rates by shrinking a tumor before surgical excision or radiation therapy.

In general, chemotherapeutic drugs prove more effective when given in higher doses, although their adverse effects commonly limit the dosage. An exception to this rule is methotrexate (Trexall), which is particularly effective against rapidly growing tumors but toxic to normal tissues that

Intraperitoneal chemotherapy: An alternative approach

Administering chemotherapeutic drugs into the peritoneal cavity has several benefits for the patient with malignant ascites or ovarian cancer that has spread to the peritoneum. This technique passes drugs directly to the tumor area in the peritoneal cavity, exposing malignant cells to high concentrations of chemotherapy—up to 1,000 times the amount that could be safely given systemically. Furthermore, the semipermeable peritoneal membrane permits prolonged exposure of malignant cells to the drug.

Typically, intraperitoneal chemotherapy is performed using a peritoneal dialysis kit, but drugs can also be administered directly to the peritoneal cavity by way of a Tenckhoff catheter (as shown in the illustration below). This method can be performed on an outpatient basis, if necessary, and uses equipment that's readily available on most units with oncology patients.

In this technique, the chemotherapy bag is connected directly to the Tenckhoff catheter with a length of I.V. tubing, the solution is infused, and the catheter and I.V. tubing are clamped. Then the patient is asked to change positions every 10 to 15 minutes for 1 hour. After the prescribed dwell time, the chemotherapeutic drugs are drained into an I.V. bag. The patient is encouraged to change positions. Then the I.V. tubing and catheter are clamped, the I.V. tubing is removed, and a new intermittent infusion cap is fitted to the catheter. Finally, the catheter is flushed with a syringe of heparin flush solution.

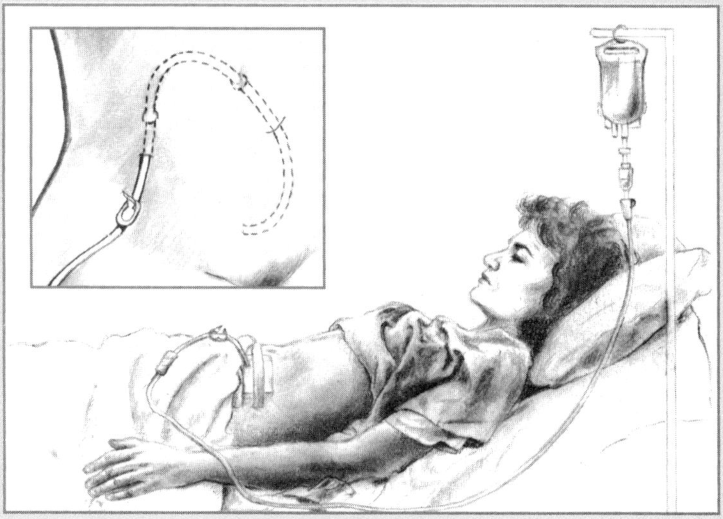

grow and divide rapidly. Folinic acid halts the effects of methotrexate; therefore, it's administered after the methotrexate has destroyed the cancer cells but before it damages vital organs.

Equipment

Prescribed drug ♦ aluminum foil or a brown paper bag (if the drug is photosensitive) ♦ normal saline solution ♦ syringes and needleless adapters ♦ infusion pump ♦ gloves ♦ impervious containers labeled CAUTION: BIOHAZARD

Preparation

- Verify the drug, dosage, and administration route by checking the medication record against the practitioner's order.

Risks of tissue damage

To administer chemotherapy safely, you need to know each drug's potential for damaging tissue. In this regard, chemotherapeutic drugs are classified as vesicants, nonvesicants, or irritants.

Vesicants

Vesicants cause a reaction so severe that blisters form and tissue is damaged or destroyed. Chemotherapeutic vesicants include:

- dactinomycin (Cosmegen)
- daunorubicin (Cerubidine)
- doxorubicin (Adriamycin)
- idarubicin (Indamycin)
- mechlorethamine (Mustargen)
- mitomycin (Mutamycin)
- mitoxantrone (Novantrone)
- vinblastine (Velban)
- vincristine (Oncovin)
- vinorelbine (Navelbine).

Nonvesicants

Nonvesicants don't cause irritation or damage. Chemotherapeutic nonvesicants include:

- asparaginase (Elspar)
- bleomycin (Blenoxane)
- cyclophosphamide (Cytoxan)
- cytarabine (Cytosar-u)
- floxuridine (FUDR)
- fluorouracil (Efudex).

Irritants

Irritants can cause a local venous response, with or without a skin reaction. Chemotherapeutic irritants include:

- carboplatin (Paraplatin)
- carmustine (BiCNU)
- dacarbazine (DTIC-Dome)
- etoposide (VePesid)
- ifosfamide (Ifex)
- irinotecan (Camptosar)
- streptozocin (Zanosar)
- topotecan (Hycamtin).

- Make sure that you know the immediate and delayed adverse effects of the ordered drug.
- Follow administration guidelines for appropriate procedures.

Key steps

- Confirm the patient's identity using two patient identifiers according to your facility's policy.
- Assess the patient's physical condition and review his medical history.
- Make sure that you understand what needs to be given and by what route, and provide the necessary teaching and support to the patient and his family.
- Determine the best site to administer the drug. When selecting the site, consider drug compatibility, frequency of administration, and the vesicant potential of the drug. (See *Risks of tissue damage*.) For example, if the practitioner has ordered the intermittent administration of a vesicant drug, you can give it by either instilling the drug into the side port of an infusing I.V. line or by direct I.V. push. If the vesicant drug is to be infused continuously, you should administer it only through a CV line or vascular access device. On the other hand, nonvesicant agents (including irritants) may be given by direct I.V. push, through the side port of an infusing I.V. line, or as a continuous infusion.
- Check your facility's policy before administering a vesicant. Because vein integrity decreases with time, some facilities require that vesicants be administered before other drugs. Conversely, because vesicants increase vein fragility, other facilities require that vesicants be given after other drugs.
- Evaluate your patient's condition, paying particular attention to the results of recent laboratory studies, specifically the complete blood count, blood urea nitrogen level, platelet count, urine creatinine level, and liver function studies.

- Determine whether the patient has received chemotherapy before, and note the severity of any adverse effects.
- Check his drug history for medications that might interact with chemotherapy. As a rule, you shouldn't mix chemotherapeutic drugs with other medications. If you have questions or concerns about giving the chemotherapeutic drug, talk with the practitioner or pharmacist before you give the drug.
- Next, double-check the patient's chart for the complete chemotherapy protocol order, including the patient's name, drug's name and dosage, and the route, rate, and frequency of administration. See if the drug's dosage depends on certain laboratory values. Be aware that some facilities require two nurses to read the dosage order and to check the drug and the amount being administered.
- Check to see whether the practitioner has ordered an antiemetic, fluids, a diuretic, or electrolyte supplements to be given before, during, or after chemotherapy administration.
- Evaluate the patient's and his family's understanding of chemotherapy, and make sure that the patient or a responsible family member has signed the consent form.
- Next, put on gloves. Keep them on through all stages of handling the drug, including preparation, priming the I.V. tubing, and administration.
- Before administering the drug, perform a new venipuncture proximal to the old site. Avoid giving chemotherapeutic drugs through an existing I.V. line. To identify an administration site, examine the patient's veins, starting with his hand and proceeding to his forearm.
- After an appropriate line is in place, infuse 10 to 20 ml of normal saline solution to test vein patency. Never test vein patency with a chemotherapeutic drug. Next, administer the drug as appropriate: nonvesicants by I.V. push or admixed in a bag of I.V. fluid; vesicants by I.V. push through a piggyback set connected to a rapidly infusing I.V. line.
- During I.V. administration, closely monitor the patient for signs of a hypersensitivity reaction or extravasation. Check for adequate blood return after 5 ml of the drug has been infused or according to your facility's guidelines.
- After infusion of the medication, infuse 20 ml of normal saline solution. Do this between administrations of different chemotherapeutic drugs and before discontinuing the I.V. line.

DEVICE SAFETY

Dispose of used needles and syringes carefully. To prevent aerosol dispersion of chemotherapeutic drugs, don't clip needles. Place them intact in an impervious container for incineration. Dispose of I.V. bags, bottles, gloves, and tubing in a properly labeled and covered trash container.

- Wash your hands thoroughly with soap and warm water after giving a chemotherapeutic drug, even though you've worn gloves.

Special considerations

- Observe the I.V. site frequently for signs of extravasation and allergic reaction (swelling, redness, urticaria). If you suspect extravasation, stop the infusion immediately. Leave the I.V. catheter in place and notify the practitioner. A conservative method for treating extravasation involves aspirating any residual drug from the tubing and I.V. catheter, instilling an I.V. antidote, and then removing the I.V. catheter. Afterward, you may apply heat or cold to the site and elevate the affected limb. (See *Managing extravasation,* page 106.)
- During infusion, some drugs need protection from direct sunlight to avoid possible drug breakdown. If this is the case, cover the vial with a brown paper bag or aluminum foil.
- When giving vesicants, avoid sites where damage to underlying tendons or nerves may occur (for example, veins in the antecubital fossa, near the wrist, or in the dorsal surface of the hand).
- If you can't stay with the patient during the entire infusion, use an infusion pump to ensure drug delivery within the prescribed time and rate.

ACTION STAT!

Managing extravasation

Extravasation—the infiltration of a vesicant drug into the surrounding tissue—can result from a punctured vein or leakage around a venipuncture site. If vesicant drugs or fluids extravasate, severe local tissue damage may result. This may cause prolonged healing, infection, cosmetic disfigurement, and loss of function and may necessitate multiple debridements and, possibly, amputation.

Extravasation of vesicant drugs requires emergency treatment. Follow your facility's protocol. Essential steps include:

- Stop the I.V. flow, aspirate the remaining drug in the catheter, and remove the I.V. line, unless you need the needle to infiltrate the antidote.
- Estimate the amount of extravasated solution and notify the practitioner.
- Instill the appropriate antidote according to your facility's protocol.
- Elevate the extremity.
- Record the extravasation site, patient's symptoms, estimated amount of infiltrated solution, and treatment. Include the time you notified the practitioner and the practitioner's name. Continue documenting the appearance of the site and associated symptoms.
- Depending on your facility's protocol, apply either ice packs or warm compresses to the affected area. Ice is applied to all extravasated areas for 15 to 20 minutes every 4 to 6 hours for about 3 days. For etoposide and vinca alkaloids, heat is applied.
- If skin breakdown occurs, apply dressings as ordered.
- If severe tissue damage occurs, plastic surgery and physical therapy may be needed.

- Observe the patient at regular intervals and after treatment for adverse reactions. Monitor his vital signs throughout the infusion to assess any changes during chemotherapy administration.
- Maintain a list of the types and amounts of drugs the patient has received. This is especially important if he has received drugs that have a cumulative effect and that can be toxic to such organs as the heart or kidneys.

Complications

- Nausea and vomiting ranging from mild to debilitating
- Bone marrow suppression leading to neutropenia and thrombocytopenia
- Intestinal irritation, stomatitis, pulmonary fibrosis, cardiotoxicity, nephrotoxicity, neurotoxicity, hearing loss, anemia, alopecia, urticaria, radiation recall (if drugs are given with, or soon after, radiation therapy), anorexia, esophagitis, diarrhea, and constipation
- Extravasation, causing inflammation, ulceration, necrosis, and loss of vein patency due to I.V. administration

Patient teaching

- Teach the patient about possible adverse reactions to chemotherapy.
- Let the patient know that drugs can be given to treat some of the adverse reactions.
- Explain to the patient the type and sequence of drugs he'll receive.

Documentation

Record the location and description of the I.V. site before treatment, or the presence of blood return during bolus administration. Also record the drugs and dosages administered, sequence of drug administration, needle type and size used, amount and type of flushing solution, and the site's condition after treatment. Document adverse reactions, the patient's tolerance of the treatment, and the topics discussed with the patient and his family.

Chemotherapeutic drug preparation

Preparation of chemotherapeutic drugs requires extra care for the safety of the patient and the health care provider. The patient receiving chemotherapy and the people who prepare and handle the drugs are at risk for teratogenic, mutagenic, and carcinogenic effects of the drugs.

Occupational Safety and Health Administration (OSHA) guidelines for handling chemotherapeutic drugs have two basic requirements; first, all health care workers who handle chemotherapeutic drugs must be educated and trained. A key element of such training involves learning how to reduce your exposure when handling the drugs. The second requirement states that the drugs should be prepared in a class II biological safety cabinet. If a biological safety cabinet isn't available, OSHA recommends that a respirator be worn while mixing the drugs.

OSHA guidelines recommend that chemotherapeutic drugs be mixed in a properly enclosed and ventilated work area and that respiratory and skin protection be worn. Smoking, drinking, applying cosmetics, and eating where these drugs are prepared, stored, or used should be strictly prohibited, and sterile technique should be used while mixing the drugs.

Gloves, gowns, syringes or vials, and other materials that have been used in chemotherapy preparation and administration present a possible source of exposure or injury to the facility's staff, patients, and visitors. Therefore, use of properly labeled, sealed, and covered containers, handled only by trained and protected personnel, should be routine practice. Spills also represent a hazard, and all employees should be familiar with appropriate spill procedures for their own protection.

Equipment

Prescribed drug or drugs ♦ patient's medication record and chart ♦ long-sleeved gown ♦ latex surgical gloves ♦ face shield or goggles ♦ eyewash ♦ plastic absorbent pad ♦ alcohol pads ♦ sterile gauze pads ♦ shoe covers ♦ impervious container with the label CAUTION: BIOHAZARD for the disposal of unused drugs or equipment ♦ I.V. solution ♦ diluent (if necessary) ♦ compatibility reference source ♦ medication labels ♦ class II biological safety cabinet ♦ disposable towel ♦ hydrophobic filter or dispensing pin ♦ 18G needle ♦ syringes and needles of various sizes ♦ I.V. tubing with luer-lock fittings ♦ I.V. pump (if available)

Chemotherapeutic spill kit: water-resistant, nonpermeable, long-sleeved gown with cuffs and back closure ♦ shoe covers ♦ two pairs of gloves (for double gloving) ♦ goggles ♦ mask ♦ disposable dustpan ♦ plastic scraper (for collecting broken glass) ♦ plastic-backed or absorbent towels ♦ container of desiccant powder or granules (to absorb wet contents) ♦ two disposable sponges ♦ punctureproof, leakproof container labeled biohazard waste ♦ container of 70% alcohol for cleaning the spill area

Key steps

- Remember to wash your hands before and after drug preparation and administration.
- Prepare the drugs in a class II biological safety cabinet.
- Wear protective garments (such as a long-sleeved gown, gloves, a face shield or goggles, and shoe covers), as indicated by your facility's policy. Don't wear the garments outside the preparation area.

DO'S & DON'TS

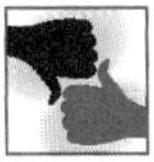

Don't eat, drink, smoke, or apply cosmetics in the drug preparation area.

- Before you prepare the drug (and after you finish), clean the internal surfaces of the cabinet with 70% alcohol and a disposable towel. Discard the towel in a leakproof chemical waste container.
- Cover the work surface with a clean plastic absorbent pad to minimize contamination by droplets or spills. Change the pad at the end of the shift or whenever a spill occurs.

■ Consider all of the equipment used in drug preparation as well as any unused drug as hazardous waste. Dispose of them according to your facility's policy.
■ Place all chemotherapeutic waste products in labeled, leakproof, sealable plastic bags or other appropriate impervious containers.

Special considerations

■ Prepare the drugs according to current product instructions, paying attention to compatibility, stability, and reconstitution technique. Label the prepared drug with the patient's name, dosage, strength, and date and time of preparation.
■ Take precautions to reduce your exposure to chemotherapeutic drugs. Systemic absorption can occur through ingestion of contaminated materials, contact with the skin, or inhalation. You can inhale a drug without realizing it, such as while opening a vial, clipping a needle, expelling air from a syringe, or discarding excess drug. You can also absorb a drug from handling contaminated stools or body fluids.
■ For maximum protection, mix all chemotherapeutic drugs in an approved class II biological safety cabinet. Also, prime all I.V. bags that contain chemotherapeutic drugs under the hood. Leave the hood blower on 24 hours per day, 7 days per week.
■ If a hood isn't available, prepare drugs in a well-ventilated work space, away from heating or cooling vents and other personnel. Vent vials with a hydrophobic filter, or use negative-pressure techniques. Also, use a needle with a hydrophobic filter to remove the solution from a vial. To break an ampule, wrap a sterile gauze pad or alcohol pad around the neck of the ampule to decrease the risk of contamination.
■ Make sure that the biological safety cabinet is examined every 6 months, or any time the cabinet is moved by a company specifically qualified to perform this work. If the cabinet passes certification, the certifying company will affix a sticker to the cabinet attesting to its approval.
■ Use only syringes and I.V. sets that have luer-lock fittings. Label all chemotherapeutic drugs with a chemotherapy hazard label.

DO'S & DON'TS

Don't clip needles, break syringes, or remove the needles from the syringes. Use a gauze pad when removing chemotherapy syringes and needles from I.V. bags of chemotherapeutic drugs.

■ Place used syringes or needles in a puncture-proof container, along with other sharp or breakable items.
■ When mixing chemotherapeutic drugs, wear latex surgical gloves and a gown of low-permeability fabric with a closed front and cuffed long sleeves. When working steadily with chemotherapeutic drugs, change gloves every 30 minutes. If you spill a drug solution or puncture or tear a glove, remove your gloves immediately. Wash your hands before putting on new gloves and any time you remove your gloves.
■ If some of the drug comes in contact with your skin, wash the involved area thoroughly with soap (not a germicidal agent) and water. If eye contact occurs, flood the eye with water or an isotonic eyewash for at least 5 minutes while holding the eyelid open. Obtain a medical evaluation as soon as possible after accidental exposure.
■ If a major spill occurs, use a chemotherapeutic spill kit to clean the area.
■ Discard disposable gowns and gloves in an appropriately marked, waterproof receptacle when contaminated or when you leave the work area.

DO'S & DON'TS

Don't place food or beverages in the same refrigerator as chemotherapeutic drugs.

■ Become familiar with drug excretion patterns, and take appropriate precautions when handling a chemotherapy patient's body fluids.
■ Provide male patients with a urinal with a tightfitting lid. Wear disposable latex surgical gloves when handling body fluids.

Before flushing the toilet, place a waterproof pad over the toilet bowl to avoid splashing. Wear gloves and a gown when handling linens soiled with body fluids. Place soiled linens in isolation linen bags designated for separate laundering.

- Women who are pregnant, trying to conceive, or breast-feeding should exercise caution when handling chemotherapeutic drugs.

Complications

- Drugs' mutagenic effects causing liver or chromosome damage due to chronic exposure
- Burns and damage to the skin from direct exposure

Patient teaching

- If the patient will be receiving chemotherapy at home, teach him how to handle the drugs and discuss appropriate safety measures such as disposing of contaminated equipment. Tell the patient and his family to wear gloves whenever handling chemotherapy equipment or contaminated linens or gowns and pajamas. Instruct them to place soiled linens in a separate washable pillowcase and to launder the pillowcase twice, with the soiled linens inside, separately from other linens.
- Instruct the patient to empty waste products into the toilet close to the water to minimize splashing. Close the lid and flush three times.
- All materials used for the treatment should be placed in a leak-proof container and taken to a designated disposal area. The patient or his family should make arrangements with either a hospital or a private company for pickup and proper disposal of contaminated waste.

Documentation

Document each incident of exposure according to your facility's policy.

Chest physiotherapy

Chest physiotherapy includes postural drainage, chest percussion and vibration, and coughing and deep-breathing exercises. Together, these techniques mobilize and eliminate secretions, reexpand lung tissue, and promote efficient use of respiratory muscles. Of critical importance to the bedridden patient, chest physiotherapy helps prevent or treat atelectasis and may also help prevent pneumonia—two respiratory complications that can seriously impede recovery.

Postural drainage, or sequential repositioning of the patient, encourages peripheral pulmonary secretions to empty by gravity into the major bronchi or trachea when performed in conjunction with percussion and vibration. Secretions usually drain best with the patient positioned so that the bronchi are perpendicular to the floor. Lower and middle lobe bronchi usually empty best with the patient in the head-down position; upper lobe bronchi, in the head-up position. (See *Postural drainage positions,* pages 110 and 111.)

Percussing the chest with cupped hands mechanically dislodges thick, tenacious secretions from the bronchial walls. Vibration can be used with percussion, or as an alternative to it, in the patient who's frail, in pain, or recovering from thoracic surgery or trauma.

Candidates for chest physiotherapy include patients who expectorate large amounts of sputum (if sputum production is less than 25 ml/day, chest physiotherapy isn't needed), such as those with bronchiectasis and cystic fibrosis. The procedure hasn't proved effective in treating patients with status asthmaticus, lobar pneumonia, or acute exacerbations of chronic bronchitis when the patient has scant secretions and is being mechanically ventilated. Chest physiotherapy has little value for treating patients with stable, chronic bronchitis.

Contraindications for chest physiotherapy include active pulmonary bleeding with hemoptysis and the immediate posthemorrhage stage, fractured ribs or an unstable chest wall, lung contusions, pulmonary tuberculosis, untreated pneumothorax, acute asthma or bronchospasm, lung abscess or tumor, bony metastasis, head injury, recent myocardial infarction, and vomiting or immediately after eating.

Postural drainage positions

The following illustrations show the various postural drainage positions and the areas of the lungs affected by each.

Lower lobes: Posterior basal segments

Elevate the foot of the bed 30 degrees. Have the patient lie prone with his head lowered. Position pillows under his chest and abdomen. Percuss his lower ribs on both sides of his spine.

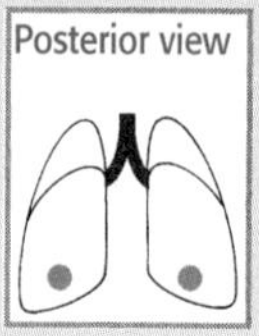

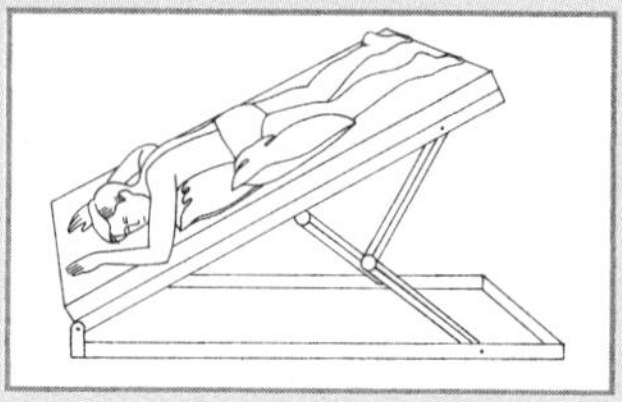

Lower lobes: Lateral basal segments

Elevate the foot of the bed 30 degrees. Instruct the patient to lie on his abdomen with his head lowered and his upper leg flexed over a pillow for support. Then have him rotate a quarter turn upward. Percuss his lower ribs on the uppermost portion of his lateral chest wall.

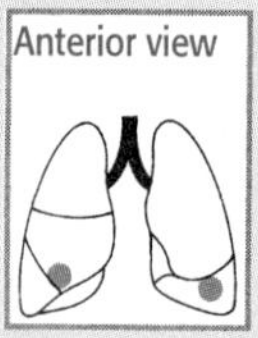

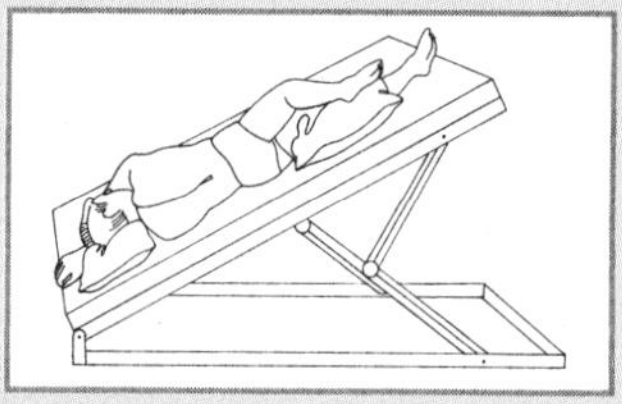

Lower lobes: Anterior basal segments

Elevate the foot of the bed 30 degrees. Instruct the patient to lie on his side with his head lowered. Then place pillows as shown. Percuss with a slightly cupped hand over his lower ribs just beneath the axilla. If an acutely ill patient has trouble breathing in this position, adjust the bed to an angle he can tolerate. Then begin percussion.

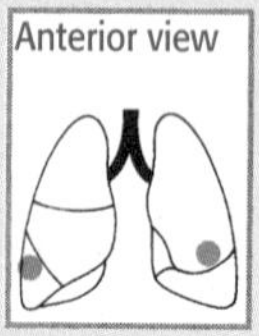

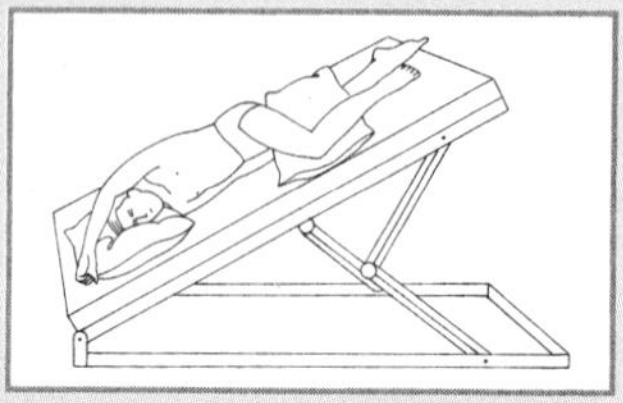

Lower lobes: Superior segments

With the bed flat, have the patient lie on his abdomen. Place two pillows under his hips. Percuss on both sides of his spine at the lower tips of his scapulae.

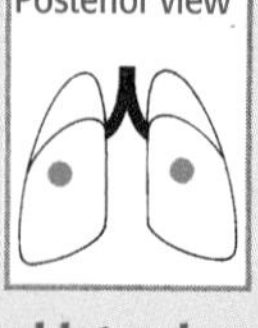

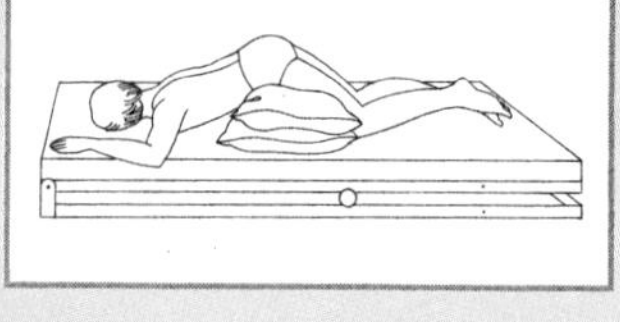

Right middle lobe: Medial and lateral segments

Elevate the foot of the bed 15 degrees. Have the patient lie on his left side with his head down and his knees flexed. Then have him rotate a quarter turn backward. Place a pillow beneath him. Percuss with your hand moder-

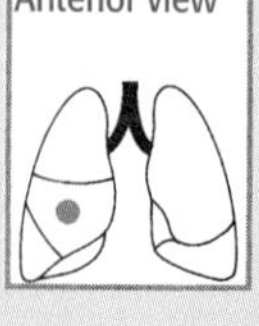

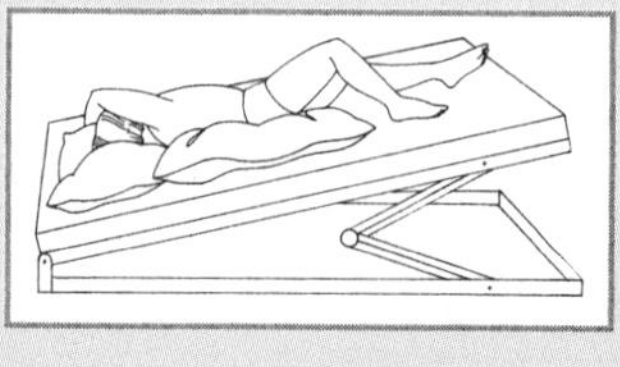

Postural drainage positions *(continued)*

ately cupped over the right nipple. For a woman, cup your hand so that its heel is under the armpit and your fingers extend forward beneath the breast.

Left upper lobe: Superior and inferior segments, lingular portion

Elevate the foot of the bed 15 degrees. Have the patient lie on his right side with his head down and knees flexed. Then have him rotate a quarter turn backward. Place a pillow behind him, from shoulders to hips. Percuss with your hand moderately cupped over his left nipple. For a woman, cup your hand so that its heel is beneath the armpit and your fingers extend forward beneath the breast.

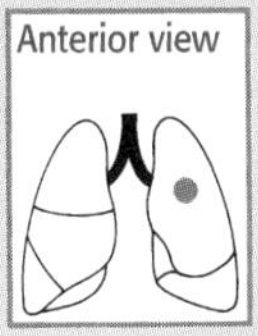

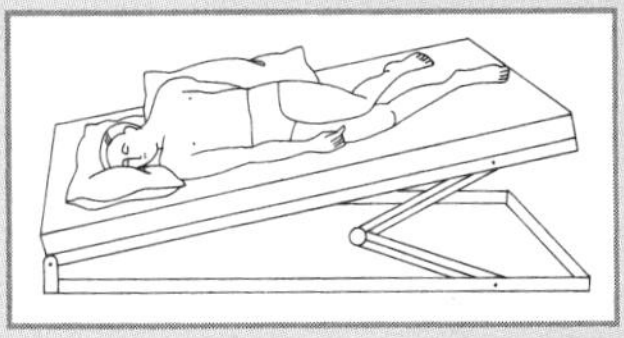

Upper lobes: Anterior segments

Make sure the bed is flat. Have the patient lie on his back with a pillow folded under his knees. Then have him rotate slightly away from the side being drained. Percuss between his clavicle and nipple.

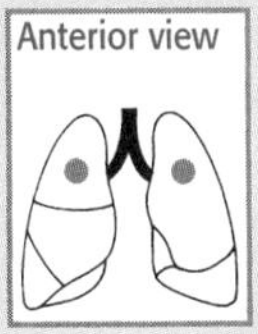

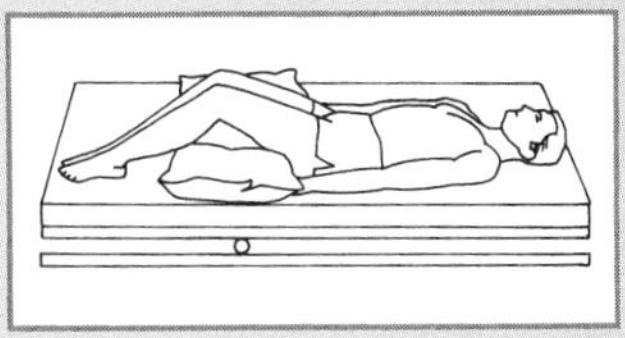

Upper lobes: Apical segments

Keep the bed flat. Have the patient lean back at a 30-degree angle against you and a pillow. Percuss with a cupped hand between his clavicles and the top of each scapula.

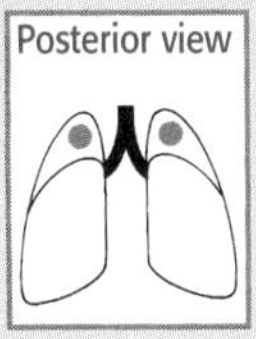

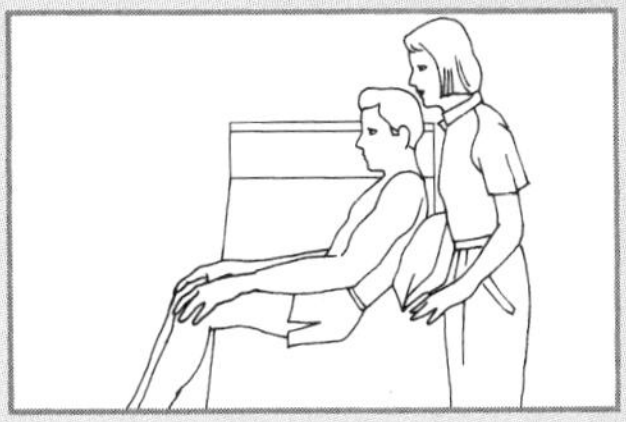

Upper lobes: Posterior segments

Keep the bed flat. Have the patient lean over a pillow at a 30-degree angle. Percuss and clap his upper back on each side.

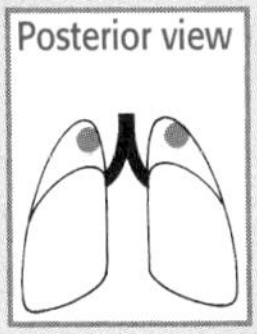

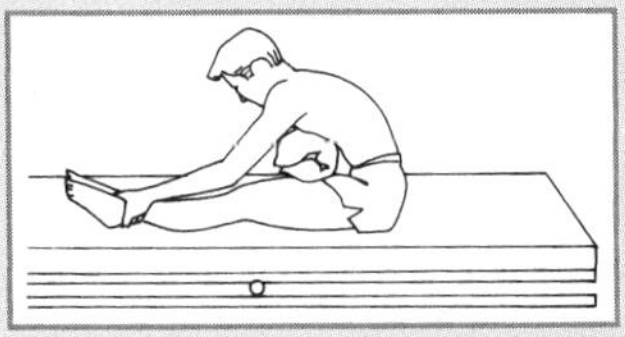

Equipment

Stethoscope ♦ pillows ♦ tilt or postural drainage table (if available) or adjustable hospital bed ♦ emesis basin ♦ facial tissues ♦ suction equipment as needed ♦ equipment for oral care ♦ trash bag ♦ optional: sterile specimen container, mechanical ventilator, supplemental oxygen

Preparation

- Gather the equipment at the patient's bedside.
- Set up suction equipment, if needed, and test its function.

Performing percussion and vibration

To perform percussion, instruct the patient to breathe slowly and deeply, using the diaphragm, to promote relaxation. Hold your hands in a cupped shape, with fingers flexed and thumbs pressed tightly against your index fingers (as shown below). Percuss each segment for 1 to 2 minutes by alternating your hands against the patient in a rhythmic manner. Listen for a hollow sound on percussion to verify correct performance of the technique.

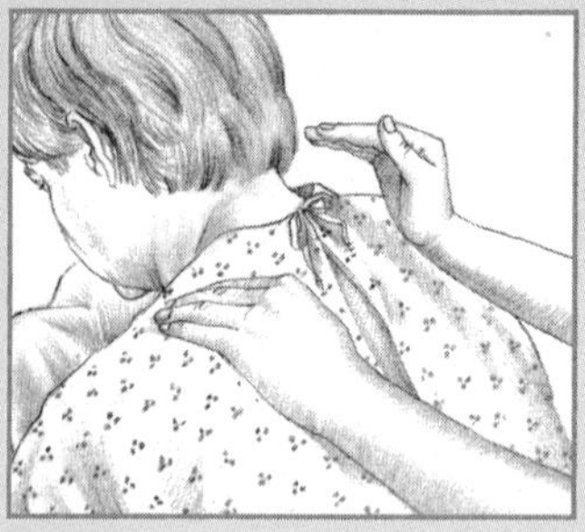

To perform vibration, ask the patient to inhale deeply and then exhale slowly through pursed lips. During exhalation, firmly press your fingers and the palms of your hands against the chest wall (as shown below). Tense the muscles of your arms and shoulders in an isometric contraction to send fine vibrations through the chest wall. Vibrate during five exhalations over each chest segment.

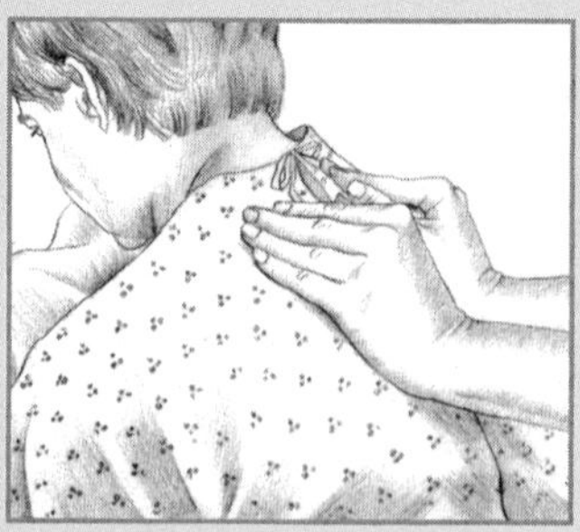

Key steps

- Confirm the patient's identity using two patient identifiers according to your facility's policy.
- Explain the procedure to the patient, provide privacy, and wash your hands.
- Auscultate the patient's lungs to determine baseline respiratory status.
- Position the patient as ordered. In generalized disease, drainage usually begins with the lower lobes, continues with the middle lobes, and ends with the upper lobes. In localized disease, drainage begins with the affected lobes and then proceeds to the other lobes to avoid spreading the disease to uninvolved areas.
- Instruct the patient to remain in each position for 3 to 15 minutes. During this time, perform percussion and vibration as ordered. (See *Performing percussion and vibration*.)
- Explain coughing and deep-breathing exercises preoperatively so that the patient can practice them when he's pain-free and better able to concentrate.
- After postural drainage therapy, percussion, or vibration, instruct the patient to cough to remove loosened secretions. First, tell him to inhale deeply through his nose and then exhale in three short huffs. Then have him inhale deeply again and cough through a slightly open mouth. Three consecutive coughs are highly effective. An effective cough sounds deep, low, and hollow; an ineffective one, high-pitched. Have the patient perform exercises for about 1 minute and then have him rest for 2 minutes. Gradually progress to a 10-minute exercise period, four times daily.
- Provide oral hygiene because secretions may have a foul taste or a stale odor.
- Auscultate the patient's lungs to evaluate the effectiveness of therapy.

Special considerations

- For optimal effectiveness and safety, modify chest physiotherapy according to the patient's condition. For example, initiate or increase the flow of supplemental oxygen, if indicated. Also, suction the patient who has an ineffective cough reflex. If the patient tires quickly during therapy, shorten the sessions because fatigue leads to shallow respirations and increased hypoxia.

- Maintain adequate hydration in the patient receiving chest physiotherapy to prevent mucus dehydration and promote easier mobilization. Avoid performing postural drainage immediately before or within 1½ hours after meals to avoid nausea and aspiration of food or vomitus.
- Because chest percussion can induce bronchospasm, any adjunct treatment (for example, intermittent positive-pressure breathing or aerosol or nebulizer therapy) should precede chest physiotherapy.
- Refrain from percussing over the spine, liver, kidneys, or spleen to avoid injury to the spine or internal organs. Also, avoid performing percussion on bare skin or the female patient's breasts. Percuss over soft clothing (but not over buttons, snaps, or zippers), or place a thin towel over the chest wall. Remember to remove jewelry that might scratch or bruise the patient.

Complications

- Impaired respiratory excursion leading to hypoxia or orthostatic hypotension due to postural drainage therapy in the head-down position that causes pressure on the diaphragm by abdominal contents
- Increased intracranial pressure, which precludes the use of chest physiotherapy in a patient with acute neurologic impairment, in the head-down position
- Rib fracture, especially in the patient with osteoporosis, from vigorous percussion or vibration
- Pneumothorax caused by coughing in the patient with emphysema who has blebs

Patient teaching

- Teach a caregiver how to perform chest physiotherapy, as necessary, and have them provide a return demonstration.

Documentation

Record the frequency, date, and time of chest physiotherapy; positions for postural drainage and length of time each is maintained; chest segments percussed or vibrated; the color, amount, odor, and viscosity of secretions produced and presence of any blood; any complications and interventions taken, and the patient's tolerance of treatment.

Closed-wound drain management

Typically inserted during surgery in anticipation of substantial postoperative drainage, a closed-wound drain promotes healing and prevents swelling by suctioning the serosanguineous fluid that accumulates at the wound site. By removing this fluid, the closed-wound drain helps reduce the risk of infection and skin breakdown as well as the number of dressing changes. Hemovac and Jackson-Pratt closed drainage systems are used most commonly.

A closed-wound drain consists of perforated tubing connected to a portable vacuum unit. The distal end of the tubing lies within the wound and usually leaves the body from a site other than the primary suture line to preserve the integrity of the surgical wound. The tubing exit site is treated as an additional surgical wound; the drain is usually sutured to the skin.

If the wound produces heavy drainage, the closed-wound drain may be left in place for longer than 1 week. Drainage must be emptied and measured frequently to maintain maximum suction and prevent strain on the suture line.

Equipment

Graduated biohazard cylinder ♦ sterile laboratory container, if needed ♦ alcohol pads ♦ gloves ♦ gown ♦ face shield ♦ trash bag ♦ sterile gauze pads ♦ antiseptic cleaning agent

Key steps

- Check the practitioner's order, and assess the patient's condition.
- Explain the procedure to the patient, provide privacy, and wash your hands.
- Unclip the vacuum unit from the patient's bed or gown.
- Using aseptic technique, release the vacuum by removing the spout plug on the

Using a closed-wound drainage system

The portable closed-wound drainage system draws drainage from a wound site, such as the chest wall postmastectomy (as shown top right), by means of a Y tube. To empty the drainage, remove the plug and empty it into a graduated cylinder. To reestablish suction, compress the drainage unit against a firm surface to expel air and, while holding it down, replace the plug with your other hand (as shown bottom left). The same principle is used for the Jackson-Pratt bulb drain (as shown bottom right).

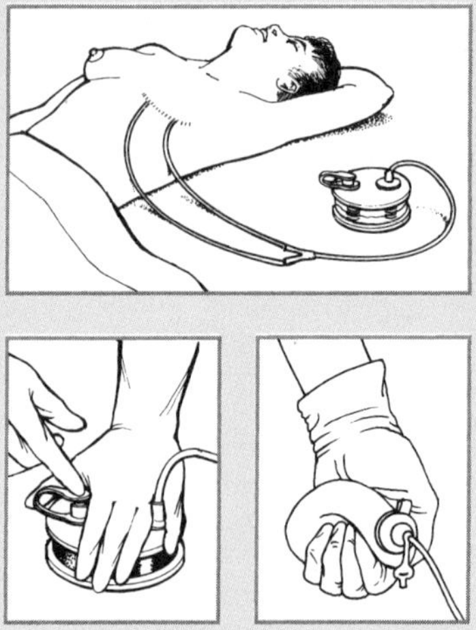

collection chamber. The container expands completely as it draws in air.

- Empty the unit's contents into a graduated biohazard cylinder, and note the amount and appearance of the drainage. If diagnostic tests will be performed on the fluid specimen, pour the drainage directly into a sterile laboratory container, note the amount and appearance, and send it to the laboratory.
- Maintaining aseptic technique, use an alcohol pad to clean the unit's spout and plug.
- To reestablish the vacuum that creates the drain's suction power, fully compress the vacuum unit. With one hand holding the unit compressed to maintain the vacuum, replace the spout plug with your other hand. (See *Using a closed-wound drainage system*.)
- Check the patency of the equipment. Make sure the tubing is free of twists, kinks, and leaks because the drainage system must be airtight to work properly. The vacuum unit should remain compressed when you release manual pressure; rapid reinflation indicates an air leak. If this occurs, recompress the unit and make sure the spout plug is secure.
- Secure the vacuum unit to the patient's gown. Fasten it below wound level to promote drainage. Don't apply tension on drainage tubing when fastening the unit to prevent possible dislodgment. Remove and discard your gloves, and wash your hands thoroughly.
- Observe the sutures that secure the drain to the patient's skin; look for signs of pulling or tearing and for swelling or infection of surrounding skin. Gently clean the sutures with an antiseptic cleaning solution.
- Properly dispose of drainage, solutions, and trash bag, and clean or dispose of soiled equipment and supplies according to your facility's policy.

Special considerations

- Empty the drain and measure its contents once during each shift if drainage has accumulated, more often if drainage is excessive. Removing excess drainage maintains maximum suction and avoids straining the drain's suture line.
- If the patient has more than one closed drain, number the drains so you can record drainage from each site.

ALERT

Be careful not to mistake chest tubes with water seal drainage devices for closed-wound drains because the care of these devices differs from closed-wound drainage systems, and the vacuum of a chest tube should never be released.

Complications

- Reduction or obstruction of drainage due to occlusion of the tubing by fibrin, clots, or other particles

Documentation

Record the date and time you empty the drain, appearance of the drain site and presence of swelling or signs of infection, equipment malfunction and consequent nursing action, and the patient's tolerance of the treatment. On the intake and output sheet, record drainage color, consistency, type, and amount. If the patient has more than one closed-wound drain, number the drains and record the information above separately for each drainage site.

Code management

The goals of any code are to restore the patient's spontaneous heartbeat and respirations and to prevent hypoxic damage to the brain and other vital organs. Fulfilling these goals requires a team approach. Ideally, the team should consist of health care workers trained in advanced cardiac life support (ACLS), although nurses trained in basic life support (BLS) may also be a part of the team. Sponsored by the American Heart Association, the ACLS course incorporates BLS skills with advanced resuscitation techniques. BLS and ACLS procedures and protocols should be performed according to the 2005 AHA guidelines.

In most health care facilities, ACLS-trained nurses provide the first resuscitative efforts to cardiac arrest patients, often administering cardiac medications and performing defibrillation before the physician's arrival. Because ventricular fibrillation commonly precedes sudden cardiac arrest, initial resuscitative efforts focus on rapid recognition of arrhythmias and, when indicated, defibrillation. If monitoring equipment isn't available, you should simply perform BLS measures. Of course, the scope of your responsibilities in any situation depends on your facility's policies and procedures and your state's nurse practice act.

A code may be called for patients with absent pulse, apnea, ventricular fibrillation, ventricular tachycardia, or asystole. Some facilities allow family members to be present during a code; check you facility's policy regarding this issue.

Equipment

Oral, nasal, and endotracheal (ET) airways ♦ one-way valve masks ♦ oxygen source ♦ oxygen flowmeter ♦ intubation supplies ♦ handheld resuscitation bag ♦ suction supplies ♦ nasogastric (NG) tube ♦ goggles, masks, and gloves ♦ cardiac arrest board ♦ peripheral I.V. supplies, including 14G and 18G peripheral I.V. catheters ♦ central I.V. supplies, including an 18G thin-wall catheter, a 6-cm needle catheter, and a 16G 15- to 20-cm catheter ♦ I.V. administration sets (including microdrip and minidrip) ♦ I.V. fluids, including dextrose 5% in water (D_5W), normal saline solution, and lactated Ringer's solution ♦ electrocardiogram (ECG) monitor and leads ♦ cardioverter-defibrillator ♦ conductive medium ♦ cardiac drugs, including adenosine, epinephrine, lidocaine, procainamide (Procan), vasopressin, amiodarone (Cordarone), atropine, isoproterenol (Isuprel), dopamine, calcium chloride, and dobutamine ♦ optional: external pacemaker, percutaneous transvenous pacer, cricothyrotomy kit, end-tidal carbon dioxide detector

Preparation

- Because effective emergency care depends on reliable and accessible equipment, the equipment as well as the personnel, must be ready for a code at any time. You should also be familiar with the cardiac drugs you may have to administer.
- Always be aware of your patient's code status as defined by the practitioner's orders, the patient's advance directives, and

family wishes. If the practitioner has ordered a "no code," make sure he has written and signed the order. If possible, have the patient or a responsible family member cosign the order.

- In some cases, you may need to consider whether the family wishes to be present during a code. If they do want to be present, and if a nurse or clergyman can remain with them, consider allowing them to remain during the code.

Key steps

- If you're the first to arrive at the site of a code, call for help and instruct another person to retrieve the emergency equipment. Then assess the patient's level of consciousness (LOC), airway, breathing, and circulation, and then begin cardiopulmonary resuscitation (CPR). Use a pocket mask, if available, to ventilate the patient.
- When the emergency equipment arrives, have the second BLS provider place the cardiac arrest board under the patient and assist with two-rescuer CPR. Meanwhile, have the nurse assigned to the patient relate the patient's medical history and describe the events leading to cardiac arrest.
- A third person, either a nurse certified in BLS or a respiratory therapist, will then attach the handheld resuscitation bag to the oxygen source and begin to ventilate the patient with 100% oxygen.
- When the ACLS-trained nurse arrives, she'll expose the patient's chest and apply defibrillator pads. She'll then apply the paddles to the patient's chest to obtain a "quick look" at the patient's cardiac rhythm. If the patient is in ventricular fibrillation, ACLS protocol calls for defibrillation as soon as possible with 360 joules. Then, resume CPR immediately. A rhythm check isn't done at this time. The ACLS-trained nurse will act as code leader until the practitioner arrives.
- If not already in place, apply ECG electrodes and attach the patient to the defibrillator's cardiac monitor. Avoid placing electrodes on bony prominences or hairy areas. Also avoid the areas where the defibrillator pads will be placed and where chest compressions will be given.
- After 5 cycles of CPR, the patient's rhythm will be checked and, if necessary, another shock will be given at the same dose; then continue CPR while the defibrillator is charging. After another 5 cycles of CPR, the patient's rhythm will be checked and another shock will be given at the same dose, if necessary.
- As CPR and defibrillation is occurring, you or an ACLS-trained nurse will then start two peripheral I.V. lines with large-bore I.V. catheters. Be sure to use only a large vein, such as the antecubital vein, to allow for rapid fluid administration and to prevent drug extravasation.
- As soon as the I.V. catheter is in place, begin an infusion of normal saline solution or lactated Ringer's solution to help prevent circulatory collapse. D_5W continues to be acceptable but the latest ACLS guidelines encourage the use of normal saline solution or lactated Ringer's solution because D_5W can produce hyperglycemic effects during a cardiac arrest.
- While one nurse starts the I.V. lines, the other nurse will set up portable or wall suction equipment and suction the patient's oral secretions, as necessary, to maintain an open airway.
- The ACLS-trained nurse will then prepare and administer emergency cardiac drugs as needed. (See *ACLS pulseless arrest algorithm,* pages 118 and 119.) Keep in mind that drugs administered through a central line reach the myocardium more quickly than those administered through a peripheral line.
- The ACLS pulseless arrest algorithm shows the timing of drug administration and shock administration. Drug doses should be given immediately after a rhythm check.
- If the patient doesn't have an accessible I.V. line, you may administer such medications as epinephrine, lidocaine, vasopressin, and atropine through an ET tube. To do so, dilute the drugs in 10 ml of normal saline solution or sterile water and then instill them into the patient's ET tube. Afterward, ventilate the patient manually to improve absorption by distributing the drug throughout the bronchial tree.

- The ACLS-trained nurse will also prepare for, and assist with, ET intubation or other advanced airway. Compression interruption should be minimized during advanced airway placement.
- Suction the patient as needed. After the patient has been intubated, the health care provider should use clinical assessment and confirmation devices to check ET tube placement. Assessment includes visualizing chest expansion, auscultation of equal breath sounds, and auscultation of no breath sounds over the epigastrium. Devices used to check tube placement include exhaled carbon-dioxide detectors and esophageal detectors. When the tube is correctly positioned, tape it securely. To serve as a reference, mark the point on the tube that's level with the patient's lips.
- Meanwhile, other members of the code team should keep a written record of the events. Other duties include prompting participants about when to perform certain activities (such as when to check a pulse or take vital signs), overseeing the effectiveness of CPR, and keeping track of the time between therapies. Each team member should know what each participant's role is to prevent duplicating effort. Finally, someone from the team should make sure the primary nurse's other patients are reassigned to another nurse.
- If the family is present during the code, have someone, such as a clergy member or social worker, remain with them. Be sure to keep the family regularly informed of the patient's status.
- If the family isn't at the facility, contact them as soon as possible. Encourage them not to drive to the facility, but offer to call someone who can give them a ride.

Special considerations

- When the patient's condition has stabilized, assess his LOC, breath sounds, heart sounds, peripheral perfusion, bowel sounds, and urine output. Measure his vital signs every 15 minutes, and monitor his cardiac rhythm continuously.
- Make sure the patient receives an adequate supply of oxygen, whether through a mask or a ventilator.
- Check the infusion rates of all I.V. fluids, and use infusion pumps to deliver vasoactive drugs. To evaluate the effectiveness of fluid therapy, insert an indwelling catheter if the patient doesn't already have one. Also insert an NG tube to relieve or prevent gastric distention.
- If appropriate, reassure the patient and explain what's happening. Allow the patient's family to visit as soon as possible. If the patient dies, notify the family and allow them to see the patient as soon as possible.
- To make sure your code team performs optimally, schedule a time to review the code.

Complications

- Fractured ribs, liver laceration, lung puncture, and gastric distention
- Electric shock caused by defibrillation
- Esophageal or tracheal laceration, subcutaneous emphysema, or accidental right mainstem bronchus intubation caused by emergency intubation
- Accidental right mainstem bronchus intubation causing decreased or absent breath sounds on the left side of the chest and normal breath sounds on the right

Documentation

During the code, document the events in as much detail as possible. Note whether the arrest was witnessed or unwitnessed, the time of the arrest, the time CPR was begun, the time the ACLS-trained nurse arrived, and the total resuscitation time. Also document the number of defibrillations, the times they were performed, the joule level, the patient's cardiac rhythm before and after the defibrillation, and whether the patient had a pulse.

Document all drug therapy, including dosages, routes of administration, and patient response. You'll also want to record all procedures, such as peripheral and central line insertion, pacemaker insertion, and ET tube insertion, as well as the time they were performed and the patient's tolerance of the procedures. Also keep track of all arterial blood gas results.

(Text continues on page 120.)

ACLS pulseless arrest algorithm

This American Heart Association algorithm outlines the steps an advanced cardiac life support (ACLS)-certified nurse should take to treat rhythms that produce cardiac arrest, such as ventricular fibrillation (VF), rapid ventricular tachycardia (VT), pulseless electrical activity (PEA), and asystole. If you aren't ACLS-certified, the algorithm will help you know what to expect in such an emergency.

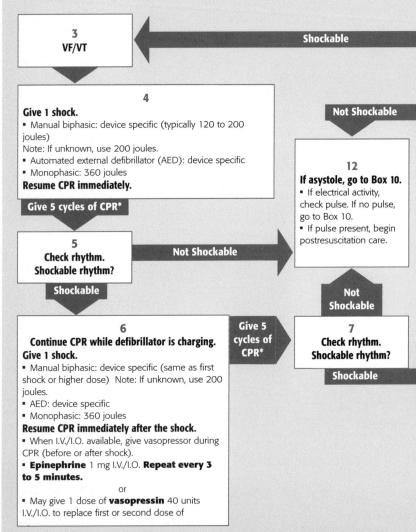

Shockable →

3
VF/VT

↓

4
Give 1 shock.
- Manual biphasic: device specific (typically 120 to 200 joules)
Note: If unknown, use 200 joules.
- Automated external defibrillator (AED): device specific
- Monophasic: 360 joules

Resume CPR immediately.

Give 5 cycles of CPR*

↓

5
Check rhythm.
Shockable rhythm?

Not Shockable → Box 12

Shockable ↓

6
Continue CPR while defibrillator is charging.
Give 1 shock.
- Manual biphasic: device specific (same as first shock or higher dose) Note: If unknown, use 200 joules.
- AED: device specific
- Monophasic: 360 joules

Resume CPR immediately after the shock.
- When I.V./I.O. available, give vasopressor during CPR (before or after shock).
- **Epinephrine** 1 mg I.V./I.O. **Repeat every 3 to 5 minutes.**

or

- May give 1 dose of **vasopressin** 40 units I.V./I.O. to replace first or second dose of

Give 5 cycles of CPR* →

7
Check rhythm.
Shockable rhythm?

Not Shockable ↑ Box 12

Shockable

Not Shockable ↓

12
If asystole, go to Box 10.
- If electrical activity, check pulse. If no pulse, go to Box 10.
- If pulse present, begin postresuscitation care.

*After an advanced airway is placed, rescuers no longer deliver "cycles" of CPR. Give continuous chest compressions without pauses for breaths. Give 8 to 10 breaths/minute. Check rhythm every 2 minutes.

1

PULSELESS ARREST

- Basic life support algorithm: Call for help, give cardiopulmonary resuscitation (CPR).
- Give oxygen when available.
- Attach monitor/defibrillator when available.

2
Check rhythm.
Shockable rhythm?

Not Shockable

9
Asystole/pulseless electrical activity (PEA)

10

Resume CPR immediately for 5 cycles.

- When I.V./I.O. available, give vasopressor.
- **Epinephrine** 1 mg I.V./I.O.

Repeat every 3 to 5 minutes.

or

- May give 1 dose of **vasopressin** 40 units I.V./I.O. to replace first or second dose of **epinephrine**.
- Consider **atropine** 1 mg I.V./I.O. for asystole or slow PEA rate.

Repeat every 3 to 5 minutes (up to 3 doses).

Give 5 cycles of CPR*

11
Check rhythm.
Shockable rhythm?

Shockable

13
Go to Box 4.

8

Continue CPR while defibrillator is charging.

Give 1 shock.

- Manual biphasic: device specific (same as first shock or higher dose)

Note: If unknown, use 200 joules.

- AED: device specific
- Monophasic: 360 joules

Resume CPR immediately after the shock.

- Consider antiarrhythmics; give during CPR (before or after shock); amiodarone (300 mg I.V./I.O. once, then consider additional 150 mg I.V./I.O. once) or lidocaine (1 to 1.5 mg/kg first dose, then 0.5 to 0.75 mg/kg I.V./I.O., maximum 3 doses or 3 mg/kg)
- Consider magnesium, loading dose 1 to 2 g I.V./I.O. for torsades de pointes

After 5 cycles of CPR,* go to Box 5 above.

During CPR

- **Push hard and fast (100/minute).**
- **Ensure full chest recoil.**
- **Minimize interruptions in chest compressions.**
- One cycle of CPR: 30 compressions then 2 breaths; 5 cycles = 2 minutes.
- Avoid hyperventilation.
- Secure airway and confirm placement.
- Rotate compressors every 2 minutes with rhythm checks.
- Search for and treat possible contributing factors:
  - Hypovolemia
  - Hypoxia
  - Hydrogen ion (acidosis)
  - Hypokalemia/hyperkalemia
  - Hypoglycemia
  - Hypothermia
  - Toxins
  - Tamponade, cardiac
  - Tension pneumothorax
  - Thrombosis (coronary or pulmonary)
  - Trauma

Record whether the patient is transferred to another unit or facility along with his condition at the time of transfer and whether his family was notified. Finally, document any complications and the measures taken to correct them. When your documentation is complete, have the practitioner and ACLS nurse review and then sign the document.

Colostomy and ileostomy care

The patient with an ascending or transverse colostomy or an ileostomy must wear an external pouch to collect emerging fecal matter, which will be watery or pasty. Besides collecting waste matter, the pouch helps to control odor and to protect the stoma and peristomal skin. Most disposable pouching systems can be used for 2 to 7 days; some models last even longer.

All pouching systems need to be changed immediately if a leak develops, and every pouch needs emptying when it's one-third to one-half full. The patient with an ileostomy may need to empty his pouch four or five times daily.

Naturally, the best time to change the pouching system is when the bowel is least active, usually between 2 and 4 hours after meals. After a few months, most patients can predict the best changing time.

The selection of a pouching system should take into consideration which system provides the best adhesive seal and skin protection for the individual patient. The type of pouch selected also depends on the stoma's location and structure, availability of supplies, wear time, consistency of effluent, personal preference, and finances.

Equipment

Pouching system ♦ stoma measuring guide ♦ stoma paste (if drainage is watery to pasty or stoma secretes excess mucus) ♦ scissors ♦ washcloth and towel ♦ closure clamp ♦ toilet or bedpan ♦ water or pouch cleaning solution ♦ gloves ♦ facial tissues ♦ optional: paper tape, mild nonmoisturizing soap, electric clippers, liquid skin sealant, and pouch deodorant

Pouching systems may be drainable or closed-bottomed, disposable or reusable, adhesive-backed, and one-piece or two-piece.

Key steps

- Provide privacy and emotional support.

Fitting the pouch and skin barrier

- For a pouch with an attached skin barrier, measure the stoma with the stoma measuring guide. Select the opening size that matches the stoma.
- For an adhesive-backed pouch with a separate skin barrier, measure the stoma with the measuring guide and select the opening that matches the stoma. Trace the selected size opening onto the paper back of the skin barrier's adhesive side. Cut out the opening. (If the pouch has precut openings, which can be handy for a round stoma, select an opening that's $1/8''$ larger than the stoma. If the pouch comes without an opening, cut the hole $1/8''$ wider than the measured tracing.) The cut-to-fit system works best for an irregularly shaped stoma.
- For a two-piece pouching system with flanges, see *Applying a skin barrier and pouch.*
- Avoid fitting the pouch too tightly because the stoma has no pain receptors. A constrictive opening could injure the stoma or skin tissue without the patient feeling warning discomfort. Avoid cutting the opening too big because this may expose the skin to fecal matter and moisture.
- The patient with a descending or sigmoid colostomy who has formed stools and whose ostomy doesn't secrete much mucus may choose to wear only a pouch. In this case, make sure the pouch opening closely matches the stoma size.
- Between 6 weeks and 1 year after surgery, the stoma will shrink to its permanent size. At that point, pattern-making preparations will be unnecessary unless the patient gains weight, has additional surgery, or injures the stoma.

Applying a skin barrier and pouch

Fitting a skin barrier and ostomy pouch properly can be done in a few steps. Shown below is a two-piece pouching system with flanges, which is in common use.

1. Measure the stoma using a measuring guide.

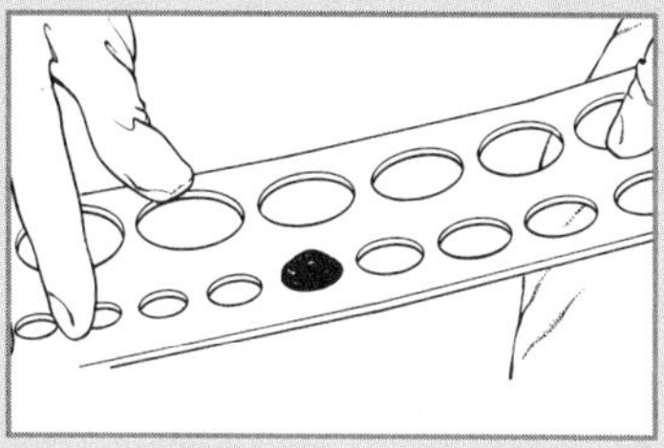

2. Trace the appropriate circle carefully on the back of the skin barrier.

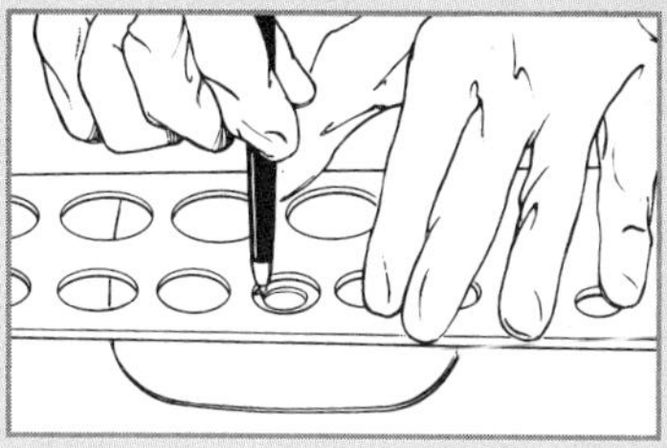

3. Cut the circular opening in the skin barrier. Bevel the edges to keep them from irritating the patient.

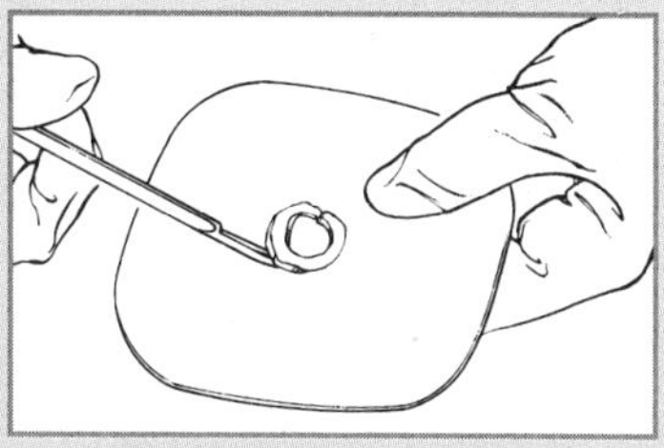

4. Remove the backing from the skin barrier and moisten it or apply barrier paste, as needed, along the edge of the circular opening.

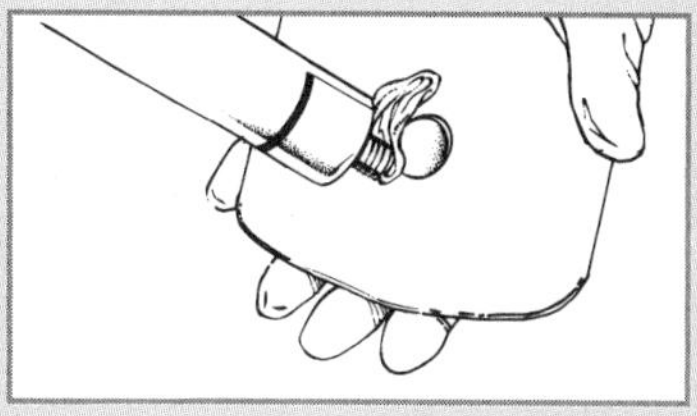

5. Center the skin barrier over the stoma, adhesive side down, and gently press it to the skin.

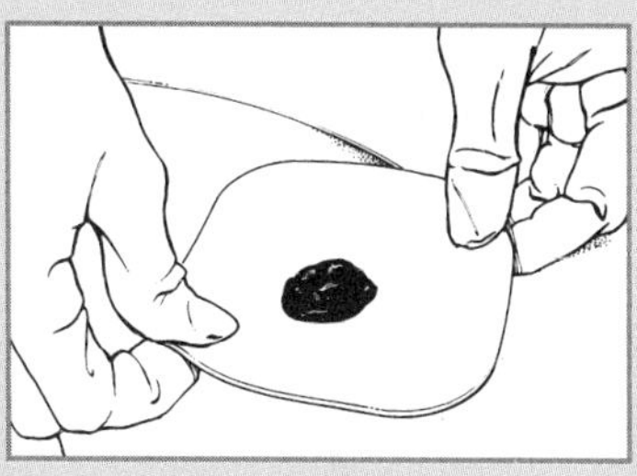

6. Gently press the pouch opening onto the ring until it snaps into place.

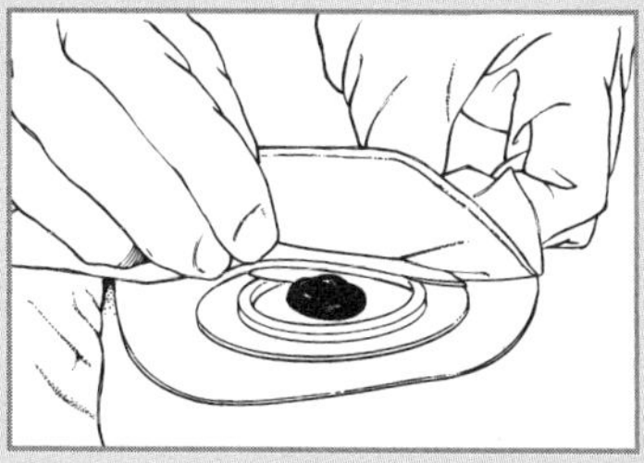

Applying or changing the pouch

- Collect all equipment.
- Provide privacy, wash your hands, and put on gloves.
- Confirm the patient's identity using two patient identifiers according to your facility's policy.
- Explain the procedure to the patient. As you perform each step, explain what you're doing and why because the patient

will eventually perform the procedure himself.

- Remove and discard the old pouch. Wipe the stoma and peristomal skin gently with a facial tissue.
- Carefully wash with mild soap and water and dry the peristomal skin by patting gently. Allow the skin to dry thoroughly. Inspect the peristomal skin and stoma. If necessary, clip surrounding hair to promote a better seal and avoid skin irritation from hair pulling against the adhesive.
- If applying a separate skin barrier, peel off the paper backing of the prepared skin barrier, center the barrier over the stoma, and press gently to ensure adhesion.
- You may want to outline the stoma on the back of the skin barrier (depending on the product) with a thin ring of stoma paste to provide extra skin protection. (Skip this step if the patient has a sigmoid or descending colostomy, formed stools, and little mucus.)
- Remove the paper backing from the adhesive side of the pouching system and center the pouch opening over the stoma. Press gently to secure.
- For a pouching system with flanges, align the lip of the pouch flange with the bottom edge of the skin barrier flange. Gently press around the circumference of the pouch flange, beginning at the bottom, until the pouch securely adheres to the barrier flange. (The pouch will click into its secured position.) Holding the barrier against the skin, gently pull on the pouch to confirm the seal between flanges.
- Encourage the patient to stay quietly in position for about 5 minutes to improve adherence. The patient's body warmth also helps to improve adherence and soften a rigid skin barrier.
- Leave a bit of air in the pouch to allow drainage to fall to the bottom.
- Apply the closure clamp, if necessary.
- If desired, apply paper tape in a picture-frame fashion to the pouch edges for additional security.

Emptying the pouch

- Put on gloves.
- Tilt the bottom of the pouch upward and remove the closure clamp.
- Turn up a cuff on the lower end of the pouch and allow it to drain into the toilet or bedpan.
- Wipe the bottom of the pouch and reapply the closure clamp.
- If desired, the bottom portion of the pouch can be rinsed with cool tap water.

DO'S & DON'TS

Don't aim water up near the top of the pouch because this may loosen the seal on the skin.

- A two-piece flanged system can also be emptied by unsnapping the pouch. Let the drainage flow into the toilet.
- Release flatus through the gas release valve if the pouch has one. Otherwise, release flatus by tilting the pouch bottom upward, releasing the clamp, and expelling the flatus. To release flatus from a flanged system, loosen the seal between the flanges. (Some pouches have gas release valves.)
- Never make a pinhole in a pouch to release gas. This destroys the odor-proof seal.
- Remove and discard gloves.

Special considerations

- Use adhesive solvents and removers only after patch-testing the patient's skin because some products may irritate the skin or produce hypersensitivity reactions. Consider using a liquid skin sealant, if available, to give skin tissue additional protection from drainage and adhesive irritants.
- Remove the pouching system if the patient reports burning or itching beneath it or purulent drainage around the stoma. Notify the practitioner or therapist of any skin irritation, breakdown, rash, or unusual appearance of the stoma or peristomal area.
- Use commercial pouch deodorants if desired. However, most pouches are odor-free, and odor should be evident only when you empty the pouch or if it leaks.
- If the patient wears a reusable pouching system, suggest that he obtain two or more systems so he can wear one while the other dries after cleaning with soap and water

or a commercially prepared cleaning solution.

Complications

- Injury to the stoma due to failure to fit the pouch properly over the stoma
- Allergic reaction to adhesives and other ostomy products

Patient teaching

- After performing and explaining the procedure to the patient, teach the patient self-care.
- Before discharge, suggest that the patient avoid odor-causing foods, such as fish, eggs, onions, and garlic.

Documentation

Record the date and time of the pouching system change and note the character of drainage, including color, amount, type, and consistency. Describe the appearance of the stoma and the peristomal skin. Document patient teaching. Describe the teaching content. Record the patient's response to self-care, and evaluate his learning progress.

Contact precautions

Contact precautions prevent the spread of infectious diseases transmitted by direct or indirect contact with the patient (skin-to-skin), patient-care items (bedpans, urinals), or indirect contact with surfaces in the patient's room that are contaminated with the infectious microorganism. Contact precautions apply to patients who are known or suspected to be infected or colonized (presence of microorganism without obvious clinical signs and symptoms of infection) with epidemiologically important organisms that can be transmitted by direct or indirect contact. (See *Indications for contact precautions,* pages 124 and 125.)

Effective contact precautions require a private room. If no private room is available, two patients infected with the same (but no other) microorganism can share a room. Anyone having contact with the patient, the patient's support equipment, or items soiled with the patient's bodily fluids should wear clean, nonsterile gowns and gloves. Gloves should be changed after contact with infective material that may contain high concentrations of the microorganism, such as fecal material or wound drainage. A gown and gloves should be removed before leaving the patient's room. Thorough hand washing with an antimicrobial agent or waterless antiseptic agent and proper handling and disposal of contaminated items are also essential in maintaining contact precautions.

Patient transport should be limited to essential purposes only. If the patient is transported, make sure that precautions are maintained to decrease the risk of transmission to other patients and contamination of environmental surfaces.

When possible, medical and noncritical patient-care equipment (I.V. pumps, monitors) should be used for only one patient. If sharing equipment is unavoidable, then items must be properly cleaned or disinfected before use with another patient.

Equipment

Gloves ♦ gowns or aprons ♦ masks, if necessary ♦ isolation door card ♦ plastic bags

Gather additional supplies, such as a thermometer, stethoscope, and blood pressure cuff.

Preparation

- Keep contact precaution supplies outside the patient's room in a cart or anteroom.

Key steps

- Inform the patient of the need for contact precautions and instruct him that he isn't to leave his room.
- Situate the patient in a single room with private toilet facilities and an anteroom, if possible. If necessary, two patients with the same (but no other) infection may share a room. Explain isolation procedures to the patient and his family.
- Instruct visitors to wear gloves and a gown while visiting the patient and to wash their hands after removing the gown and gloves.
- Place a contact precautions card on the door to notify anyone entering the room.

Indications for contact precautions

Contact precautions are designed to reduce the risk of transmitting infectious agents by direct or indirect contact. This list presents the diseases that spread infectious agents along with the precautionary periods.

Disease	Precautionary period
Acute viral (acute hemorrhagic) conjunctivitis	Duration of illness
Clostridium difficile enteric infection	Duration of illness
Diphtheria (cutaneous)	Duration of illness
Enteroviral infection, in diapered or incontinent patient	Duration of illness
Escherichia coli disease, in diapered or incontinent patient	Duration of illness
Hepatitis A, in diapered or incontinent patient	Duration of illness
Herpes simplex virus infection (neonatal or mucocutaneous)	Duration of illness
Impetigo	Until 24 hours after initiation of effective therapy
Infection or colonization with multidrug-resistant bacteria	Until off antibiotics and culture is negative
Major abscesses, cellulitis, or decubiti	Until 24 hours after initiation of effective therapy
Parainfluenza virus infection, in diapered or incontinent patient	Duration of illness
Pediculosis (lice)	Until 24 hours after initiation of effective therapy
Respiratory syncytial virus infection, in infants and young children	Duration of illness
Rotavirus infection, in diapered or incontinent patient	Duration of illness

Indications for contact precautions *(continued)*

Disease	Precautionary period
Rubella, congenital syndrome	Precautions during any admission until infant is age 1, unless nasopharyngeal and urine cultures negative for virus after age 3 months
Scabies	Until 24 hours after initiation of effective therapy
Shigellosis, in diapered or incontinent patient	Duration of illness
Smallpox	Duration of illness; requires airborne precautions
Staphylococcal furunculosis in infants and young children	Duration of illness
Viral hemorrhagic infections (Ebola, Lassa, Marburg)	Duration of illness
Zoster (chickenpox, disseminated zoster, or localized zoster in immunodeficient patient)	Until all lesions are crusted; requires airborne precautions

- Wash your hands before entering and after leaving the patient's room and after removing gloves.
- Place laboratory specimens in impervious, labeled containers, and send them to the laboratory at once. Attach requisition slips to the outside of the container.
- Place items that have come in contact with the patient in a single impervious bag, and arrange for disposal or disinfection and sterilization.
- Limit the patient's movement from the room. If the patient must be moved, cover draining wounds with clean dressings. Notify the receiving department or area of the patient's isolation precautions so that the precautions will be maintained and the patient can be returned to the room promptly.

Special considerations

- Clean and disinfect equipment between uses by different patients.
- Try to dedicate certain reusable equipment (thermometer, stethoscope, blood pressure cuff) for the patient in contact precautions to reduce the risk of transmitting infection to other patients.
- Remember to change gloves during patient care as indicated by the procedure or task. Wash your hands after removing gloves and before putting on new gloves.

Complications

- None known

Documentation

Record the need for contact precautions on the nursing care plan and as otherwise indicated by your facility. Document initiation and maintenance of the precautions, the patient's tolerance of the procedure, and patient or family teaching. Also document the date contact precautions were discontinued.

Continuous positive airway pressure

Continuous positive airway pressure (CPAP) is used to provide low flow pressure into the airways to help hold the airway open. This prevents the palate and tongue from collapsing and obstructing the airways. CPAP is used to treat patients who are having respiratory distress by easing the work of breathing. It's also commonly used to treat obstructive sleep apnea. Many patients are started on CPAP in the hospital, and then continue CPAP use at home. CPAP has traditionally been administered through a face mask, but newer, more comfortable methods include the face pillow and nasal mask.

Equipment

Nasal mask, nasal pillows, or face mask properly sized ♦ permanent marker ♦ CPAP machine ♦ oxygen delivery tubing ♦ washcloth ♦ water ♦ optional: oxygen source, oxygen tubing, pulse oximetry

Key steps

- Check the practitioner's order.
- Confirm the patient's identity using two patient identifiers according to facility policy.

Setting up the CPAP machine

- Position the CPAP machine so the tubing easily reaches the patient and plug in the machine.

DEVICE SAFETY

Don't plug the CPAP machine into an outlet with another plug in it; don't use an extension cord to reach the outlet.

- Connect the oxygen delivery tubing to the air outlet valve on the CPAP unit.

Applying the headgear

- Have the patient wash his face with the washcloth and water to remove facial oils and help achieve a better fit.
- Check the face mask, nasal mask, or nasal pillow to make sure the cushion is not hard or broken. If it is, replace it.

Applying the nasal mask

- Place the nasal mask so the longer straps are located at the top of the mask (as shown below).

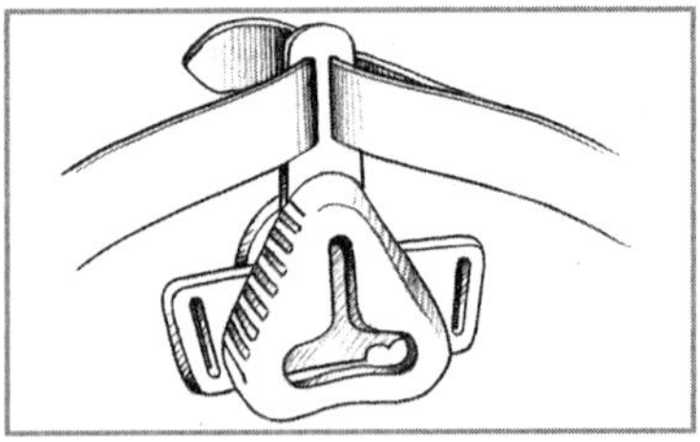

- Make sure that the Velcro is facing away from you and thread the four tabs through the tabs on the side and top of the mask (as shown below).

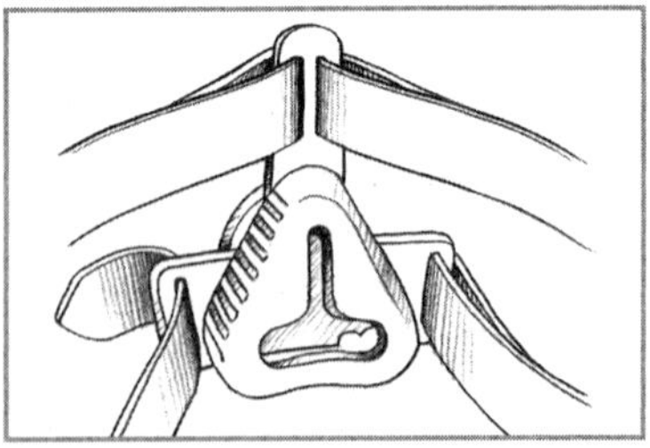

- Pull the straps through the slots and fasten them using the Velcro.
- Place the mask over the patient's nose and position the headgear over his head (as shown below).
- Gradually tighten all the straps on the mask until a seal is obtained. The mask doesn't have to be tight to fit correctly—it just has to have a seal.

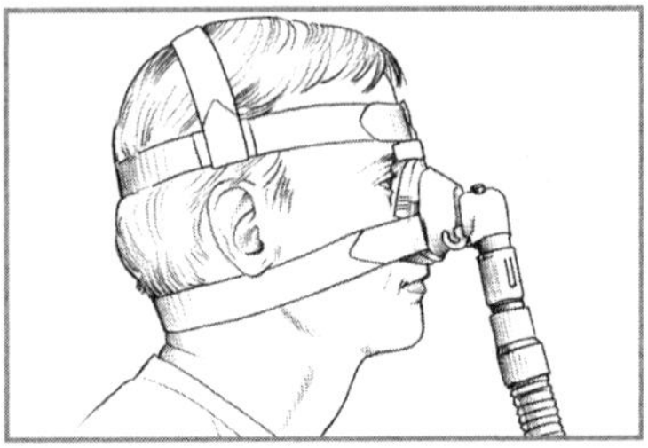

■ Use the permanent marker to mark the straps and the final position to eliminate having to fit the mask each time the patient wears it.

Applying the nasal pillow

■ Insert the nasal pillows into the shell making sure they fit correctly and there's no air leaking around them (as shown below).

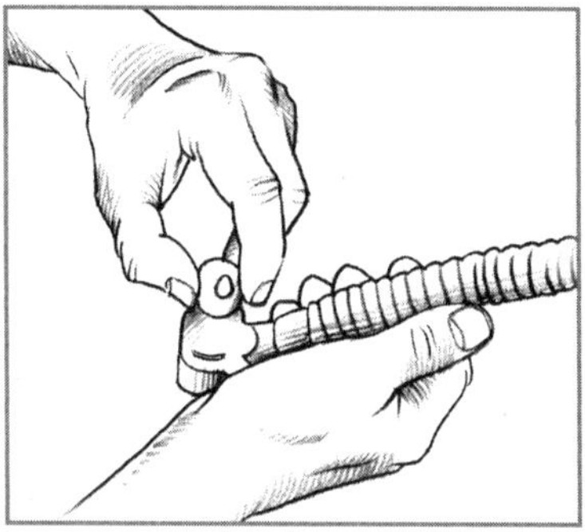

■ Place the headgear around the patient's head and use the Velcro straps to achieve the proper fit. Once the straps are in the correct place, remove the headgear without undoing the straps.

■ Attach the nasal pillow to the headgear by wrapping the Velcro around the tubing, leaving room for rotation (as shown below).

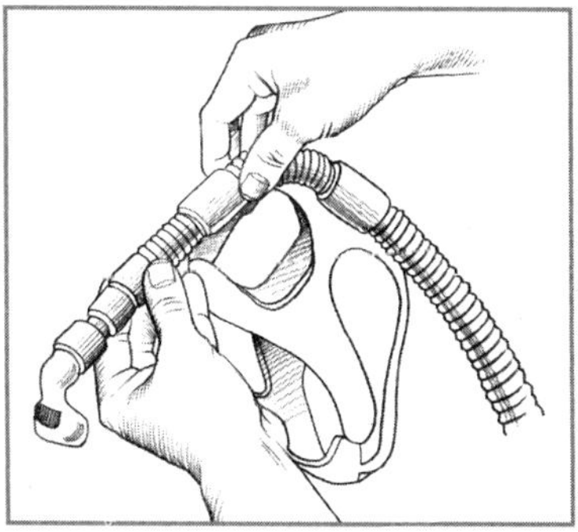

■ Place the completely assembled headgear back on the patient and position the nasal pillows comfortably.

■ Attach the shell strap across the shell and adjust the tension of the strap until there's a seal in both nostrils (as shown below).

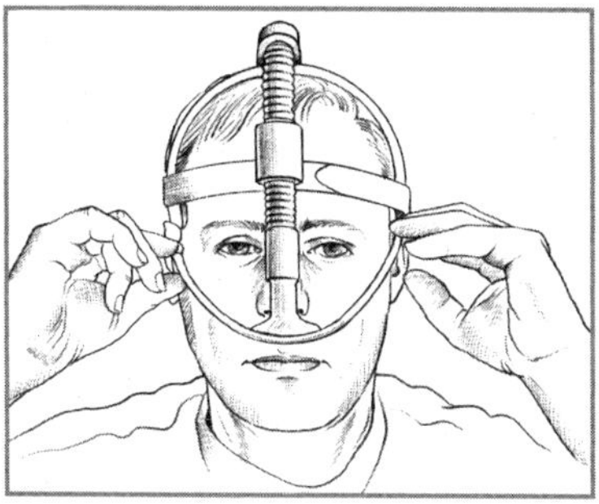

DO'S & DON'TS

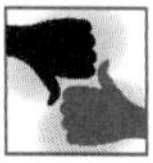

Don't block the exhalation port on the backside of the shell.

Applying the face mask

■ Hold the mask against the patient's face and position the head gear over his head.

■ Using the Velcro straps, adjust them as with the nasal mask until there are no leaks present (as shown below).

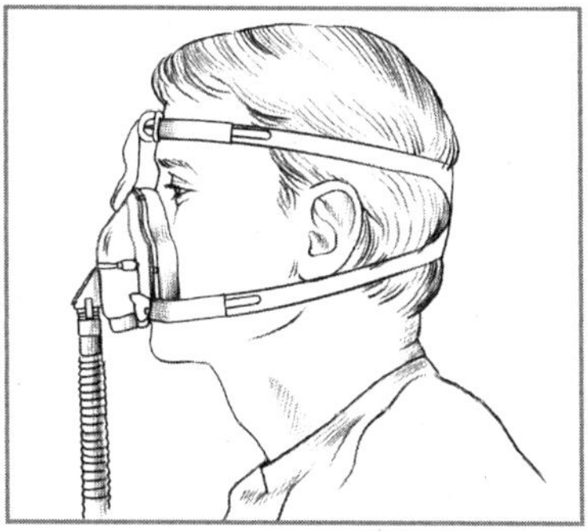

■ Connect the flexible tubing to the mask and turn on the airflow.

Using oxygen with CPAP

■ Connect the oxygen tubing to the CPAP unit. There are a variety of different types of adapters that may be used to do this.

■ Turn on the CPAP unit before turning on the oxygen flow.

Administering CPAP

- After the administration device is correctly fitted on the patient, turn on the pressure generator.
- If ordered, monitor the patient's pulse oximetry during the treatment.
- When the treatment is over, in the morning or upon discontinuation of the order, turn off the pressure generator and remove the headgear and appliance from the patient.

Special considerations

- If the mask isn't properly fitted, the patient may complain of dry or sore eyes. If this is the case, remove the mask and headgear and readjust them to minimize leaks.
- The patient may need to use a humidifier with the CPAP unit if he complains of a runny nose, or dryness or burning in his nose and throat. Discuss this with the practitioner and obtain an order for humidification.
- Always make sure there's air coming out of the unit when the power is turned on.

Complications

- Dry eyes, runny or dry nose, burning in the throat or nose due to ill-fitting masks
- Allergy or skin irritation from the mask (If this happens, apply a barrier between the mask and the skin.)
- Nose bleeds, abdominal bloating, headaches, and nightmares

Patient teaching

- Teach the patient how to use the machine at home, including fitting the mask and care of the equipment.
- Make sure the patient has the name and phone number of the company that will be supplying the machine and a contact number for him to ask questions.

Documentation

Document the CPAP settings, the length of time the patient was on the CPAP, how the patient tolerated the CPAP, and if there were any complications.

Continuous renal replacement therapy

Continuous renal replacement therapy (CRRT) is used to treat patients who suffer from acute renal failure. Unlike the more traditional intermittent hemodialysis (IHD), CRRT is administered around the clock, providing patients with continuous therapy and sparing them the destabilizing hemodynamic and electrolyte changes characteristic of IHD. CRRT is used for the patients with hypotension who can't tolerate traditional hemodialysis. For such patients, CRRT is usually the only choice of treatment; however, it can also be used on many patients who can tolerate IHD. CRRT methods vary in complexity. The techniques include the following:

- Slow continuous ultrafiltration (SCUF) uses arteriovenous (AV) access and the patient's blood pressure to circulate blood through a hemofilter. Because this therapy's goal is the removal of fluids, the patient doesn't receive replacement fluids.
- Continuous arteriovenous hemofiltration (CAVH) uses the patient's blood pressure and AV access to circulate blood through a flow resistance hemofilter. However, to maintain the patency of the filter and systemic blood pressure, the patient receives replacement fluids.
- Continuous venovenous hemofiltration (CVVH) uses SCUF and CAVH. A double-lumen catheter is used to provide access to a vein, and a pump moves blood through the hemofilter.
- Continuous arteriovenous hemodialysis (CAVH-D) combines hemofiltration with hemodialysis. In this technique, the infusion pump moves dialysate solution concurrent to blood flow, adding the ability to continuously remove solute while removing fluid. Like CAVH, it can also be performed in patients with hypotension and fluid overload.
- Continuous venovenous hemodialysis (CVVH-D) is similar to CAVH-D, except that a vein provides the access while a pump is used to move dialysate solution concurrent with blood flow.

ALERT

CVVH or CVVH-D is used instead of CAVH or CAVH-D in many facilities to treat critically ill patients. CVVH has several advantages over CAVH: It doesn't require arterial access, can be performed in patients with low mean arterial pressures, and has a better solute clearance than CAVH.

Equipment

CRRT equipment ♦ heparin flush solution ♦ occlusive dressings for catheter insertion sites ♦ sterile gloves ♦ sterile mask ♦ antiseptic solution ♦ sterile 4″ × 4″ gauze pads ♦ tape ♦ filtration replacement fluid (FRF) as ordered ♦ infusion pump

Preparation

- Prime the hemofilter and tubing according to the manufacturer's instructions.

Key steps

- Confirm the patient's identity using two patient identifiers according to your facility's policy.
- Wash your hands. Assemble the equipment at the patient's bedside, and explain the procedure. (See *CAVH setup,* page 130.)
- If necessary, assist with inserting the catheters into the femoral artery and vein, using strict sterile technique. (In some cases, an internal AV fistula or external AV shunt may be used instead of the femoral route.) If ordered, flush both catheters with heparin flush solution to prevent clotting.
- Apply occlusive dressings to the insertion sites, and mark the dressings with the date and time. Secure the tubing and connections with tape.
- Before starting therapy, weigh the patient, take his baseline vital signs, make sure that necessary laboratory studies have been done (usually, electrolyte levels, coagulation factors, complete blood count, blood urea nitrogen, and creatinine studies), and assess the patient's risk of bleeding.
- Monitor the patient's vital signs, cardiac rhythm and rate, level of consciousness, intravascular and extravascular volume status, respiratory status, biochemical profile, and coagulation and hematologic status throughout CRRT.
- Assess the patient for disequilibrium, including headache, nausea and vomiting, hypertension, decreased sensorium, seizures, and coma.
- Assess the patient for hyperglycemia.
- Put on sterile gloves and the mask. Prepare the connection sites by cleaning them with gauze pads soaked in antiseptic solution, and then connect them to the exit port of each catheter.
- Using sterile technique, connect the arterial and venous lines to the hemofilter.
- Turn on the hemofilter and monitor the blood flow rate through the circuit. The flow rate is usually kept between 500 and 900 ml/hour.
- Inspect the ultrafiltrate during the procedure. It should remain clear yellow, with no gross blood. Pink-tinged or bloody ultrafiltrate may signal a blood leak in the hemofilter, which permits bacterial contamination. If a leak occurs, follow your facility's policy for termination of treatment.
- Assess the affected leg for signs of obstructed blood flow, such as coolness, pallor, and a weak pulse. Check the groin area on the affected side for signs of hematoma. Ask the patient if he has pain at the insertion sites.
- Calculate the amount of FRF every hour, or as ordered, according to your facility's policy. Infuse the prescribed amount and type of FRF through the infusion pump into the arterial side of the circuit.

Special considerations

- Because blood flows through an extracorporeal circuit during CAVH and CVVH, blood in the hemofilter may need to be anticoagulated. To do this, infuse heparin in low doses (starting at 500 units/hour) into an infusion port on the arterial side of the setup. Measure thrombin clotting time or the activated clotting time (ACT). This ensures that the circuit, not the patient, is anticoagulated. A normal ACT is 100 seconds; during CRRT, keep it between 100 and 300 seconds, depending on the pa-

CAVH setup

During continuous arteriovenous hemofiltration (CAVH), the patient's arterial blood pressure serves as a natural pump, driving blood through the arterial line. A hemofilter removes water and toxic solutes (ultrafiltrate) from the blood. Filter replacement fluid is infused into a port on the arterial side; this same port can be used to infuse heparin. The venous line carries the replacement fluid, along with purified blood, to the patient. This illustration shows one of several CAVH setups.

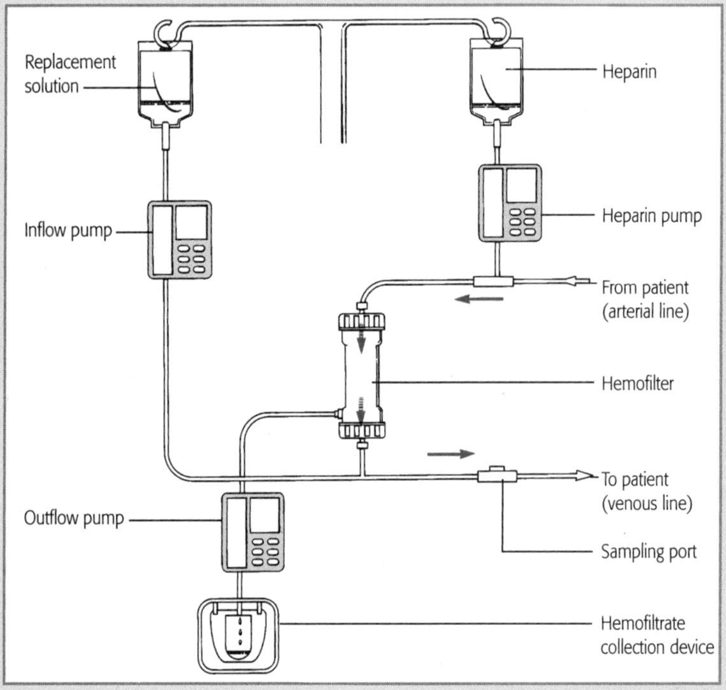

tient's clotting times. If the ACT is too high or too low, the practitioner will adjust the heparin dose.

- Another way to prevent clotting in the hemofilter is to infuse medications or blood through another line.
- A third way to help prevent clots in the hemofilter, and also to prevent kinks in the catheter, is to make sure that the patient doesn't bend the affected leg more than 30 degrees at the hip.
- To prevent infection, perform skin care at the catheter insertion sites every 48 hours using sterile technique. Cover the sites with an occlusive dressing.
- If the ultrafiltrate flow rate decreases, raise the bed to increase the distance between the collection device and the hemofilter. Lower the bed to decrease the flow rate.

Device safety

Clamping the ultrafiltrate line is contraindicated with some types of hemofilters because pressure may build up in the filter, clotting it and collapsing the blood compartment.

Preventing complications in CRRT

Listed below are some possible complications of continuous renal replacement therapy (CRRT) and measures to prevent them from occurring.

Complication	Interventions
Hypotension	▪ Monitor blood pressure. ▪ Decrease the speed of the blood pump temporarily for any transient hypotension. ▪ Increase the vasopressor support.
Hypothermia	▪ Use an inline fluid warmer placed on the blood return line to the patient or an external warming blanket.
Fluid and electrolyte imbalances	▪ Monitor fluid levels every 4 to 6 hours. ▪ Monitor sodium, lactate, potassium, and calcium levels and replace as necessary.
Acid-base imbalances	▪ Monitor bicarbonate levels and arterial blood gas values.
Air embolism	▪ Observe for air in the system. ▪ Use luer-lock devices on catheter openings.
Hemorrhage	▪ Keep all connections tight and the dialysis lines visible.
Infection	▪ Perform sterile dressing changes.

Complications

▪ Hypotension, hemorrhage, hypothermia, infection, fluid and electrolyte imbalances, acid-base imbalances, air embolism, and thrombosis (see *Preventing complications in CRRT*)

Documentation

Record the time the treatment began and ended, fluid balance information, times of dressing changes, complications, medications given, and the patient's tolerance.

D

Defibrillation

The standard treatment for ventricular fibrillation, defibrillation involves using electrode paddles to direct an electric current through the patient's heart. The current causes the myocardium to depolarize, which in turn encourages the sinoatrial node to resume control of the heart's electrical activity. This current may be delivered by a monophasic or biphasic defibrillator. The electrode paddles delivering the current may be placed on the patient's chest or, during cardiac surgery, directly on the myocardium.

Because ventricular fibrillation leads to death if not corrected, the success of defibrillation depends on early recognition and quick treatment of this arrhythmia. In addition to treating ventricular fibrillation, defibrillation may also be used to treat ventricular tachycardia that doesn't produce a pulse.

Patients with a history of ventricular fibrillation may be candidates for an implantable cardioverter-defibrillator (ICD), a sophisticated device that automatically discharges an electric current when it senses a ventricular tachyarrhythmia. (See *Understanding the ICD*.)

Equipment

Defibrillator (monophasic or biphasic) ♦ external paddles ♦ internal paddles (sterilized for cardiac surgery) ♦ conductive medium pads ♦ electrocardiogram (ECG) monitor with recorder ♦ oxygen therapy equipment ♦ handheld resuscitation bag ♦ airway equipment ♦ emergency pacing equipment ♦ emergency cardiac medications

Key steps

- Assess the patient to determine if he lacks a pulse. Call for help and perform cardiopulmonary resuscitation (CPR) until the defibrillator and other emergency equipment arrive.
- Refer to the sequence for defibrillation as described under "Code management," page 115, and "Automated external defibrillation," page 21.
- If defibrillation restores a normal rhythm, check the patient's central and peripheral pulses and obtain a blood pressure reading, heart rate, and respiratory rate. Assess the patient's level of consciousness, cardiac rhythm, breath sounds, skin color, and urine output. Obtain baseline arterial blood gas levels and a 12-lead ECG. Provide supplemental oxygen, ventilation, and medications, as needed. Check the patient's chest for electrical burns and treat them, as ordered, with corticosteroids or lanolin-based creams
- Prepare the defibrillator for immediate reuse.

Special considerations

- When applying conductive pads, make sure to place them 1″ (2.5 cm) away from any implantable device the patient may have.

DEVICE SAFETY

Defibrillators vary from one manufacturer to the next, so familiarize yourself with your facility's

Understanding the ICD

The implantable cardioverter-defibrillator (ICD) has a programmable pulse generator and lead system that monitors the heart's activity, detects ventricular bradyarrhythmias and tachyarrhythmias, and responds with appropriate therapies. The range of therapies includes antitachycardia and bradycardia pacing, cardioversion, and defibrillation. Newer defibrillators also have the ability to pace both the atrium and the ventricle.

Implantation of the ICD is similar to that of a permanent pacemaker. The cardiologist positions the lead (or leads) transvenously in the endocardium of the right ventricle (and the right atrium, if both chambers require pacing). The lead connects to a generator box, which is implanted in the right or left upper chest near the clavicle.

ICD implantation has the same complications that may occur with permanent pacemaker insertion. In addition, inappropriate cardioversion, ineffective cardioversion/defibrillation, and device deactivation may occur. Causes may include T-wave oversensing, lead fracture, lead insulation breakage, electrocautery, magnetic resonance imaging, and electromagnetic interference. Use of a magnet over the ICD will inhibit further shocks, until the underlying cause is diagnosed and treated. The bradycardiac pacing function will still activate should the patient require it.

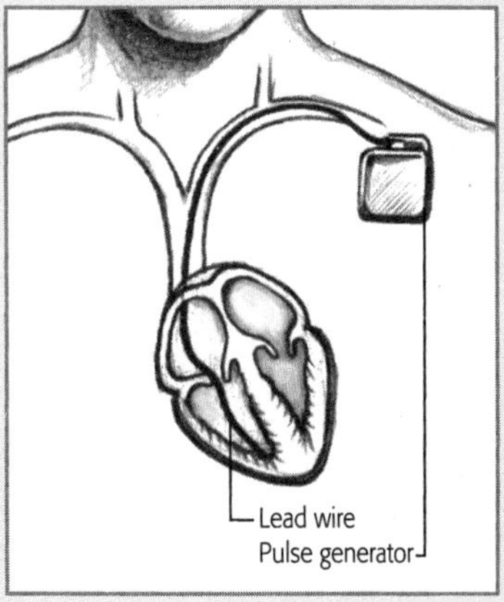

equipment. Defibrillator operation should be checked at least every 8 hours and after each use.

- Defibrillation can be affected by several factors, including paddle size and placement, condition of the patient's myocardium, duration of the arrhythmia, chest resistance, and the number of countershocks.

Complications

- Accidental electric shock to those providing care
- Skin burns due to use of an insufficient amount of conductive medium

Documentation

Document the procedure, including the patient's ECG rhythms both before and after defibrillation; the number of times defibrillation was performed; the voltage used during each attempt; whether a pulse returned; the dosage, route, and time of drug administration; whether CPR was used; how the airway was maintained; and the patient's outcome.

Diabetic ulcer care

Diabetic foot ulcers are usually caused by peripheral neuropathy, both sensory (lack of sensation) and motor (decreased function of the motor nerves in the foot), but may also be the result of peripheral vascular disease. Arterial insufficiency can be another cause of a nonhealing ulcer in the patient with diabetes. An ulcer can also result from trauma or excess pressure undetected by the patient because of neuropathy. The border is undefined and may be small at the surface, although the wound may have a large subcutaneous abscess. Drainage usually is absent unless the ulcer is infected.

Diabetic neuropathic ulcers should be treated like pressure ulcers, with debridement of necrotic tissue, moist wound healing and off-loading of pressure.

Equipment

Bedside table ♦ piston-type irrigating system ♦ two pairs of gloves ♦ normal saline solution, as ordered ♦ sterile 4″ × 4″ gauze pads and sterile cotton swabs ♦ selected topical dressing ♦ linen-saver pads ♦ impervious plastic trash bag ♦ disposable wound-measuring device (a square, transparent card with concentric circles arranged in bull's-eye fashion and bordered with a straight-edge ruler)

Preparation

- Assemble equipment at the patient's bedside.
- Cut tape into strips for securing dressings.
- Loosen lids on cleaning solutions and medications for easy removal.
- Loosen existing dressing edges and tapes before putting on gloves.
- Attach an impervious plastic trash bag to the bedside table to hold used dressings and refuse.

Key steps

- Premedicate the patient before dressing change as needed.
- Wash your hands and put on sterile gloves. Be sure to review your facility's policy on standard precautions.
- Remove the previous dressing and place it into the impervious trash bag. If the old dressing is dry, soak it with normal saline solution before removing it so that granulating tissue isn't removed when the dressing is pulled off.
- Inspect the wound. Note the location, pain, shape, size of the wound, wound base and edges, presence of necrosis, periwound skin and the color, amount, and odor of any drainage and necrotic debris. Measure the wound perimeter with the disposable wound-measuring device.
- Irrigate the wound, using a piston-style syringe containing normal saline solution.
- Remove and discard your soiled gloves, and put on a fresh pair.
- Insert a cotton-tipped swab into the wound to assess for tunneling. Gauge the tunnel depth by how far you can insert your finger or cotton swab.
- Clean the ulcer with normal saline solution or commercially prepared noncytotoxic cleanser. When applying the gauze, use a moist dressing to promote a moist wound environment.
- To apply a moist dressing, squeeze out the excess saline from the gauze layers. Place the layer of moist gauze into the wound. If there's tunneling, make sure the dressing is tucked loosely into the tunneled areas. Make sure that there's a moist dressing next to all of the tissue in the wound, filling up all of the wound's dead space. Avoid overpacking the wound. Your patient may need absorbent dressings if the ulcer has moderate to heavy drainage.
- Notify the practitioner of your assessment findings. The patient may need ulcer debridement or surgical intervention. Debridement helps ulcer healing by removing necrotic tissue that acts as a physical barrier to wound repair. If you suspect infection, the patient may need a wound culture or tissue biopsy. If the ulcer is caused by arterial insufficiency, the patient may need surgery.
- Check the patient's laboratory results, and notify the practitioner if any findings deviate from the norm.
- If the patient's wound is infected, prepare him for a tissue biopsy—the gold standard to confirm the diagnosis of infection and the possibility of systemic antibiotics.
- Prepare the patient for tests that may be performed to determine ulcer severity and the presence of complications. Radiographic imaging is used to rule out gas formation, the presence of foreign objects, and bony abnormalities. Magnetic resonance imaging is used to diagnose osteomyelitis. A transcutaneous oxygen tension measurement determines skin perfusion. If the ulcer is in an atypical location or doesn't respond to treatment, a biopsy may be performed.

■ Apply growth factors as ordered after necrotic tissue and infection have been eliminated and there's adequate perfusion to the wound.
■ Assess the patient's level of pain and refer to a pain specialist if necessary.

Complications

■ Gangrene of the feet (In many cases, amputation is necessary to control the spread of infection.)

Patient teaching

■ Tell the patient to thoroughly inspect his feet daily, wear proper-fitting shoes and socks, avoid walking barefoot in the home, and not to test the temperature of bath water with his feet.
■ Instruct the patient to keep his legs elevated above the level of his heart while sitting or sleeping. Suggest that he place phone books in between his mattress and box spring so that his legs are elevated above his head.

Documentation

Document the ulcer's anatomic location and its length, width, and depth. Record the extent of tunneling or undermining, if present. Reassess the wound at specified intervals and document the date and time of dressing changes. If the wound is infected, its dimensions may change rapidly. Document ulcer-related pain by asking the patient about it, teaching him to use a pain-rating scale, and looking for nonverbal indicators. Photograph the wound to supplement your comprehensive wound care documentation.

Doppler use

The Doppler ultrasound blood flow detector is more sensitive than palpation for determining pulse rate. It's especially useful when a pulse is faint or weak. Doppler ultrasound detects the motion of red blood cells (RBCs), unlike palpation, which detects arterial wall expansion and retraction.

Equipment

Doppler ultrasound blood flow detector ♦ coupling or transmission gel ♦ soft cloth ♦ antiseptic solution or soapy water ♦ surgical marker

Key steps

■ Apply a small amount of coupling gel or transmission gel (not water-soluble lubricant) to the ultrasound probe.
■ Position the probe on the skin directly over the selected artery. (See *Pulse points,* page 136.)
■ When using a Doppler model with a speaker, turn the instrument on and, moving counter-clockwise, set the volume control to the lowest setting.
■ If your model doesn't have a speaker, plug in the earphones and slowly raise the volume.
■ The Doppler ultrasound stethoscope is basically a stethoscope fitted with an audio unit, volume control, and transducer, which amplifies the movement of RBCs.
■ To obtain the best signals with either device, tilt the probe 45 degrees from the artery, making sure you put gel between the skin and the probe.
■ Slowly move the probe in a circular motion to locate the center of the artery and the Doppler signal, which will produce a hissing noise at the heartbeat.
■ Avoid rapid movements of the probe because this distorts the signal.
■ Count the signals for 60 seconds to determine the pulse rate.
■ Mark the location of the pulses with the surgical marker to easily relocate.
■ Clean the probe with a soft cloth soaked in antiseptic solution or soapy water.

Special considerations

■ Don't immerse the probe in the water or solution or bump it against a hard surface.

Complications

■ None known

Documentation

Record the location and quality of the pulse as well as the pulse rate and time of measurement.

Pulse points

Shown below are the locations where an artery crosses bone or firm tissue and can be palpated for a pulse or assessed by using a Doppler ultrasound device.

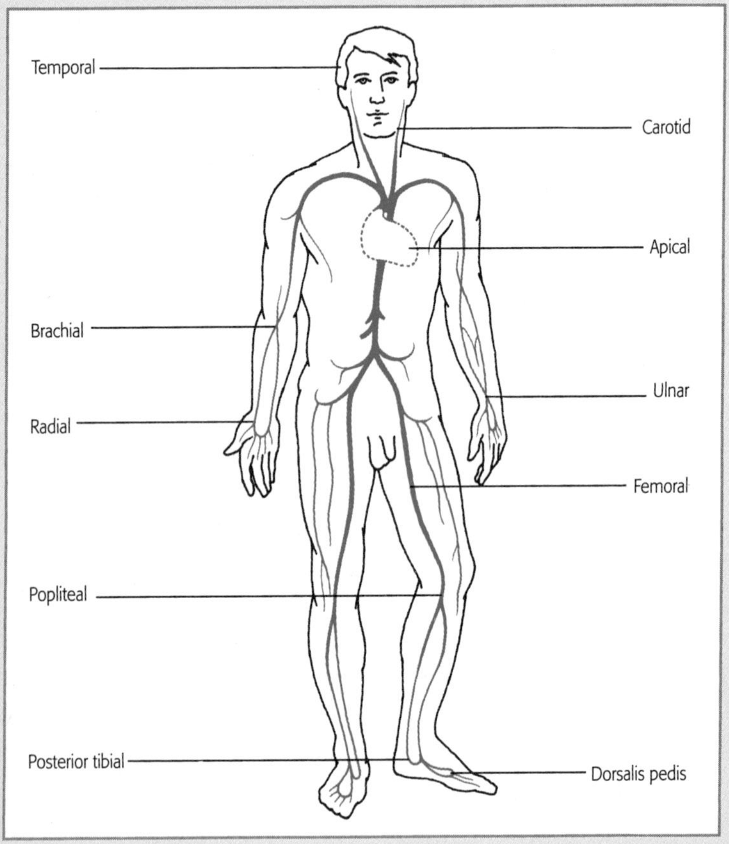

Droplet precautions

Droplet precautions prevent the transmission and spread of infectious diseases caused by large-particle droplets (larger than 5 mm in size) from the infected patient to the susceptible host. Infection occurs when droplets come in contact with the mucous membranes of a host. (See *Indications for droplet precautions.*)

Effective droplet precautions require a private room (the door may remain open). If a private room isn't available, the Centers for Disease Control and Prevention and the Occupational Safety and Health Administration guidelines state that the patient may be placed in a room with another patient who has the same active (but no other) infection. All persons—including visitors—who may be in close contact with the patient should maintain a distance of at least 3′ (1 m) from the patient and should wear a surgical mask covering the nose and mouth.

During handling of infants and young children who require droplet precautions,

Indications for droplet precautions

Droplet precautions are designed to reduce the risk of droplet transmission of the diseases that are listed here with their precautionary periods.

Disease	Precautionary period
Adenovirus infection in infants and young children	Duration of illness
Diphtheria (pharyngeal)	Until off antibiotics and two cultures taken at least 24 hours apart are negative
Influenza	Duration of illness
Invasive *Haemophilus influenzae* type b disease, including meningitis, pneumonia, and sepsis	Until 24 hours after initiation of effective therapy
Invasive *Neisseria meningitidis* disease, including meningitis, pneumonia, epiglottitis, and sepsis	Until 24 hours after initiation of effective therapy
Mumps	For 9 days after onset of swelling
Mycoplasma pneumoniae infection	Duration of illness
Parvovirus B19	Maintain precautions for duration of hospitalization when chronic disease occurs in an immunodeficient patient; patients with transient aplastic crisis or red-cell crisis, maintain precautions for 7 days
Pertussis	Until 5 days after initiation of effective therapy
Pneumonic plague	Until 72 hours after initiation of effective therapy
Rubella (German measles)	Until 7 days after onset of rash
Streptococcal pharyngitis, pneumonia, or scarlet fever in infants and young children	Until 24 hours after initiation of effective therapy

gloves and a gown should be worn to prevent soiling clothing from nasal and oral secretions.

Equipment

Masks ♦ gowns, if necessary ♦ gloves ♦ plastic bags droplet precautions door card

Gather additional supplies needed for routine patient care, such as a thermometer, stethoscope, and blood pressure cuff.

Preparation

- Keep droplet precaution supplies outside the patient's room in a cart or anteroom.

Key steps

- Situate the patient in a single room with private toilet facilities and an anteroom, if possible. If necessary, two patients with the same infection (but no other infections) may share a room. Explain isolation procedures to the patient and his family.
- Make sure that visitors wear masks (and, if necessary, gowns and gloves) within 3′ (1 m) of the patient.
- Put a droplet precautions sign on the door to notify anyone entering the room.
- Wash your hands before entering and after leaving the room and during patient care, as indicated.
- Pick up your mask by the top strings, adjust it around your nose and mouth, and tie the strings for a comfortable fit. If the mask has a flexible metal nose strip, adjust it to fit firmly but comfortably.
- Instruct the patient to cover his nose and mouth with a facial tissue while coughing or sneezing.
- Tape a plastic bag to the patient's bedside so the patient can dispose of facial tissues correctly.
- Limit the patient's movement from the room. If he must leave the room for essential procedures, make sure that he wears a surgical mask over his nose and mouth. Notify the receiving department or area of the patient's isolation precautions so that the precautions will be maintained and the patient can be returned to the room promptly.
- Some health care facilities have added contact precautions to droplet precautions because the patient's environment is contaminated.

Special considerations

- Before removing your mask, remove your gloves (if worn), and wash your hands.
- Untie the strings and dispose of the mask, handling it by the strings only.

Complications

- None known

Patient teaching

- Instruct the patient to cover his nose and mouth with facial tissue while coughing or sneezing

Documentation

Record the need for droplet precautions on the nursing care plan and as otherwise indicated by your facility. Document initiation and maintenance of the precautions, the patient's tolerance of the procedure, and patient or family teaching. Also document the date droplet precautions were discontinued.

Drug implants

A method of advanced drug delivery involves implanting drugs beneath the skin—subdermally or subcutaneously—as well as targeting specific tissues with radiation implants.

With subdermal implants, flexible capsules are placed under the skin. Small Silastic capsules are placed under the skin of the patient's upper arm, and the drug then diffuses through the capsule walls continuously.

With subcutaneous implants, drug pellets are injected into the skin's subcutaneous layer. The drug is then stored in one area of the body, called a depot. A treatment for prostate cancer cells calls for implants of goserelin, a synthetic form of luteinizing hormone. By inhibiting pituitary gland secretion, goserelin implants reduce testosterone levels to those previously achieved only through castration. This reduction causes tumor regression and suppression of symptoms.

Radiation drug implants with a short half-life may be placed inside a body cavity, within a tumor or on its surface, or in the area from which a tumor has been removed. Implants that contain iodine 125 are used for lung and prostate tumors; gold 198, for oral and ocular tumors; and radium 226 and cesium 137, for tongue, lip, and skin therapy. These implants are usually inserted by a physician with a nurse assisting. Some specially trained nurses may insert or inject intradermal implants. Radiation implants are usually put in place in an operating room or a radiation oncology suite.

Equipment

Subdermal implants

Sterile surgical drapes ♦ sterile gloves ♦ antiseptic solution ♦ local anesthetic ♦ set of implants ♦ needles ♦ 5-ml syringe ♦ #11 scalpel ♦ #10 trocar ♦ forceps ♦ sutures ♦ sterile gauze ♦ tape

Subcutaneous implants

Alcohol pad ♦ drug implant in a preloaded syringe ♦ local anesthetic (for some patients)

Radiation implants

RADIATION PRECAUTION sign for the patient's door ♦ warning labels for the patient's wristband and personal belongings ♦ film badge or pocket dosimeter ♦ lead-lined container ♦ long-handled forceps ♦ masking tape ♦ portable lead shield

Key steps

- Explain the procedure and its benefits and risks to the patient, and show her the set of implants.

Inserting subdermal implants

- Assist the patient into a supine position on the examination table. During the procedure, stay and provide support as necessary.

The steps below describe how subdermal implants are inserted:

- Have the patient lie supine on the examination table and flex the elbow of his nondominant arm so that his hand is opposite his head.
- Swab the insertion site with antiseptic solution. (The ideal insertion site is inside the upper arm about 3″ to 4″ [7.5 to 10 cm] above the elbow.)
- Cover the arm above and below the insertion site with sterile surgical drapes.
- The physician fills a 5-ml syringe with a local anesthetic, inserts the needle under the skin, and injects a small amount of anesthetic into several areas, each about 1½″ to 2″ (4 to 5 cm) deep, in a fanlike pattern.
- The physician uses the scalpel to make a small, shallow incision (about 2 mm) through the skin.
- Next, he inserts the tip of the trocar through the incision at a shallow angle beneath the skin. He makes sure the trocar bevel is up so that he can place the capsules in a superficial plane. He advances the trocar slowly to the first mark near the hub of the trocar. The tip of the trocar should now be about 1½″ to 2″ from the incision site. The physician then removes the obturator and loads the first capsule into the trocar.
- He gently advances the capsule with the obturator toward the tip of the trocar until he feels resistance. Next, he inserts each succeeding capsule beside the last one in a fanlike pattern. With the forefinger and middle finger of his free hand, he fixes the position of the previous capsule, advancing the trocar along the tips of his fingers. This ensures a suitable distance of about 15 degrees between capsules and keeps the trocar from puncturing the previously inserted capsules.
- After insertion, he'll remove the trocar and palpate the area. He'll then close the incision and cover it with a dry compress and sterile gauze.

Inserting subcutaneous implants

- Help the patient into the supine position, and drape him so that his abdomen is accessible. Remove the syringe from the package, and make sure you can see the drug in the chamber. Clean a small area on the patient's upper abdominal wall with the alcohol pad.
- As you stretch the skin at the injection site with one hand, grip the needle with the fingers of your other hand around the barrel of the syringe. Insert the needle into subcutaneous fat at a 45-degree angle. Don't attempt to aspirate. If blood appears in the syringe, withdraw the needle and inject a new preloaded syringe and needle at another site.
- Next, change the direction of the needle so that it's parallel to the abdominal wall. With the barrel hub touching the patient's skin, push the needle in. Then withdraw it

about ½″ (1.3 cm) to create a space for the drug. Depress the plunger. Withdraw the needle and bandage the site.

- Inspect the tip of the needle. If you can see the metal tip of the plunger, the drug has been discharged.

Inserting radiation implants

- To prepare for a radiation implant, first place the lead-lined container and long-handled forceps in a corner of the patient's room. With masking tape, mark a safe line on the floor 6′ (2 m) from the bed to warn visitors of the danger of radiation exposure. Place the lead shield in the back of the room to wear when providing care.
- Place an emergency tracheotomy tray in the room if an implant will be inserted in the patient's mouth or neck.
- To insert the implant, the physician makes a small incision in the skin and creates a pocket in the tissue. He inserts the implant and closes the incision. If the patient is being treated for tonsillar cancer, he'll undergo a bronchoscopy, during which radioactive pellets are implanted in tonsillar tissue.
- Your role in the implant procedure is to explain the treatment and its goals to the patient. Review radiation safety procedures and visitation policies. Talk with the patient about long-term physical and emotional aspects of the therapy, and discuss home care.

Special considerations

Special care may be necessary, depending on the type of implant used.

Subdermal implants

- Tell the patient to resume normal activities but to protect the site during the first few days after implantation. Advise her not to bump the insertion site and to keep the area dry and covered with a gauze bandage for 3 days.
- Tell the patient to report signs of bleeding or infection at the insertion site.
- Tell the patient to notify the physician immediately if one of the implanted capsules falls out before the skin heals over the implants.

Subcutaneous implants

- Be aware that if a subcutaneous implant must be removed, a physician will order an X-ray to locate it.
- Tell the patient to check the administration site for signs of infection or bleeding.
- Goserelin implants must be changed every 28 days.

Radiation implants

- Know that if laboratory work is required during treatment, a technician wearing a film badge will obtain the specimen, affix a RADIATION PRECAUTION label to the specimen container, and alert laboratory personnel. If urine tests are needed, ask the radiation oncology department or laboratory technician how to transport the specimens safely.
- Minimize your own exposure to radiation. Wear a personal, nontransferable film badge or dosimeter at waist level during your entire shift. Turn in the film badge regularly. Pocket dosimeters measure immediate exposure.
- Use the three principles of time, distance, and shielding. Time: Plan to give care in the shortest time possible. Less time equals less exposure. Distance: Work as far away from the radiation source as possible. Give care from the side opposite the implant or from a position that allows the greatest working distance possible. Prepare the patient's meal trays outside his room. Shielding: Wear a portable shield, if necessary.
- Make sure that the patient's room is monitored daily by the radiation oncology department and that disposable items are monitored and removed according to your facility's policy.
- Keep away staff members and visitors who are pregnant or trying to conceive or father a child. The gonads and a developing embryo or fetus are highly susceptible to the damaging effects of ionizing radiation.
- If you must take the patient out of his room, notify the appropriate department of the patient's status to allow time for the necessary preparations.
- Collect a dislodged implant with long-handled forceps, and place it in a lead-lined container.

- A patient with a permanent implant may not be released until his radioactivity level is less than 5 millirems per hour at a distance of about 3′ (1 m).
- If a patient with an implant dies while on the unit, notify the radiation oncology staff so that a temporary implant can be properly removed and stored. If the implant was permanent, the staff will also determine which precautions should be followed after postmortem care measures.

Complications

Subdermal implants

- Hyperpigmentation at the insertion site, menstrual irregularities, headache, nervousness, nausea, dizziness, adnexal enlargement, dermatitis, acne, and appetite and weight changes.
- Breast abnormalities, mammographic changes, diabetes, elevated cholesterol or triglyceride levels, hypertension, seizures, and depression

Subcutaneous implants

- Anemia, lethargy, pain, dizziness, insomnia, anxiety, depression, headache, chills, fever, edema, heart failure, arrhythmias, stroke, hypertension, peripheral vascular disease, nausea, vomiting, diarrhea, impotence, renal insufficiency, urinary obstruction, rash, sweating, hot flashes, gout, hyperglycemia, weight increase, and breast swelling and tenderness (from goserelin implants)

Radiation implants

- Implant dislodgment, tissue fibrosis, xerostomia, radiation pneumonitis, airway obstruction, muscle atrophy, sterility, vaginal dryness or stenosis, fistulas, altered bowel habits, diarrhea, hypothyroidism, infection, cystitis, myelosuppression, neurotoxicity, and secondary cancers depending on the implant site and dosage

Patient teaching

- If the patient is being discharged with drug implants, instruct him when to return to have the implants removed.

Documentation

For subdermal and subcutaneous implants, document the name of the drug, insertion or administration site, date and time of insertion, and patient's response to the procedure. Note the date that implants should be removed and a new set inserted or the date of the next administration, as appropriate.

For radiation implants, document radiation precautions taken during treatment, adverse reactions, patient and family teaching and their responses, patient's tolerance of isolation procedures and the family's compliance with procedures, and referrals to local cancer services.

Drug infusion through a secondary I.V. line

A secondary I.V. line is a complete I.V. set—container, tubing, and microdrip or macrodrip system—connected to the lower Y port (secondary port) of a primary line instead of to the I.V. catheter or needle. It can be used for continuous or intermittent drug infusion. When used continuously, a secondary I.V. line permits drug infusion and titration while the primary line maintains a constant total infusion rate.

When used intermittently, a secondary I.V. line is commonly called a *piggyback set.* In this case, the primary line maintains venous access between drug doses. Typically, a piggyback set includes a small I.V. container, short tubing, and a macrodrip system. This set connects to the primary line's upper Y port, also called a *piggyback port.* Antibiotics are most commonly administered by intermittent (piggyback) infusion. To make this set work, the primary I.V. container must be positioned below the piggyback container. (The manufacturer provides an extension hook for this purpose.)

I.V. pumps may be used to maintain constant infusion rates, especially with a drug such as lidocaine. A pump allows more accurate titration of drug dosage and helps maintain venous access because the drug is delivered under sufficient pressure to prevent clot formation in the I.V. cannula.

Equipment

Patient's medication record and chart ♦ prescribed I.V. medication ♦ prescribed I.V. solution ♦ administration set with secondary injection port ♦ needleless adapter ♦ alcohol pads ♦ 1″ adhesive tape ♦ time tape ♦ labels ♦ infusion pump ♦ extension hook and appropriate solution for intermittent piggyback infusion ♦ optional: normal saline solution for infusion with incompatible solutions

For intermittent infusion, the primary line typically has a piggyback port with a backcheck valve that stops the flow from the primary line during drug infusion and returns to the primary flow after infusion. A volume-control set can also be used with an intermittent infusion line.

Preparation

- Verify the order on the patient's medication record by checking it against the practitioner's order.
- Wash your hands.
- Inspect the I.V. container for cracks, leaks, and contamination, and check drug compatibility with the primary solution. Verify the expiration date. Check to see whether the primary line has a secondary injection port. If it doesn't and the medication is to be given regularly, replace the I.V. set with one that has a secondary injection port.
- If necessary, add the drug to the secondary I.V. solution. To do so, remove any seals from the secondary container and wipe the main port with an alcohol pad. Inject the prescribed medication, and gently agitate the solution to mix the medication thoroughly. Properly label the I.V. mixture. Insert the administration set spike and attach the needle. Open the flow clamp and prime the line. Then close the flow clamp.
- Some medications are available in vials that are suitable for hanging directly on an I.V. pole. Instead of preparing medication and injecting it into a container, you can inject diluent directly into the medication vial. Then you can spike the vial, prime the tubing, and hang the set, as directed.

Key steps

- Explain the particular I.V. therapy, its purpose, the procedure, and what drug is being given to the patient.
- Confirm the patient's identity using two patient identifiers according to your facility's policy. If you're hanging an antibiotic, confirm that the patient has no history of an allergic reaction to the drug.
- If the drug is incompatible with the primary I.V. solution, replace the primary solution with a fluid that's compatible with both solutions, such as normal saline solution, and flush the line before starting the drug infusion. Many facility protocols require that the primary I.V. solution be removed and that a sterile I.V. plug be inserted into the container until it's ready to be rehung. This maintains the sterility of the solution and prevents someone else from inadvertently restarting the incompatible solution before the line is flushed with normal saline solution.
- Hang the secondary set's container and wipe the injection port of the primary line with an alcohol pad.
- Insert the needleless adapter from the secondary line into the injection port and secure it to the primary line.
- To run the secondary set's container by itself, lower the primary set's container with an extension hook. To run both containers simultaneously, place them at the same height. (See *Assembling a piggyback set.*)
- Open the clamp and adjust the drip rate. For continuous infusion, set the secondary solution to the desired drip rate; then adjust the primary solution to achieve the desired total infusion rate.
- For intermittent infusion, adjust the primary drip rate, as required, on completion of the secondary solution. If the secondary solution tubing is being reused, close the clamp on the tubing and follow your facility's policy: Either remove the needleless adapter and replace it with a new one, or leave it securely taped in the injection port and label it with the time it was first used. In this case, also leave the empty container

Assembling a piggyback set

A piggyback set is useful for intermittent drug infusion. To work properly, the secondary set's container must be positioned higher than the primary set's container.

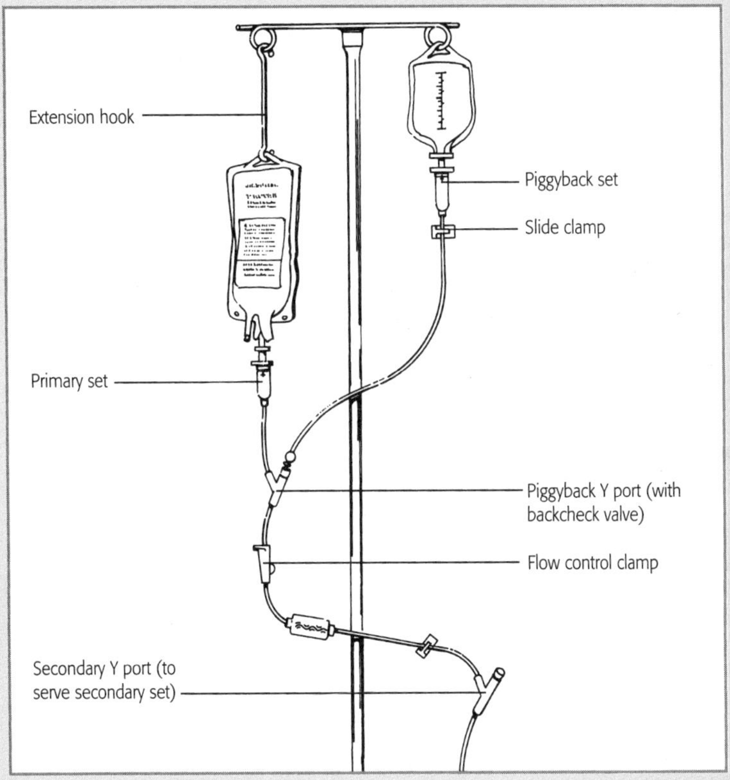

in place until you replace it with a new dose of medication at the prescribed time. If the tubing won't be reused, discard it appropriately with the I.V. container.

Special considerations

- If your facility's policy allows, use a pump for drug infusion. Put a time tape on the secondary container to help prevent an inaccurate administration rate.
- When reusing secondary tubing, change it according to your facility's policy, usually every 48 to 72 hours. Similarly, inspect the injection port for leakage with each use and change it more often if needed.
- Unless you're piggybacking lipids, don't piggyback a secondary I.V. line to a total parenteral nutrition line because of the risk of contamination. Check your facility's policy for possible exceptions.
- After adding a medication to an administration set, the solution should be infused or discarded within a 24-hour period.

Complications

- Adverse reaction to the infused drug
- Leakage or contamination of the secondary injection port from damage to the seal due to repeated punctures

Documentation

Record the amount and type of drug and the amount of I.V. solution on the intake and output and medication records. Note the date, duration and rate of infusion, and the patient's response, when applicable.

Dying patient care

As a patient approaches death, he needs intensive physical support, and he and his family require emotional comfort. Signs and symptoms of impending death include reduced respiratory rate and depth, decreased or absent blood pressure, weak or erratic pulse rate, lowered skin temperature, decreased level of consciousness (LOC), diminished sensorium and neuromuscular control, diaphoresis, pallor, cyanosis, and mottling. Emotional support for the dying patient and his family typically means simple reassurance and the nurse's physical presence to help ease fear and loneliness. More intense emotional support is important at much earlier stages, especially for the patient with a long-term progressive illness, who can work through the stages of dying. (See *Five stages of dying.*)

Respect the patient's wishes about extraordinary means or supporting life. The patient may have signed a living will. This document, legally binding in most states, declares the patient's desire for a death unimpeded by the artificial support of such equipment as defibrillators, respirators, life-sustaining drugs, or auxiliary hearts. Nurses should know if a living will is legal in their state and their facility's policy regarding a signed living will. If the patient has signed such a document, the nurse must respect his wishes and communicate the practitioner's "no code" order to all staff members.

Equipment

Clean bed linens ♦ clean gowns ♦ gloves ♦ water-filled basin ♦ soap ♦ washcloth ♦ towels ♦ lotion ♦ linen-saver pads ♦ petroleum jelly ♦ suction equipment, as necessary ♦ optional: indwelling urinary catheter

Key steps

- Assemble equipment at the patient's bedside, as needed.
- Fully explain all care and treatments to the patient even if he's unconscious because he may still be able to hear. Answer questions as candidly as possible, without sounding callous.

Meeting physical needs

- Take the patient's vital signs often, and observe for pallor, diaphoresis, and decreased LOC.
- Reposition the patient in bed at least every 2 hours because sensation, reflexes, and mobility diminish first in the legs and gradually in the arms. Make sure the bed sheets cover him loosely to reduce discomfort caused by pressure on his arms and legs.
- When the patient's vision and hearing start to fail, turn his head toward the light and speak to him from near the head of the bed. Because hearing may be acute despite loss of consciousness, avoid whispering or speaking inappropriately about the patient in his presence.
- Change the bed linens and the patient's gown as needed. Provide skin care during gown changes, and adjust the room temperature for patient comfort, as necessary.
- Observe for incontinence or anuria, the result of diminished neuromuscular control or decreased renal function. If necessary, obtain an order to catheterize the patient, or place linen-saver pads beneath the patient's buttocks. Put on gloves and provide perineal care with soap, a washcloth, and towels to prevent irritation.
- Suction the patient's mouth and upper airway to remove secretions. Elevate the head of the bed to decrease respiratory resistance. As the patient's condition deteriorates, he may breathe mostly through his mouth.
- Offer fluids frequently, and lubricate the patient's lips and mouth with petroleum jelly to counteract dryness.
- If the comatose patient's eyes are open, provide appropriate eye care to prevent corneal ulceration.
- Provide mouth care for the comatose patient.

Five stages of dying

Elisabeth Kübler-Ross, author of *On Death and Dying,* explained that the dying patient progresses through five psychological stages in preparation for death. Further research has shown that not all patients experience these emotional states in the same order or in the same way. However, knowing about the five stages allows you to more accurately assess the emotional needs of the dying patient.

Denial

The patient refuses to accept the diagnosis. He may experience physical symptoms similar to a stress reaction—shock, fainting, pallor, sweating, tachycardia, nausea, or GI disorders. During this stage, be honest with the patient but not blunt or callous. Maintain communication with him, so he can discuss his feelings when he accepts the reality of death. Don't force the patient to confront this reality.

Anger

When a patient stops denying his impending death, he may show deep resentment toward those who will live on after he dies—you, the facility staff, and his own family. Although you may instinctively draw back from the patient or even resent this behavior, it may help if you understand it as a normal reaction to the loss of control in his life rather than a personal attack. Maintaining a calm manner will help to diffuse the anger and allow you to help him find different ways to express it.

Bargaining

Although the patient acknowledges his impending death, he attempts to bargain for more time with God or fate for more time. He'll probably strike this bargain secretly. If he does confide in you, don't urge him to keep his promises.

Depression

In this stage, the patient may first experience regrets about his past and then grieve about his current condition. He may withdraw from his friends, family, physician, and you. He may suffer from anorexia, increased fatigue, or self-neglect. You may find him sitting alone, in tears. Accept the patient's sorrow, and if he talks to you, listen. Provide comfort by touch, as appropriate. Resist the temptation to make optimistic remarks or cheerful small talk.

Acceptance

In this last stage, the patient accepts the inevitability and imminence of his death—without emotion. The patient may simply desire the quiet company of a family member or friend. If, for some reason, a family member or friend can't be present, stay with the patient to satisfy his final need. Remember, however, that many patients die before reaching this stage.

- Provide ordered pain medication as needed. Keep in mind that, as circulation diminishes, medications given I.M. will be poorly absorbed. Medications should be given I.V., if possible, for optimum results.

Meeting emotional needs

- Allow the patient and his family to express their feelings, which may range from anger to loneliness. Take time to talk with the patient. Sit near the head of the bed, and avoid looking rushed or unconcerned.
- Notify family members, if they're absent, when the patient wishes to see them. Let the patient and his family discuss death at their own pace.
- Offer to contact a member of the clergy or social services department, if appropriate.
- If a living will and advance directives have been completed, make sure that the documents can be easily located. Notify all relevant care providers of their existence

Understanding organ and tissue donation

A federal regulation enacted in 1998 requires health care facilities to report all deaths to the regional organ procurement organization. This regulation was enacted so that no potential donor is missed and the family of every potential donor understands the option to donate. Although organ donor requirements vary, the typical donor must be between the ages of a neonate and 60 and free from transmissible disease. Tissue donations are less restrictive, and some tissue banks will accept skin from donors up to age 75.

According to the American Medical Association, about 25 kinds of organs and tissues are being transplanted. Collection of most organs, such as the heart, liver, kidney, or pancreas, requires that the patient be pronounced brain dead and kept physically alive until the organs are harvested. Tissue such as eyes, skin, bone, and heart valves may be taken after death. Contact your regional organ procurement organization for specific organ donation criteria or to identify a potential donor. If you don't know the regional organ procurement organization in your area, call the United Network for Organ Sharing at (804) 330-8500.

and review them to be sure you understand the patient's wishes.

- If no living will has been executed, provide the patient and significant others with information regarding end-of-life issues. Remember to be sensitive, yet straightforward, taking into account cultural, ethnic, and religious issues for the patient and his family. Respect the patient's or his family's right not to complete advance directives if they choose, and inform them that you won't abandon them or provide substandard care because of their choice.

Special considerations

- If the patient has signed a living will, the practitioner will write a "no code" order on his progress notes and order sheets. Know your state's policy regarding living wills. If living wills are legal, transfer the "no code" order to the patient's chart or Kardex and, at the end of your shift, inform the incoming staff of this order.
- At an appropriate time, ask the patient's family if they have considered organ and tissue donation. Check the patient's records to determine whether he completed an organ donor card. (See *Understanding organ and tissue donation*.)
- If family members remain with the patient, show them the location of bathrooms, lounges, and cafeterias. Explain the patient's needs, treatments, and care plan to them. If appropriate, offer to teach them specific skills so they can take part in nursing care. Emphasize that their efforts are important and effective. As the patient's death approaches, give them emotional support.

Complications

- None known

Documentation

Record changes in the patient's vital signs, intake and output, and LOC. Note the times of cardiac arrest and the end of respiration, and notify the practitioner when these occur.

E

Eardrop instillation

Eardrops may be instilled to treat infection and inflammation, soften cerumen for later removal, produce local anesthesia, or facilitate removal of an insect trapped in the ear by immobilizing and smothering it.

Instillation of eardrops is usually contraindicated if the patient has a perforated eardrum, but it may be permitted with certain medications and adherence to sterile technique. Other conditions may also prohibit instillation of certain medications into the ear. For example, instillation of drops containing hydrocortisone is contraindicated if the patient has herpes, another viral infection, or a fungal infection.

Equipment

Prescribed eardrops ♦ patient's medication record and chart ♦ light source ♦ facial tissue or cotton-tipped applicator ♦ optional: cotton ball, bowl of warm water

Preparation

- Verify the order on the patient's medication record by checking it against the practitioner's order.
- To avoid adverse effects (such as vertigo, nausea, and pain) resulting from instillation of eardrops that are too cold, warm the medication to body temperature in the bowl of warm water or carry it in your pocket for 30 minutes before administration. If necessary, test the temperature of the medication by placing a drop on your wrist. (If the medication is too hot, it may burn the patient's eardrum.)

Key steps

- Wash your hands.
- Confirm the patient's identity using two patient identifiers according to your facility's policy.
- If your facility utilizes a bar code scanning system, be sure to scan your ID badge, the patient's ID bracelet, and the medication's bar code.
- Provide privacy if possible. Explain the procedure to the patient.
- Have the patient lie on the side opposite the affected ear.
- Straighten the patient's ear canal. For an adult, pull the auricle of the ear up and back. For an infant or a child younger than age 3, gently pull the auricle down and back because the ear canal is straighter at this age. (See *Positioning the patient for eardrop instillation,* page 148.)
- Using a light source, examine the ear canal for drainage. If you find any, clean the canal with a tissue or cotton-tipped applicator because drainage can reduce the medication's effectiveness.
- Compare the label on the eardrops with the order on the patient's medication record. Check the label again while drawing the medication into the dropper. Check the label for the final time before returning the eardrops to the shelf or drawer.
- To avoid damaging the ear canal with the dropper, gently support the hand holding the dropper against the patient's head. Straighten the patient's ear canal once again, and instill the ordered number of drops. To avoid patient discomfort, aim the dropper so that the drops fall against the sides of the ear canal, not on the

Positioning the patient for eardrop instillation

Before instilling eardrops, have the patient lie on his side. Then straighten the patient's ear canal to help the medication reach the eardrum. For an adult, gently pull the auricle *up and back;* for an infant or a young child, gently pull *down and back.*

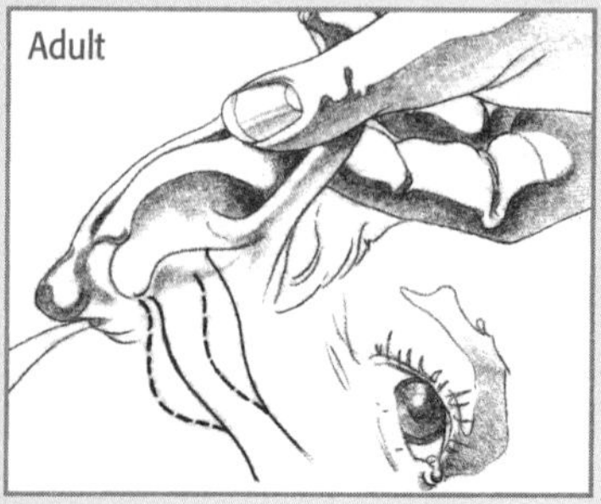

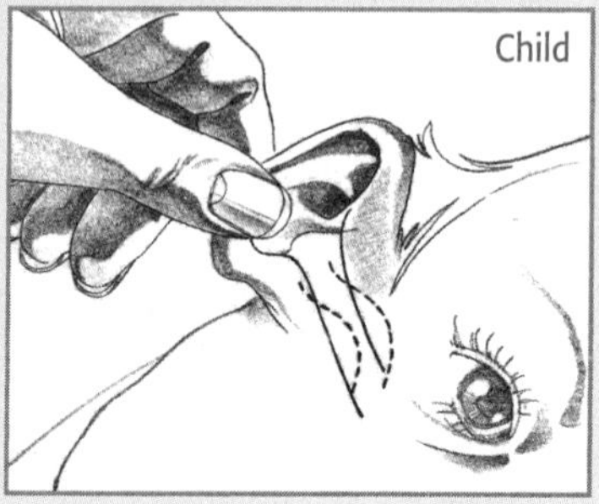

eardrum. Hold the ear canal in position until you see the medication disappear down the canal. Then release the ear.

- Instruct the patient to remain on his side for 5 to 10 minutes to let the medication run down into the ear canal.
- If ordered, tuck the cotton ball loosely into the opening of the ear canal to prevent the medication from leaking out. Be careful not to insert it too deeply into the canal because this would prevent drainage of secretions and increase pressure on the eardrum.
- Clean and dry the outer ear.
- If ordered, repeat the procedure in the other ear after 5 to 10 minutes.
- Assist the patient into a comfortable position.
- Wash your hands.

Special considerations

- Remember that some conditions make the normally tender ear canal even more sensitive, so be especially gentle when performing this procedure. Wash your hands before and after caring for the patient's ear and between caring for each ear.
- To prevent injury to the eardrum, never insert a cotton-tipped applicator into the ear canal past the point where you can see the tip. After applying eardrops to soften the cerumen, irrigate the ear as ordered to facilitate its removal.
- If the patient has vertigo, keep the side rails of his bed up and help him during the procedure as needed. Also, move slowly and unhurriedly to avoid exacerbating his vertigo.
- If both an ointment and drop have been ordered, the drops should be administered first.

Complications

- None known

Patient teaching

- Teach the patient to instill the eardrops correctly so that he can continue treatment at home, if necessary. Review the procedure and let the patient try it himself while you observe.

Documentation

Record the medication used, the ear treated, and the date, time, and number of eardrops instilled. Also document any signs or symptoms that the patient experienced during the procedure, such as drainage, redness, vertigo, nausea, and pain.

Electrocardiography

One of the most valuable and frequently used diagnostic tools, electrocardiography measures the heart's electrical activity as waveforms. Impulses moving through the heart's conduction system create electric currents that can be monitored on the body's surface. Electrodes attached to the skin can detect these electric currents and transmit them to an instrument that produces a record (the electrocardiogram [ECG]) of cardiac activity.

An ECG can be used to identify myocardial ischemia and infarction, rhythm and conduction disturbances, chamber enlargement, electrolyte imbalances, and drug toxicity.

The standard 12-lead ECG uses a series of electrodes placed on the extremities and the chest wall to assess the heart from 12 different views (leads). The 12 leads consist of three standard bipolar limb leads (designated I, II, III), three unipolar augmented leads (aV_R, aV_L, aV_F), and six unipolar precordial leads (V_1 to V_6). The limb leads and augmented leads show the heart from the frontal plane. The precordial leads show the heart from the horizontal plane.

The ECG device measures and averages the differences between the electrical potential of the electrode sites for each lead and graphs them over time. This creates the standard ECG complex, called PQRST. The P wave represents atrial depolarization; the QRS complex, ventricular depolarization; and the T wave, ventricular repolarization. (See *Reviewing ECG waveforms and components,* page 150.)

Variations of the standard ECG include the exercise ECG (stress ECG) and ambulatory ECG (Holter monitoring). The exercise ECG monitors heart rate, blood pressure, and ECG waveforms as the patient walks on a treadmill or pedals a stationary bicycle. For an ambulatory ECG, the patient wears a portable Holter monitor to record heart activity continually over 24 hours.

Today, the ECG is typically accomplished using a multichannel method. All electrodes are attached to the patient at once, and the machine prints a simultaneous view of all leads.

Equipment

ECG machine ♦ recording paper ♦ disposable pregelled electrodes ♦ 4″ × 4″ gauze pads ♦ optional: clippers, marking pen

Preparation

- Place the ECG machine close to the patient's bed, and plug the power cord into the wall outlet.
- If the patient is already connected to a cardiac monitor, remove the electrodes to accommodate the precordial leads and minimize electrical interference on the ECG tracing.
- Keep the patient away from objects that might cause electrical interference, such as equipment, fixtures, and power cords.

Key steps

- Confirm the patient's identity using two patient identifiers according to your facility's policy.
- As you set up the machine to record a 12-lead ECG, explain the procedure to the patient. Tell him that the test records the heart's electrical activity and it may be repeated at certain intervals. Emphasize that no electrical current will enter his body. Also, tell him that the test typically takes about 5 minutes.
- Have the patient lie in a supine position in the center of the bed with his arms at his sides. You may raise the head of the bed to promote his comfort. Expose his arms and legs, and drape him appropriately. His arms and legs should be relaxed to minimize muscle trembling, which can cause electrical interference.
- If the bed is too narrow, place the patient's hands under his buttocks to prevent muscle tension. Also use this technique if the patient is shivering or trembling. Make sure his feet aren't touching the bed board.
- Select flat, fleshy areas to place the electrodes. Avoid muscular and bony areas. If the patient has an amputated limb, choose a site on the stump.
- If an area is excessively hairy, clip it. Clean excess oil or other substances from the skin to enhance electrode contact.
- Peel off the contact paper of the disposable electrodes and apply them directly to

Reviewing ECG waveforms and components

An electrocardiogram (ECG) waveform has three basic components: P wave, QRS complex, and T wave. These elements can be further divided into PR interval, J point, ST segment, U wave, and QT interval.

P wave and PR interval

The P wave represents atrial depolarization. The PR interval represents the time it takes an impulse to travel from the atria through the atrioventricular nodes and bundle of His. The PR interval measures from the beginning of the P wave to the beginning of the QRS complex.

QRS complex

The QRS complex represents ventricular depolarization (the time it takes for the impulse to travel through the bundle branches to the Purkinje fibers). The Q wave appears as the first negative deflection in the QRS complex; the R wave, as the first positive deflection. The S wave appears as the second negative deflection or the first negative deflection after the R wave.

J point and ST segment

Marking the end of the QRS complex, the J point also indicates the beginning of the ST segment. The ST segment represents part of ventricular repolarization.

T wave and U wave

Usually following the same deflection pattern as the P wave, the T wave represents ventricular repolarization. The U wave follows the T wave, but isn't always seen.

QT interval

The QT interval represents ventricular depolarization and repolarization. It extends from the beginning of the QRS complex to the end of the T wave.

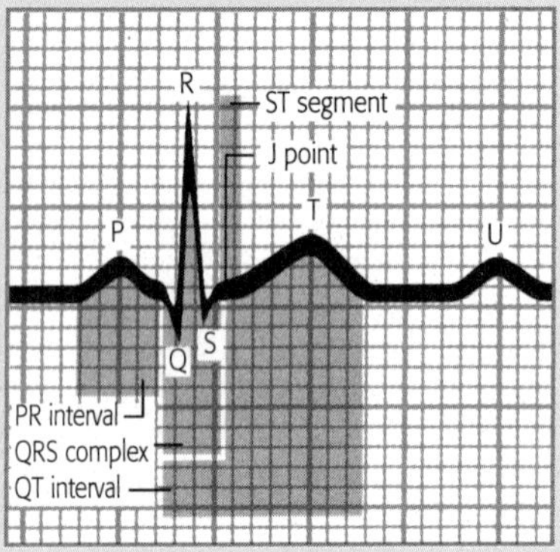

the prepared site, as recommended by the manufacturer's instructions. To guarantee the best connection to the leadwire, position disposable electrodes on the patient's legs with the lead connection pointing superiorly.

- Connect the limb leadwires to the electrodes. Make sure the metal parts of the electrodes are clean and bright. Dirty or corroded electrodes prevent a good electrical connection.
- You'll see that the tip of each leadwire is lettered and color-coded for easy identification. The white or RA leadwire goes to the right arm; the green or RL leadwire, to the right leg; the red or LL leadwire, to the left leg; the black or LA leadwire, to the left arm; and the brown or V_1 to V_6 leadwires, to the chest.
- Expose the patient's chest. Put a small amount of electrode gel or paste on a disposable electrode at each electrode position. (See *Positioning chest electrodes*.)
- If your patient is a woman, be sure to place the chest electrodes below the breast tissue. In a large-breasted woman, you may need to displace the breast tissue laterally.
- Check to see that the paper speed selector is set to the standard 25 mm/second and that the machine is set to full voltage. The machine will record a normal stan-

dardization mark—a square that's the height of two large squares or 10 small squares on the recording paper. Then, if necessary, enter the appropriate patient identification data.

- If any part of the waveform extends beyond the paper when you record the ECG, adjust the normal standardization to half-standardization. Note this adjustment on the ECG strip because this will need to be considered in interpreting the results.
- Now you're ready to begin the recording. Ask the patient to relax and breathe normally. Tell him to lie still and not to talk when you record his ECG. Then press the AUTO button. Observe the tracing quality. The machine will record all 12 leads automatically, recording three consecutive leads simultaneously. Some machines have a display screen so you can preview waveforms before the machine records them on paper.
- When the machine finishes recording the 12-lead ECG, remove the electrodes and clean the patient's skin. After disconnecting the leadwires from the electrodes, dispose of or clean the electrodes, as indicated.
- If serial ECGs are expected, consider marking the electrode positions on the patient's skin. Consistent lead placement enhances the comparison of serial ECGs and eliminates inaccuracy due to lead placement.

Special considerations

- Small areas of hair on the patient's chest or extremities may be clipped, but this usually isn't necessary.
- If the patient's skin is exceptionally oily, scaly, or diaphoretic, rub the electrode site with a dry 4" × 4" gauze or alcohol pad before applying the electrode to help reduce interference in the tracing. During the procedure, ask the patient to breathe normally. If his respirations distort the recording, ask him to hold his breath briefly to reduce baseline wander in the tracing.
- If the patient has a pacemaker, you can perform an ECG with or without a magnet, according to the practitioner's orders. Be sure to note the presence of a pacemaker and the use of the magnet on the strip.

Positioning chest electrodes

To ensure accurate test results, position chest electrodes as follows:

V_1: Fourth intercostal space at right sternal border

V_2: Fourth intercostal space at left sternal border

V_3: Halfway between V_2 and V_4

V_4: Fifth intercostal space at midclavicular line

V_5: Fifth intercostal space at anterior axillary line (halfway between V and V_6)

V_6: Fifth intercostal space at midaxillary line, level with V_4

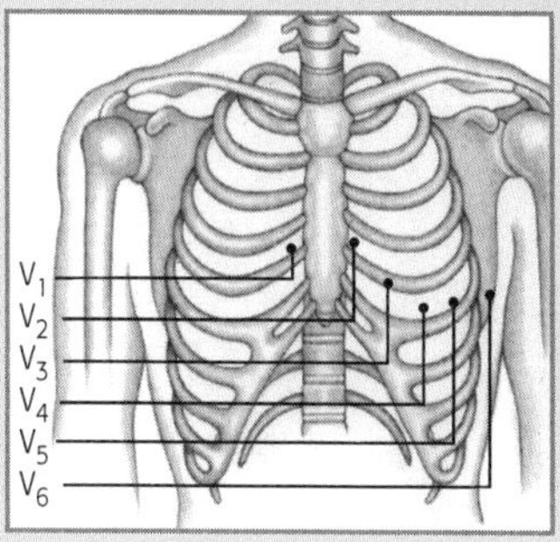

Complications

- None known

Documentation

Label the ECG recording with the patient's name, room number, and facility identification number. Document in your notes the test's date and time as well as significant responses by the patient as well. Note any appropriate clinical information on the ECG.

Electrocardiography, posterior chest lead

Because of the location of the heart's posterior surface, changes associated with myocardial damage aren't apparent on a standard 12-lead electrocardiogram (ECG). To

Placing electrodes for posterior ECG

To ensure an accurate electrocardiogram (ECG) reading, make sure the posterior electrodes V_7, V_8, and V_9 are placed at the same level horizontally as the V_6 lead at the fifth intercostal space. Place lead V_7 at the posterior axillary line, lead V_9 at the paraspinal line, and lead V_8 halfway between leads V_7 and V_9.

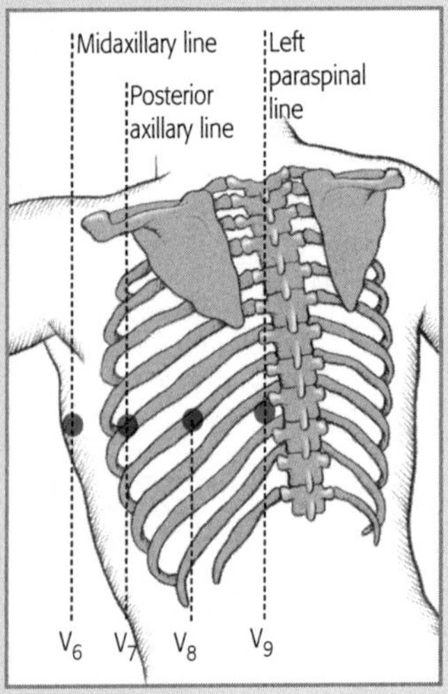

help identify posterior involvement, some practitioners recommend adding posterior leads to the 12-lead ECG. Despite lung and muscle barriers, posterior leads may provide clues to posterior wall infarction so that appropriate treatment can begin.

Usually, the posterior lead ECG is performed with a standard ECG and only involves recording the additional posterior leads: V_7, V_8, and V_9.

Equipment

Multichannel ECG machine with recording paper ♦ disposable pregelled electrodes ♦ 4″ × 4″ gauze pads ♦ optional: electric clippers

Key steps

- Confirm the patient's identity using two patient identifiers according to your facility's policy.
- Prepare the electrode sites according to the manufacturer's instructions. To ensure good skin contact, clip the site if the patient has considerable back hair.
- These leads are placed opposite the anterior leads, V_4, V_5, and V_7, on the left side of the patient's back, following the same horizontal line. Begin by attaching a disposable electrode to the lead V_7 position on the left posterior midaxillary line at the same horizontal level as lead V_6 at the fifth intercostal space. Then attach the V_4 leadwire to the V_7 electrode.
- Next, attach a disposable electrode to the patient's back at the V_8 position on the left midscapular line, fifth intercostal space, and attach the V_8 leadwire to this electrode.
- Finally, attach a disposable electrode to the patient's back at the V_9 position, just left of the spinal column at the fifth intercostal space. Then attach the V_6 leadwire to the V_9 electrode. (See *Placing electrodes for posterior ECG*.)
- Turn on the machine and make sure the paper speed is set for 25 mm/second. If necessary, standardize the machine. Press AUTO and the machine will record.
- When the ECG is complete, remove the electrodes and clean the patient's skin with a gauze pad or moist cloth. If you think you may need more than one posterior lead ECG, use a marking pen to mark the electrode sites on his skin to permit accurate comparison for future tracings.

Special considerations

- The number of leads may vary according to the cardiologist's preference. (If right posterior leads are requested, position the patient on his left side. These leads, known as V_{7R}, V_{8R}, and V_{9R}, are located at the same landmarks on the right side of the patient's back.)

DEVICE SAFETY

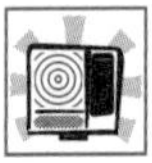

Some ECG machines won't operate unless you connect all leadwires. In that case, you may need to connect the limb leadwires and the leadwires for V_1, V_2, and V_3.

Complications

- None known

Documentation

Document the procedure in your nurse's notes. Make sure the patient's name, age, room number, time, date, and practitioner's name are clearly written on the ECG along with the relabeled lead tracings. Document any patient teaching you may have performed as well as the patient's tolerance to the procedure.

Electrocardiography, right chest lead

Unlike a standard 12-lead electrocardiogram (ECG), used primarily to evaluate left ventricular function, a right chest lead ECG reflects right ventricular function and provides clues to damage or dysfunction in this chamber.

Right ventricular infarction should be suspected in the patient with acute inferior wall myocardial infarction (MI). Between 25% and 50% of patients with this type of MI have right ventricular involvement.

Early identification of a right ventricular infarction is essential because it's associated with significant morbidity and mortality. An ST-segment elevation of 1 mm or more in the right precordial lead V_{4R} indicates a right ventricular MI.

Treatment for this condition differs from other types of MI. Instead of judiciously hydrating the patient to prevent heart failure, the patient requires I.V. fluids administration to maintain adequate filling pressures on the right side of the heart. This helps the right ventricle eject an adequate volume of blood at a sufficient pressure and supports left ventricular filling.

If a right chest lead ECG isn't routinely performed at your facility, consider the need for this test in the patient with an inferior wall MI who shows signs of poor left ventricular output and clear lung sounds on auscultation.

Equipment

Multichannel ECG machine ♦ paper ♦ pregelled disposable electrodes ♦ several 4″ × 4″ gauze pads

Key steps

- Confirm the patient's identity using two patient identifiers according to your facility's policy.
- Take the equipment to the patient's bedside, and explain the procedure to him. Inform him that the practitioner has ordered a right chest lead ECG, a procedure that involves placing electrodes on his wrists, ankles, and chest and that the gel may feel cold. Reassure him that the test is painless and takes only a few minutes, during which he'll need to lie quietly on his back.
- Tell the patient to lie still, relax, not talk, and breathe normally.
- Make sure the paper speed is set at 25 mm/second and the amplitude at 1 mV/10 mm.
- Place the patient in a supine position or, if he has difficulty lying flat, in semi-Fowler's position. Provide privacy and expose his arms, chest, and legs. (Cover a female patient's chest with a drape until you apply the chest leads.)
- Examine the patient's wrists and ankles for the best areas to place the electrodes. Choose flat and fleshy (not bony or muscular), hairless areas such as the inner aspects of the wrists and ankles. Clean the sites with the gauze pads to promote good skin contact.
- Connect the leadwires to the electrodes. The leadwires are color-coded and lettered. Place the white or right arm (RA) wire on the right arm; the black or left arm (LA) wire on the left arm; the green or right leg (RL) wire on the right leg; and the red or left leg (LL) wire on the left leg.
- Then examine the patient's chest to locate the correct sites for chest lead placement (as shown top of next page). If the patient is a woman, place the electrodes under the breast tissue.

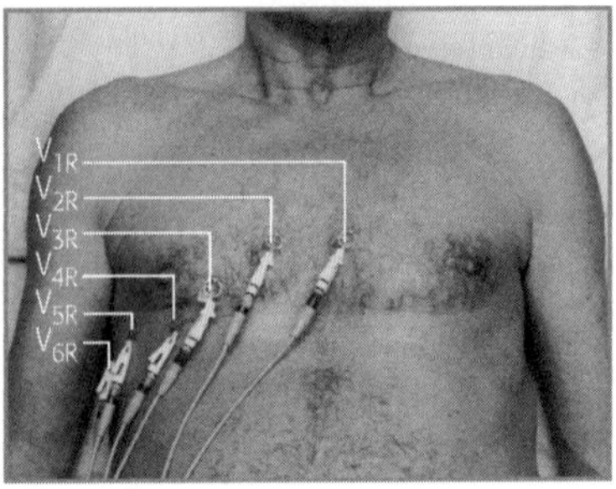

- Use your fingers to feel between the patient's ribs (the intercostal spaces). Start at the second intercostal space on the left (the notch felt at the top of the sternum, where the manubrium joins the body of the sternum). Count down two spaces to the fourth intercostal space. Then apply a disposable electrode to the site and attach leadwire V_{1R} to that electrode.
- Move your fingers across the sternum to the fourth intercostal space on the right side of the sternum. Apply a disposable electrode to that site and attach lead V_{2R}.
- Move your finger down to the fifth intercostal space and over to the midclavicular line. Place a disposable electrode here and attach lead V_{4R}.
- Visually draw a line between V_{2R} and V_{4R}. Apply a disposable electrode midway on this line and attach lead V_{3R}.
- Move your finger horizontally from V_{4R} to the right midaxillary line. Apply a disposable electrode to this site and attach lead V_{6R}.
- Move your fingers along the same horizontal line to the midpoint between V_{4R} and V_{6R}. This is the right anterior midaxillary line. Apply a disposable electrode to this site and attach lead V_{5R}.
- Turn on the ECG machine. Ask the patient to breathe normally but to refrain from talking during the recording so that muscle movement won't distort the tracing. Enter any appropriate patient information required by the machine you're using. If necessary, standardize the machine. This will cause a square tracing of 10 mm (two large squares) to appear on the ECG paper when the machine is set for 1 mV (1 mV = 10 mm).
- Press the AUTO key. The ECG machine will record all 12 leads automatically. Check your facility's policy for the number of readings to obtain. (Some facilities require at least two ECGs so that one copy can be sent out for interpretation while the other remains at the bedside.)
- When you're finished recording the ECG, turn off the machine. Clearly label the ECG with the patient's name, the date, and the time. Also label the tracing "Right chest ECG" to distinguish it from a standard 12-lead ECG. Remove the electrodes and help the patient get comfortable.
- If serial right-chest lead ECGs are anticipated, consider marking the electrode sites on the patient's skin to facilitate consistent lead placement.

Special considerations

- For best results, place the electrodes symmetrically on the limbs. If the patient's wrist or ankle is covered by a dressing, or if the patient is an amputee, choose an area that's available on both sides.

Complications

- None known

Documentation

Document the procedure in your nurse's notes, and document the patient's tolerance to the procedure. Place a copy of the tracing on the patient's chart.

Electrocardiography, signal-averaged

Signal-averaged electrocardiography helps to identify the patient at risk for sustained ventricular tachycardia. Because this cardiac arrhythmia can be a precursor of sudden death after a myocardial infarction (MI), the results of signal-averaged electrocardiography can allow appropriate preventive measures.

Through a computer-based electrocardiogram (ECG), signal averaging detects low-amplitude signals or late electrical potentials, which reflect slow conduction or disorganized ventricular activity through abnormal or infarcted regions of the ventricles. The signal-averaged ECG is developed by recording the noise-free surface ECG in three specialized leads for several hundred beats.

Signal averaging enhances signals that would otherwise be missed because of increased amplitude and sensitivity to ventricular activity. For example, on the standard 12-lead ECG, "noise" created by muscle tissue, electronic artifacts, and electrodes masks late potentials, which have a low amplitude.

This procedure identifies the risk for sustained ventricular tachycardia in patients with malignant ventricular tachycardia, a history of MI, unexplained syncope, nonischemic congestive cardiomyopathy, or nonsustained ventricular tachycardia.

Equipment

Signal-averaged ECG machine ♦ signal-averaged computer ♦ record of patient's surface ECG for 200 to 300 QRS complexes ♦ three bipolar electrodes or leads ♦ alcohol pads ♦ clippers

Key steps

- Confirm the patient's identity using two patient identifiers according to your facility's policy.
- Inform the patient that this procedure will take 10 to 30 minutes and will help the practitioner determine his risk for a certain type of arrhythmia. If appropriate, mention that it may be done along with other tests, such as echocardiography, Holter monitoring, and a stress test.
- Place the patient in the supine position, and tell him to lie as still as possible. Tell him he shouldn't speak and should breathe normally during the procedure.
- If the patient has hair on his chest, clip the hair, then rub the patient's chest with alcohol and dry it before placing the electrodes on it.
- Place the leads in the X, Y, and Z orthogonal positions. (See *Placing electrodes for signal-averaged ECG.*)
- The ECG machine gathers input from these leads and amplifies, filters, and samples the signals. The computer collects and stores data for analysis. The crucial values are those showing QRS complex duration, duration of the portion of the QRS complex with an amplitude under 40 microvolts, and the root mean square voltage of the last 40 msec.

Special considerations

- Because muscle movements may cause a false-positive result, patients who are rest-

Placing electrodes for signal-averaged ECG

To prepare your patient for a signal-averaged electrocardiogram (ECG), place the electrodes in the X, Y, and Z orthogonal positions (as shown). These positions bisect one another to provide a three-dimensional, composite view of ventricular activation.

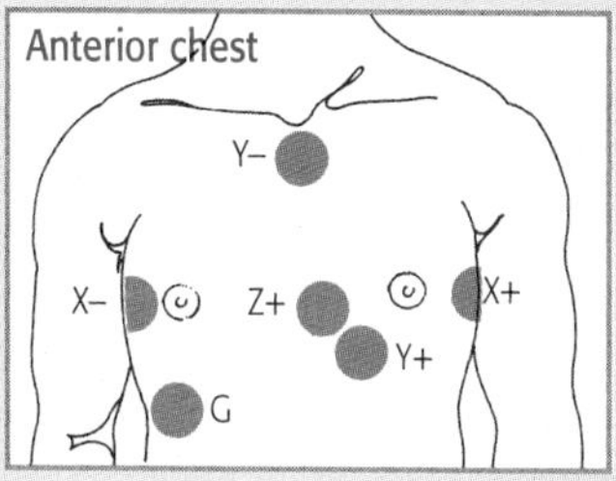

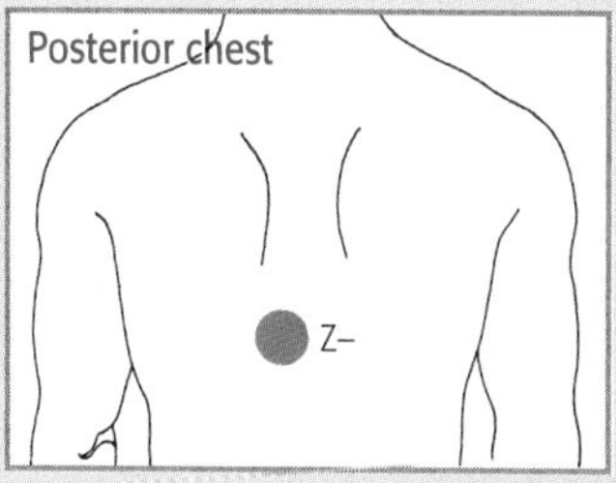

KEY

X+ Fourth intercostal space, midaxillary line, left side

X– Fourth intercostal space, midaxillary line, right side

Y+ Standard V_3 position (or proximal left leg)

Y– Superior aspect of manubrium

Z+ Standard V_2 position

Z– V_2 position, posterior

G Ground; eighth rib on right side

less or in respiratory distress are poor candidates for a signal-averaged ECG. Proper electrode placement and skin preparation are essential to this procedure.

- Results indicating low-amplitude signals include a QRS complex duration greater than 110 msec; a duration of more than 40 msec for the amplitude portion under 40 μV; and a root mean square voltage of less than 25 μV during the last 40 msec of the QRS complex. However, all three factors need not be present to consider the result positive or negative. The final interpretation hinges on individualized patient factors.
- Results of a signal-averaged ECG help the practitioner determine whether the patient is a candidate for invasive procedures, such as electrophysiologic testing or angiography.
- Keep in mind that the significance of a signal-averaged ECG results in patients with bundle-branch heart block is unknown because myocardial activation doesn't follow the usual sequence in these patients.

Complications

- None known

Documentation

Document the time of the procedure, why the procedure was done, and how the patient tolerated it.

Electroconvulsive therapy

In electroconvulsive therapy (ECT), an electric shock is delivered to the patient's brain by way of electrodes placed on his temples. Electrodes may be placed bilaterally or unilaterally. ECT is an effective way to treat patients with affective disorders and selected schizophrenias or related psychoses.

A physician is primarily responsible for administering ECT, but safe and effective therapy requires an interdisciplinary approach and cooperation. The nurse's role is to provide care during the assessment, preparation, treatment, and recovery. The treatment team also includes a certified registered nurse-anesthetist (CRNA) and, possibly, a nurse practitioner (NP).

The physician's role is to obtain appropriate consent, order pretreatment and posttreatment regimens, titrate drug doses, administer treatment, and determine when the patient may be released from the post-ECT recovery unit. The CRNA is responsible for ensuring a patent airway, administering positive pressure oxygen during the treatment and until the patient is breathing well on his own, and administering specific drugs during the procedure. If an NP is part of the team, she's responsible for making sure all equipment, drugs, and emergency equipment are available, preparing the patient by attaching electrocardiogram (ECG) and EEG monitors, explaining the procedure to the patient, and completing a preprocedure assessment.

Equipment

EEG/ECG machine ♦ five connection wires (three ECG and two EEG) ♦ rubber headband ♦ two stimulus electrodes ♦ conduction gel ♦ ECG monitor and disposable ECG electrodes ♦ crash cart with emergency drug kit and defibrillator ♦ suction machine with sterile pharyngeal catheters ♦ endotracheal intubation tray ♦ rubber mouthpiece ♦ electronic blood pressure monitor ♦ oxygen source and tubing with positive pressure equipment ♦ two pairs of gloves ♦ alcohol pads ♦ 21G needles ♦ butterfly infusion set ♦ sterile 3-cc, 5-cc, and 10-cc syringes ♦ methohexital ♦ succinylcholine (Anectine) ♦ glycopyrrolate (Robinul) ♦ dantrolene (Dantrium) ♦ tape ♦ sterile water or normal saline solution for injection ♦ tourniquet ♦ patient's medical record ♦ documentation records ♦ stretcher ♦ optional: protective equipment such as gloves, gowns, masks, and eye protectors

Preparation

- Plug the EEG/ECG machine into a 120-volt wall socket. Plug the stimulus output electrode leads into the machine's outlet, marked STIMULUS OUTPUT. Plug the stimulus monitor electrode leads into the machine's receptacle, labeled PATIENT MONITOR INPUT, which monitors the EEG and ECG.

- Check the dual channel chart recorder to ensure that it's properly loaded with heat sensitive graph paper. The paper will show a red warning line when a new roll of paper is needed.
- Press the master power switch to activate the display panels and chart recorder. The panel switches light up when the power switch is pressed.
- Briefly turn on the chart recorder using the manual switch to advance the paper to ensure that the machine is working properly.
- Set the treatment parameters as ordered for pulse width (ms), frequency (Hz), duration (sec), and current (amp). These parameters represent the total volume of electrical stimulus applied, which differs depending on the patient's age, medication use, seizure threshold, and other factors.
- Plug in the electronic blood pressure monitor.
- Make sure the crash cart, with emergency drug kit, defibrillator, suction equipment, an endotracheal intubation tray, and oxygen is readily available and that needed medications are properly prepared. (See *Preparing medications for ECT,* page 158.)

Key steps

- Check the order.
- Gather the appropriate equipment.
- After arrival in the ECT room, identify the patient and check his nothing-by-mouth status.
- Explain the procedure to the patient to allay his anxiety.
- Make sure the physician has obtained a signed informed consent form.
- Make sure the patient's history (including allergies to medications or latex), physical examination, and dental evaluation are documented in his chart.
- Make sure the following diagnostic tests have been completed and assessed: complete blood count, thyroid profile, urinalysis, ECG, pseudocholinesterase activity determination (especially in patients with severe liver disease, malnutrition, or a history of sensitivity to muscle relaxants or similar substances), chest X-ray, spine radiographs, EEG, and cranial computed tomography scan.
- Wash your hands and put on gloves. Help the patient remove dentures, partial plates, or other foreign objects from his mouth to prevent choking.
- Remove and dispose of gloves.
- Make sure the patient removes all jewelry, metal objects, and prosthetic devices before the procedure to prevent injury.
- Have the patient dress in a hospital gown and ask him to void to prevent incontinence during the procedure.
- Help the patient onto the stretcher.
- Put on gloves, attach the patient to an electronic blood pressure monitor, and check his baseline vital signs.
- Attach the patient to a pulse oximeter to monitor his respiratory status during the procedure because the drugs used cause respiratory depression.
- Insert an I.V. catheter using sterile technique.
- Attach the patient to the ECG monitor.
- Attach the EEG electrodes and stimulus electrodes to the rubber headband. Coat the electrodes with conduction gel and place the band around the patient's head. Place the large, silver-colored stimulus electrodes on each temple at about eye-level. Space the small, brown-colored EEG electrodes across the forehead.
- Connect the stimulus electrodes to the stimulus output receptacle on the machine.
- Run the EEG/ECG machine in the self-test mode. When the machine is ready, it displays the message "Self Test Passed" and prints the date, time, treatment parameters, a brief ECG strip, and EEG monitors.
- The CRNA or physician will then administer glycopyrrolate, followed by methohexital. Methohexital acts very rapidly. Expect an abrupt loss of consciousness when the appropriate dose is infused.
- After the patient is unconscious, succinylcholine is administered. A tremor or fasciculation of various muscle groups occurs due to the depolarizing effect of this drug. Succinylcholine also causes complete flaccid paralysis, so mechanical ventilation is started at this time. A rubber mouth-

Preparing medications for ECT

Even though the physician or certified registered nurse-anesthetist administers medications during electroconvulsive therapy (ECT), you should become familiar with the medications that can be used so you can assess the patient for adverse effects. Brief descriptions of the most commonly used drugs are provided here.

Drug	Actions	Adverse effects
Dantrolene (Dantrium)	Dantrolene is a direct-acting skeletal muscle relaxant that's effective against malignant hyperthermia.	▪ Seizures ▪ Muscle weakness ▪ Drowsiness ▪ Fatigue ▪ Headache ▪ Hepatitis ▪ Nervousness ▪ Insomnia
Glycopyrrolate (Robinul)	Glycopyrrolate has desirable cholinergic blocking effects because it reduces secretions in the respiratory system as well as oral and gastric secretions. It also prevents a drop in heart rate caused by vagal nerve stimulation during anesthesia.	▪ Dilated pupils ▪ Tachycardia ▪ Urine retention ▪ Anaphylaxis ▪ Confusion (in elderly patients) ▪ Dry mouth
Methohexital	Methohexital is a rapid, ultra-short-acting barbiturate anesthetic agent.	▪ Hypotension ▪ Tachycardia ▪ Respiratory arrest ▪ Bronchospasm ▪ Anxiety ▪ Hypersensitivity reaction ▪ Emergence delirium
Succinylcholine (Anectine)	Succinylcholine is an ultra-short-acting depolarizing skeletal muscle relaxant. Given I.V., it causes rapid, flaccid paralysis.	▪ Bradycardia ▪ Arrhythmias ▪ Cardiac arrest ▪ Prolonged respiratory depression ▪ Malignant hyperthermia ▪ Anaphylaxis

piece is inserted and positive pressure oxygen is given.

- The physician initiates the stimulus, and mild seizure like activity occurs for about 30 seconds. The patient's jaw and extremities must be supported while avoiding contact with metal.
- Monitor vital signs as well as ECG and EEG rhythm strips. Assess the patient's skin for burns.
- When spontaneous ventilation returns, usually in 3 to 5 minutes, discontinue the I.V. infusion. Continue to monitor vital signs.

- As the patient becomes more alert, speak quietly and explain what's happening. Remove the rubber mouthpiece.
- Place the patient on his side to maintain a patent airway. Measure and document his vital signs every 15 minutes until they stabilize.
- Discharge the patient from the recovery area when he's able to move all four extremities voluntarily, can breathe and cough adequately, is roused and oriented when called, has an Aldrete score of 7 or greater, has stable vital signs and temperature within 1° F (0.6° C) of the pretreatment value, and has a normal swallowing reflex. A physician's order is required to release the patient from the recovery area.
- One hour after treatment, obtain and record the patient's vital signs. Check the patient's temperature to assess for malignant hyperthermia. Then continue to check vital signs every hour as necessary until stable.

Special considerations

- If the patient is taking benzodiazepines before the procedure, obtain an order to begin tapering and discontinue the drugs 3 to 4 days before the procedure. Benzodiazepines (such as lorazepam [Ativan]) and anticonvulsant drugs (such as phenytoin [Dilantin]) negatively affect the patient's response to treatment.
- Contraindications to ECT include brain tumors, space-occupying lesions, and other brain diseases that cause increased intracranial pressure. The seriousness of any physical illness, such as heart, liver, or kidney disease as well as that of the psychiatric disorder, must be weighed against each other before ECT is initiated.

ACTION STAT!

Malignant hyperthermia is an uncommon but potentially life-threatening complication that can follow the administration of anesthetic agents or depolarizing muscle relaxant such as succinylcholine. An oral temperature above 100° F (37.8° C) within 1 hour after treatment should be reported to the physician immediately. Malignant hyperthermia is a medical emergency that requires multiple personnel to care for the patient and administer dantrolene (Dantrium) to treat the disorder. Follow your facility's policy and procedure for a malignant hyperthermia crisis.

Complications

- None known

Documentation

Document using flow sheets or progress notes. Include the patient's vital signs and responses during the treatment sequence, recovery, and post-recovery. Assess and document the patient's physical and mental status and any behavioral changes or lack of such changes.

Endotracheal drug administration

When an I.V. line isn't readily available, drugs can be administered into the respiratory system through an endotracheal (ET) tube. This route allows uninterrupted resuscitation efforts and can save precious moments in an emergency while waiting for venous access. This route also avoids complications from direct cardiac administration of drugs, such as cardiac tamponade, pneumothorax, and coronary artery laceration.

Drugs given endotracheally usually have a longer duration of action than when given I.V. because they're absorbed in the alveoli. For this reason, repeat doses and continuous infusions must be adjusted to prevent adverse effects.

Epinephrine, lidocaine, atropine, naloxone (Narcan), and vasopressin (Pitressin) can be absorbed via the trachea, I.V. route, or intraosseous route, which is preferred. The American Heart Association recommends administering all ET medication at 2 to 2½ times the recommended I.V. dose.

In an emergency, a physician, a critical care nurse, or an emergency medical technician usually administers these drugs. Although guidelines may vary, depending on state, county, or city regulations, the basic

Administering ET drugs

In an emergency, some drugs may be given through an endotracheal (ET) tube if I.V. access isn't available. The syringe method or the adapter method may be used.

Before injecting any drug, use your stethoscope to check for proper placement of the ET tube. Make sure the patient is supine and that her head is level with or slightly higher than her trunk.

Syringe method

Remove the needle before injecting medication into the ET tube. Insert the tip of the syringe into the ET tube, and inject the drug deep into the tube (as shown below).

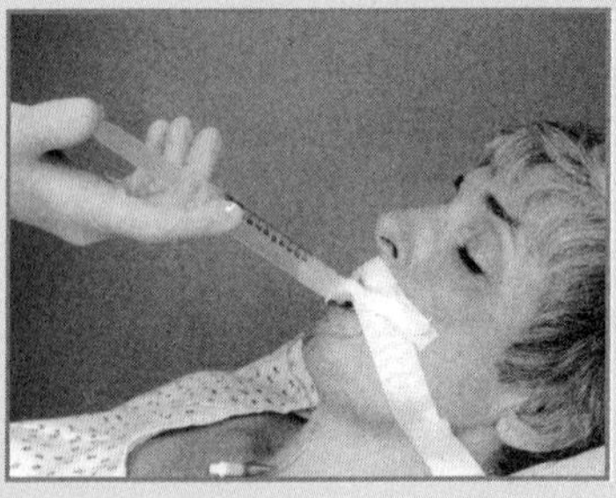

Adapter method

A device developed for ET drug administration provides a more closed system of drug delivery than the syringe method. A special adapter placed on the end of the ET tube (as shown below) allows insertion and drug delivery through the closed stopcock.

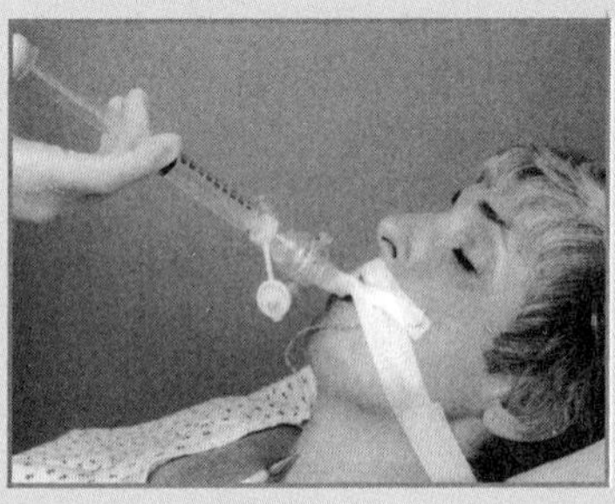

administration method is the same. (See *Administering ET drugs*.)

ET drugs may be given using the syringe method or adapter method. Usually used for bronchoscopy suctioning, the swivel adapter can be placed on the end of the ET tube and, while ventilation continues through a bag-valve device, the drug can be delivered through the closed stopcock.

Equipment

ET tube or swivel adapter ♦ gloves ♦ carbon dioxide (CO_2) detector or an esophageal detector device ♦ handheld resuscitation bag ♦ prescribed drug ♦ syringe or adapter ♦ sterile water or normal saline solution

Preparation

- Verify the order on the patient's medication record by checking it against the prescriber's order. Wash your hands. Check ET tube placement by using an exhaled CO_2 detector or an esophageal detector device.
- Calculate the drug dose. Adult advanced cardiac life support guidelines recommend that the drugs be administered at 2 to 2½ times the recommended I.V. dose. Next, draw the drug up into a syringe. Dilute the dose in 5 to 10 ml of distilled water or normal saline solution. Dilution increases drug volume and contact with the lung.

Key steps

- Put on gloves.
- Move the patient into the supine position, and make sure that his head is level with or slightly higher than his trunk.
- Ventilate the patient three to five times with the resuscitation bag, and then remove the bag.
- Remove the needle from the syringe and insert the tip of the syringe into the ET

tube or swivel adapter. Inject the drug deep into the tube.

- After injecting the drug, reattach the resuscitation bag and ventilate the patient briskly to propel the drug into the lungs, oxygenate the patient, and clear the tube.
- Discard the syringe in the sharps container.
- Remove and discard your gloves.

Special considerations

- Be aware that the drug's onset of action may be quicker than it would be by I.V. administration.
- If the patient doesn't respond quickly, the prescriber may order a repeat dose.

Complications

- Vary, depending on the drug administered

Documentation

Record the date and time of the drug administered and the patient's response.

Endotracheal intubation

Endotracheal (ET) intubation involves the oral or nasal insertion of a flexible tube through the larynx into the trachea for the purpose of controlling the airway and mechanically ventilating the patient. Performed by a physician, anesthetist, respiratory therapist, or nurse educated in the procedure, ET intubation usually occurs in emergencies, such as cardiopulmonary arrest, or in diseases such as epiglottiditis. However, intubation may also occur under more controlled circumstances such as just before surgery. In such instances, ET intubation requires patient teaching and preparation.

Advantages of ET intubation include establishing and maintaining a patent airway, protecting against aspiration by sealing off the trachea from the digestive tract, permitting removal of tracheobronchial secretions in the patient who can't cough effectively, and providing a route for mechanical ventilation. Disadvantages include bypassing normal respiratory defenses against infection, reducing cough effectiveness, and preventing the patient from communicating.

Oral ET intubation is contraindicated in the patient with acute cervical spinal injury and degenerative spinal disorders, while nasal intubation is contraindicated in the patient with apnea, bleeding disorders, chronic sinusitis, or nasal obstructions.

Equipment

Two ET tubes (one spare) in appropriate size ♦ 10-ml syringe ♦ stethoscope ♦ gloves ♦ lighted laryngoscope with a handle and blades of various sizes, curved and straight ♦ sedative ♦ local anesthetic spray ♦ mucosal vasoconstricting agent (for nasal intubation) ♦ overbed or other table ♦ water-soluble lubricant ♦ adhesive or other strong tape or Velcro tube holder (see *Securing an ET tube,* pages 162 and 163) ♦ compound benzoin tincture ♦ oral airway or bite block (for oral intubation) ♦ suction equipment ♦ handheld resuscitation bag with sterile swivel adapter ♦ humidified oxygen source ♦ optional: prepackaged intubation tray, sterile gauze pad, stylet, Magill forceps, sterile water, sterile basin

Preparation

- Gather the individual supplies, or use a prepackaged intubation tray that typically contains most of the necessary supplies.
- Select an ET tube of the appropriate size—typically, 2.5 to 5.5 mm, uncuffed, for children and 6 to 10 mm, cuffed, for adults. The typical size of an oral tube is 7.5 mm for women and 9 mm for men. Select a slightly smaller tube for nasal intubation.
- Check the light in the laryngoscope by snapping the appropriate-size blade into place; if the bulb doesn't light, replace the batteries or the laryngoscope, whichever is quicker.
- Using sterile technique, open the package containing the ET tube and, if desired, open the other supplies on an overbed table.
- Pour the sterile water into the sterile basin. Then, to ease insertion, lubricate the

Securing an ET tube

Before taping an endotracheal (ET) tube in place, make sure the patient's face is clean, dry, and free of beard stubble. If possible, suction his mouth and dry the tube just before taping. Check the reference mark on the tube to ensure correct placement. After taping, always check for bilateral breath sounds to ensure that the tube hasn't been displaced by manipulation. To tape the tube securely, use one of the following three methods.

Method 1

Cut two 2″ (5.1-cm) strips and two 15″ (38.1-cm) strips of 1″ cloth adhesive tape. Then cut a 13″ (33-cm) slit in one end of each 15″ strip (as shown below).

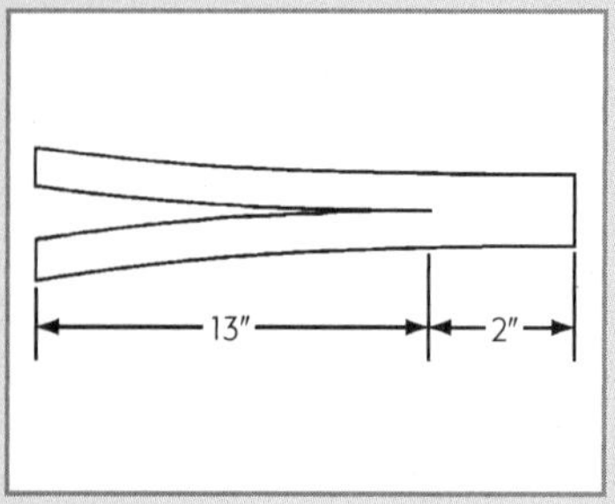

Apply compound benzoin tincture to the patient's cheeks. Place the 2″ strips on his cheeks, creating a new surface on which to anchor the tape securing the tube. If the patient's skin is excoriated or at risk, you can use a transparent semipermeable dressing to protect the skin.

Apply compound benzoin tincture to the tape on the patient's face and to the part of the tube where you will be applying the tape. On the side of the mouth where the tube will be anchored, place the unslit end of the long tape on top of the tape on the patient's cheek.

Wrap the top half of the tape around the tube twice, pulling the tape tightly around the tube. Then, directing the tape over the patient's upper lip, place the end of the tape on his other cheek.

Cut off any excess tape. Use the lower half of the tape to secure an oral airway, if necessary (as shown top of next column).

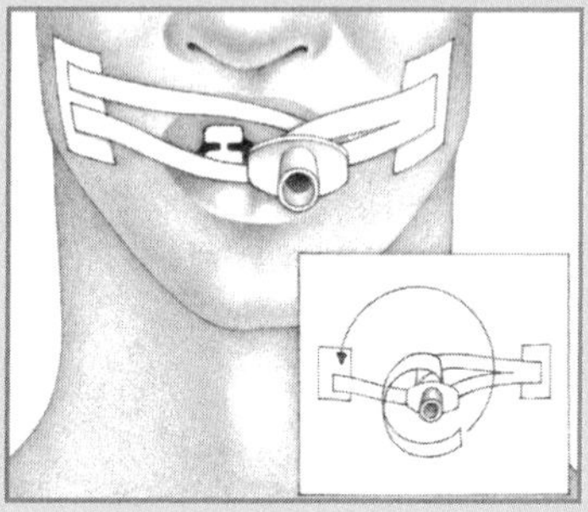

Alternatively, twist the lower half of the tape around the tube twice, and attach it to the original cheek (as shown below).

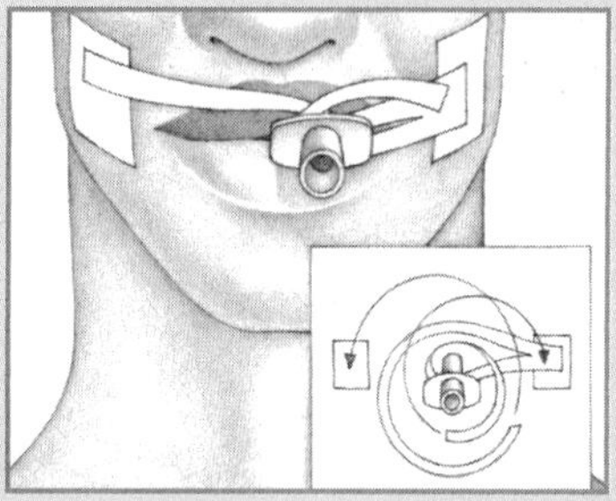

If you've taped in an oral airway or are concerned about the tube's stability, apply the other 15″ strip of tape in the same manner, starting on the other side of the patient's face. If the tape around the tube is too bulky, use only the upper part of the tape and cut off the lower part. If the patient has copious oral secretions, seal the tape by cutting a 1″ piece of paper tape, coating it with compound benzoin tincture, and placing the paper tape over the adhesive tape.

Securing an ET tube *(continued)*

Method 2

Cut one piece of 1" cloth adhesive tape long enough to wrap around the patient's head and overlap in front. Then cut an 8" (20.3-cm) piece of tape and center it on the longer piece, sticky sides together. Next, cut a 5" (12.7-cm) slit in each end of the longer tape (as shown below).

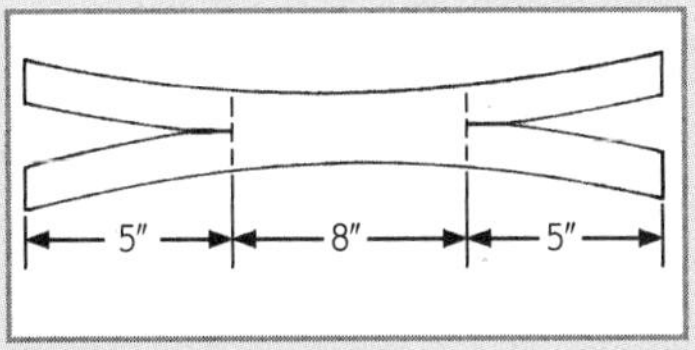

Apply compound benzoin tincture to the patient's cheeks, under his nose, and under lower lip. (Don't spray benzoin directly on the patient's face.)

Place the top half of one end of the tape under the patient's nose and wrap the lower half around the ET tube. Place the lower half of the other end of the tape along his lower lip and wrap the top half around the tube (as shown below).

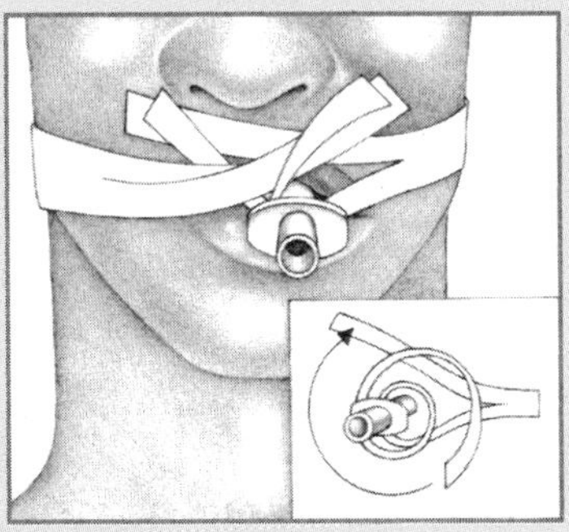

Method 3

Cut a tracheostomy tie in two pieces, one a few inches longer than the other, and cut two 6" (15.2-cm) pieces of 1" cloth adhesive tape. Then cut a 2" (5.1-cm) slit in one end of both pieces of tape. Fold back the other end of the tape ½" (1.3 cm) so that the sticky sides are together, and cut a small hole in it (as shown below).

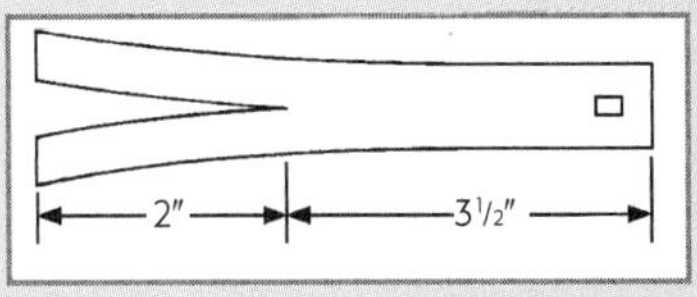

Apply compound benzoin tincture to the part of the ET tube that will be taped. Wrap the split ends of each piece of tape around the tube, one piece on each side. Overlap the tape to secure it.

Apply the free ends of the tape to both sides of the patient's face. Then insert tracheostomy ties through the holes in the tape and knot the ties (as shown below).

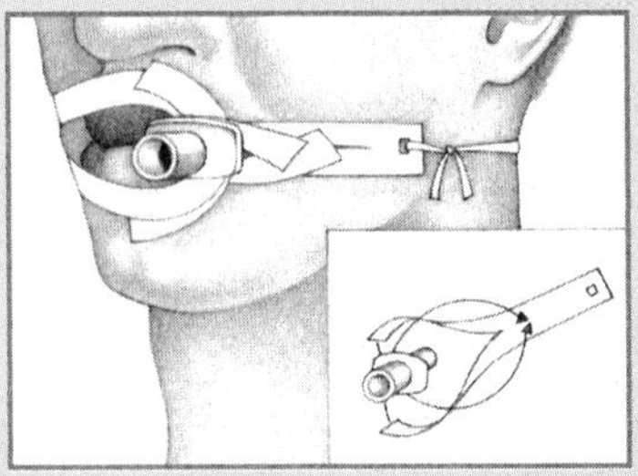

Bring the longer tie behind the patient's neck.

first 1" (2.5 cm) of the distal end of the ET tube with the water-soluble lubricant, using aseptic technique. Do this by squeezing the lubricant directly onto the tube. Use only water-soluble lubricant because it can be absorbed by mucous membranes.

- Attach the syringe to the port on the tube's exterior pilot cuff.
- Slowly inflate the cuff, observing for uniform inflation. If desired, submerge the tube in the sterile water and watch for air bubbles. Use the syringe to deflate the cuff.
- A stylet may be used in oral intubation to stiffen the tube. Lubricate the entire stylet. Insert the stylet into the tube so that its distal tip lies about ½" (1.3 cm) inside the

distal end of the tube. Make sure that the stylet doesn't protrude from the tube to avoid vocal cord trauma.

- Prepare the humidified oxygen source and the suction equipment for immediate use.
- If the patient is in bed, remove the headboard to provide easier access.

Key steps

- Tell the patient that the tube will help him breathe easier and that he'll be given an anesthetic to numb his throat.
- Administer sedatives, as ordered, to induce amnesia or analgesia, and help calm and relax the conscious patient. Remove dentures and bridgework, if present.
- Administer oxygen until the ET tube is inserted to prevent hypoxia.
- Place the patient supine in the sniffing position so that his mouth, pharynx, and trachea are extended. For a blind intubation, place the patient's head and neck in a neutral position.
- Put on gloves.
- For oral intubation, spray a local anesthetic, such as lidocaine (Xylocaine), deep into the posterior pharynx to diminish the gag reflex and reduce patient discomfort. For nasal intubation, spray a local anesthetic and a mucosal vasoconstrictor into the nasal passages to anesthetize the nasal turbinates and reduce the chance of bleeding.
- If necessary, suction the patient's pharynx just before ET tube insertion to improve visualization of the patient's pharynx and vocal cords.
- Time each intubation attempt, limiting attempts to less than 30 seconds to prevent hypoxia.

Intubation with direct visualization

- Stand at the head of the patient's bed. Using your right hand, hold the patient's mouth open by crossing your index finger over your thumb, placing your thumb on the patient's upper teeth and your index finger on his lower teeth. This technique provides greater leverage.
- Grasp the laryngoscope handle in your left hand, and gently slide the blade into the right side of the patient's mouth. Center the blade, and push the patient's tongue to the left. Hold the patient's lower lip away from his teeth to prevent the lip from being traumatized.
- Advance the blade to expose the epiglottis. When using a straight blade, insert the tip under the epiglottis; when using a curved blade, insert the tip between the base of the tongue and the epiglottis.
- Lift the laryngoscope handle upward and away from your body at a 45-degree angle to reveal the vocal cords. Avoid pivoting the laryngoscope against the patient's teeth to avoid damaging them.
- If desired, have an assistant apply pressure to the cricoid ring to occlude the esophagus and minimize gastric regurgitation.
- When performing oral intubation, insert the ET tube into the right side of the patient's mouth. When performing nasotracheal intubation, insert the ET tube through the nostril and into the pharynx. Then use Magill forceps to guide the tube through the vocal cords.
- Guide the tube into the vertical openings of the larynx between the vocal cords, being careful not to mistake the horizontal opening of the esophagus for the larynx. If the vocal cords are closed because of a spasm, wait a few seconds for them to relax, and then gently guide the tube past them to avoid traumatic injury.
- Advance the tube until the cuff disappears beyond the vocal cords. Avoid advancing the tube further to avoid occluding a major bronchus or precipitate lung collapse.
- Holding the ET tube in place, quickly remove the stylet, if present.

Blind nasotracheal intubation

- Pass the ET tube along the floor of the nasal cavity. If necessary, use gentle force to pass the tube through the nasopharynx and into the pharynx.
- Listen and feel for air movement through the tube as it's advanced to ensure that the tube is properly placed in the airway.
- Slip the ET tube between the vocal cords when the patient inhales because the vocal cords separate on inhalation.

- When the tube is past the vocal cords, the breath sounds should become louder. If at any time during tube advancement breath sounds disappear, withdraw the tube until they reappear.

After intubation

- Inflate the tube's cuff with 5 to 10 cc of air, until you feel resistance. When the patient is mechanically ventilated, you'll use the minimal-leak technique or the minimal occlusive volume technique to establish correct inflation of the cuff.
- Remove the laryngoscope. If the patient was intubated orally, insert an oral airway or bite block to prevent the patient from obstructing airflow or puncturing the tube with his teeth.
- Confirm ET tube placement by listening for bilateral breath sounds, observing chest expansion, and using techniques, such as capnography or capnometry.
- If you determine that the tube isn't in the trachea, immediately deflate the cuff and remove the tube. After reoxygenating the patient to prevent hypoxia, repeat insertion using a sterile tube to prevent contamination of the trachea.
- Auscultate bilaterally to exclude the possibility of endobronchial intubation. If you fail to hear breath sounds on both sides of the chest, you may have inserted the tube into one of the mainstem bronchi (usually the right one because of its wider angle at the bifurcation); such insertion occludes the other bronchus and lungs and results in atelectasis on the obstructed side. The tube may also be resting on the carina, resulting in dry secretions that obstruct both bronchi. (The patient's coughing and fighting the ventilator will alert you to the problem.) To correct these situations, deflate the cuff, withdraw the tube 1 to 2 mm, auscultate for bilateral breath sounds, and reinflate the cuff.
- When you've confirmed correct ET tube placement, administer oxygen or initiate mechanical ventilation, and suction, if indicated.
- To secure tube position, apply compound benzoin tincture to each cheek and let it dry. Tape the tube firmly with adhesive or another strong tape or use a Velcro tube holder.
- Inflate the cuff with the minimal-leak or minimal occlusive volume technique. For the minimal-leak technique, attach a 10-ml syringe to the port on the tube's exterior pilot cuff, and place a stethoscope on the side of the patient's neck. Inject small amounts of air with each breath until you hear no leak. Then aspirate 0.1 cc of air from the cuff to create a minimal air leak. Record the amount of air needed to inflate the cuff. For the minimal occlusive volume technique, follow the first two steps of the minimal-leak technique, but place the stethoscope over the trachea instead. Aspirate until you hear a small leak on inspiration, and add just enough air to stop the leak. Record the amount of air needed to inflate the cuff for subsequent monitoring of tracheal dilation or erosion.
- Clearly note the centimeter marking on the tube where it exits the patient's mouth or nose. By periodically monitoring this mark, you can detect tube displacement.
- Make sure a chest X-ray is taken to verify tube position.
- Place a swivel adapter between the ET tube and the humidified oxygen source to allow for intermittent suctioning and to reduce tube tension
- Place the patient on his side with his head in a comfortable position to avoid tube kinking and airway obstruction.
- Auscultate both sides of the chest, and watch chest movement as indicated by the patient's condition to ensure correct tube placement and full lung ventilation. Provide frequent oral care to the orally intubated patient, and position the ET tube to prevent the formation of pressure ulcers and to avoid excessive pressure on the sides of the mouth. Provide frequent nasal and oral care to the nasally intubated patient to prevent formation of pressure ulcers and drying of oral mucous membranes.
- Suction secretions through the ET tube as the patient's condition indicates to clear secretions and to prevent mucus plugs from obstructing the tube.

Special considerations

- Orotracheal intubation is preferred in emergencies because insertion is easier and faster than with nasotracheal intubation. However, maintaining exact tube placement is more difficult, and the tube must be well secured to avoid kinking and prevent bronchial obstruction or accidental extubation. Orotracheal intubation is also poorly tolerated by conscious patients because it stimulates salivation, coughing, and retching.
- Nasotracheal intubation is preferred for elective insertion when the patient is capable of spontaneous ventilation for a short period. Blind intubation is typically used in conscious patients who risk imminent respiratory arrest or who have cervical spinal injury.
- Although nasotracheal intubation is more comfortable than oral intubation, it's also more difficult to perform. Because the tube passes blindly through the nasal cavity, the procedure causes greater tissue trauma, increases the risk of infection by nasal bacteria introduced into the trachea, and risks pressure necrosis of the nasal mucosa. However, exact tube placement is easier, and the risk of dislodgment is lower. The cuff on the ET tube maintains a closed system that permits positive-pressure ventilation and protects the airways from aspiration of secretions and gastric contents.
- Although low-pressure cuffs have significantly reduced the incidence of tracheal erosion and necrosis caused by cuff pressure on the tracheal wall, overinflation of a low-pressure cuff can negate the benefit. Use the minimal-leak technique to avoid these complications. Inflating the cuff a bit more to make a complete seal with the least amount of air is the next most desirable method.
- Always record the volume of air needed to inflate the cuff. A gradual increase in this volume indicates tracheal dilation or erosion. A sudden increase in volume indicates rupture of the cuff and requires immediate reintubation if the patient is being ventilated or if he requires continuous cuff inflation to maintain a high concentration of delivered oxygen. When the cuff has been inflated, measure its pressure at least every 8 hours to avoid overinflation. Normal cuff pressure is about 18 mm Hg.
- Reassure the patient and provide a message board so he can communicate.

Complications

ET intubation

- Apnea caused by reflex breath-holding or interruption of oxygen delivery; bronchospasm; tooth damage or loss; aspiration of blood, secretions, or gastric contents; and injury to the lips, mouth, pharynx, or vocal cords
- Laryngeal edema and erosion and tracheal stenosis, erosion, and necrosis

Nasotracheal intubation

- Nasal bleeding, laceration, sinusitis, and otitis media

Documentation

Record the date and time of the procedure, its indication and success or failure, tube type and size, cuff size, depth of ET tube as marked at the front teeth, amount of inflation and inflation technique, administration of medication, initiation of supplemental oxygen or ventilation therapy, results of chest auscultation and the chest X-ray, any complications and interventions, and the patient's reaction to the procedure.

Endotracheal tube care

The intubated patient requires meticulous care to ensure airway patency and prevent complications until he can maintain independent ventilation. This care includes frequent assessment of his airway status, maintenance of proper cuff pressure to prevent tissue ischemia and necrosis, repositioning the tube to avoid traumatic manipulation, and constant monitoring for complications. Endotracheal (ET) tubes are repositioned for patient comfort or if a chest X-ray shows improper placement. Move the tube from one side of the mouth to the other to prevent pressure ulcers.

Equipment

Maintaining the airway

Stethoscope ♦ suction equipment ♦ gloves

Repositioning the ET tube

10-ml syringe ♦ compound benzoin tincture ♦ stethoscope ♦ adhesive or hypoallergenic tape or Velcro tube holder ♦ suction equipment ♦ sedative or 2% lidocaine ♦ gloves ♦ handheld resuscitation bag with mask in case of accidental extubation

Removing the ET tube

10-ml syringe ♦ suction equipment ♦ supplemental oxygen source with mask ♦ cool-mist large-volume nebulizer ♦ handheld resuscitation bag with mask ♦ gloves ♦ equipment for reintubation

Preparation

Repositioning the ET tube

- Assemble all equipment at the patient's bedside.
- Using sterile technique, set up the suction equipment.

Removing the ET tube

- Assemble all equipment at the patient's bedside.
- Set up the suction and supplemental oxygen equipment.
- Have ready all equipment for emergency reintubation.

Key steps

- Confirm the patient's identity using two patient identifiers according to your facility's policy.
- Explain the procedure to the patient even if he doesn't appear to be alert. Provide privacy, wash your hands thoroughly, and put on gloves.

Maintaining airway patency

- Auscultate the patient's lungs regularly and at any sign of respiratory distress. If you detect an obstructed airway, determine the cause and treat it accordingly. If secretions are obstructing the ET tube lumen, suction the secretions from the tube. (See "Tracheal suction," page 525.)

ALERT

Ongoing monitoring of ET tube placement is recommended, especially when transporting the patient.

- If the ET tube has slipped from the trachea into the right or left mainstem bronchus, breath sounds will be absent over one lung. Obtain a chest X-ray as ordered to verify tube placement and, if necessary, reposition the tube.

Repositioning the ET tube

- Tell the patient why the ET tube is being repositioned and how it will be done.
- Tell the patient to keep his head still during repositioning.
- Get help from a respiratory therapist or another nurse to prevent accidental extubation during the procedure if the patient coughs.
- Hyperoxygenate the patient and then suction the patient's trachea through the ET tube to remove secretions, which can cause the patient to cough during the procedure. Then suction the patient's pharynx to remove secretions that may have accumulated above the ET tube cuff. This helps to prevent aspiration of secretions during cuff deflation.
- To prevent traumatic manipulation of the tube, instruct the assisting nurse to hold it as you carefully untape the tube or unfasten the Velcro tube holder. When freeing the tube, locate a landmark, such as a number on the tube, or measure the distance from the patient's mouth to the top of the tube so that you have a reference point when moving the tube.
- Deflate the cuff by attaching a 10-ml syringe to the pilot balloon port and aspirating air until you meet resistance and the pilot balloon deflates. Deflate the cuff before moving the ET tube because the cuff forms a seal within the trachea and movement of an inflated cuff can damage the tracheal wall and vocal cords.
- Reposition the ET tube as necessary, noting new landmarks or measuring the length. Immediately reinflate the cuff; instruct the patient to inhale, and slowly inflate the cuff using a 10-ml syringe at-

tached to the pilot balloon port. As you do this, use your stethoscope to auscultate the patient's neck to determine the presence of an air leak. When air leakage ceases, stop cuff inflation and, while still auscultating the patient's neck, aspirate a small amount of air until you detect a slight leak. This creates a minimal air leak, which indicates that the cuff is inflated at the lowest pressure possible to create an adequate seal. If the patient is being mechanically ventilated, aspirate to create a minimal air leak during the inspiratory phase of respiration because the positive pressure of the ventilator during inspiration will create a larger leak around the cuff. Note the number of cubic centimeters of air required to achieve a minimal air leak.

- Measure cuff pressure, and compare the reading with previous pressure readings to prevent overinflation. Then use benzoin and hypoallergenic tape to secure the ET tube in place, or refasten the Velcro tube holder.
- The ET tube also can be secured with a backboard commercial device. Studies show that using backboard commercial devices better prevent tube displacement when compared to using tape.
- Make sure that the patient is comfortable and the airway is patent. Properly clean or dispose of equipment.
- When the cuff is inflated, measure pressure at least every 8 hours to avoid overinflation.
- Auscultate the lungs to ensure bilateral breath sounds.

Removing the ET tube

- Explain to the patient how the ET tube will be removed and what he can do to help to reduce his anxiety.
- When you're authorized to remove the tube, obtain another nurse's assistance to prevent traumatic manipulation of the tube when it's untaped or unfastened.
- Elevate the head of the patient's bed to high Fowler's position, unless contraindicated.
- Suction the patient's oropharynx and nasopharynx to remove accumulated secretions and to help prevent aspiration of secretions when the cuff is deflated.
- Using a handheld resuscitation bag or the mechanical ventilator, give the patient several deep breaths through the ET tube to hyperinflate his lungs and to increase his oxygen reserve.
- Attach a 10-ml syringe to the pilot balloon port, and aspirate air until you meet resistance and the pilot balloon deflates. If you fail to detect an air leak around the deflated cuff, notify the practitioner immediately and don't proceed with extubation. Absence of an air leak may indicate marked tracheal edema, which can result in total airway obstruction if the ET tube is removed.
- If you detect the proper air leak, untape or unfasten the ET tube while the assisting nurse stabilizes the tube.
- Insert a sterile suction catheter through the ET tube. Then apply suction and ask the patient to take a deep breath and to open his mouth fully and pretend to cry out. This causes abduction of the vocal cords and reduces the risk of laryngeal trauma during withdrawal of the tube.
- Simultaneously remove the ET tube and the suction catheter in one smooth, outward and downward motion, following the natural curve of the patient's mouth. Suctioning during extubation removes secretions retained at the end of the tube and prevents aspiration.
- Give the patient supplemental oxygen. For maximum humidity, use a cool-mist, large-volume nebulizer to help decrease airway irritation, patient discomfort, and laryngeal edema.
- Encourage the patient to cough and deep-breathe. Remind him that a sore throat and hoarseness are to be expected and will gradually subside.
- Make sure that the patient is comfortable and the airway is patent. Clean or dispose of equipment.
- After extubation, auscultate the patient's lungs frequently and watch for signs of respiratory distress. Stay especially alert for stridor or other evidence of upper airway obstruction. If ordered, obtain a sample for arterial blood gas analysis.

Special considerations

- When repositioning an ET tube, be especially careful in patients with highly sensitive airways. Sedation or direct instillation of 2% lidocaine to numb the airway may be indicated in such patients. Because the lidocaine is absorbed systemically, you must have a practitioner's order to use it.
- After extubation of a patient who has been intubated for an extended time, keep reintubation supplies readily available for at least 12 hours or until you're sure he can tolerate extubation.
- Never extubate a patient unless someone skilled at intubation is readily available.
- If you inadvertently cut the pilot balloon on the cuff, immediately call the person responsible for intubation in your facility, who will remove the damaged ET tube and replace it with one that's intact. Don't remove the tube because a tube with an air leak is better than no airway.

Complications

- Traumatic injury to the larynx or trachea resulting from tube manipulation, accidental extubation, or tube slippage into the right bronchus
- Ventilatory failure and airway obstruction due to laryngospasm or marked tracheal edema

Documentation

After ET tube repositioning, record the date and time of the procedure, reason for repositioning (such as malposition shown by chest X-ray), new tube position, total amount of air in the cuff after the procedure, any complications and interventions, and the patient's tolerance of the procedure. Document the physical findings and nonphysical examination to confirm tube placement.

After extubation, record the date and time of extubation, presence or absence of stridor or other signs of upper airway edema, type of supplemental oxygen administered, any complications and required subsequent therapy, and the patient's tolerance of the procedure.

End-tidal carbon dioxide monitoring

Monitoring end-tidal carbon dioxide ($ETCO_2$) determines the carbon dioxide (CO_2) concentration in exhaled gas. In this technique, a photodetector measures the amount of infrared light absorbed by airway gas during inspiration and expiration. (Light absorption increases along with the CO_2 concentration.) A monitor converts these data to a CO_2 value and a corresponding waveform, or capnogram, if capnography is used. (See *How $ETCO_2$ monitoring works,* page 170.)

$ETCO_2$ monitoring provides information about the patient's pulmonary, cardiac, and metabolic status that aids patient management and helps prevent clinical compromise. This technique has become standard during anesthesia administration and mechanical ventilation.

The sensor, which contains an infrared light source and a photodetector, is positioned at one of two sites in the monitoring setup. With a mainstream monitor, it's positioned directly at the patient's airway with an airway adapter, between the endotracheal (ET) tube and the breathing circuit tubing. With a sidestream monitor, the airway adapter is positioned at the airway (regardless of whether the patient is intubated) to allow aspiration of gas from the patient's airway back to the sensor, which lies either within or close to the monitor.

Some CO_2 detection devices provide semiquantitative indications of CO_2 concentrations, supplying an approximate range rather than a specific value for $ETCO_2$. Other devices simply indicate whether CO_2 is present during exhalation. (See *Analyzing CO_2 levels,* page 171.)

$ETCO_2$ monitoring may be used to help wean a patient with a stable acid-base balance from mechanical ventilation. It also reduces the need for frequent arterial blood gas (ABG) measurements, especially when combined with pulse oximetry. Other uses for $ETCO_2$ monitoring include assessing resuscitation efforts and identifying the return of spontaneous circulation. This

How $ETco_2$ monitoring works

The optical portion of an end-tidal carbon dioxide ($ETco_2$) monitor contains an infrared light source, a sample chamber, a special carbon dioxide (CO_2) filter, and a photodetector. The infrared light passes through the sample chamber and is absorbed in varying amounts, depending on the amount of CO_2 the patient has just exhaled. The photodetector measures CO_2 content and relays this information to the microprocessor in the monitor, which displays the CO_2 value and waveform.

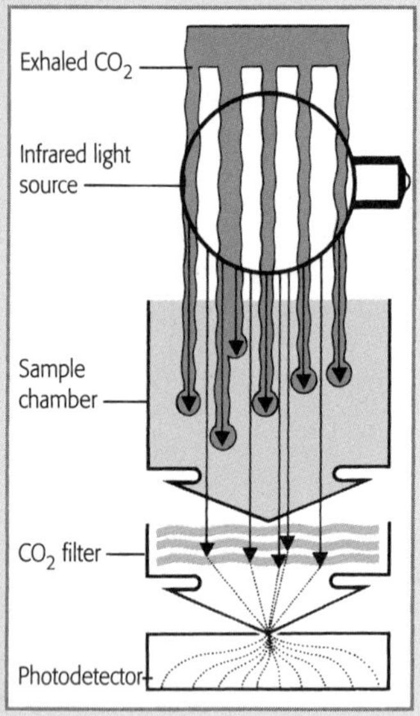

technique also detects apnea because no CO_2 is exhaled when breathing stops.

When used during ET intubation, $ETco_2$ monitoring can avert neurologic injury and even death by confirming correct ET tube placement and detecting accidental esophageal intubation because CO_2 isn't normally produced by the stomach. Ongoing $ETco_2$ monitoring throughout intubation also can prove valuable because an ET tube may become dislodged during manipulation or patient movement or transport.

Equipment

Gloves ♦ mainstream or sidestream CO_2 monitor ♦ CO_2 sensor ♦ airway adapter as recommended by the manufacturer (a neonatal adapter may have a much smaller dead space, making it appropriate for a smaller patient) ♦ $ETco_2$ sensor

Preparation

- If the monitor you're using isn't self-calibrating, calibrate it as the manufacturer directs.
- If you're using a sidestream CO_2 monitor, be sure to replace the water trap between patients, if directed. The trap allows humidity from exhaled gases to be condensed into an attached container. Newer sidestream models don't require water traps.

Key steps

- Tell the patient why $ETco_2$ monitoring is needed and explain the procedure.
- Confirm the patient's identity using two patient identifiers according to your facility's policy.
- If the patient requires ET intubation, an $ETco_2$ detector or monitor is usually applied immediately after the tube is inserted. If he doesn't require intubation or is already intubated and alert, explain the purpose and expected duration of monitoring. Tell an intubated patient that the monitor will painlessly measure the amount of CO_2 he exhales. Inform a nonintubated patient that the monitor will track his CO_2 concentration to make sure that his breathing is effective.
- Wash your hands. After turning on the monitor and calibrating it (if necessary), position the airway adapter and CO_2 sensor as the manufacturer directs. For an intubated patient, position the adapter directly on the ET tube. For a nonintubated patient, place the adapter at or near the patient's airway. (An oxygen-delivery cannula may have a sample port through which gas can be aspirated for monitoring.)

Analyzing CO_2 levels

Depending on the end-tidal carbon dioxide ($ETCO_2$) detector you use, the meaning of color changes within the detector dome may differ from the analysis for the Easy Cap detector described below.

- The rim of the Easy Cap is divided into four segments (clockwise from the top): CHECK, A, B, and C. The CHECK segment is solid purple, signifying the absence of carbon dioxide (CO_2).
- The numbers in the other sections range from 0.03 to 5 and indicate the percentage of exhaled CO_2. The color should fluctuate during ventilation from purple (in section A) during inspiration to yellow (in section C) at the end of expiration. This indicates that the $ETCO_2$ levels are adequate: above 2%.
- An end-expiratory color change from the C range to the B range may be the first sign of hemodynamic instability.
- During cardiopulmonary resuscitation (CPR), an end-expiratory color change from the A or B range to the C range may mean the return of spontaneous ventilation.
- During prolonged cardiac arrest, inadequate pulmonary perfusion leads to inadequate gas exchange. The patient exhales little or no CO_2, so the color stays in the purple range even with proper intubation. Ineffective CPR also leads to inadequate pulmonary perfusion.

Color indicators on $ETCO_2$ detector

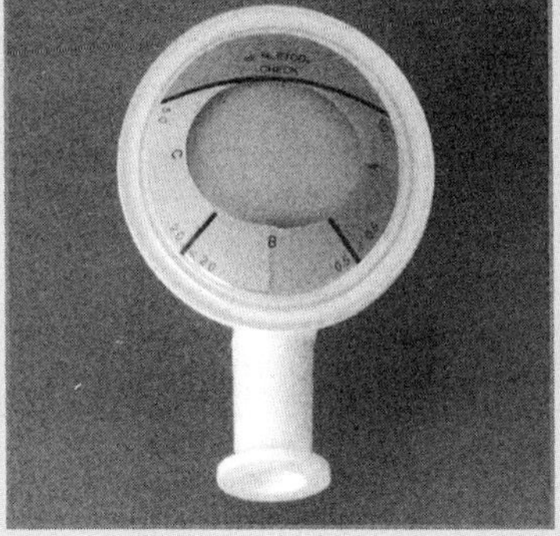

- Turn on all alarms and adjust alarm settings as appropriate for your patient. Make sure that the alarm volume is loud enough to hear.

Special considerations

- Wear gloves when handling the airway adapter to prevent cross-contamination. Make sure that the adapter is changed with every breathing circuit and ET tube change.
- Place the adapter on the ET tube to avoid contaminating exhaled gases with fresh gas flow from the ventilator. If you're using a heat and moisture exchanger, you may be able to position the airway adapter between the exchanger and breathing circuit.
- If the patient's $ETCO_2$ values differ from the partial pressure of arterial carbon dioxide level, assess him for factors that can influence $ETCO_2$—especially when the differential between arterial and $ETCO_2$ values (the arterial absolute difference of carbon dioxide [$a\text{-}ADCO_2$]) is above normal. Such factors include decreasing CO_2 production, increased CO_2 removal caused by hyperventilation, and diminished pulmonary perfusion.
- The $a\text{-}ADCO_2$ value, if correctly interpreted, provides useful information about the patient's status. For example, an increased $a\text{-}ADCO_2$ may mean that the patient has worsening dead space, especially if his tidal volume remains constant.
- Remember that $ETCO_2$ monitoring doesn't replace ABG analysis because it doesn't assess oxygenation or blood pH. Supplementing $ETCO_2$ monitoring with pulse oximetry may provide more complete information.
- If the CO_2 waveform is available, assess it for height, frequency, rhythm, baseline, and shape to help evaluate gas exchange. Make sure that you know how to recognize a normal waveform and can identify

CO_2 waveform

The carbon dioxide (CO_2) waveform, or capnogram, produced in end-tidal carbon dioxide ($ETCO_2$) monitoring reflects the course of CO_2 elimination during exhalation. A normal capnogram (shown below) consists of several segments that reflect the various stages of exhalation and inhalation.

Normally, any gas eliminated from the airway during early exhalation is dead-space gas that hasn't undergone exchange at the alveolocapillary membrane. Measurements taken during this period contain no CO_2.

As exhalation continues, CO_2 concentration rises sharply and rapidly. The sensor now detects gas that has undergone exchange, producing measurable quantities of CO_2.

The final stages of alveolar emptying occur during late exhalation. During the alveolar plateau phase, CO_2 concentration rises more gradually because alveolar emptying is more constant.

The point at which $ETCO_2$ value is derived is the end of exhalation, when CO_2 concentration peaks. Unless an alveolar plateau is present, this value doesn't accurately estimate alveolar CO_2. During inhalation, the CO_2 concentration declines sharply to zero.

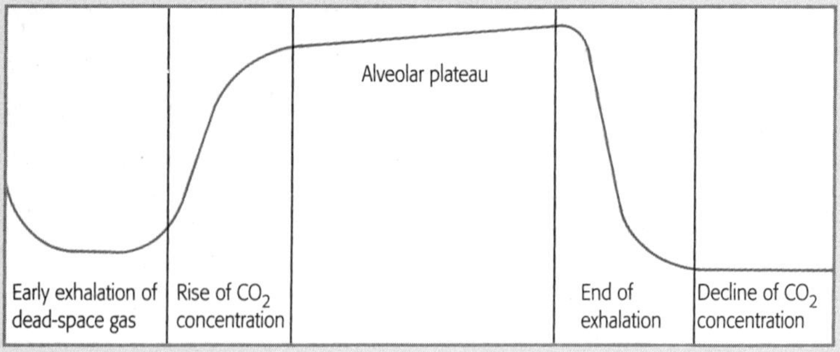

abnormal waveforms in the patient's medical record. (See *CO_2 waveform.*)

- In a nonintubated patient, use $ETCO_2$ values to establish trends. Be aware that in this patient, exhaled gas is more likely to mix with ambient air and exhaled CO_2 may be diluted by fresh gas flow from the nasal cannula.
- $ETCO_2$ monitoring is usually discontinued when the patient has been weaned effectively from mechanical ventilation or when he's no longer at risk for respiratory compromise. Carefully assess the patient's tolerance to weaning.

ALERT

After extubation, continuous $ETCO_2$ monitoring may detect the need for reintubation.

- Disposable $ETCO_2$ detectors are available. When using a disposable $ETCO_2$ detector, always check its color under fluorescent or natural light because the dome looks pink under incandescent light (light provided by ordinary light bulbs). (See *Using a disposable $ETCO_2$ detector.*)

Complications

- Misdiagnosis and improper treatment due to inaccurate measurements, such as from poor sampling technique, calibration drift, contamination of optics with moisture or secretions, or equipment malfunction
- Altered detector findings from the effects of manual resuscitation or ingestion of alcohol or carbonated beverages
- Misleading readings from color changes detected after fewer than six ventilations

DO'S & DON'TS

Using a disposable $ETco_2$ detector

Before using a disposable end-tidal carbon dioxide ($ETco_2$) detector, check the instructions and ensure ideal working conditions for the device. Additional guidelines are provided below.

Avoiding high humidity, moisture, and heat

- Watch for changes indicating that the $ETco_2$ detector's efficiency is decreasing—for example, sluggish color changes from breath to breath. A detector may be used for about 2 hours; however, using it with a ventilator that delivers high-humidity ventilation may shorten its usefulness to no more than 15 minutes.
- Don't use the detector with a heated humidifier or a nebulizer.
- Keep the detector protected from secretions, which render the device useless. If secretions enter the dome, remove and discard the detector.
- Use a heat and moisture exchanger to protect the detector. In some detectors, this filter fits between the endotracheal (ET) tube and the detector.
- If you're using a heat and moisture exchanger, remember that it will increase your patient's breathing effort. Be alert for increased resistance and breathing difficulties, and remove the exchanger, if necessary.

Taking additional precautions

- Instilling epinephrine through the ET tube can damage the detector's indicator (the color may stay yellow). If this happens, discard the device.
- Take care when using an $ETco_2$ detector in a child who weighs less than 30 lb (13.6 kg).
- Frequently spot-check the $ETco_2$ detector you're using for effectiveness. If you must transport the patient to another area for testing or treatment, use another method to verify the tube's placement.
- Never reuse a disposable $ETco_2$ detector. It's intended for one-time, one-patient use only.

Documentation

Document the initial $ETco_2$ value and all ventilator settings. Describe the waveform if one appears on the monitor. If the monitor has a printer, you may want to print out a sample waveform and include it in the patient's medical record.

Document $ETco_2$ values at least as often as vital signs, whenever significant changes in waveform or patient status occur, and before and after weaning, respiratory, and other interventions. Periodically obtain samples for ABG analysis as the patient's condition dictates, and document the corresponding $ETco_2$ values.

Enema administration

An enema is given by instilling a solution into the rectum and colon to clean the lower bowel to:

- prepare for diagnostic or surgical procedures
- relieve distention and promote expulsion of flatus
- lubricate the rectum and colon
- soften hardened stool for removal.

Enemas stimulate peristalsis by mechanically distending the colon and stimulating rectal wall nerves.

Equipment

Prescribed solution ♦ Bath thermometer ♦ enema administration bag with attached rectal tube and clamp ♦ I.V. pole ♦ gloves ♦ linen-saver pads ♦ bath blanket ♦ two bedpans with covers, or bedside commode ♦ water-soluble lubricant ♦ toilet tissue ♦ bulb syringe or funnel ♦ plastic bag for equipment ♦ water ♦ gown ♦ washcloth ♦ soap and water ♦ plastic trash bags, labels, if observing enteric precautions ♦

plastic rectal tube guard, indwelling urinary catheter or rectal catheter with 30-ml balloon and syringe (optional, for patients who can't retain solution)

Preparation

- Prepare the prescribed type and amount of solution, as indicated.
- Standard irrigating enema volume is 750 to 1,000 ml for an adult. Standard irrigating enema volumes for pediatric patients are 100 to 200 ml for infants weighing 11 to 23 lb (5 to 10.5 kg), 200 to 300 ml for children weighing 24 to 67 lb (11 to 30.5 kg), 300 to 500 ml for a child weighing 68 to 110 lb (31 to 50 kg), and 500 to 700 ml for an adolescent weighing over 110 lb.
- Some ingredients may be mucosal irritants; make sure proportions are correct and agents thoroughly mixed to avoid localized irritation.
- Warm the solution to reduce patient discomfort. Administer an adult's enema at 100° to 105° F (37.8° to 40.6° C). Administer a child's enema at 100° F to avoid burning rectal tissues.
- Check the temperature of the solution with a bath thermometer.
- Clamp the tubing and fill the solution bag with prescribed solution.
- Unclamp tubing, flush solution, and then reclamp. Flushing detects leaks and removes air that could cause discomfort.
- Hang the container on an I.V. pole and take supplies to the patient's room.
- If using an indwelling urinary catheter or rectal catheter, fill the syringe with 30 ml of water.

Key steps

- Check the practitioner's order and assess the patient's condition.
- Provide privacy and explain the procedure. If administering an enema to a child, familiarize him with the equipment and allow a parent to remain with him during the procedure.
- Discuss relaxation techniques and have the patient breathe through his mouth to relax the anal sphincter, which will facilitate catheter insertion.
- Ask if he has had previous difficulty retaining an enema to determine whether you need to use a rectal tube guard or a catheter.
- Wash your hands and put on gloves.
- Have the patient put on a hospital gown.
- Position the patient in the left-lateral Sims' position.

ALERT

If contraindicated, or if the patient reports discomfort, reposition him on his back or right side.

- Place linen-saver pads under his buttocks to prevent soiling linens.
- Replace the top bed linens with a bath blanket to provide privacy.
- Have a bedpan or commode nearby. If he can use the bathroom, make sure it's available when needed.
- Lubricate the distal tip of the rectal tube with water-soluble lubricant to facilitate rectal insertion and reduce irritation.
- Separate his buttocks and touch the anal sphincter with the rectal tube to stimulate contraction. As the sphincter relaxes, tell him to breathe deeply through the mouth as you advance the tube.

ALERT

If the patient feels pain or there's resistance, notify the practitioner. There may be an unknown stricture or abscess.

- If he has poor sphincter control, use a plastic rectal tube guard.
- You can use an indwelling urinary or rectal catheter as a rectal tube if your facility's policy permits.
- Hold the solution container slightly above bed level and release the tubing clamp.
- Raise the container gradually to start flow; usually 75 to 100 ml/minute for an irrigating enema or slowest possible rate for a retention enema to avoid stimulating peristalsis and promote retention.
- Adjust the flow rate of an irrigating enema by raising or lowering the solution container according to the patient's retention ability and comfort. Don't raise container higher than 18" (45.7 cm) for an

adult or 5″ (12.7 cm) for a child. Excessive pressure can force colon bacteria into the small intestine or rupture the colon.

ALERT

If the patient has discomfort or needs to defecate, clamp the tube and hold his buttocks together. Help him relax abdominal muscles and promote retention. Resume administration at a slower rate.

- If flow slows or stops, the catheter tip may be clogged or pressed against the rectal wall. Turn it slightly to free it. If it remains clogged, withdraw it, flush with solution, and reinsert.
- After administering most of the prescribed solution, clamp the tubing. Stop before the container empties to avoid introducing air into the bowel.
- If the patient is apprehensive, position him on a bedpan and have him hold toilet tissue or a washcloth against his anus. Place the call signal within reach.
- Provide privacy while he expels the solution. Tell him not to flush the toilet.
- Remove and discard soiled linen and linen-saver pads. Place a clean linen-saver pad under him to absorb rectal drainage.
- Check contents of the toilet or bedpan. Note fecal color, consistency, amount, and foreign matter such as blood, rectal tissue, worms, pus, or mucus.
- Send specimens to the laboratory, if ordered.
- Properly dispose of the enema equipment. If additional enemas are scheduled, store clean, reusable equipment in a closed plastic bag.

Special considerations

- For a flush enema, stop flow by lowering the container below the bed level and allowing gravity to siphon the enema from the colon. Continue to raise and lower until gas bubbles cease or abdominal distention subsides.
- For an irrigating enema, instruct the patient to retain the solution for 15 minutes, if possible.
- For a retention enema, instruct the patient not to defecate for the prescribed time or 30 minutes for oil retention; 15 to 30 minutes for anthelmintic and emollient enemas. If an indwelling catheter is in place, leave it to promote retention.
- Sodium may be absorbed from the saline enema solution; administer cautiously and monitor electrolyte status of patients with sodium restrictions.
- In patients with fluid and electrolyte disturbances, measure the amount of expelled solution to assess for retention of enema fluid.
- Give a retention enema before meals.
- Follow an oil-retention enema with a soap and water enema 1 hour later.
- Administer less solution when giving a hypertonic enema.
- If the patient has hemorrhoids, instruct him to bear down gently during tube insertion. This causes the anus to open and facilitates insertion.
- If he fails to expel solution within 1 hour you may need to remove the enema solution.

ALERT

Inform the practitioner when a patient can't expel an enema spontaneously because of possible bowel perforation or electrolyte imbalance.

- When siphoning solution have him lie on his side. Place a bedpan on a chair. Disconnect the tubing, place the distal end in the bedpan, and reinsert the rectal end. If gravity fails to drain the solution, instill 30 to 50 ml of warm water through the tube; quickly direct the distal end of the tube into the bedpan. Measure the return to make sure the solution has drained.
- Double-bag and label enema equipment "isolation" if the patient is on enteric precautions.
- If the practitioner orders enemas until returns are clear, give no more than three to avoid excessive irritation of the rectal mucosa.

Complications

- Dizziness or faintness
- Excessive irritation of colonic mucosa

- Hyponatremia or hypokalemia from repeated use of hypotonic solutions
- Cardiac arrhythmias from vasovagal reflex stimulation
- Colonic water absorption or hypervolemia from prolonged retention

Patient teaching

- Review such measures for preventing constipation as regular exercise, dietary modifications, and adequate fluid intake.

Documentation

Record the date and time of enema administration. Record the type and amount of solution administered and the length of time the patient retained the solution. Document the approximate amount of solution that was returned, along with the color, consistency, and any abnormalities. Record the patient's tolerance of the procedure.

Epidural analgesic administration

In this procedure, the practitioner injects or infuses medication into the epidural space, which lies just outside the subarachnoid space where cerebrospinal fluid (CSF) flows. The drug diffuses slowly into the subarachnoid space of the spinal canal and then into the CSF, which carries it directly into the spinal area, bypassing the blood-brain barrier. In some cases, the practitioner injects medication directly into the subarachnoid space. (See *Understanding intrathecal injections*.)

Epidural analgesia helps manage acute and chronic pain, including moderate to severe postoperative pain. It's especially useful in patients with cancer or degenerative joint disease. This procedure works well because opioid receptors are located along the entire spinal cord. Opioid drugs act directly on the receptors of the dorsal horn to produce localized analgesia without motor blockade. Opioids, such as preservative-free morphine, fentanyl, and hydromorphone, are administered as a bolus dose or by continuous infusion, either alone or in combination with bupivacaine (a local anesthetic). Infusion through an epidural catheter is preferable because it allows a smaller drug dose to be given continuously.

The epidural catheter, inserted into the epidural space, eliminates the risks of multiple I.M. injections, minimizes adverse cerebral and systemic effects, and eliminates the analgesic peaks and valleys that usually occur with intermittent I.M. injections. (See *Placement of a permanent epidural catheter,* page 178.)

Typically, epidural catheter insertion is performed by an anesthesiologist using sterile technique. When the catheter has been inserted, the nurse is responsible for monitoring the infusion and assessing the patient.

Epidural analgesia is contraindicated in patients who have local or systemic infection, neurologic disease, coagulopathy, spinal arthritis or a spinal deformity, hypotension, marked hypertension, or an allergy to the prescribed medication and in those who are undergoing anticoagulant therapy.

Equipment

Volume infusion device and epidural infusion tubing (depending on your facility's policy) ♦ patient's medication record and chart ♦ prescribed epidural solutions ♦ transparent dressing or sterile gauze pads ♦ epidural tray ♦ labels for epidural infusion line ♦ silk tape ♦ optional: monitoring equipment for blood pressure and pulse, apnea monitor, pulse oximeter ♦ for emergency use: naloxone, 0.4 mg I.V.; ephedrine, 50 mg I.V; oxygen; intubation set; handheld resuscitation bag

Preparation

- Prepare the infusion device according to the manufacturer's instructions and your facility's policy.
- Obtain an epidural tray.
- Make sure that the pharmacy has been notified ahead of time regarding the medication order because epidural solutions require special preparation.
- Check the medication concentration and infusion rate against the practitioner's order.

Key steps

- Confirm the patient's identity using two patient identifiers according to your facility's policy.
- Explain the procedure and its potential complications to the patient. Tell him that he'll feel some pain as the catheter is inserted. Answer any questions he has. Make sure that a consent form has been properly signed and witnessed.
- Position the patient on his side in the knee-chest position, or have him sit on the edge of the bed and lean over a bedside table.
- After the catheter is in place, prime the infusion device, confirm the appropriate medication and infusion rate, and then adjust the device for the correct rate.
- Help the anesthesiologist connect the infusion tubing to the epidural catheter. Then connect the tubing to the infusion pump.
- Bridge-tape all connection sites, and apply an EPIDURAL INFUSION label to the catheter, infusion tubing, and infusion pump to prevent accidental infusion of other drugs. Then start the infusion.
- Tell the patient to immediately report any pain. Instruct him to use a pain scale from 0 to 10, with 0 denoting no pain and 10 denoting the worst pain imaginable. A response of 3 or less typically indicates tolerable pain. If the patient reports a higher pain score, the infusion rate may need to be increased. Call the practitioner or change the rate within prescribed limits.
- If ordered, place the patient on an apnea monitor for the first 24 hours after beginning the infusion.
- Change the dressing over the catheter's exit site every 24 to 48 hours, as needed, or as specified by your facility's policy. The dressing is usually transparent to allow inspection of drainage and commonly appears moist or slightly blood-tinged.
- The epidural generally isn't sutured in place and it's important that you don't manipulate the catheter during a dressing change.
- Change the infusion tubing every 48 hours or as specified by your facility's policy.

Understanding intrathecal injections

An intrathecal injection allows the physician to inject medication into the subarachnoid space of the spinal canal. Certain drugs—such as anti-infectives or antineoplastics used to treat meningeal leukemia—are administered by this route because they can't readily penetrate the blood-brain barrier through the bloodstream. Intrathecal injection may also be used to deliver anesthetics, such as lidocaine, to achieve regional anesthesia (as in spinal anesthesia) and for pain management with medications such as preservative-free morphine.

An invasive procedure performed under sterile conditions by a physician with the nurse assisting, intrathecal injection requires informed patient consent. The injection site is usually between the third and fourth (or fourth and fifth) lumbar vertebrae, well below the spinal cord to avoid the risk of paralysis. This procedure may be preceded by aspiration of spinal fluid for laboratory analysis.

Contraindications to intrathecal injection include inflammation or infection at the puncture site, septicemia, and spinal deformities (especially when considered as an anesthesia route).

- Change the epidural solution every 24 hours.

Removing an epidural catheter

- Typically, the anesthesiologist orders analgesics and removes the catheter. However, your facility's policy may allow a specially trained nurse to remove the catheter.
- If you feel resistance when removing the catheter, stop and call the practitioner for further orders.
- Be sure to save the catheter. The practitioner will want to examine the catheter tip to rule out any damage during removal.

Placement of a permanent epidural catheter

An epidural catheter is implanted beneath the patient's skin and inserted near the spinal cord at the first lumbar (L1) interspace. For temporary analgesic therapy (less than 1 week), the catheter may exit directly over the spine and be taped up the patient's back to the shoulder. For prolonged therapy, the catheter may be tunneled subcutaneously to an exit site on the patient's side or abdomen or over his shoulder.

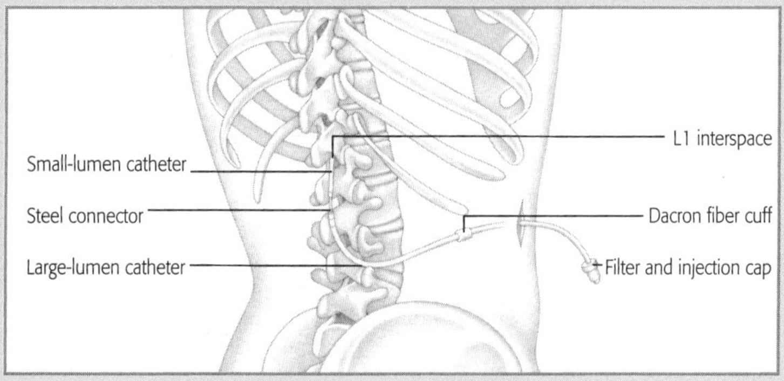

Special considerations

- Assess the patient's respiratory rate, blood pressure, and oxygen saturation every 2 hours for 8 hours and then every 4 hours for 8 hours during the first 24 hours after starting the infusion. Then assess the patient once per shift, depending on his condition or unless ordered otherwise. Your facility may require more frequent assessments.

ACTION STAT!

Notify the practitioner if the patient's respiratory rate is less than 10 breaths/minute or if his systolic blood pressure is less than 90 mm Hg.

- Assess the patient's sedation level, mental status, and pain-relief status every hour initially and then every 2 to 4 hours until adequate pain control is achieved. Notify the physician if the patient appears drowsy; experiences nausea and vomiting, refractory itching, or inability to void, which are adverse effects of certain opioid analgesics; or complains of unrelieved pain. A change in sedation level (the patient becoming somnolent) is an early indicator of the respiratory depressant effects of the opioid. Respiratory depression usually occurs during the first 24 hours and is treated with I.V. naloxone. Nausea, vomiting, and pruritus may also be treated with low-dose I.V. naloxone.
- Assess the patient's lower-extremity motor strength every 2 to 4 hours. If sensorimotor loss (numbness and leg weakness) occurs, large motor nerve fibers have been affected and the dose may need to be decreased. Notify the practitioner because he may need to titrate the dosage in order to identify the dose that provides adequate pain control without causing excessive numbness and weakness.
- Keep in mind that drugs given epidurally diffuse slowly and may cause adverse effects, including excessive sedation, up to 12 hours after the infusion has been discontinued.
- The patient should always have a peripheral I.V. line (either continuous infusion or heparin lock) open to allow immediate administration of emergency drugs.
- If CSF leaks into the dura mater at the initial puncture site, the patient usually

experiences a headache. This postanalgesia headache worsens with postural changes, such as standing and sitting. The headache can be treated with a "blood patch," in which the patient's own blood (about 10 ml) is withdrawn from a peripheral vein and then injected into the epidural space. When the epidural needle is withdrawn, the patient is instructed to sit up. Because the blood clots seal off the leaking area, the blood patch should relieve the patient's headache immediately. The patient need not restrict his activity after this procedure.

Complications

- Adverse effects from opioids or local anesthetics; catheter-related problems, such as infection, epidural hematoma, or catheter migration (Infection is treated with antibiotics. Epidural hematomas should be observed and any increase in size should be reported to the practitioner.)
- Decreased pain relief and leaking at the catheter site due to catheter migration that migrates out of the epidural space toward the skin (Notify the practitioner because the infusion needs to be stopped and the catheter removed. Contact the practitioner for further pain management orders.)
- Catheter migration occurring through the dura into the subarachnoid space if the epidural dose is too high for the smaller subarachnoid space, and the dose may eventually be toxic in high concentrations (The patient may show signs of increasing somnolence and eventually a decrease in respirations. Notify the practitioner immediately. The infusion needs to be stopped, the catheter removed, and the patient may need to be treated with I.V. naloxone and oxygen therapy.)

Patient teaching

- Home use of epidural analgesia is possible only if the patient or a family member is willing and able to learn the care needed.
- The patient also must be willing and able to abstain from alcohol and recreational drugs because these substances potentiate opioid action.

Documentation

Record the patient's response to treatment, catheter patency, condition of the dressing and insertion site, vital signs, and assessment results. Also document the labeling of the epidural catheter, changing of the infusion bags, ordered analgesics, if any, and patient's response.

Esophageal airway insertion and removal

Esophageal airways, such as the esophageal gastric tube airway (EGTA) and the esophageal obturator airway (EOA), are used temporarily (for up to 2 hours) to maintain ventilation in the comatose patient during cardiac or respiratory arrest. These devices avoid tongue obstruction, prevent air from entering the stomach, and keep stomach contents from entering the trachea. They can be inserted only after a patent airway is established.

An esophageal-tracheal tube is an alternative to esophageal airways. (See *Combitube,* page 180.) This tube has two cuffed lumens—one is sealed at the distal end and has perforations at the level of the pharynx and the other lumen is open at the distal end. If the esophageal-tracheal tube is in the trachea, it functions as an ET tube after the small distal cuff is inflated. If the tube enters the esophagus, the larger cuff on the sealed lumen is inflated and the tube functions as an EOA. This device can provide ventilations, unlike the EOA, if the tube is inserted into the trachea.

Although health care providers must have special training to insert an EGTA or EOA, insertion is much simpler than ET intubation. One reason is that these devices don't require visualization of the trachea or hyperextension of the neck. This makes them useful for treating patients with suspected spinal cord injuries.

Esophageal airways shouldn't be used unless the patient is unconscious and not breathing because conscious and semiconscious patients will reject this method. They're also contraindicated if facial trauma prevents a snug mask fit or if the patient has an absent or weak gag reflex, has

Combitube

An alternative version to esophageal airways is the esophageal-tracheal combitube, which may be inserted blindly into the victim's throat and allows ventilation through an opening located in both the esophageal or the tracheal portion of the tube (depending on which is intubated).

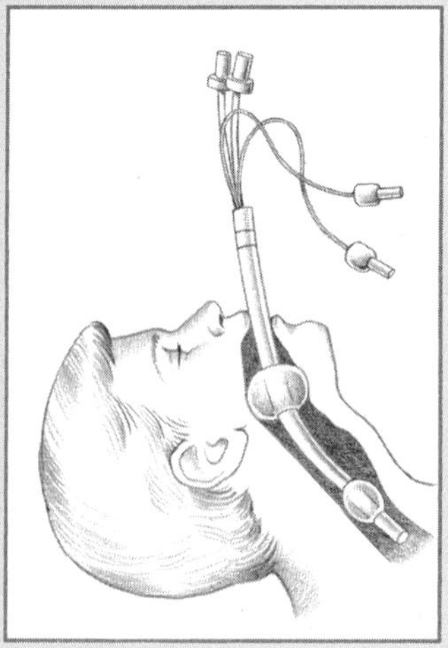

recently ingested toxic chemicals, has an esophageal disease, or has taken an overdose of opioids that can be reversed by naloxone (Narcan).

DEVICE SAFETY

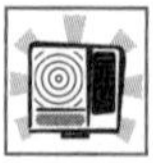

Because pediatric sizes aren't currently available, these airways shouldn't be used in patients younger than age 16.

Equipment

Esophageal tube ♦ face mask ♦ #16 or #18 French nasogastric (NG) tube (for EGTA) ♦ 35-ml syringe ♦ intermittent gastric suction equipment ♦ oral suction equipment ♦ gloves and face shield ♦ optional: handheld resuscitation bag, water-soluble lubricant

Preparation

- Gather the equipment. (See *Types of esophageal airways*.)
- Fill the face mask with air to check for leaks.
- Inflate the esophageal tube's cuff with 35 cc of air to check for leaks; then deflate the cuff.
- Connect the esophageal tube to the face mask (the lower opening on an EGTA) and listen for the tube to click to determine proper placement.

Key steps

- Lubricate the tube's distal tip with a water-soluble lubricant.
- Assess the patient's condition to determine if he's an appropriate candidate for an esophageal airway.
- If the patient's condition permits, place him in the supine position with his neck in a neutral or semiflexed position. Hyperextension of the neck may cause the tube to enter the trachea instead of the esophagus. Remove his dentures, if applicable.
- Insert your thumb deeply into the patient's mouth behind the base of his tongue. Place your index finger and middle fingers of the same hand under the patient's chin and lift his jaw straight up.
- With your other hand, grasp the esophageal tube just below the mask in the same way you would grasp a pencil. This promotes gentle maneuvering of the tube and reduces the risk of pharyngeal trauma.
- Still elevating the patient's jaw with one hand, insert the tip of the esophageal tube into the patient's mouth. Gently guide the airway over the tongue into the pharynx and then into the esophagus, following the natural pharyngeal curve. No force is required for proper insertion; the tube should easily seat itself. If you encounter resistance, withdraw the tube slightly and readvance it. When the tube is fully advanced, the mask should fit snugly over the patient's mouth and nose. When this is accomplished, the cuff will lie below the level of the carina. If the cuff is above the carina, it may, when inflated, compress the posterior membranous portion of the trachea and cause tracheal obstruction.

Types of esophageal airways

Gastric tube airway

A gastric tube airway consists of an inflatable mask and an esophageal tube, as shown below. The transparent face mask has two ports: a lower one for insertion of an esophageal tube and an upper one for ventilation, which can be maintained with a handheld resuscitation bag. The inside of the mask is soft and pliable; it molds to the patient's face and makes a tight seal, preventing air loss.

The proximal end of the esophageal tube has a one-way, nonrefluxing valve that blocks the esophagus. This valve prevents air from entering the stomach, thus reducing the risk of abdominal distention and aspiration. The distal end of the tube has an inflatable cuff that rests in the esophagus just below the tracheal bifurcation, preventing pressure on the noncartilaginous tracheal wall. During ventilation, air is directed into the upper port in the mask and, with the esophagus blocked, enters the trachea and lungs.

Obturator airway

An obturator airway consists of an adjustable, inflatable transparent face mask with a single port, attached by a snap lock to a blind esophageal tube, as shown below. When properly inflated, the transparent mask prevents air from escaping through the nose and mouth.

The esophageal tube has holes at its proximal end, through which air or oxygen introduced into the port of the mask is transferred to the trachea. The tube's distal end is closed and circled by an inflatable cuff. When the cuff is inflated, it occludes the esophagus, preventing air from entering the stomach and acting as a barrier against vomitus and involuntary aspiration.

Esophageal gastric tube airway

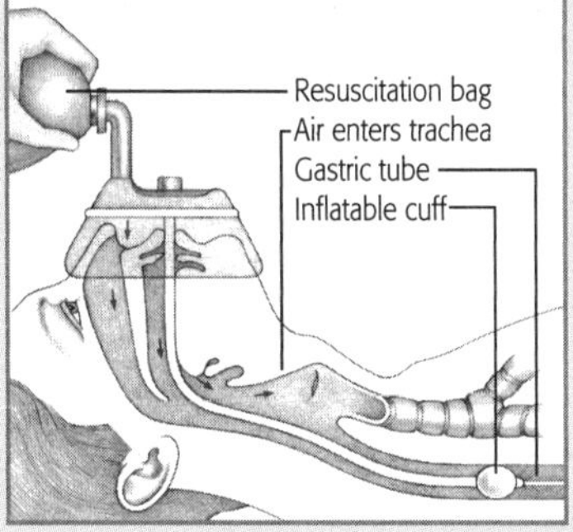

Esophageal obturator airway

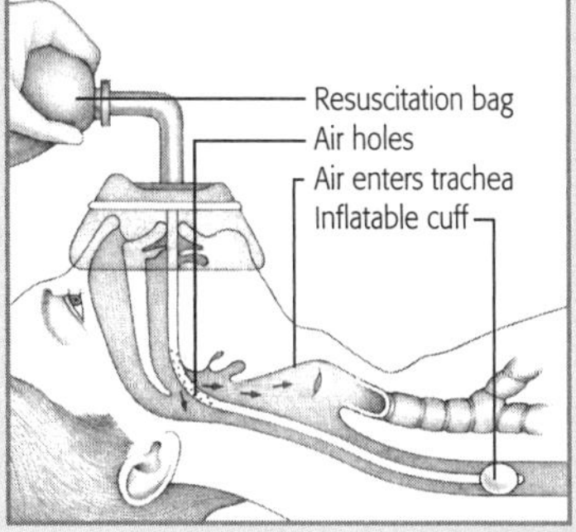

- Because the tube may enter the trachea, deliver positive-pressure ventilation before inflating the cuff. Watch for the chest to rise to confirm that the tube is in the esophagus.
- When the tube is properly in place in the esophagus, draw 35 cc of air into the syringe, connect the syringe to the tube's cuff-inflation valve, and inflate the cuff. Avoid overinflation because this can cause esophageal trauma.
- If you've inserted an EGTA, insert the NG tube through the lower port on the face mask and into the esophageal tube and advance it to the second marking, so it reaches 6″ (15.2 cm) beyond the distal end of the esophageal tube. Suction stomach contents using intermittent gastric suction

to decompress the stomach. This is particularly necessary after mouth-to-mouth resuscitation, which introduces air into the stomach. Leave the tube in place during resuscitation.

- For both airways, attach a handheld resuscitation bag or a mechanical ventilator to the face mask port (upper port) on the EGTA. Up to 100% of the fraction of inspired oxygen can be delivered this way.
- Monitor the patient to ensure adequate ventilation. Watch for chest movement, and suction the patient if mucus blocks the EOA tube perforations or in any way interrupts respiration.

Removing an esophageal airway

- Assess the patient's condition to determine if airway removal is appropriate. The airway may be removed if respirations are spontaneous and number 16 to 20 breaths/minute. If 2 hours have elapsed since airway insertion and respirations aren't spontaneous and at the normal rate, the patient must be switched to an artificial airway that can be used for long-term ventilation such as an ET tube.
- Detach the mask from the esophageal tube.
- Place the patient on his left side, if possible, to avoid aspiration during the removal of the esophageal airway. If he's unconscious and requires an ET tube, insert it or assist with its insertion and inflate the cuff of the ET tube before removing the esophageal tube. With the esophageal tube in place, the ET tube can be guided easily into the trachea, and stomach contents are less likely to be aspirated when the esophageal tube is removed.
- Deflate the cuff on the esophageal tube by removing air from the inflation valve with the syringe.

DO'S & DON'TS

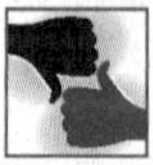

Don't try to remove the tube with the cuff inflated because it may perforate the esophagus.

- Remove the EGTA or EOA with one swift, smooth motion, following the natural pharyngeal curve to avoid esophageal trauma.
- Perform oropharyngeal suctioning to remove residual secretions.
- Assist the practitioner as required in monitoring and maintaining adequate ventilation.

Special considerations

- Store EGTAs and EOAs in the manufacturer's package to preserve their natural curve.
- To ease insertion, direct the airway along the right side of the patient's mouth because the esophagus is located to the right and behind the trachea. Alternatively, you may advance the tip upward toward the hard palate, and then invert the tip and glide it along the tongue surface and into the pharynx. This keeps the tube centered, avoids snagging on the sides of the throat, and eases insertion in the patient with clenched jaws.
- Watch the unconscious patient as he regains consciousness because activation of the gag reflex can cause retching. Evaluate the conscious patient's need for continued ventilatory support and for removal of the esophageal airway. To help prevent complications, don't leave the EOA in place for more than 2 hours.
- A mechanical ventilator attached to the ET tube or tracheostomy tube maintains more exact tidal volume than a mechanical ventilator attached to an esophageal airway.
- EOAs are a poorer choice to ET intubation in providing adequate oxygenation and ventilation; they also don't prevent aspiration of foreign material from the mouth and pharynx into the trachea and bronchi

Complications

- Esophageal injuries, including rupture, caused by esophageal airways; laryngospasm, vomiting, and aspiration (in semiconscious patients)
- Tracheal occlusion occurring if the esophageal airway is inserted in the trachea

Documentation
Record the date and time of the procedure, type of airway inserted, patient's vital signs and level of consciousness, removal of the airway, any alternative airway inserted after extubation, and any complications and interventions taken.

Esophageal tube care
Although the practitioner inserts an esophageal tube, the nurse cares for the patient during and after intubation. Typically, the patient is in the intensive care unit for close observation and constant care. The environment may help to increase the patient's tolerance for the procedure and may help to control bleeding. Sedatives may be contraindicated, especially for a patient with portal systemic encephalopathy.

Most important, the patient who has an esophageal tube in place to control variceal bleeding (typically from portal hypertension) must be observed closely for esophageal rupture because varices weaken the esophagus. Additionally, possible traumatic injury from intubation or esophageal balloon inflation increases the chance of rupture. Emergency surgery is usually performed if a rupture occurs, but the operation has a low success rate.

Equipment
Manometer ♦ two 2-L bottles of normal saline solution ♦ irrigation set ♦ water-soluble lubricant ♦ several cotton-tipped applicators ♦ mouth-care equipment ♦ nasopharyngeal suction apparatus ♦ several #12 French suction catheters ♦ intake and output record sheets ♦ gloves ♦ goggles ♦ sedatives ♦ traction weights or football helmet

Key steps
- To ease the patient's anxiety, explain the care that you'll give.
- Provide privacy. Wash your hands and put on gloves and goggles.
- Monitor the patient's vital signs every 5 minutes to 1 hour, as ordered. A change in vital signs may signal complications or recurrent bleeding.
- If the patient has a Sengstaken-Blakemore or Minnesota tube, check the pressure gauge on the manometer every 30 to 60 minutes to detect any leaks in the esophageal balloon and to verify the set pressure.
- Maintain drainage and suction on gastric and esophageal aspiration ports, as ordered. This is important because fluid accumulating in the stomach may cause the patient to regurgitate the tube, and fluid accumulating in the esophagus may lead to vomiting and aspiration.
- Irrigate the gastric aspiration port, as ordered, using the irrigation set and normal saline solution. Frequent irrigation keeps the tube from clogging. Obstruction in the tube can lead to regurgitation of the tube and vomiting.
- To prevent pressure ulcers, clean the patient's nostrils, and apply water-soluble lubricant frequently. Use warm water to loosen crusted nasal secretions before applying the lubricant with cotton-tipped applicators. Make sure the tube isn't pressing against the nostril.
- Provide mouth care often to rid the patient's mouth of foul-tasting matter and to relieve dryness from mouth breathing.
- Use #12 French catheters to provide gentle oral suctioning, if necessary, to help remove secretions.
- Offer emotional support. Keep the patient as quiet as possible, and administer sedatives if ordered.
- Make sure the traction weights hang from the foot of the bed at all times. Never rest them on the bed. Instruct housekeepers and other coworkers not to move the weights because reduced traction may change the position of the tube.
- Elevate the head of the bed about 25 degrees to ensure countertraction for the weights.
- Keep the patient on complete bed rest because exertion, such as coughing or straining, increases intra-abdominal pressure, which may trigger further bleeding.
- Keep the patient in semi-Fowler's position to reduce blood flow into the portal system and to prevent reflux into the esophagus.
- Monitor intake and output, as ordered.

Special considerations

- Observe the patient carefully for esophageal rupture indicated by signs and symptoms of shock, increased respiratory difficulties, and increased bleeding. Tape scissors to the head of the bed so you can cut the tube quickly to deflate the balloons if asphyxia develops. When performing this emergency intervention, hold the tube firmly close to the nostril before cutting.
- If using traction, be sure to release the tension before deflating any balloons. If weights and pulleys supply traction, remove the weights. If a football helmet supplies traction, untape the esophageal tube from the face guard before deflating the balloons. Deflating the balloon under tension triggers a rapid release of the entire tube from the nose, which may injure mucous membranes, initiate recurrent bleeding, and obstruct the airway.
- If the practitioner orders an X-ray study to check the tube's position or to view the chest, lift the patient in the direction of the pulley, and then place the X-ray film behind his back. Never roll him from side to side because pressure exerted on the tube in this way may shift the tube's position. Similarly, lift the patient to make the bed or to assist him with the bedpan.

Complications

- Esophageal rupture (the most life-threatening complication associated with esophageal balloon tamponade) occurring at any time but most likely occurring during intubation or inflation of the esophageal balloon
- Asphyxia resulting if the balloon moves up the esophagus and blocks the airway
- Aspiration of pooled esophageal secretions complicating this procedure

Documentation

Read the manometer hourly, and record the esophageal pressures. Note when the balloons are deflated and by whom. Document vital signs, the condition of the patient's nostrils, routine care, and any drugs administered. Also note the color, consistency, and amount of gastric returns.

Record any signs and symptoms of complications and the nursing actions taken. Document gastric port and nasogastric tube irrigations. Maintain accurate intake and output records.

Esophageal tube insertion and removal

Used to control hemorrhage from esophageal or gastric varices, an esophageal tube is inserted nasally or orally and advanced into the esophagus or stomach. Ordinarily, a physician inserts and removes the tube. In an emergency situation, a nurse may remove it.

After the tube is in place, a gastric balloon secured at the end of the tube can be inflated and drawn tightly against the cardia of the stomach. The inflated balloon secures the tube and exerts pressure on the cardia. The pressure, in turn, controls the bleeding varices.

Most tubes also contain an esophageal balloon to control esophageal bleeding. (See *Types of esophageal tubes*.) Usually, gastric or esophageal balloons are deflated after 24 hours. If the balloon remains inflated longer than 24 hours, pressure necrosis may develop and cause further hemorrhage or perforation.

Other procedures to control bleeding include irrigation with tepid or iced normal saline solution and drug therapy with a vasopressor. Used with the esophageal tube, these procedures provide effective, temporary control of acute variceal hemorrhage.

Equipment

Esophageal tube ♦ nasogastric (NG) tube (if using a Sengstaken-Blakemore tube) ♦ two suction sources ♦ basin of ice ♦ irrigation set ♦ 2 L of normal saline solution ♦ two 60-ml syringes ♦ water-soluble lubricant ♦ ½″ or 1″ adhesive tape ♦ stethoscope ♦ foam nose guard ♦ four rubber-shod clamps (two clamps and two plastic plugs for a Minnesota tube) ♦ anesthetic spray (as ordered) ♦ traction equipment (football helmet or a basic frame with traction rope, pulleys, and a 1-lb [0.5-kg] weight) ♦ mercury aneroid manometer ♦ Y-connector tube (for Sengstaken-Blake-

Types of esophageal tubes

When working with patients who have an esophageal tube, remember the advantages of the most common types.

Sengstaken-Blakemore tube

A Sengstaken-Blakemore tube is a triple-lumen, double-balloon tube that has a gastric aspiration port, which allows you to obtain drainage from below the gastric balloon and also to instill medication.

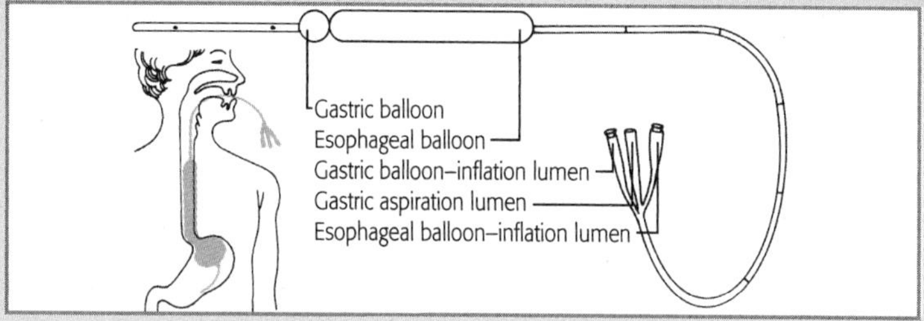

Linton tube

A Linton tube is a triple-lumen, single-balloon tube that has a port for gastric aspiration and one for esophageal aspiration, too. Additionally, the Linton tube reduces the risk of esophageal necrosis because it doesn't have an esophageal balloon.

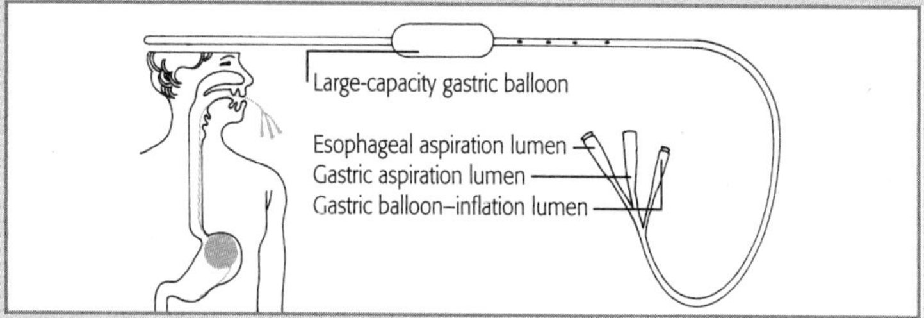

Minnesota esophagogastric tamponade tube

A Minnesota esophagogastric tamponade tube is an esophageal tube that has four lumens and two balloons. The device provides pressure-monitoring ports for both balloons without the need for Y connectors. One port is used for gastric suction, the other for esophageal suction.

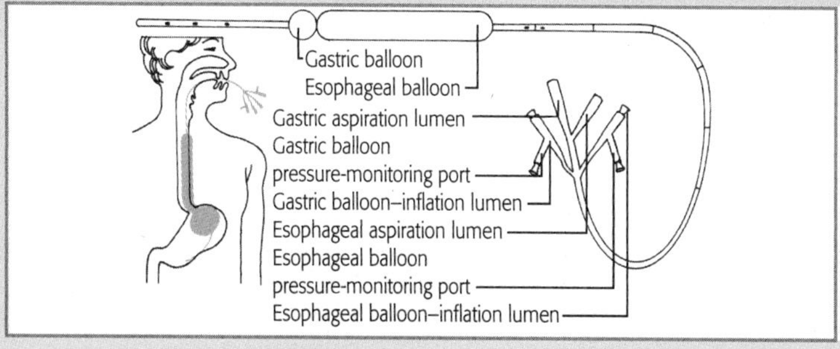

more or Linton tube) ♦ basin of water ♦ cup of water with straw ♦ scissors ♦ gloves ♦ gown ♦ waterproof marking pen ♦ goggles ♦ sphygmomanometer

Preparation

- Keep the traction helmet at the bedside or attach traction equipment to the bed so that either is readily available after tube insertion.
- Place the suction machines nearby and plug them in.
- Open the irrigation set and fill the container with normal saline solution.
- Place all equipment within reach.
- Test the balloons on the esophageal tube for air leaks by inflating them and submerging them in the basin of water. If no bubbles appear in the water, the balloons are intact.
- Remove them from the water and deflate them. Clamp the tube lumens, so that the balloons stay deflated during insertion.
- To prepare the Minnesota tube, connect the mercury manometer to the gastric pressure monitoring port. Note the pressure when the balloon fills with 100, 200, 300, 400, and 500 cc of air.
- Check the aspiration lumens for patency, and make sure they're labeled according to their purpose. If they aren't identified, label them carefully with the marking pen.
- Chill the tube in a basin of ice. This will stiffen it and facilitate insertion.

Key steps

- Explain the procedure and its purpose to the patient, and provide privacy.
- Wash your hands, and put on gloves, gown, and goggles to protect yourself from splashing blood.

Inserting the tube

- Assist the patient into semi-Fowler's position, and turn him slightly toward his left side. This position promotes stomach emptying and helps prevent aspiration.
- Explain that the physician will inspect the patient's nostrils (for patency).
- To determine the length of tubing needed, hold the balloon at the patient's xiphoid process and then, extend the tube to the patient's ear and forward to his nose. Using a waterproof pen, mark this point on the tubing.
- Inform the patient that the physician will spray his throat (posterior pharynx) and nostril with an anesthetic to minimize discomfort and gagging during intubation.
- After lubricating the tip of the tube with water-soluble lubricant to reduce friction and facilitate insertion, the physician will pass the tube through the more patent nostril. As he does, he'll direct the patient to tilt his chin toward his chest and to swallow when he senses the tip of the tube in the back of his throat. Swallowing helps to advance the tube into the esophagus and prevents intubation of the trachea. (If the physician introduces the tube orally, he'll direct the patient to swallow immediately.) As the patient swallows, the physician quickly advances the tube at least ½″ (1.3 cm) beyond the previously marked point on the tube.
- To confirm tube placement, the physician will aspirate stomach contents through the gastric port. He'll also auscultate the stomach with a stethoscope as he injects air. After partially inflating the gastric balloon with 50 to 100 cc of air, he'll order an X-ray of the abdomen to confirm correct placement of the balloon. Before fully inflating the balloon, he'll use the 60-ml syringe to irrigate the stomach with normal saline solution and empty the stomach as completely as possible. This helps the patient avoid regurgitating gastric contents when the balloon inflates.
- After confirming tube placement, the physician will fully inflate the gastric balloon (250 to 500 cc of air for a Sengstaken-Blakemore tube; 700 to 800 cc of air for a Linton tube) and clamp the tube. If he's using a Minnesota tube, he'll connect the pressure-monitoring port for the gastric balloon lumen to the mercury manometer and then inflate the balloon in 100-cc increments until it fills with up to 500 cc of air. As he introduces the air, he'll monitor the intragastric balloon pressure to make sure the balloon stays inflated. Then he'll clamp the ports. For the Sengstaken-Blakemore or Minnesota tube, the physician will gently pull on the tube until he feels resistance, which indicates

that the gastric balloon is inflated and exerting pressure on the cardia of the stomach. When he senses that the balloon is engaged, he'll place the foam nose guard around the area where the tube emerges from the nostril.

- Be ready to tape the nose guard in place around the tube. This helps to minimize pressure on the nostril from the traction and decreases the risk of necrosis.
- With the nose guard secured, traction can be applied to the tube with a traction rope and a 1-lb weight, or the tube can be pulled gently and taped tightly to the face guard of a football helmet. (See *Securing an esophageal tube*.)
- With pulley-and-weight traction, lower the head of the bed to about 25 degrees to produce countertraction.
- Lavage the stomach through the gastric aspiration lumen with normal saline solution (iced or tepid) until the return fluid is clear. The vasoconstriction thus achieved stops the hemorrhage; the lavage empties the stomach. Any blood detected later in the gastric aspirate indicates that bleeding remains uncontrolled.
- Attach one of the suction sources to the gastric aspiration lumen. This empties the stomach, helps prevent nausea and possible vomiting, and allows continuous observation of the gastric contents for blood.
- If the physician inserted a Sengstaken-Blakemore or a Minnesota tube, he'll inflate the esophageal balloon as he inflates the gastric balloon to compress the esophageal varices and control bleeding.

To do this with a Sengstaken-Blakemore tube, attach the Y-connector tube to the esophageal lumen. Then attach a sphygmomanometer inflation bulb to one end of the Y-connector and the manometer to the other end. Inflate the esophageal balloon until the pressure gauge ranges between 30 and 40 mm Hg and clamp the tube.

To do this with a Minnesota tube, attach the mercury manometer directly to the esophageal pressure-monitoring outlet. Then, using the 60-ml syringe and pushing the air slowly into the esophageal balloon port, inflate the balloon until the pressure gauge ranges from 35 to 45 mm Hg.

- Set up esophageal suction to prevent accumulation of secretions that may cause vomiting and pulmonary aspiration. This is important because swallowed secretions can't pass into the stomach if the patient has an inflated esophageal balloon in place. If the patient has a Linton or a Minnesota tube, attach the suction source to the esophageal aspiration port. If the patient has a Sengstaken-Blakemore tube, advance an NG tube through the other nostril into the esophagus to the point where the esophageal balloon begins, and attach the suction source as ordered.

Securing an esophageal tube

To reduce the risk of the gastric balloon's slipping down or away from the cardia of the stomach, secure an esophageal tube to a football helmet. Tape the tube to the face guard, as shown, and fasten the chin strap.

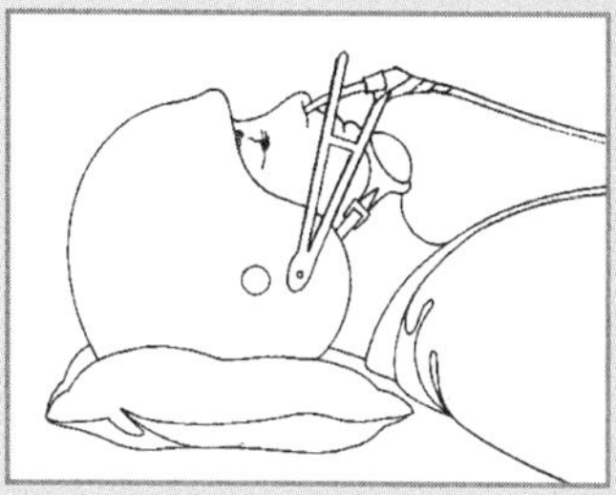

To remove the tube quickly, unfasten the chin strap and pull the helmet slightly forward. Cut the tape and the gastric balloon and esophageal balloon lumens. Be sure to hold onto the tube near the patient's nostril.

Removing the tube

- The practitioner will deflate the esophageal balloon by aspirating the air with a syringe. (He may order the esophageal balloon to be deflated at 5-mm Hg increments every 30 minutes for several hours.) Then if bleeding doesn't recur, he'll remove the traction from the gastric tube and deflate the gastric balloon (also by aspiration). The gastric balloon is always deflated just before removing the tube to prevent the balloon from riding up into the esophagus or pharynx and obstructing the airway or, possibly, causing asphyxia or rupture.

- After disconnecting all suction tubes, the practitioner will gently remove the esophageal tube. If he feels resistance, he'll aspirate the balloons again. (To remove a Minnesota tube, he'll grasp it near the patient's nostril and cut across all four lumens approximately 3" [7.5 cm] below that point. This ensures deflation of all balloons.)
- After the tube has been removed, assist the patient with mouth care.

Special considerations

ACTION STAT!

If the patient appears cyanotic or if other signs of airway obstruction develop during tube placement, remove the tube immediately because it may have entered the trachea instead of the esophagus. After intubation, keep scissors taped to the head of the bed. If respiratory distress occurs, cut across all lumens while holding the tube at the nares, and remove the tube quickly.

- Unless contraindicated, the patient can sip water through a straw during intubation to facilitate tube advancement.
- Keep in mind that the intraesophageal balloon pressure varies with respirations and esophageal contractions. Baseline pressure is the important pressure.
- The balloon on the Linton tube should stay inflated no longer than 24 hours because necrosis of the cardia may result. Usually, the practitioner removes the tube only after a trial period (lasting at least 12 hours) with the esophageal balloon deflated or with the gastric balloon tension released from the cardia to check for rebleeding. In some facilities, the practitioner may deflate the esophageal balloon for 5 to 10 minutes every hour to temporarily relieve pressure on the esophageal mucosa.

Complications

- Erosion and perforation of the esophagus and gastric mucosa resulting from the tension placed on these areas by the balloons during traction
- Esophageal rupture resulting if the gastric balloon accidentally inflates in the esophagus
- Acute airway occlusion resulting if the balloon dislodges and moves upward into the trachea
- Other erosions, nasal tissue necrosis, and aspiration of oral secretions also complicating the patient's condition

Documentation

Record the date and time of insertion and removal, the type of tube used, and the name of the physician who performed the procedure. Also document the intraesophageal balloon pressure (for Sengstaken-Blakemore and Minnesota tubes), intragastric balloon pressure (for Minnesota tube), or amount of air injected (for Sengstaken-Blakemore and Linton tubes). Also record the amount of fluid used for gastric irrigation and the color, consistency, and amount of gastric returns, both before and after lavage.

External fixation

External fixation is a system of percutaneous pins and wires that are inserted through the skin and muscle into the bone and affixed to an adjustable external frame, which maintains the bones in proper alignment. Specialized types of external fixators may be used to lengthen leg bones or immobilize the cervical spine. (See *External fixation devices.*)

An advantage of external fixation over other immobilization techniques is that it stabilizes the fracture while allowing full visualization and access to open wounds. It also facilitates early ambulation, thus reducing the risk of complications from immobilization.

The Ilizarov Fixator is a special type of external fixation device. This device is a combination of rings and tensioned transosseous wires used primarily in limb lengthening, bone transport, and limb sal-

External fixation devices

The physician's selection of an external fixation device depends on the severity of the patient's fracture and on the type of bone alignment needed.

Universal day frame

A universal day frame is used to manage tibial fractures. The frame allows the physician to readjust the position of bony fragments by angulation and rotation. The compression-distraction device allows compression and distraction of bony fragments.

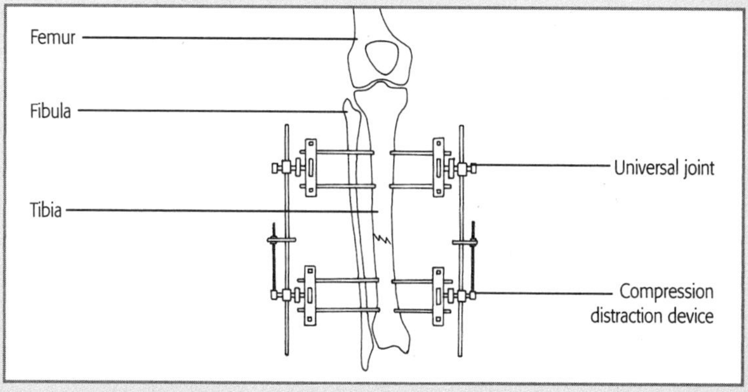

Portsmouth external fixation bar

A Portsmouth external fixation bar is used to manage complicated tibial fractures. The locking nut adjustment on the mobile carriage only allows bone compression, so the physician must accurately reduce bony fragments before applying the device.

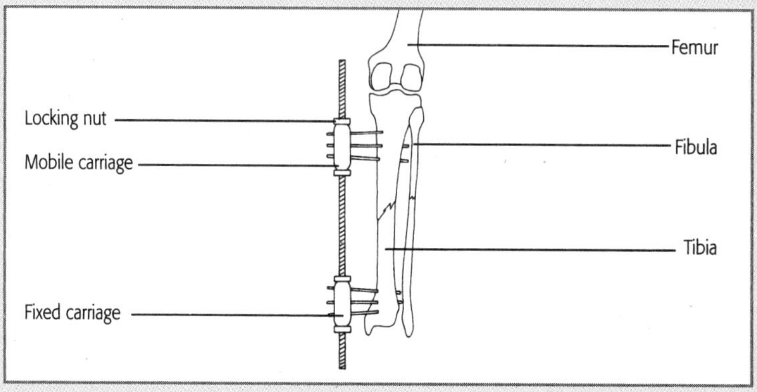

vage. Highly complex, it provides gradual distraction resulting in good-quality bone formation with minimal complications.

Equipment

Sterile cotton-tipped applicators ♦ prescribed antiseptic cleaning solution ♦ ice bag ♦ sterile gauze pads ♦ analgesic or opioid ♦ antimicrobial solution and ointment

Equipment varies with the type of fixator and the type and location of the fracture. Typically, sets of pins, stabilizing rods, and clips are available from manufacturers. Don't reuse pins.

Preparation

- Make sure that the external fixation set includes all the equipment it's supposed to include and that the equipment has been sterilized according to your facility's policy.

Key steps

- Confirm the patient's identity using two patient identifiers according to your facility's policy.
- Explain the procedure to the patient to reduce his anxiety. Emphasize that he'll feel little pain after the fixation device is in place. Assure him that his feelings of anxiety are normal.
- Tell the patient that he'll be able to move with the apparatus in place, which may help him resume normal activities more quickly.
- After the fixation device is in place, perform neurovascular checks every 2 to 4 hours for 24 hours and then every 4 to 8 hours, as appropriate, to assess for possible neurologic damage. Assess color, sensation, warmth, movement, edema, capillary refill, and pulses of the affected extremity. Compare with the unaffected side.
- Apply an ice bag to the surgical site, as ordered, to reduce swelling, relieve pain, and lessen bleeding.
- Administer analgesics or opioids, as ordered, 30 minutes to 1 hour before exercising or mobilizing the affected extremity to promote comfort.
- Monitor the patient for pain not relieved by analgesics or opioids and for burning, tingling, or numbness, which may indicate nerve damage, circulatory impairment, or compartment syndrome.
- Elevate the affected extremity, if appropriate, to minimize edema.
- Perform pin-site care, as ordered, to prevent infection. Pin-site care varies, but you'll usually follow guidelines such as these: Use sterile technique; avoid digging at pin sites with the cotton-tipped applicator; if ordered, clean the pin site and surrounding skin with a cotton-tipped applicator dipped in ordered antiseptic solution; if ordered, apply antimicrobial ointment to pin sites; and apply a loose sterile dressing, or dress with sterile gauze pads with antimicrobial solution as ordered. Perform pin-site care as often as necessary, depending on the amount of drainage.
- Check for redness, tenting of the skin, prolonged or purulent drainage from the pin site, swelling, elevated body or pin-site temperature, and any bowing or bending of pins, which may stress the skin.

Special considerations

Patient with an Ilizarov Fixator

- When the device has been placed and preliminary calluses have begun to form at the insertion sites (in 5 to 7 days), gentle distraction is initiated by turning the appropriate screws one-quarter turn (1 mm) every 4 to 6 hours as ordered.
- Teach the patient that he must be consistent in turning the screws every 4 to 6 hours around the clock. Make sure that he understands that he must be strongly committed to compliance with the protocol for the procedure to be successful. Because the treatment period may be prolonged (4 to 10 months), discuss with the patient and his family the psychological effects of long-term care.
- Don't administer nonsteroidal anti-inflammatory drugs (NSAIDs) to patients being treated with the Ilizarov Fixator. NSAIDs may decrease the necessary inflammation caused by the distraction, resulting in delayed bone formation.
- Encourage the patient to stop smoking and provide smoking-cessation materials because smoking delays bone healing.

Complications

- Loosening of pins and loss of fracture stabilization, infection of the pin tract or wound, skin breakdown, nerve damage, and muscle impingement
- Infection with Ilizarov Fixator pin sites due to the extended treatment period and pins' movement to accomplish distraction; pins also more likely to break because of their small diameter; large number of pins used increasing the patient's risk of neurovascular compromise

Patient teaching

- Before discharge, teach the patient and his family how to provide pin-site care. This is a sterile procedure in the hospital, but the patient can use clean technique at home.
- Also, provide him with written instructions and have him demonstrate the procedure before leaving the hospital.
- Teach him to recognize signs of pin-site infection.
- Tell him to keep the affected limb elevated when sitting or lying down.

Documentation

Record the patient's reaction to the apparatus. Assess and document the condition of the pin sites and skin. Document the patient's reaction to ambulation and his understanding of teaching instructions.

Eye medication application

Eye medications—drops, ointments, and disks—serve diagnostic and therapeutic purposes. During an eye examination, eyedrops can be used to anesthetize the eye, dilate the pupil to facilitate examination, and stain the cornea to identify corneal abrasions, scars, and other anomalies. Eye medications can also be used to lubricate the eye, treat certain eye conditions (such as glaucoma and infections), protect the vision of neonates, and lubricate the eye socket for insertion of a prosthetic eye.

Understanding the ocular effects of medications is important because certain drugs may cause eye disorders or have serious ocular effects. For example, anticholinergics, which are commonly used during eye examinations, can precipitate acute glaucoma in patients with a predisposition to the disorder.

Equipment

Prescribed eye medication ♦ patient's medication record and chart ♦ gloves ♦ warm water or normal saline solution ♦ sterile gauze pads ♦ facial tissues ♦ optional: ocular dressing

Preparation

- Make sure the medication is labeled for ophthalmic use. Then check the expiration date. Remember to date the container the first time you use the medication. After it's opened, an eye medication may be used for a maximum of 2 weeks to avoid contamination.
- Inspect ocular solutions for cloudiness, discoloration, and precipitation, but remember that some eye medications are suspensions and normally appear cloudy. Don't use any solution that appears abnormal. If the tip of an eye ointment tube has crusted, turn the tip on a sterile gauze pad to remove the crust.

Key steps

- Verify the order on the patient's medication record by checking it against the prescriber's order on his chart.
- Wash your hands.
- Check the medication label against the patient's medication record.

ALERT

Make sure you know which eye to treat because different medications or doses may be ordered for each eye.

- Confirm the patient's identity using two patient identifiers according to your facility's policy.
- If your facility utilizes a bar code scanning system, be sure to scan your ID badge, the patient's ID bracelet, and the medication's bar code.
- Explain the procedure to the patient and provide privacy. Put on gloves.
- If the patient is wearing an eye dressing, remove it by gently pulling it down and away from his forehead. Take care not to contaminate your hands.
- Remove any discharge by cleaning around the eye with sterile gauze pads moistened with warm water or normal saline solution. With the patient's eye closed, clean from the inner to the outer canthus, using a fresh sterile gauze pad for each stroke.
- To remove crusted secretions around the eye, moisten a gauze pad with warm water

or normal saline solution. Ask the patient to close the eye, and then place the gauze pad over it for 1 or 2 minutes. Remove the pad, and then reapply moist sterile gauze pads, as necessary, until the secretions are soft enough to be removed without traumatizing the mucosa.

- Have the patient sit or lie in the supine position. Instruct him to tilt his head back and toward the side of the affected eye so that excess medication can flow away from the tear duct, minimizing systemic absorption through the nasal mucosa.

Instilling eyedrops

- Remove the dropper cap from the medication container, if necessary, and draw the medication into it. Be careful to avoid contaminating the dropper tip or bottle top.
- Before instilling the eyedrops, instruct the patient to look up and away. This moves the cornea away from the lower lid and minimizes the risk of touching the cornea with the dropper if the patient blinks.
- You can steady the hand holding the dropper by resting it against the patient's forehead. Then, with your other hand, gently pull down the lower lid of the affected eye and instill the drops in the conjunctival sac. Try to avoid placing the drops directly on the eyeball to prevent the patient from experiencing discomfort.
- If you're instilling more than one drop agent, you should wait 5 or more minutes between agents.

Applying eye ointment

- Squeeze a small ribbon of medication on the edge of the conjunctival sac from the inner to the outer canthus. Cut off the ribbon by turning the tube. You can steady the hand holding the medication tube by bracing it against the patient's forehead or cheek. If you're applying more than one ribbon of medication, wait 10 minutes before applying the second medication.

Using a medication disk

- A medication disk can release medication in the eye for up to 1 week before needing to be replaced. Pilocarpine, for example, can be administered this way to treat glaucoma. (See *Inserting and removing an eye medication disk.*)

After instilling eyedrops or eye ointment

- Instruct the patient to close his eyes gently, without squeezing the lids shut. If you instilled drops, tell the patient to blink. If you applied ointment, tell him to roll his eyes behind closed lids to help distribute the medication over the surface of the eyeball.
- Use a clean tissue to remove any excess solution or ointment leaking from the eye. Remember to use a fresh tissue for each eye to prevent cross-contamination.
- Apply a new eye dressing if necessary.
- Return the medication to the storage area. Make sure you store it according to the label's instructions.
- Wash your hands.

Special considerations

- When administering an eye medication that may be absorbed systemically (such as atropine), gently press your thumb on the inner canthus for 1 to 2 minutes after instilling drops while the patient closes his eyes. This helps prevent medication from flowing into the tear duct.
- To maintain the drug container's sterility, never touch the tip of the bottle or dropper to the patient's eyeball, lids, or lashes. Discard any solution remaining in the dropper before returning the dropper to the bottle. If the dropper or bottle tip has become contaminated, discard it and obtain another sterile dropper. To prevent cross-contamination, never use a container of eye medication for more than one patient.
- If an ointment and drops have been ordered, the drops should be instilled first.

Complications

- Transient burning, itching, and redness
- Rarely, systemic effects

Patient teaching

- Teach the patient to instill eye medications so that he can continue treatment at home, if necessary.

Inserting and removing an eye medication disk

Small and flexible, an oval eye medication disk consists of three layers: two soft outer layers and a middle layer that contains the medication. Floating between the eyelids and the sclera, the disk stays in the eye while the patient sleeps and even during swimming and athletic activities. The disk frees the patient from having to remember to instill his eyedrops. When the disk is in place, ocular fluid moistens it, releasing the medication. Eye moisture or contact lenses don't adversely affect the disk. The disk can release medication for up to 1 week before needing replacement. Pilocarpine, for example, can be administered this way to treat glaucoma.

Contraindications include conjunctivitis, keratitis, retinal detachment, and any condition in which constriction of the pupil should be avoided.

Inserting an eye medication disk

Arrange to insert the disk before the patient goes to bed.

- Wash your hands and put on gloves.
- Press your fingertip against the oval disk so that it lies lengthwise across your fingertip. It should stick to your finger. Lift the disk out of its packet.
- Gently pull the patient's lower eyelid away from the eye and place the disk in the conjunctival sac. It should lie horizontally, not vertically. The disk will adhere to the eye naturally.

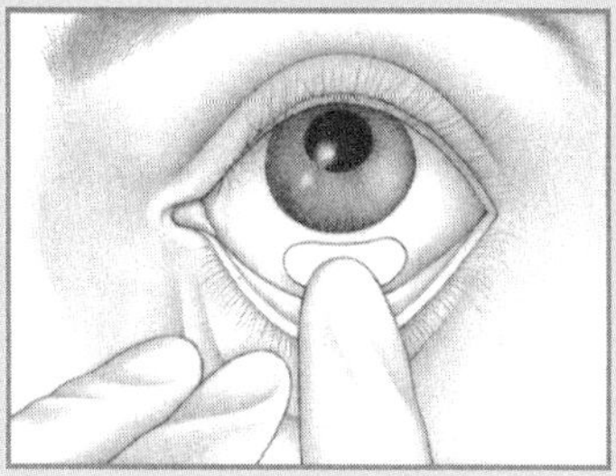

- Pull the lower eyelid out, up, and over the disk. Tell the patient to blink several times. If the disk is still visible, pull the lower lid out and over the disk again. Tell the patient that when the disk is in place, he can adjust its position by *gently* pressing his finger against his closed lid. Caution him against rubbing his eye or moving the disk across the cornea.
- If the disk falls out, wash your hands, rinse the disk in cool water, and reinsert it. If the disk appears bent, replace it.
- If both of the patient's eyes are being treated with medication disks, replace both disks at the same time.
- If the disk repeatedly slips out of position, reinsert it under the upper eyelid. To do this, gently lift and evert the upper eyelid and insert the disk in the conjunctival sac. Then gently pull the lid back into position, and tell the patient to blink several times. Again, the patient may press gently on the closed eyelid to reposition the disk. The more the patient uses the disk, the easier it should be for him to retain it. If he can't retain it, notify the practitioner.
- If the patient will continue therapy with an eye medication disk after discharge, teach him how to insert and remove it himself. To check his mastery of these skills, have him demonstrate insertion and removal for you.
- Also, teach the patient about possible adverse reactions. Foreign-body sensation in the eye, mild tearing or redness, increased mucous discharge, eyelid redness, and itchiness can occur with the use of disks. Blurred vision, stinging, swelling, and headaches can occur with pilocarpine, specifically. Mild symptoms are common but should subside within the first 6 weeks of use. Tell the patient to report persistent or severe symptoms to his practitioner.

Removing an eye medication disk

- You can remove an eye medication disk with one or two fingers. To use one finger, put on gloves and evert the lower eyelid to expose the disk. Then use the

(continued)

Inserting and removing an eye medication disk *(continued)*

forefinger of your other hand to slide the disk onto the lid and out of the patient's eye. To use two fingers, evert the lower lid with one hand to expose the disk. Then pinch the disk with the thumb and forefinger of your other hand and remove it from the eye.

- If the disk is located in the upper eyelid, apply long circular strokes to the patient's closed eyelid with your finger until you can see the disk in the corner of the patient's eye. When the disk is visible, you can place your finger directly on the disk and move it to the lower sclera. Then remove it as you would a disk located in the lower lid.

- Review the procedure and ask for a return demonstration.

Documentation

Record the medication instilled or applied, eye or eyes treated, and the date, time, and dose. Note any adverse effects and the patient's response.

F

Fall prevention and management

Falls are a major cause of injury and death among elderly people. In fact, the older the person, the more likely he is to die of a fall or its complications. In people age 75 and older, falls account for three times as many accidental deaths as motor vehicle accidents.

Factors that contribute to falls among elderly patients include lengthy convalescent periods, a greater risk of incomplete recovery, medications, increasing physical disability, and impaired vision or hearing. Injuries from falls can also trigger psychological problems, leading to a loss of self-confidence and hastening dependence and a move to a long-term care facility or nursing home.

Falls may be caused by extrinsic or environmental factors, such as poor lighting, slippery throw rugs, highly waxed floors, unfamiliar surroundings, or misuse of assistive devices. However, they usually result from intrinsic or physiologic factors, such as temporary muscle paralysis, vertigo, orthostatic hypotension, central nervous system lesions, dementia, failing eyesight, and decreased strength or coordination.

In a hospital or other health care facility, an accidental fall can change a short stay for a minor problem into a prolonged stay for serious—and possibly life-threatening—problems. The risk of falling is highest during the first week of a stay in a hospital or nursing home. (See *Who's at risk for a fall?* page 196.)

Equipment

Stethoscope ♦ sphygmomanometer ♦ analgesics ♦ cold and warm compresses ♦ pillows ♦ blankets ♦ emergency resuscitation equipment (crash cart) if needed ♦ electrocardiograph (ECG) monitor if needed

Preparation

- If you're helping a fallen patient, send an assistant to collect the assessment or resuscitation equipment you need.

Key steps

- Whether your care plan focuses on preventing a fall or managing one in an elderly patient, you'll need to proceed with patience and caution.

Preventing falls

- Assess your patient's risk of falling at least once each shift (or at least every 3 months if the patient is in a long-term care facility). Your facility may require more frequent assessments. Note any changes in his condition—such as decreased mental status—that increase his chances of falling. If you decide that he's at risk, take steps to reduce the danger.
- Correct potential dangers in the patient's room. Position the call light so that he can reach it. Provide adequate nighttime lighting.
- Place the patient's personal belongings and aids (purse, wallet, books, tissues, uri-

Who's at risk for a fall?

Preventing falls begins with identifying the patients at greatest risk. Consider a patient with one or more of the following characteristics to be at risk:
- age 65 or older
- poor general health with a chronic disease
- a history of falls
- altered mental status
- decreased mobility
- improperly fitted shoes or slippers
- inappropriate use of restraints or assistive devices
- urinary frequency or diarrhea
- sensory deficits—particularly visual deficits
- neurologic deficits
- certain drug use, such as diuretics, strong analgesics, antipsychotics, and hypnotics.

nal, commode, cane, or walker) within easy reach.
- Instruct him to rise slowly from a supine position to avoid possible dizziness and loss of balance.
- Keep the bed in its lowest position so the patient can easily reach the floor when he gets out of bed. This position also reduces the distance to the floor in case he falls. Lock the bed's wheels. If side rails are to be raised, observe the patient frequently.
- Advise the patient to wear nonskid footwear.
- Respond promptly to the patient's call light to help limit the number of times he gets out of bed without help.
- Check the patient at least every 2 hours. Check a high-risk patient every 30 minutes.
- Alert other caregivers to the patient's risk of falling and to the interventions you've implemented.
- Consider other precautions, such as placing two high-risk patients in the same room and having someone with them at all times.
- Encourage the patient to perform active range-of-motion (ROM) exercises to improve flexibility and coordination.

Managing falls

- If you're with a patient as he falls, try to break his fall with your body.
- As you gently guide him to the floor, support his body, particularly his head and trunk. If possible, help him to a supine position.
- While guiding the patient, concentrate on maintaining proper body alignment yourself to keep the center of gravity within your support base. Spread your feet to widen your support base. Remember, the wider the base, the better your balance will be. Bend your knees—rather than your back—to support the patient and to avoid injuring yourself.
- Remain calm and stay with the patient to prevent any further injury.
- Ask another nurse to collect any tools you may need, such as a stethoscope, a sphygmomanometer and, if necessary, an ECG monitor.
- Assess the patient's airway, breathing, and circulation to be sure the fall wasn't caused by respiratory or cardiac arrest. If you don't detect respirations or a pulse, call a code and begin emergency resuscitation measures. Also note his level of consciousness (LOC), and assess pupil size, equality, and reaction to light.
- To determine the extent of the patient's injuries, look for lacerations, abrasions, and obvious deformities. Note any deviations from the patient's baseline condition. Notify the practitioner. Determine if there was head trauma, which requires further diagnostic evaluation to rule out subdural hematoma.

ALERT

Patients taking anticoagulants or aspirin therapy, who experience head trauma, are at increased risk for subdural hematoma.

- If you weren't present during the fall, ask the patient or a witness what happened. Ask if the patient experienced pain or a change in LOC.

- Don't move the patient until you evaluate his status fully. Provide reassurance as needed, and observe for such signs and symptoms as confusion, tremor, weakness, pain, and dizziness.
- Assess the patient's limb strength and motion. Don't perform ROM exercises if you suspect a fracture or if the patient complains of any odd sensations or limited movement. If you suspect a disorder, don't move the patient until a practitioner examines him.
- While the patient lies on the floor until the practitioner arrives, offer pillows and blankets for comfort. If you suspect a spinal cord injury, however, don't place a pillow under his head.
- If you don't detect any problems, return the patient to his bed with the help of another staff member. Never try to lift a patient alone because you may injure yourself or the patient.
- Take steps to control bleeding (if indicated) and to obtain an X-ray if you suspect a fracture. Provide first aid for minor injuries as needed. Then monitor the patient's status for the next 24 hours or as per your facility's protocol.
- Even if the patient shows no signs of distress or has sustained only minor injuries, monitor his vital signs every 15 minutes for 1 hour, then every 30 minutes for 1 hour, then every hour for 2 hours or until his condition stabilizes. Monitor neurologic assessments with vital signs as per your facility's protocol. Notify the practitioner if you note any change from the baseline.
- Perform necessary measures to relieve the patient's pain and discomfort. Give analgesics as ordered. Apply cold compresses for the first 24 hours and warm compresses thereafter.
- Reassess the patient's environment and his risk of falling. Talk to him about the fall. Discuss why it occurred and how he thinks it could have been prevented. Refer patients to physical therapy as indicated by the practitioner for gait retraining. Review the events that preceded the fall. Did the patient change his position abruptly? Does he wear corrective lenses, and was he wearing them when he fell? Review medications that may have contributed to the fall, such as tranquilizers and opioids. (See *Medications associated with falls*, page 198.) In addition, assess gait disturbances or improper use of canes, crutches, or a walker.

Special considerations

- After a fall, review the patient's medical history to determine whether he's at risk for other complications. For example, if he hit his head, check his history to see whether he takes anticoagulants. If he does, he's at greater risk for intracranial bleeding, and you'll need to monitor him accordingly.
- Consider beginning a fall prevention program in your facility if you don't have one.

ALERT

Perform a risk assessment for falls on all admitted patients.

- Devise an alternative to restraints for a high-risk patient. For example, consider using a device such as a pressure-pad alarm used in chairs and beds. The pressure sensor pad lies under the bed linens or the chair pad. The reduced pressure that results as the patient gets out of bed triggers an alarm at the nurses' station. One such system consists of a lightweight plastic sensor sheet and a control unit. The system adapts to both a bed and chair, and setting it up according to the manufacturer's directions prevents false alarms. An alternative alarm device can be worn by the patient just above the knee. The alarm sounds when the patient moves his leg to a vertical position.
- To promote patient safety, add an appropriate notation (such as "Risk for falls") to the Kardex and chart.
- Provide emotional support, whether you're managing a fall or preventing one. Let the elderly patient know that you recognize his limitations and acknowledge his fears. Point out measures that you'll take to provide a safe environment.
- Teach the patient how to fall safely. Show him how to protect his hands and face. If he uses a walker or a wheelchair, demonstrate how to cope with and recover from a

Medications associated with falls

This chart highlights some classes of drugs that are commonly prescribed for older patients—as well as alcohol consumption—and the possible adverse effects of each that may increase the risk of falls.

Drug class	Adverse effects
Alcohol	Intoxication Motor incoordination Agitation Sedation Confusion
Antidiabetic drugs	Acute hypoglycemia
Antihypertensives	Hypotension
Antipsychotics	Orthostatic hypotension Muscle rigidity Sedation
Benzodiazepines and antihistamines	Excessive sedation Confusion Paradoxical agitation Loss of balance
Diuretics	Hypovolemia Orthostatic hypotension Electrolyte imbalance Urinary incontinence
Hypnotics	Excessive sedation Ataxia Poor balance Confusion Paradoxical agitation
Opioids	Hypotension Sedation Motor incoordination Agitation
Tricyclic antidepressants	Orthostatic hypotension

fall. Instruct him to survey the room for a low, sturdy, supportive piece of furniture (such as a coffee table). Then review the proper procedure for lifting himself off the floor and either standing up with the walker or getting into the wheelchair.

Complications

- None known

Patient teaching

- Before discharge, teach the patient and his family how to prevent accidental falls at home by correcting common household hazards. Encourage them to take steps to ensure safety.
- If the patient will use a walker or wheelchair at home, demonstrate how to cope with and recover from a fall. Instruct the patient to look for a low, sturdy, supportive piece of furniture to help himself up with; review the proper procedure for lifting himself and standing up with the walker or getting into the wheelchair.
- As needed, refer the patient to the local visiting nurse association so that nursing services can continue after discharge and during convalescence.

Documentation

After a fall, complete a detailed incident report to help track frequent patient falls so that prevention measures can be used with high-risk patients. Primarily for your facility's insurance carrier, this report isn't considered part of the patient's record. A copy, however, will go to the facility's administrator, who will evaluate care given on the unit and propose new safety policies as appropriate. It may also go to other patient care teams, such as fall prevention teams.

The incident report should note where and when the fall occurred, how the patient was found, and in what position. Include the events preceding the fall, the names of witnesses, the patient's reaction to the fall, and a detailed description of his condition based on assessment findings. The patient's statement of the event is also included. Note any interventions taken and the names of other staff members who helped care for him after the fall. Record the practitioner's name, and the date and time that he was notified as well as the patient's power of attorney's name and the date and time notified. Include a copy of the practitioner's report. Note too whether the patient was sent for diagnostic tests or transferred to another unit.

Include all of the information about the fall in the patient's record. Also, document his vital signs. If you're monitoring the patient for a severe complication, record this as well.

Fecal occult blood test

Fecal occult blood tests are valuable for determining the presence of occult blood (hidden GI bleeding) and for distinguishing between true melena and melena-like stools. Certain medications, such as iron supplements and bismuth compounds, can darken stools so that they resemble melena.

Two common occult blood screening tests are Hematest (an orthotolidine reagent tablet) and the Hemoccult slide (filter paper impregnated with guaiac). Both tests produce a blue reaction in a fecal smear if occult blood loss exceeds 5 ml in 24 hours. Another test, ColoCARE, requires no fecal smear.

Occult blood tests are particularly important for early detection of colorectal cancer because 80% of patients with this disorder test positive. However, a single positive test result doesn't necessarily confirm GI bleeding or indicate colorectal cancer. To confirm a positive result, the test must be repeated at least three times while the patient follows a special diet according to the manufacturers' recommendations for the occult blood test being used. Even then, a confirmed positive test doesn't necessarily indicate colorectal cancer. It does indicate the need for further diagnostic studies because GI bleeding can result from many causes other than cancer, such as ulcers and diverticula. These tests are easily performed on collected specimens or smears from a digital rectal examination.

Equipment

Occult blood screening test kit ♦ gloves ♦ glass or porcelain plate ♦ tongue blade or other wooden applicator

Key steps

- Confirm the patient's identity using two patient identifiers according to your facility's policy.
- Put on gloves and collect a stool specimen.

Hematest reagent tablet test

- Use a wooden applicator to smear a bit of the stool specimen on the filter paper supplied with the test kit. Or, after performing a digital rectal examination, wipe the finger you used for the examination on a square of the filter paper.
- Place the filter paper with the stool smear on a glass plate.
- Remove a reagent tablet from the bottle, and immediately replace the cap tightly. Then place the tablet in the center of the stool smear on the filter paper.
- Add one drop of water to the tablet, and allow it to soak in for 5 to 10 seconds. Add a second drop, letting it run from the tablet onto the specimen and filter paper. If necessary, tap the plate gently to dislodge any water from the top of the tablet.
- After 2 minutes, the filter paper will turn blue if the test is positive. Don't read the color that appears on the tablet itself or that develops on the filter paper after the 2-minute period.
- Note the results and discard the filter paper.
- Remove and discard your gloves, and wash your hands thoroughly.

Hemoccult slide test

- Open the flap on the slide packet, and use a wooden applicator to apply a thin smear of the stool specimen to the guaiac-impregnated filter paper exposed in box A. Or, after performing a digital rectal examination, wipe the finger you used for the examination on a square of the filter paper.
- Apply a second smear from another part of the specimen to the filter paper exposed in box B because some parts of the specimen may not contain blood.

- Allow the specimens to dry for 3 to 5 minutes.
- Open the flap on the reverse side of the slide package, and place two drops of Hemoccult developing solution on the paper over each smear. A blue reaction will appear in 30 to 60 seconds if the test is positive.
- Record the results and discard the slide package.
- Remove and discard your gloves, and wash your hands thoroughly.

Special considerations

- Make sure stool specimens aren't contaminated with urine, soap solution, or toilet tissue, and test them as soon as possible after collection.
- Test samples from several portions of the same specimen because occult blood from the upper GI tract isn't always evenly dispersed throughout the formed stool; likewise, blood from colorectal bleeding may occur mostly on the outer stool surface.

DEVICE SAFETY

Check the condition of the reagent tablets and note their expiration date. Use only fresh tablets and discard outdated ones. Protect Hematest tablets from moisture, heat, and light.

- If repeat testing is necessary after a positive screening test, explain the test to the patient. Instruct him to maintain a high-fiber diet and to refrain from eating red meat, poultry, fish, turnips, and horseradish for 48 to 72 hours before the test as well as throughout the collection period because these substances may alter test results.
- As ordered, have the patient discontinue use of iron preparations, bromides, iodides, rauwolfia derivatives, indomethacin, colchicine, salicylates, potassium, phenylbutazone, bismuth compounds, steroids, and ascorbic acid for 48 to 72 hours before the test and during it to ensure accurate test results and avoid possible bleeding, which some of these compounds may cause.

Complications

- None known

Patient teaching

- If the patient will be using the Hemoccult slide packet at home, advise him to complete the label on the slide packet before specimen collection.
- If he'll be using a ColoCARE test packet, inform him that this test is a preliminary screen for occult blood in his stool.

Documentation

Record the time and date of the test, the result, and any unusual characteristics of the stool tested. Report positive results to the practitioner.

Feeding tube insertion and removal

Inserting a feeding tube nasally or orally into the stomach or duodenum allows a patient who can't or won't eat to receive nourishment. The feeding tube also permits supplemental feedings in the patient who has very high nutritional requirements, such as an unconscious patient or one with extensive burns. Typically, the procedure is done by a nurse, as ordered. The preferred feeding tube route is nasal, but the oral route may be used for patients with such conditions as a head injury, deviated septum, or other nose injury.

The practitioner may order duodenal feeding when the patient can't tolerate gastric feeding or when he expects gastric feeding to produce aspiration. Absence of bowel sounds or possible intestinal obstruction contraindicates using a feeding tube.

Feeding tubes differ somewhat from standard nasogastric tubes. Made of silicone, rubber, or polyurethane, feeding tubes have small diameters and great flexibility. These features reduce oropharyngeal irritation, necrosis from pressure on the tracheoesophageal wall, distal esophageal irritation, and discomfort from swallowing. To facilitate passage, some feeding tubes are weighted with tungsten, and some need a guide wire to keep them from curling in the back of the throat.

These small-bore tubes usually have radiopaque markings and a water-activated coating, which provides a lubricated surface.

Equipment

Insertion

Feeding tube (#6 to #18 French, with or without guidewire) ♦ linen-saver pad ♦ gloves ♦ hypoallergenic tape ♦ water-soluble lubricant ♦ cotton-tipped applicators ♦ skin preparation (such as compound benzoin tincture) ♦ facial tissues ♦ penlight ♦ small cup of water with straw, or ice chips ♦ emesis basin ♦ 60-ml syringe ♦ pH test strip ♦ water

During use

Mouthwash or normal saline solution ♦ toothbrush

Removal

Linen-saver pad ♦ tube clamp

Preparation

- Have the proper size tube available. Usually, the practitioner orders the smallest-bore tube that will allow free passage of the liquid feeding formula.

DEVICE SAFETY

Read the instructions on the tubing package carefully because tube characteristics vary according to the manufacturer. (For example, some tubes have marks at the appropriate lengths for gastric, duodenal, and jejunal insertion.)

- Examine the tube to make sure it's free from defects, such as cracks or rough or sharp edges.
- Next, run water through the tube. This checks for patency, activates the coating, and facilitates removal of the guide.

Key steps

- Confirm the patient's identity using two patient identifiers according to your facility's policy.
- Explain the procedure to the patient and show him the tube so he knows what to expect and can cooperate more fully.
- Provide privacy. Wash your hands and put on gloves.
- Assist the patient into semi-Fowler's or high Fowler's position.
- Place a linen-saver pad across the patient's chest to protect him from spills.
- To determine the tube length needed to reach the stomach, first extend the distal end of the tube from the tip of the patient's nose to his earlobe. Coil this portion of the tube around your fingers so the end stays curved until you insert it. Then extend the uncoiled portion from the earlobe to the xiphoid process. Use a small piece of hypoallergenic tape to mark the total length of the two portions.

Inserting the tube nasally

- Using the penlight, assess nasal patency. Inspect nasal passages for a deviated septum, polyps, or other obstructions. Occlude one nostril, then the other, to determine which has the better airflow. Assess the patient's history of nasal injury or surgery.
- Lubricate the curved tip of the tube (and the feeding tube guide, if appropriate) with a small amount of water-soluble lubricant to ease insertion and prevent tissue injury.
- Ask the patient to hold the emesis basin and facial tissues in case he needs them.
- To advance the tube, insert the curved, lubricated tip into the more patent nostril and direct it along the nasal passage toward the ear on the same side. When it passes the nasopharyngeal junction, turn the tube 180 degrees to aim it downward into the esophagus. Instruct the patient to lower his chin to his chest to close the trachea. Then give him a small cup of water with a straw or ice chips. Direct him to sip the water or suck on the ice and swallow frequently. This will ease the tube's passage. Advance the tube as he swallows.

Inserting the tube orally

- Have the patient lower his chin to close his trachea, and ask him to open his mouth.

- Place the tip of the tube at the back of the patient's tongue, give water, and instruct the patient to swallow, as above. Remind him to avoid clamping his teeth down on the tube. Advance the tube as he swallows.

Positioning the tube

- Keep passing the tube until the tape marking the appropriate length reaches the patient's nostril or lips. Tube placement should be confirmed by X-ray.
- After confirming proper tube placement, remove the tape marking the tube length.
- Tape the tube to the patient's nose and remove the guide wire.
- To advance the tube to the duodenum, especially a tungsten-weighted tube, position the patient on his right side. This lets gravity assist tube passage through the pylorus. Move the tube forward 2″ to 3″ (5 to 7.5 cm) hourly until X-ray studies confirm duodenal placement. (An X-ray must confirm placement before feeding begins because duodenal feeding can cause nausea and vomiting if accidentally delivered to the stomach.)
- Apply a skin preparation to the patient's cheek before securing the tube with tape. This helps the tube adhere to the skin and prevents irritation.
- Tape the tube securely to the patient's cheek to avoid excessive pressure on his nostrils.

Removing the tube

- Protect the patient's chest with a linen-saver pad.
- Flush the tube with air, clamp or pinch it to prevent fluid aspiration during withdrawal, and withdraw it gently but quickly.
- Promptly cover and discard the used tube.

Special considerations

- Check gastric residual contents before each feeding. Feeding should be withheld if residual volumes are greater than 200 ml on two successive assessments. Successful aspiration also confirms correct tube placement before feeding by testing the pH of the gastric aspirate. Attach the syringe to the tube and gently aspirate stomach contents. Examine the aspirate and place a small amount on the pH test strip. Probability of gastric placement is increased if the aspirate has a typical gastric fluid appearance (grassy-green, clear and colorless with mucus shreds, or brown) and the pH is less than or equal to 5.
- Ideally, tube tip placement should be confirmed by X-ray.
- If no gastric secretions return, the tube may be in the esophagus. You'll need to advance the tube or reinsert it and check placement again before proceeding.
- Flush the feeding tube every 4 hours with up to 20 to 30 ml of normal saline solution or warm water to maintain patency. Retape the tube at least daily and as needed. Alternate taping the tube toward the inner and outer side of the nose to avoid constant pressure on the same nasal area. Inspect the skin for redness and breakdown.
- Provide nasal hygiene daily using the cotton-tipped applicators and water-soluble lubricant to remove crusted secretions. Help the patient brush his teeth, gums, and tongue with mouthwash or saline solution at least twice daily.
- If the patient can't swallow the feeding tube, use a guide to aid insertion.
- Precise feeding-tube placement is especially important because small-bore feeding tubes may slide into the trachea without causing immediate signs or symptoms of respiratory distress, such as coughing, choking, gasping, or cyanosis. However, the patient will usually cough if the tube enters the larynx. To make sure the tube clears the larynx, ask the patient to speak. If he can't, the tube is in the larynx. Withdraw the tube immediately and reinsert.
- When aspirating gastric contents to check tube placement, pull gently on the syringe plunger to prevent trauma to the stomach lining or bowel. If you meet resistance during aspiration, stop the procedure because resistance may result simply from the tube lying against the stomach wall. If the tube coils above the stomach, you'll be unable to aspirate stomach contents. To rectify tube coiling, change the patient's position or withdraw the tube a few inches, readvance it, and try to aspi-

Managing tube feeding problems

Complication	Interventions
Aspiration of gastric secretions	▪ Discontinue feeding immediately. ▪ Perform tracheal suction of aspirated contents if possible. ▪ Notify the practitioner. Prophylactic antibiotics and chest physiotherapy may be ordered. ▪ Check tube placement before feeding.
Tube obstruction	▪ Flush the tube with warm water. If necessary, replace the tube. ▪ Flush the tube with 50 ml of water after each feeding. ▪ When possible, use liquid forms of medications. Otherwise, crush medications well, if not contraindicated.
Oral, nasal, or pharyngeal irritation or necrosis	▪ Provide frequent oral hygiene using mouthwash or sponge-tipped swabs. Use petroleum jelly on cracked lips. ▪ Change the tube's position. If necessary, replace the tube.
Vomiting, bloating, diarrhea, or cramps	▪ Reduce the flow rate. ▪ Verify tube placement. ▪ Administer metoclopramide (Reglan). ▪ Warm the formula. ▪ For 30 minutes after feeding, position the patient on his right side with his head elevated. ▪ Notify the practitioner. He may want to reduce the amount of formula being given during each feeding.
Constipation	▪ Provide additional fluids if the patient can tolerate them. ▪ Have the patient participate in an exercise program if possible. ▪ Administer a bulk-forming laxative. ▪ Review medications. Discontinue medications that have a tendency to cause constipation. ▪ Increase fruit, vegetable, or sugar content of the feeding.
Electrolyte imbalance	▪ Monitor serum electrolyte levels. ▪ Notify the practitioner. He may want to adjust the formula content to correct the deficiency.
Hyperglycemia	▪ Monitor blood glucose levels. ▪ Notify the practitioner of elevated levels. ▪ Administer insulin if ordered. ▪ The practitioner may adjust the sugar content of the formula.

rate again. If the tube was inserted with a guide wire, don't use the guide wire to reposition the tube. The physician may do so, using fluoroscopic guidance.

Complications

- Skin erosion at the nostril, sinusitis, esophagitis, esophagotracheal fistula, gastric ulceration, and pulmonary and oral infection from prolonged intubation (See *Managing tube feeding problems,* page 203.)

Patient teaching

- If your patient will use a feeding tube at home, make appropriate home care nursing referrals and teach the patient and caregivers how to use and care for a feeding tube.
- Teach them how to obtain equipment, insert and remove the tube, prepare and store feeding formula, and solve problems with tube position and patency.

Documentation

For tube insertion, record the date, time, tube type and size, insertion site, area of placement, confirmation of proper placement. Record the name of the person performing the procedure. For tube removal, record the date and time and the patient's tolerance of the procedure.

Femoral compression

Femoral compression is used to maintain hemostasis at the puncture site following a procedure involving an arterial access site (such as cardiac catheterization or angiography). For the patient with this type of condition, a femoral compression device is used to apply direct pressure to the arterial access site.

The femoral compression device has an inflatable plastic dome that's attached to the patient with a nylon strap that's placed under his buttocks. After the dome is positioned correctly over the puncture site, it's inflated to the recommended pressure, according to the manufacturer's instructions. A practitioner or a specially trained nurse may apply the device.

Equipment

Femoral compression device strap ♦ compression arch with dome and three-way stopcock ♦ pressure inflation device ♦ sterile transparent dressing ♦ gloves (nonsterile and sterile) ♦ protective eyewear

Key steps

- Obtain a practitioner's order for the femoral compression device, including the amount of pressure to be applied and the length of time the device should remain in place.
- Explain the reason for using the device and the possible complications of the procedure. Answer the patient's questions.
- Advise the patient to use caution when moving in bed to avoid malpositioning the device.
- Instruct the patient not to bend the involved extremity.
- Position the patient on the stretcher or bed; don't flex the involved extremity.
- Assess the condition of the puncture site, obtain vital signs, perform neurovascular checks, and assess pain, according to your facility's policy for arterial access procedures.

Applying the femoral compression device

- Put on nonsterile gloves and protective eyewear, and place the device strap under the patient's hips before sheath removal (in cases that warrant the use of a sheath).
- With the assistance of another nurse, position the compression arch over the puncture site. Apply manual pressure over the dome area while the straps are secured to the arch.
- When the dome is properly positioned over the puncture site, connect the pressure inflation device to the stopcock that's attached to the device. Turn the stopcock to the open position and inflate the dome with the pressure inflation device to the ordered pressure. Turn the stopcock off and remove the pressure inflation device.
- Assess the puncture site for proper placement of the device and for signs of bleeding or hematoma. Assess distal pulses and perform neurovascular assessments according to your facility's policy. Confirm

distal pulses after any adjustments of the device.

Maintaining the device

- When the patient is transferred to the nursing unit, assess the distal pulses, the puncture site and placement of the device, and confirm the ordered amount of pressure.
- Check device placement, assess vital signs and the puncture site, and perform neurovascular checks according to your facility's policy.
- Deflate the device hourly and assess the puncture site for bleeding or hematoma. Assess for proper placement of the dome over the puncture site. Put on gloves and protective eyewear and reposition the compression arch and dome as necessary. Reinflate the device to the ordered pressure using the pressure inflation device.

Removing the device

- Explain the removal procedure to the patient.
- Put on nonsterile gloves and protective eyewear, remove the air from the dome, loosen the straps, and remove the device.
- Assess the puncture site for bleeding or hematoma.
- After achieving hemostasis, put on sterile gloves and apply a sterile transparent dressing over the puncture site, using sterile technique.
- Change the sterile transparent dressing according to your facility's policy.
- Check the puncture site and distal pulses, and perform neurovascular assessments every 15 minutes for the first hour and every 30 minutes for the next 2 hours. Your facility may require more frequent monitoring. Observe for signs of bleeding, hematoma, or infection.
- Dispose of the device according to your facility's policy.

Special considerations

- If you note external bleeding or signs of internal bleeding, remove the device, apply manual pressure, and notify the practitioner.
- Change the dressing at the puncture site every 24 to 48 hours or according to your facility's policy. (The sterile transparent dressing permits inspection of the site for bleeding, drainage, or hematoma.)

Complications

- Bleeding, hematoma, retroperitoneal bleeding, and pseudoaneurysm
- Infection and deep vein thrombosis
- Tissue damage occurring with prolonged pressure

Documentation

Document initial application of the device, sheath removal, and the patient's tolerance of the procedure. Document vital signs, puncture site checks, distal pulses, neurovascular assessments, hourly deflation, repositioning of the device, length of time the device was in place, and removal of the device. Document patient and family teaching, complications, and interventions.

Fetal monitoring, external

External fetal monitoring is an indirect, noninvasive procedure that uses two devices strapped to the mother's abdomen to evaluate fetal well-being during labor. One device, an ultrasound transducer, transmits high-frequency sound waves through soft body tissues to the fetal heart. The waves rebound from the heart, and the transducer relays them to a monitor. The other, a pressure-sensitive tocotransducer, responds to the pressure exerted by uterine contractions and simultaneously records their duration and frequency. (See *Applying an external electronic fetal monitor,* page 206.) The monitoring apparatus traces fetal heart rate (FHR) and uterine contraction data onto the same paper.

Indications for external fetal monitoring include high-risk pregnancy, oxytocin-induced labor, maternal medical illness (gestational diabetes, hypertension, asthma) and antepartal nonstress, contraction stress tests, and psychosocial factors, such as tobacco, alcohol, drug use, and lack of prenatal care. Many labor and delivery units use external fetal monitoring for all patients. The procedure has no contraindi-

Applying an external electronic fetal monitor

To ensure clear tracings that define fetal status and labor progress, be sure to precisely position external monitoring devices, such as an ultrasound transducer and a tocotransducer.

Fetal heart monitor

Palpate the uterus to locate the fetus's back. If possible, place the ultrasound transducer over the site where the fetal heartbeat sounds the loudest. Then tighten the belt. Use the fetal heart tracing on the monitor strip to confirm the transducer's position.

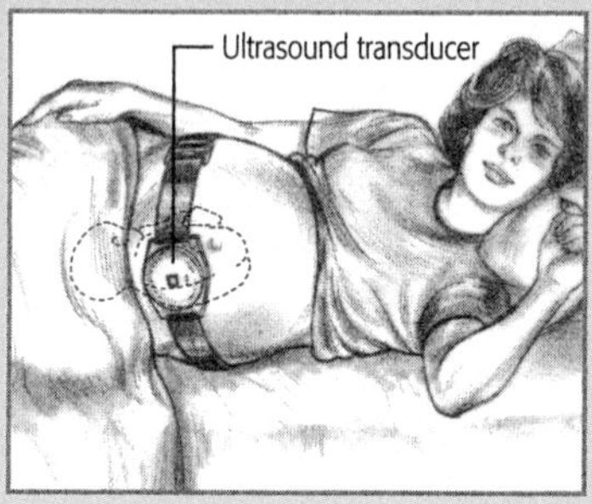

Labor monitor

A tocotransducer records uterine motion during contractions. Place the tocotransducer over the uterine fundus where it contracts, either midline or slightly to one side. Place your hand on the fundus, and palpate a contraction to verify proper placement. Secure the tocotransducer's belt, and then adjust the pen set so that the baseline values read between 5 and 15 mm Hg on the monitor strip.

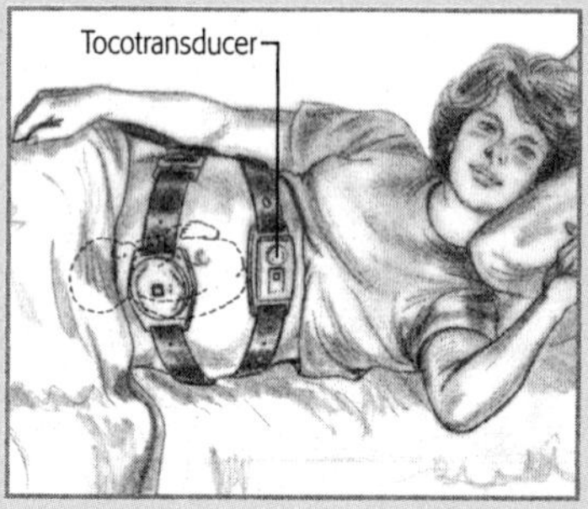

cations, but it may be difficult to perform on patients with hydramnios, on obese patients, or on hyperactive or premature fetuses.

Equipment

Electronic fetal monitor ♦ ultrasound transducer ♦ tocotransducer ♦ conduction gel ♦ transducer strap ♦ damp cloth ♦ printout paper

Monitoring devices, such as phonotransducers and abdominal electrocardiogram transducers, are commercially available. However, facilities use these devices less frequently than the ultrasound transducer.

Preparation

- Because fetal monitor features and complexity vary, review the manufacturer's manual before proceeding. If the monitor has two paper speeds, select the higher speed (typically 3 cm/minute) to ensure an easy-to-read tracing. At slower speeds (for example, 1 cm/minute), the printed tracings are difficult to decipher and interpret accurately.
- Plug the tocotransducer cable into the uterine activity jack and the ultrasound transducer cable into the phono-ultrasound jack. Attach the straps to the tocotransducer and the ultrasound transducer.
- Label the printout paper with the patient's identification number or birth date and name, the date, maternal vital signs and position, the paper speed, and the number of the strip paper to maintain accurate, consecutive monitoring records.
- If your facility has central monitoring capabilities, enter the patient data into the

central computer to ensure accurate labeling of monitor strips.

Key steps

- Explain the procedure to the patient, and provide emotional support. Inform her that the monitor may make noise if the pen set tracer moves above or below the printed paper. Reassure her that this doesn't indicate fetal distress. As appropriate, explain other aspects of the monitor to help reduce maternal anxiety about fetal well-being.
- Make sure the patient has signed a consent form, if required.
- Wash your hands, and provide privacy.

Beginning the procedure

- Assist the patient to the semi-Fowler or a left-lateral position with her abdomen exposed. Don't let her lie in a supine position because pressure from the gravid uterus on the maternal inferior vena cava may cause maternal hypotension and decreased uterine perfusion and may induce fetal hypoxia.
- Palpate the patient's abdomen to locate the fundus—the area of greatest muscle density in the uterus. Using transducer straps, secure the tocotransducer over the fundus.
- Adjust the pen set tracer controls so that the baseline values read between 5 and 15 mm Hg on the monitor strip. This prevents triggering the alarm that indicates the tracer has dropped below the paper's margins. The proper setting varies among tocotransducers.
- Apply conduction gel to the ultrasound transducer crystals to promote an airtight seal and optimal sound-wave transmission.
- Use Leopold's maneuvers to palpate the fetal back, through which fetal heart tones resound most audibly.
- Start the monitor. Apply the ultrasound transducer directly over the site having the strongest heart tones.
- Activate the control that begins the printout. On the printout paper, note coughing, position changes, drug administration, vaginal examinations, and blood pressure readings that may affect interpretation of the tracings.
- Explain to the patient and her support person how to time and anticipate contractions with the monitor. Inform them that the distance from one dark vertical line to the next on the printout grid represents 1 minute. The support person can use this information to prepare the patient for the onset of a contraction and to guide and slow her breathing as the contraction subsides.

Monitoring the patient

- Observe the tracings to identify the frequency and duration of uterine contractions, but palpate the uterus to determine intensity of contractions.
- Mentally note the baseline FHR—the rate between contractions—to compare with suspicious-looking deviations. FHR normally ranges from 110 to 160 beats/minute.
- Assess periodic accelerations or decelerations from the baseline FHR. Compare FHR patterns with those of the uterine contractions. Note the time relationship between the onset of an FHR deceleration and the onset of a uterine contraction, the time relationship of the lowest level of an FHR deceleration to the peak of a uterine contraction, and the range of FHR deceleration. These data help distinguish fetal distress from benign head compression.
- Move the tocotransducer and the ultrasound transducer to accommodate changes in maternal or fetal position. Readjust both transducers every hour, and assess the patient's skin for reddened areas caused by the strap pressure. Document skin condition.
- Clean the ultrasound transducer periodically with a damp cloth to remove dried conduction gel, which can interfere with ultrasound transmission. Apply fresh gel as necessary. After using the ultrasound transducer, replace the cover over it.

Special considerations

- If the monitor fails to record uterine activity, palpate for contractions. Check for equipment problems as the manufacturer directs and readjust the tocotransducer.
- If the patient reports discomfort in the position that provides the clearest signal,

try to obtain a satisfactory 5- or 10-minute tracing with the patient in this position before assisting her to a more comfortable position. As the patient progresses through labor and abdominal pressure increases, the pen set tracer may exceed the alarm boundaries.

Complications

- None known

Documentation

Make sure you numbered each monitor strip in sequence and labeled each printout sheet with the patient's identification number or birth date and name, the date, the time, and the paper speed. Record the time of vaginal examinations, membrane rupture, drug administration, and maternal or fetal movements. Record maternal vital signs and the intensity of uterine contractions. Document each time that you moved or readjusted the tocotransducer and ultrasound transducer, and summarize this information in your notes.

Fetal monitoring, internal

Also called *direct fetal monitoring,* this sterile, invasive procedure uses a spiral electrode and an intrauterine catheter to evaluate fetal status during labor. By providing an electrocardiogram (ECG) of the fetal heart rate (FHR), internal electronic fetal monitoring assesses fetal response to uterine contractions more accurately than external fetal monitoring. Internal FHR monitoring allows evaluation of short- and long-term FHR variability. The intrauterine catheter measures uterine pressure during contraction and relaxation.

Internal fetal monitoring is indicated whenever direct, beat-to-beat FHR monitoring is required. Specific indications include maternal diabetes or hypertension, fetal postmaturity, suspected intrauterine growth retardation, and meconium-stained fluid. However, internal monitoring is performed only if the amniotic sac has ruptured, the cervix is dilated at least 2 cm, and the presenting part of the fetus is at least at the –1 station.

Contraindications for internal fetal monitoring include maternal blood dyscrasias, suspected fetal immune deficiency, placenta previa, face presentation or uncertainty about the presenting part, maternal human immunodeficiency virus-positive status, and cervical or vaginal herpetic lesions.

A spiral electrode is the most commonly used device for internal fetal monitoring. Shaped like a corkscrew, the electrode is attached to the presenting fetal part (usually the scalp). It detects the fetal heartbeat and then transmits it to the monitor, which converts the signals to a fetal ECG waveform.

A pressure-sensitive catheter, though not as widely used as the tocotransducer, is the most accurate method of determining the true intensity of contractions. It's especially helpful in dysfunctional labor and in preventing or rapidly determining the need for a cesarean birth. But the risk of infection or uterine perforation associated with this device is high.

Equipment

Electronic fetal monitor ♦ spiral electrode and a drive tube ♦ disposable leg plate pad or reusable leg plate with Velcro belt ♦ conduction gel ♦ antiseptic solution ♦ hypoallergenic tape ♦ two pairs of sterile gloves ♦ intrauterine catheter connection cable and pressure-sensitive catheter ♦ graph paper ♦ optional: sterile drape

Preparation

Device safety

Be sure to review the operator's manual before using the equipment.

- If the monitor has two paper speeds, set the speed at 3 cm/minute to ensure a readable tracing. A tracing at 1 cm/minute is more condensed and harder to interpret accurately.
- Connect the intrauterine cable to the uterine activity outlet on the monitor.

Wash your hands and open the sterile equipment, maintaining sterile technique.

Key steps

- Describe the procedure to the patient and her partner, if present, and explain how the equipment works. Tell the patient that a practitioner will perform a vaginal examination to identify the position of the fetus.
- Make sure the patient is fully informed about the procedure and that a signed consent form has been obtained.
- Label the printout paper with the patient's identification number or name and birth date, the date, the paper speed, and the number on the monitor strip.

Monitoring contractions

- Assist the patient into the lithotomy position for a vaginal examination. The practitioner puts on sterile gloves.
- Attach the connection cable to the appropriate outlet on the monitor marked UA (uterine activity). Connect the cable to the intrauterine catheter. Next, zero the catheter with a gauge provided on the distal end of the catheter. This helps to determine the resting tone of the uterus, usually 5 to 15 mm Hg.
- Cover the patient's perineum with a sterile drape, if your facility's policy dictates. Clean the perineum with antiseptic solution, according to your facility's policy. Using sterile technique, the practitioner inserts the catheter into the uterine cavity while performing a vaginal examination. The catheter is advanced to the black line on the catheter and secured with hypoallergenic tape along the inner thigh.
- Observe the monitoring strip to verify proper placement of the catheter guide and to ensure a clear tracing. Periodically evaluate the monitoring strip to determine the exact amount of pressure exerted with each contraction. Note all such data on the monitoring strip and on the patient's medical record.
- The intrauterine catheter is usually removed during the second stage of labor or at the practitioner's discretion. Dispose of the catheter, and clean and store the cable according to facility policy. (See *Applying an internal electronic fetal monitor,* page 210.)

Monitoring FHR

- Apply conduction gel to the leg plate. Secure the leg plate to the patient's inner thigh with Velcro straps or 2" tape. Connect the leg plate cable to the ECG outlet on the monitor.
- Inform the patient that she'll undergo a vaginal examination to identify the fetal presenting part (which is usually the scalp or buttocks), to determine the level of fetal descent, and to apply the electrode. Explain that this examination is done to ensure that the electrode isn't attached to the suture lines, fontanels, face, or genitalia of the fetus. The spiral electrode will be placed in a drive tube and advanced through the vagina to the fetal presenting part. To secure the electrode, mild pressure will be applied and the drive tube will be turned clockwise 360 degrees.
- After the electrode is in place and the drive tube has been removed, connect the color-coded electrode wires to the corresponding color-coded leg plate posts.
- Turn on the recorder, and note the time on the printout paper.
- Assist the patient to a comfortable position, and evaluate the strip to verify proper placement and a clear FHR tracing.

Monitoring the patient

- Begin by noting the frequency, duration, and intensity of uterine contractions. Normal intrauterine pressure ranges from 8 to 12 mm Hg. (See *Reading a fetal monitor strip,* page 211.)
- Next, check the baseline FHR. Assess periodic accelerations or decelerations from the baseline FHR.
- Compare the FHR pattern with the uterine contraction pattern. Note the interval between the onset of an FHR deceleration and the onset of a uterine contraction, the interval between the lowest level of an FHR deceleration and the peak of a uterine contraction, and the range of FHR deceleration.
- Check for FHR variability, which is a measure of fetal oxygen reserve and neurologic integrity and stability.

Applying an internal electronic fetal monitor

During internal electronic fetal monitoring, a spiral electrode monitors the fetal heart rate (FHR), and an internal catheter monitors uterine contractions.

Monitoring FHR

The spiral electrode is inserted after a vaginal examination that determines the position of the fetus. As shown at right, the electrode is attached to the presenting fetal part, usually the scalp or buttocks.

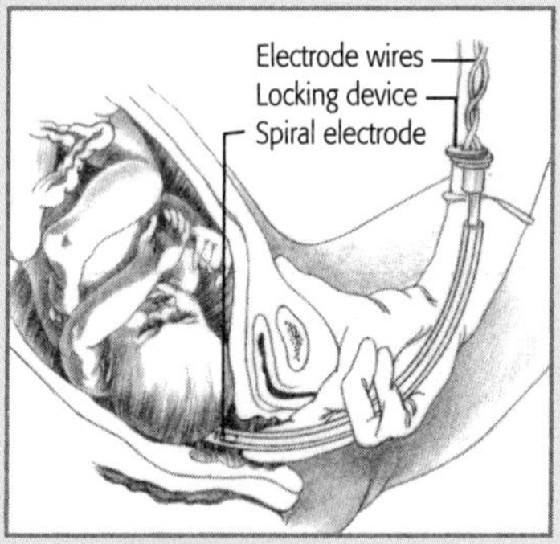

Monitoring uterine contractions

The intrauterine catheter is inserted up to a premarked level on the tubing and then connected to a monitor that interprets uterine contraction pressure.

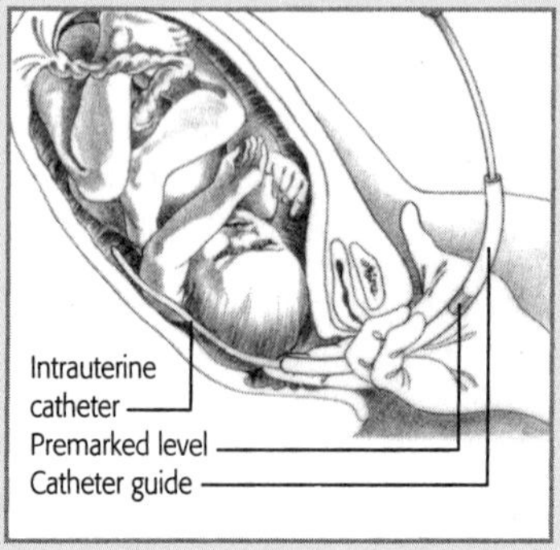

- When removing the spiral electrode, perform a vaginal examination and turn the electrode counterclockwise or until it releases from the fetal presenting part.

DO'S & DON'TS

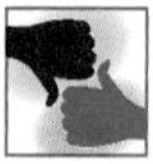

Don't pull on the electrode. If it won't disconnect easily from the presenting part, it may be removed after delivery under direct visualization.

- The electrode should be removed just before a cesarean birth. It should be brought through the uterine incision. If unable to detach, cut the wire at the perineum and notify the practitioner.

Special considerations

- Interpret the FHR and uterine contractions at regular intervals.
- First, determine the baseline FHR within 10 beats/minute, and then assess the degree of baseline variability. Note the presence or absence of short-term or long-term variability. Identify periodic FHR changes, such as decelerations (early, late, variable, or mixed), or nonperiodic changes such as a sinusoidal pattern.
- Keep in mind that acute fetal distress can result from any change in the baseline FHR that causes fetal compromise. If necessary, take steps to counteract FHR changes. (See *Identifying baseline FHR irregularities,* pages 212 to 215.)

Reading a fetal monitor strip

Presented in two parallel recordings, the fetal monitor strip records the fetal heart rate (FHR) in beats per minute in the top recording and uterine activity (UA) in mm Hg in the bottom recording. You can obtain information on fetal status and labor progress by reading the strips horizontally and vertically.

Reading horizontally on the FHR or the UA strip, each small block represents 10 seconds. Six consecutive small blocks, separated by a dark vertical line, represent 1 minute.

Reading vertically on the FHR strip, each block represents an amplitude of 10 beats/minute. Reading vertically on the UA strip, each block represents 5 mm Hg of pressure.

Assess the baseline FHR—the "resting" heart rate—between uterine contractions when fetal movement diminishes. This baseline FHR (normal range, 110 to 160 beats/minute) pattern serves as a reference for subsequent FHR tracings produced during contractions.

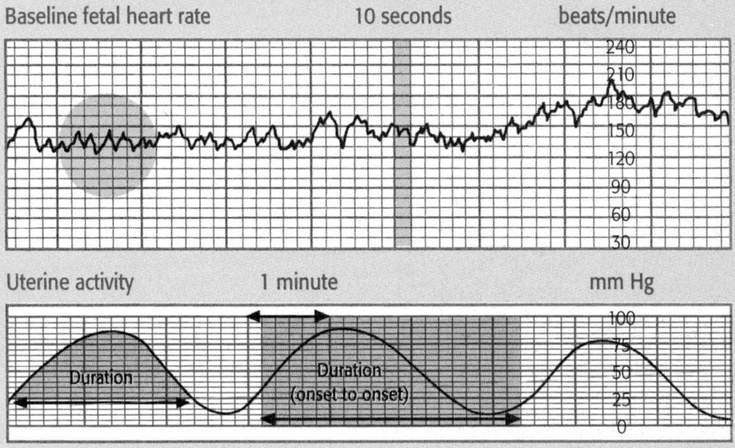

ACTION STAT!

If vaginal delivery isn't imminent (within 30 minutes) and fetal distress patterns don't improve, cesarean birth is necessary.

Complications

- Uterine perforation and intrauterine infection in the mother
- Abscess, hematoma, and infection in the fetus

Documentation

Document all activity related to monitoring. (A fetal monitoring strip becomes part of the patient's permanent record, so it's considered a legal document.) Be sure to record the type of monitoring your patient received as well as all interventions. Identify the monitoring strip with the patient's name, her practitioner's name, your name, and the date and time. Document the paper speed and electrode placement.

Record the patient's vital signs as per the standard of practice. Note her pushing efforts and record changes in her position. Document I.V. line insertion and changes in the I.V. solution or infusion rate. Note the use of oxytocin, regional anesthetics, or other medications.

After a vaginal examination, document cervical dilation and effacement as well as fetal station, presentation, and position.

Identifying baseline FHR irregularities

Irregularity	Possible causes
Baseline tachycardia Beats/minute 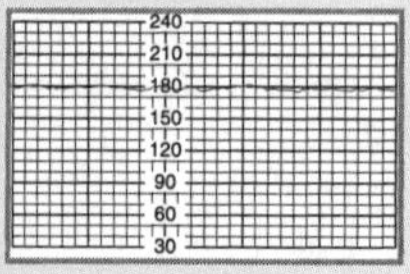	▪ Early fetal hypoxia ▪ Maternal fever ▪ Parasympathetic agents, such as atropine and scopolamine ▪ Beta-adrenergics such as terbutaline ▪ Amnionitis (inflammation of inner layer of fetal membrane, or amnion) ▪ Maternal hyperthyroidism ▪ Fetal anemia ▪ Fetal heart failure ▪ Fetal arrhythmias
Baseline bradycardia Beats/minute 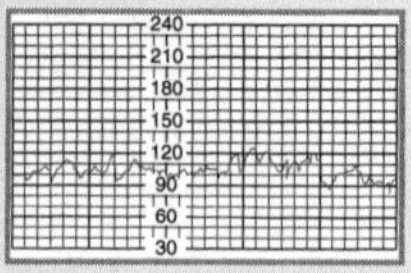	▪ Late fetal hypoxia ▪ Beta-adrenergic blocking agents, such as propranolol, and anesthetics ▪ Maternal hypotension ▪ Prolonged umbilical cord compression ▪ Fetal congenital heart block
Early decelerations Beats/minute 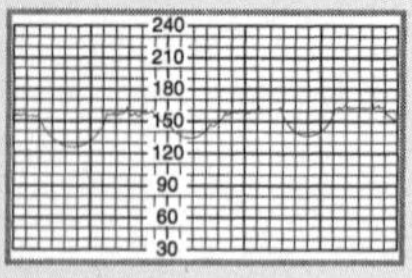 mm Hg 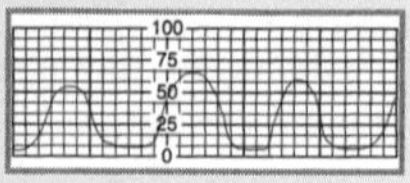	▪ Fetal head compression

Document membrane rupture, including the time it occurred and whether it was spontaneous or artificial. Note the amount, color, and odor of the fluid. If internal electronic fetal monitoring was used, document electrode placement.

Foreign body airway obstruction

Severe airway obstruction is an uncommon but preventable emergency that can result in death within minutes if not treated. Sudden airway obstruction may occur

Clinical significance	Nursing interventions
Persistent tachycardia without periodic changes usually doesn't adversely affect fetal well-being—especially when associated with maternal fever. However, tachycardia is an ominous sign when associated with late decelerations, severe variable decelerations, or lack of variability.	▪ Intervene to alleviate the cause of fetal distress and provide supplemental oxygen, as ordered. Also administer I.V. fluids, as prescribed. ▪ Discontinue oxytocin infusion to reduce uterine activity. ▪ Turn the patient onto her left side and elevate her legs. ▪ Continue to observe the fetal heart rate (FHR). ▪ Document interventions and outcomes. ▪ Notify the practitioner; further medical intervention may be necessary.
Bradycardia with good variability and no periodic changes doesn't signal fetal distress if FHR remains above 80 beats/minute. But bradycardia caused by hypoxia and acidosis is an ominous sign when associated with loss of variability and late decelerations.	▪ Intervene to correct the cause of fetal distress. Administer supplemental oxygen, as ordered. ▪ Start an I.V. line and administer fluids, as prescribed. ▪ Discontinue oxytocin infusion to reduce uterine activity. ▪ Turn the patient onto her left side and elevate her legs. ▪ Continue observing the FHR. ▪ Document interventions and outcomes. ▪ Notify the practitioner; further medical intervention may be necessary.
Early decelerations are benign, indicating fetal head compression at dilation of 4 to 7 cm.	▪ Reassure the patient that the fetus isn't at risk. ▪ Observe the FHR. ▪ Document the frequency of decelerations.

(continued)

when a foreign body lodges in the throat or bronchus, when the tongue blocks the pharynx, when the patient experiences traumatic injury, or when the patient aspirates blood, mucus, or vomitus. An obstructed airway can also occur from bronchoconstriction or bronchospasm.

An obstructed airway causes anoxia, which in turn leads to brain damage and death in 4 to 6 minutes. The Heimlich maneuver uses an upper-abdominal thrust to create sufficient diaphragmatic pressure in the static lung below the foreign body to expel the obstruction. It's used in conscious adult patients and in children older

Identifying baseline FHR irregularities *(continued)*

Irregularity	Possible causes
Late decelerations Beats/minute 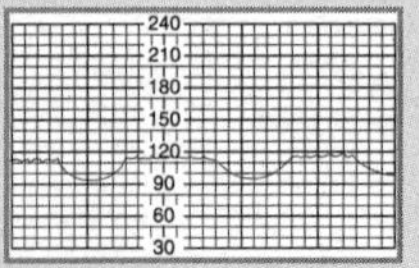 mm Hg 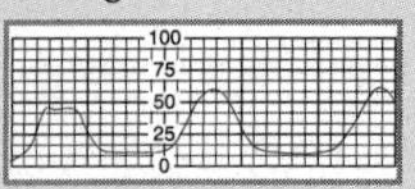 	▪ Uteroplacental circulatory insufficiency (placental hypoperfusion) caused by decreased intervillous blood flow during contractions or a structural placental defect such as abruptio placentae ▪ Uterine hyperactivity caused by excessive oxytocin infusion ▪ Maternal hypotension ▪ Maternal supine hypotension
Variable decelerations Beats/minute 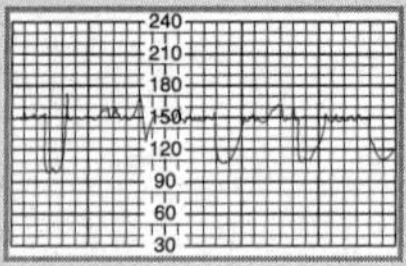 mm Hg 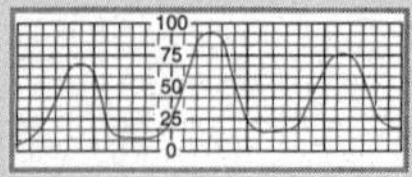 	▪ Umbilical cord compression causing decreased fetal oxygen perfusion

than age 1. However, the abdominal thrust is contraindicated in pregnant women, markedly obese patients, and infants younger than age 1. For such patients, a chest thrust, which forces air out of the lungs to create an artificial cough, should be used.

These maneuvers are contraindicated in the patient with mild airway obstruction, when the patient can maintain adequate ventilation to dislodge the foreign body by effective coughing, and in an infant. However, if the patient has poor air exchange and increased breathing difficulty, a silent cough, cyanosis, or the inability to speak or breathe, immediate action to dislodge the obstruction should be taken. (See also "Cardiopulmonary resuscitation," page 64.)

Equipment

No specific equipment needed

Clinical significance	Nursing interventions
Late decelerations indicate uteroplacental circulatory insufficiency and may lead to fetal hypoxia and acidosis if the underlying cause isn't corrected.	■ Turn the patient onto her left side to increase placental perfusion and decrease contraction frequency. ■ Increase the I.V. fluid rate to boost intravascular volume and placental perfusion, as prescribed. ■ Administer oxygen by mask to increase fetal oxygenation, as ordered. ■ Assess for signs of the underlying cause, such as hypotension or uterine tachysystole. ■ Take other appropriate measures, such as discontinuing oxytocin, as prescribed. ■ Document interventions and outcomes. ■ Notify the practitioner; further medical intervention may be necessary.
Variable decelerations are the most common deceleration pattern in labor because fetal movement during contractions compresses the umbilical cord.	■ Help the patient change position to relieve pressure on the cord. No other intervention is necessary unless you detect fetal distress. ■ Assure the patient that the fetus tolerates cord compression well. Explain that cord compression affects the fetus the same way that breath holding affects her. ■ Assess the deceleration pattern for reassuring signs: a baseline FHR that isn't increasing, short-term variability that isn't decreasing, abruptly beginning and ending decelerations, and decelerations lasting less than 50 seconds. If assessment doesn't reveal reassuring signs, notify the practitioner. ■ Start I.V. fluids and administer oxygen by mask at 10 to 12 L/minute, as prescribed. ■ Document interventions and outcomes. ■ Discontinue oxytocin infusion to decrease uterine activity.

Key steps

Conscious adult with mild airway obstruction

■ Ask the person who's coughing or using the universal distress sign (clutching the neck between the thumb and fingers) if she's choking. If she indicates that she is but can speak and cough forcefully, she has good air exchange and should be encouraged to continue to cough. Remain with the person and monitor her.

Conscious adult with severe airway obstruction

■ Ask the person, "Are you choking?" If the patient nods yes and has signs of severe airway obstruction, tell her that you'll help dislodge the foreign body.

■ Standing behind the patient, wrap your arms around her waist. Make a fist with one hand, and place the thumb side against her abdomen in the midline, slightly above the umbilicus and well below the xiphoid process. Then grasp your fist with the other hand (as shown below).

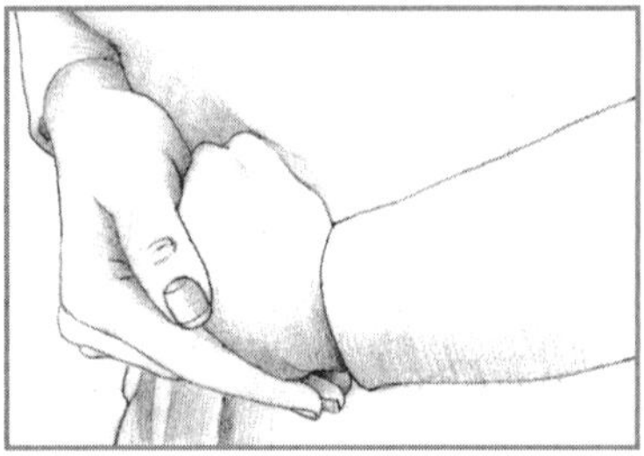

▪ Squeeze the patient's abdomen with quick inward and upward thrusts. Each thrust should be a separate and distinct movement, forceful enough to create an artificial cough that will dislodge an obstruction (as shown below).

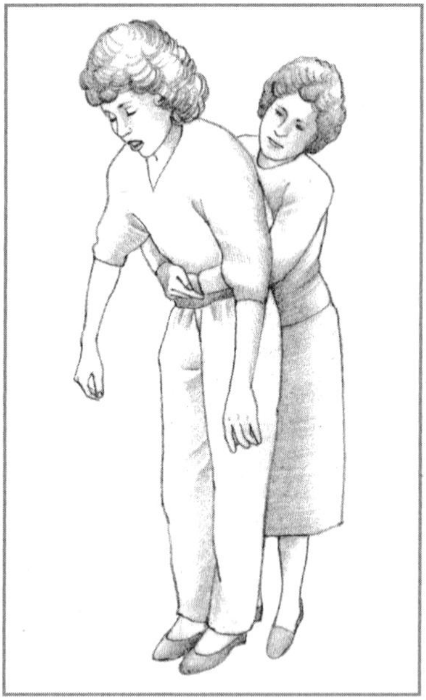

▪ Make sure that you have a firm grasp on the patient because she may lose consciousness and need to be lowered to the floor. Support her head and neck to prevent injury, and continue as described below.

▪ Repeat the thrusts until the foreign body is expelled or if the patient becomes unconscious. At this point, contact the emergency medical service (EMS) and follow the interventions for relieving an obstructed airway in an unconscious person.

ALERT

If the victim of an airway obstruction becomes unconscious, the lay rescuer should lower the patient to the ground and immediately contact EMS and begin cardiopulmonary resuscitation (CPR).

Unresponsive adult

▪ Lower the patient to the ground and immediately contact EMS.
▪ Begin CPR.
▪ Each time the airway is opened using a head tilt-chin lift, look for an object in the patient's mouth.
▪ Remove the object if present.
▪ Attempt to ventilate the patient and follow with 30 chest compressions.

ALERT

The blind finger-sweep is no longer being taught by the American Heart Association. A finger-sweep should only be used when a foreign body can be seen in the mouth. Studies have shown that blind finger-sweeps may result in injury to the patient's mouth and throat or to the rescuer's fingers, and there's no evidence of its effectiveness. In addition, the tongue-jaw lift is no longer used. The patient's mouth should be opened using a head tilt-chin lift.

Obese or pregnant adult

▪ If the patient is conscious, stand behind her and place your arms under her armpits and around her chest.
▪ Place the thumb side of your clenched fist against the middle of the sternum, avoiding the margins of the ribs and the xiphoid process. Grasp your fist with your other hand and perform a chest thrust with enough force to expel the foreign body. Continue until the patient expels the obstruction or loses consciousness (as shown top of next page).

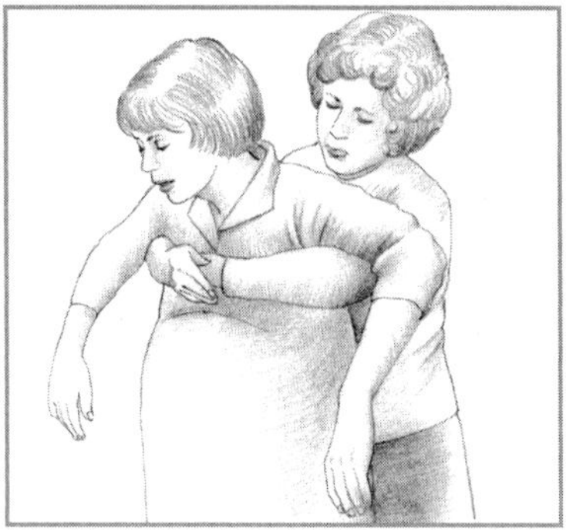

■ If the patient loses consciousness, carefully lower her to the floor.
■ Then, follow the same steps you would use for the unresponsive adult (as shown below).

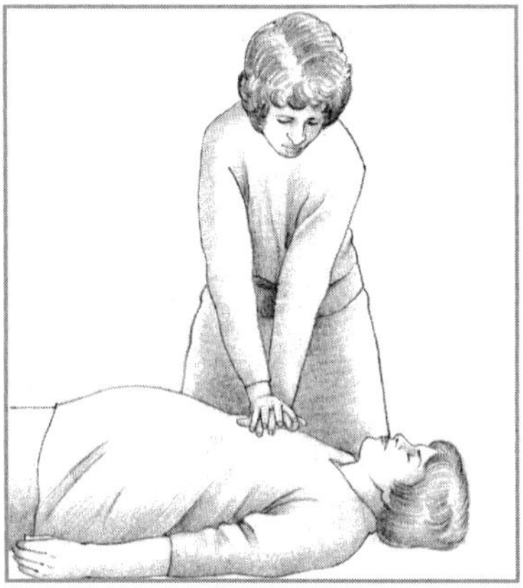

Conscious child with severe airway obstruction

■ If the child is conscious and can stand but can't cough or make a sound, perform abdominal thrusts using the same technique as you would with an adult.

Unresponsive child

■ Use the same techniques you would for the unresponsive adult.

Conscious infant

■ Place the conscious infant face down so that he's straddling your arm with his head lower than his trunk. Rest your forearm on your thigh and deliver five forceful back blows with the heel of your hand between the infant's shoulder blades (as shown below).

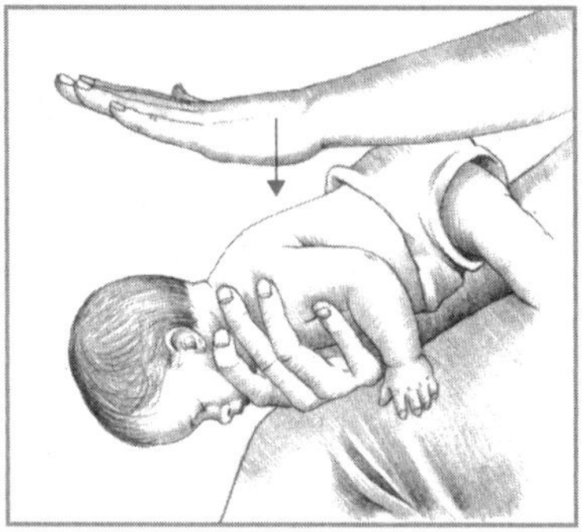

■ If you haven't removed the obstruction, place your free hand on the infant's back. Supporting his neck, jaw, and chest with your other hand, turn him over onto your thigh. Keep his head lower than his trunk.
■ Position your fingers. To do so, imagine a line between the infant's nipples and place the index finger of your free hand on his sternum, just below this imaginary line. Then place your middle and ring fingers next to your index finger and lift the index finger off his chest. Deliver five quick chest thrusts as you would for chest compression at a rate of approximately one per second.

ALERT

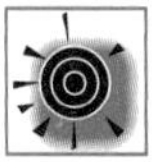

Never perform a blind finger-sweep on a child or an infant because you risk pushing the foreign body farther back into the airway. Also, abdominal thrusts aren't recommended for infants because they may damage the liver.

■ If the airway obstruction persists, repeat the five back blows and five chest thrusts until the obstruction is relieved or the infant becomes unresponsive.

Unresponsive infant

■ Use the same techniques you would for the unresponsive adult.

Special considerations

■ If the patient vomits during abdominal thrusts, quickly wipe out his mouth with your fingers and resume the maneuver as necessary.

- Even if your efforts to clear the airway don't seem to be effective, keep trying. As oxygen deprivation increases, smooth and skeletal muscles relax, making your maneuvers more likely to succeed.
- The patient who has received abdominal thrusts should be evaluated by a practitioner to detect possible complications.

Complications

- Nausea, regurgitation, and achiness developing after the patient regains consciousness and can breathe independently
- Damage to the internal organs of the abdomen or chest by laceration or rupture
- Increased risk of fracture due to incorrect placement of the rescuer's hands, or osteoporosis or metastatic lesions

Documentation

Record the date and time of the procedure, the patient's actions before the obstruction, signs and symptoms of airway obstruction, approximate length of time it took to clear the airway, and the type and size of the object removed. Note his vital signs after the procedure, any complications that occurred and interventions taken, and his tolerance of the procedure. Note the time, name of the practitioner notified, any orders given, and your interventions.

G

Gastric lavage

After poisoning or a drug overdose, especially in the patient who has central nervous system depression or an inadequate gag reflex, gastric lavage flushes the stomach and removes ingested substances through a gastric lavage tube. The procedure is also used to empty the stomach in preparation for endoscopic examination. For the patient with gastric or esophageal bleeding, lavage with tepid or iced water or normal saline solution may be used to stop bleeding.

Gastric lavage can be continuous or intermittent. Typically, this procedure is done in the emergency department or intensive care unit by a physician, gastroenterologist, or nurse; a side-bore lavage tube is almost always inserted by a gastroenterologist.

Gastric lavage is contraindicated after ingestion of a corrosive substance (such as lye, petroleum distillates, ammonia, alkalis, or mineral acids) because the lavage tube may perforate the already compromised esophagus.

Equipment

Lavage setup (two graduated containers for drainage, three pieces of large-lumen rubber tubing, Y-connector, and a clamp or hemostat) ♦ 2 to 3 L of normal saline solution, tap water, or appropriate antidote as ordered ♦ I.V. pole ♦ basin of ice, if ordered ♦ Ewald tube or any large-lumen gastric tube, typically #36 to #40 French (see *Using wide-bore gastric tubes,* page 220) ♦ water-soluble lubricant or anesthetic ointment ♦ stethoscope ♦ 1/2″ hypoallergenic tape ♦ 50-ml bulb or catheter-tip syringe ♦ gloves ♦ face shield ♦ linen-saver pad or towel ♦ Yankauer or tonsil-tip suction device ♦ suction apparatus ♦ labeled specimen container ♦ laboratory request form ♦ norepinephrine (Levophed) ♦ optional: patient restraints, charcoal tablets

A prepackaged, syringe-type irrigation kit may be used for intermittent lavage. For poisoning or a drug overdose, however, the continuous lavage setup may be more appropriate to use because it's a faster and more effective means of diluting and removing the harmful substance.

Preparation

- Set up the lavage equipment.
- If iced lavage is ordered, chill the desired irrigant (water or normal saline solution) in a basin of ice.
- Lubricate the end of the lavage tube with the water-soluble lubricant or anesthetic ointment.

Key steps

DEVICE SAFETY

Correct lavage tube placement is essential for patient safety because accidental misplacement (in the lungs, for example) followed by lavage can be fatal.

- Explain the procedure to the patient, provide privacy, and wash your hands.
- Put on gloves and a face shield.
- Drape the towel or linen-saver pad over the patient's chest to protect him from spills.

Using wide-bore gastric tubes

If you need to deliver a large volume of fluid rapidly through a gastric tube (when irrigating the stomach of the patient with profuse gastric bleeding or poisoning, for example), a wide-bore gastric tube usually serves best. Typically inserted orally, these tubes remain in place only long enough to complete the lavage and evacuate stomach contents.

Ewald tube

In an emergency, using the Ewald tube (a single-lumen tube with several openings at the distal end) allows you to aspirate large amounts of gastric contents quickly.

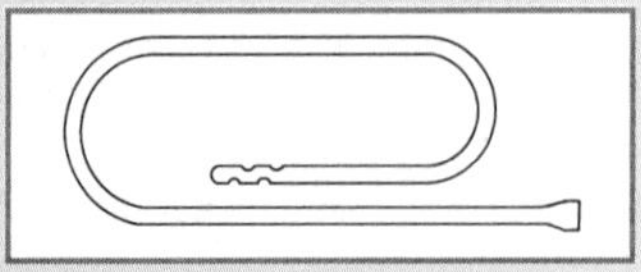

Lavacuator tube

The lavacuator tube has two lumens. Use the larger lumen for evacuating gastric contents; the smaller, for instilling an irrigant.

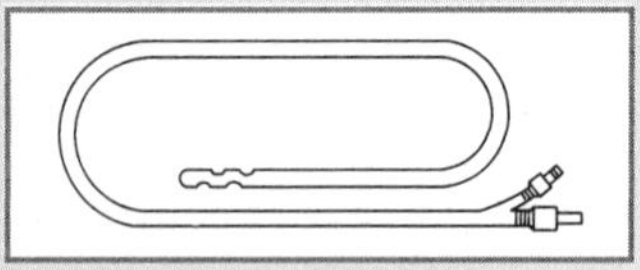

Edlich tube

The Edlich tube is a single-lumen tube that has four openings near the closed distal tip. A funnel or syringe may be connected at the proximal end. Like the Ewald tube, the Edlich tube lets you withdraw large quantities of gastric contents quickly.

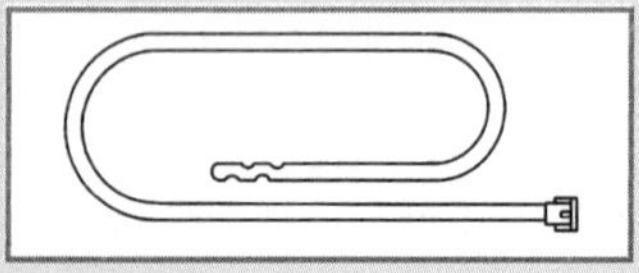

- The physician inserts the lavage tube nasally or orally and advances it slowly and gently because forceful insertion may injure tissues and cause epistaxis. He checks the tube's placement by injecting about 30 cc of air into the tube with the bulb syringe and then auscultating the patient's abdomen with a stethoscope. If the tube is in place, he'll hear the sound of air entering the stomach.
- Because the patient may vomit when the lavage tube reaches the posterior pharynx during insertion, be prepared to suction the airway immediately with either a Yankauer or a tonsil-tip suction device.
- After the lavage tube passes the posterior pharynx, assist the patient into Trendelenburg's position and turn him toward his left side in a three-quarter prone posture. This position minimizes passage of gastric contents into the duodenum and may prevent the patient from aspirating vomitus.
- After securing the lavage tube nasally or orally with tape and making sure the irrigant inflow tube on the lavage setup is clamped, connect the unattached end of this tube to the lavage tube. Check tube placement by injecting air into the tube while listening over the stomach or by testing the pH of the aspirate. Allow the stomach contents to empty into the drainage container before instilling any irrigant. This confirms proper tube placement and decreases the risk of overfilling the stomach with irrigant and inducing vomiting. If you're using a syringe irrigation set, aspirate stomach contents with a 50-ml bulb or catheter-tip syringe before instilling the irrigant.
- After you confirm proper tube placement, begin gastric lavage by instilling about 200 to 300 ml of fluid for an adult. Water or normal saline solution should be used, preferably warmed to 68.4° F (20.2° C) to avoid the risk of hypothermia.
- Clamp the inflow tube and unclamp the outflow tube to allow the irrigant to flow out. If you're using the syringe irrigation kit, aspirate the irrigant with the syringe and empty it into a calibrated container. Measure the outflow amount to make sure it equals at least the amount of irrigant you instilled. This prevents accidental stomach

distention and vomiting. If the drainage amount falls significantly short of the instilled amount, reposition the tube until sufficient solution flows out. Gently massage the abdomen over the stomach to promote outflow.

- Repeat the inflow-outflow cycle until returned fluids appear clear. This signals that the stomach no longer holds harmful substances or that bleeding has stopped.
- Assess the patient's vital signs, urine output, and level of consciousness (LOC) every 15 minutes. Notify the practitioner of any changes.
- If ordered, remove the lavage tube.

Special considerations

- To control GI bleeding, the practitioner may order continuous irrigation of the stomach with an irrigant and a vasoconstrictor such as norepinephrine. After the stomach absorbs norepinephrine, the portal system delivers the drug directly to the liver, where it's metabolized. This prevents the drug from circulating systemically and initiating a hypertensive response. Or the practitioner may direct you to clamp the outflow tube for a prescribed period after instilling the irrigant and the vasoconstrictive medication and before withdrawing it. This allows the mucosa time to absorb the drug.
- Never leave the patient alone during gastric lavage. Observe continuously for any changes in LOC, and monitor vital signs frequently because the natural vagal response to intubation can depress the patient's heart rate.
- If you need to restrain the patient, secure restraints on the same side of the bed or stretcher so you can free him quickly without moving to the other side of the bed.
- Remember also to keep tracheal suctioning equipment nearby and watch closely for airway obstruction caused by vomiting or excess oral secretions. Throughout gastric lavage, you may need to suction the oral cavity frequently to ensure an open airway and prevent aspiration. For the same reasons, and if the patient doesn't exhibit an adequate gag reflex, he may require an endotracheal tube before the procedure.
- When aspirating the stomach for ingested poisons or drugs, save the contents in a labeled container to send to the laboratory for analysis along with a laboratory request form. If ordered, after lavage to remove poisons or drugs, mix charcoal tablets with the irrigant (water or normal saline solution) and administer the mixture through the nasogastric (NG) tube. The charcoal will absorb remaining toxic substances. The tube may be clamped temporarily, allowed to drain via gravity, attached to intermittent suction, or removed.
- When performing gastric lavage to stop bleeding, keep precise intake and output records to determine the amount of bleeding. When large volumes of fluid are instilled and withdrawn, serum electrolyte and arterial blood gas levels may be measured during or at the end of lavage.

Complications

- Vomiting and subsequent aspiration typically occurring in the groggy patient
- Bradyarrhythmias
- Cardiac arrhythmias, triggered especially after iced lavage, due to the patient's dropping body temperature

Documentation

Record the date and time of lavage, the size and type of NG tube used, the volume and type of irrigant, and the amount of drained gastric contents. Record this information on the intake and output record sheet, and include your observations, including the color and consistency of drainage. Keep precise records of the patient's vital signs and LOC, any drugs instilled through the tube, the time the tube was removed, and how well the patient tolerated the procedure.

Gastrostomy feeding button care

A gastrostomy feeding button serves as an alternative feeding device for the ambulatory patient who's receiving long-term enteral feedings.

Approved by the U.S. Food and Drug Administration for 6-month implantation, feeding buttons can be used to replace gastrostomy tubes if necessary.

The button has a mushroom dome at one end and two wing tabs and a flexible safety plug at the other. When inserted into an established stoma, the button lies almost flush with the skin, with only the top of the safety plug visible.

The button can usually be inserted into a stoma in less than 15 minutes. Besides its cosmetic appeal, the device is easily maintained, reduces skin irritation and breakdown, and is less likely to become dislodged or migrate than an ordinary feeding tube. A one-way, antireflux valve mounted just inside the mushroom dome prevents accidental leakage of gastric contents. The device usually requires replacement after 3 to 4 months, typically because the antireflux valve wears out.

Equipment

Gastrostomy feeding button of the correct size (all three sizes, if the correct one isn't known) ♦ obturator ♦ water-soluble lubricant ♦ gloves ♦ feeding accessories, including adapter, feeding catheter, food syringe or bag, and formula ♦ catheter clamp ♦ cleaning equipment, including water, a syringe, cotton-tipped applicator, pipe cleaner, and mild soap or antiseptic cleaning solution ♦ optional: I.V. pole, pump to provide continuous infusion over several hours

Key steps

- Confirm the patient's identity using two patient identifiers according to your facility's policy.
- Explain the insertion, reinsertion, and feeding procedure to the patient. Tell him the physician will perform the initial insertion.
- Wash your hands and put on gloves. (See *Reinserting a gastrostomy feeding button.*)
- Elevate the head of the bed 30 to 45 degrees.
- Check for residual with the syringe. If greater than 50 to 100 cc, report to the practitioner and hold feeding until reassessment.
- Attach the adapter and feeding catheter to the syringe or feeding bag. Clamp the catheter and fill the syringe or bag and catheter with formula. Refill the syringe before it's empty. These steps prevent air from entering the stomach and distending the abdomen.
- Open the safety plug and attach the adapter and feeding catheter to the button. Elevate the syringe or feeding bag above stomach level, and gravity-feed the formula for 15 to 30 minutes, varying the height as needed to alter the flow rate. Use a pump for continuous infusion or for feedings lasting several hours.
- After the feeding, flush the button with 10 ml of water and clean the inside of the feeding catheter with a cotton-tipped applicator and water to preserve patency and to dislodge formula or food particles, and lower the syringe or bag below stomach level to allow burping. Remove the adapter and feeding catheter. The antireflux valve should prevent gastric reflux. Then snap the safety plug in place to keep the lumen clean and prevent leakage if the antireflux valve fails. If the patient feels nauseated or vomits after the feeding, vent the button with the adapter and feeding catheter to control emesis.
- Maintain the head of the bed elevated at 30 to 45 degrees for at least 1 hour after feeding.
- Wash the catheter and syringe or feeding bag in warm soapy water and rinse thoroughly. Clean the catheter and adapter with a pipe cleaner. Rinse well before using for the next feeding. Soak the equipment once per week according to manufacturer's recommendations.

Special considerations

- If the button pops out while feeding, reinsert it, estimate the formula already delivered, and resume feeding.
- Once daily, clean the peristomal skin with mild soap and water or povidone-iodine, and let the skin air-dry for 20 minutes to avoid skin irritation. Clean the site whenever spillage from the feeding bag occurs.
- As the patient's weight or body mass index increases, monitor the site for embedded bumper (external). Report skin irrita-

Reinserting a gastrostomy feeding button

If your patient's gastrostomy feeding button pops out (with coughing, for instance), either you or he will need to reinsert the device. Here are some steps to follow.

Prepare the equipment

Collect the feeding button, an obturator, and water-soluble lubricant. If the button will be reinserted, wash it with soap and water and rinse it thoroughly.

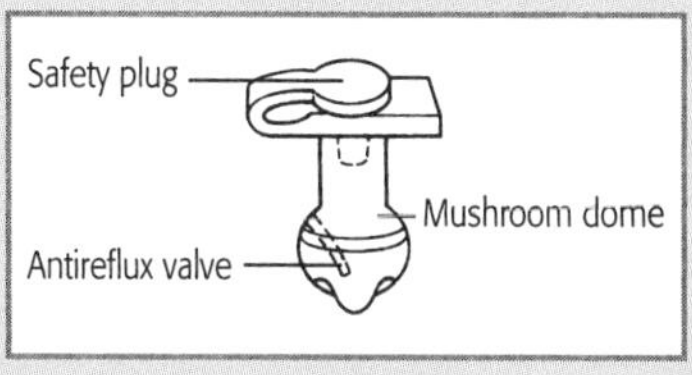

Insert the button

- Check the depth of the patient's stoma to make sure you have a feeding button of the correct size. Then clean around the stoma.
- Lubricate the obturator with a water-soluble lubricant, and distend the button several times.
- Lubricate the mushroom dome and the stoma. Gently push the button through the stoma into the stomach.

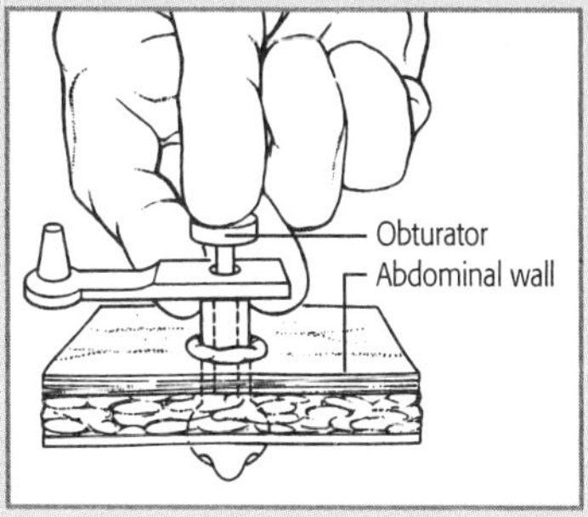

- Remove the obturator by gently rotating it as you withdraw it. If the valve sticks, gently push the obturator back into the button until the valve closes.
- After removing the obturator, make sure the valve is closed. Then close the flexible safety plug, which should be relatively flush with the skin surface.

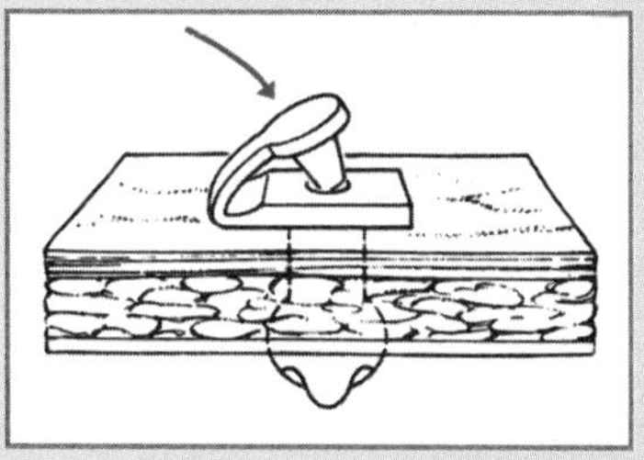

- If you need to administer a feeding right away, open the safety plug and attach the feeding adapter and feeding tube. Deliver the feeding as ordered.

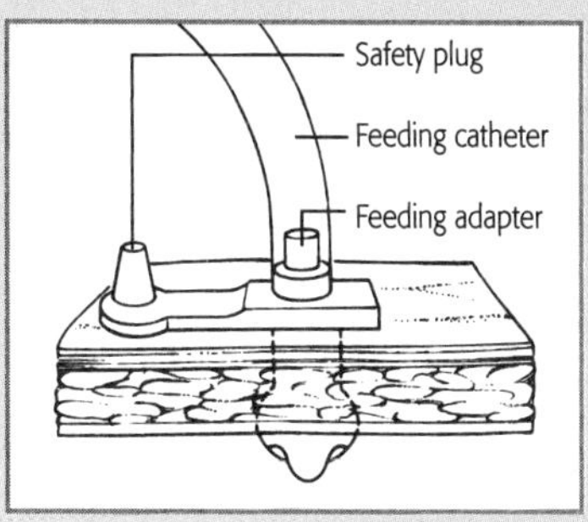

tion and increased tension between exit site and bumper to the practitioner.

Complications

- Nausea and vomiting, abdominal distention, exit-site infection, exit-site leakage, and peritonitis

Patient teaching

- Before discharge, make sure the patient can insert and care for the gastrostomy feeding button.
- If necessary, teach him or a family member how to reinsert the button by first practicing on a model.

- Explain to the patient how to care for the skin around the button.
- Offer written instructions and answer his questions about obtaining replacement supplies.
- Tell the patient when and whom to call for questions.

Documentation

Record the feeding time and duration, amount and type of feeding formula used, and the patient's tolerance. Maintain intake and output records as necessary. Note the appearance of the stoma and surrounding skin.

H

Halo-vest traction

Halo-vest traction immobilizes the head and neck after traumatic injury to the cervical vertebrae, the most common of all spinal injuries. This procedure, which can prevent further injury to the spinal cord, is performed by a neurosurgeon or an orthopedic surgeon, with nursing assistance, in the emergency department, at the patient's bedside, or in the operating room after surgical reduction of vertebral injuries. The halo-vest traction device consists of a metal ring that fits over the patient's head and metal bars that connect the ring to a plastic vest that distributes the weight of the entire apparatus around the chest. (See *Comparing halo-vest traction devices,* page 226.)

When in place, halo-vest traction allows the patient greater mobility than does traction with skull tongs. It also carries less risk of infection because it doesn't require skin incisions and drill holes to position skull pins.

Equipment

Halo-vest traction unit ♦ halo ring ♦ cervical collar or sandbags (if needed) ♦ plastic vest ♦ board or padded headrest ♦ tape measure ♦ halo ring conversion chart ♦ scissors ♦ 4″ × 4″ gauze pads ♦ antiseptic cleaning solution ♦ sterile gloves ♦ Allen wrench ♦ four positioning pins ♦ multiple-dose vial of 1% lidocaine ♦ alcohol pads ♦ 3-ml syringe ♦ 25G needles ♦ five sterile skull pins (one more than needed) ♦ torque screwdriver ♦ sheepskin liners ♦ cotton-tipped applicators ♦ ordered cleaning solution ♦ medicated powder or cornstarch ♦ sterile water or normal saline solution ♦ optional: pain medication (such as an analgesic)

Most facilities supply packaged halo-vest traction units that include software (jacket and sheepskin liners), hardware (halo, head pins, upright bars, and screws), and tools (torque screwdriver, two conventional wrenches, Allen wrench, and screws and bolts). These units don't include sterile gloves, antiseptic solution, sterile drapes, cervical collars, or equipment for local anesthetic injection.

Preparation

- Obtain a halo-vest traction unit with halo rings and plastic vests in several sizes. Vest sizes are based on the patient's head and chest measurements.
- Check the expiration date of the prepackaged tray, and check the outside covering for damage to ensure the sterility of the contents.
- Then assemble the equipment at the patient's bedside.

Key steps

- Check the support that was applied to the patient's neck on the way to the hospital. If necessary, apply the cervical collar immediately or immobilize the head and neck with sandbags. Keep the cervical collar or sandbags in place until the halo is applied. This support will then be carefully removed to facilitate application of the vest. Because the patient is likely to be frightened, try to reassure him.

Comparing halo-vest traction devices

Type	Description	Advantages
Low profile (standard) 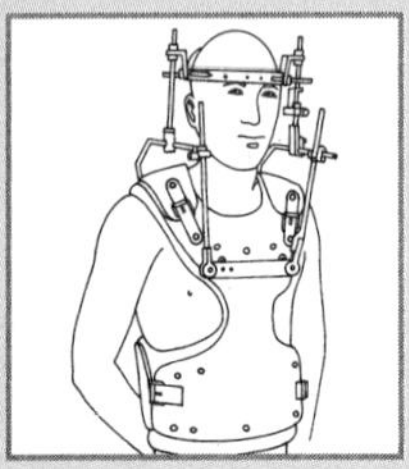	■ Traction and compression are produced by threaded support rods on either side of the halo ring. ■ Flexion and extension are obtained by moving the swivel arm to an anterior or posterior position, depending on the location of the skull pins.	■ Immobilizes cervical spine fractures while allowing patient mobility ■ Facilitates surgery of the cervical spine and permits flexion and extension ■ Allows airway intubation without losing skeletal traction ■ Facilitates necessary alignment by an adjustment at the junction of the threaded support rods and horizontal frame
Mark II (type of low profile) 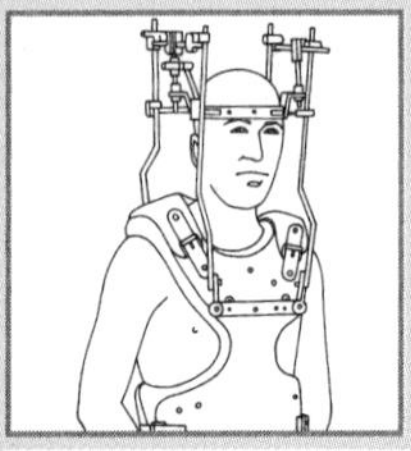	■ Traction and compression are produced by threaded support rods on either side of the halo ring. ■ Flexion and extension are obtained by swivel clamps, which allow the bars to intersect and hold at any angle.	■ Enables the physician to assemble the metal framework more quickly ■ Allows unobstructed access for anteroposterior and lateral X-rays of the cervical spine ■ Allows the patient to wear his usual clothing because uprights are shaped closer to the body
Mark III (update of Mark II) 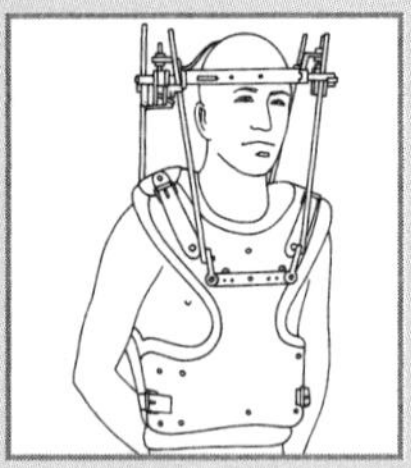	■ Traction and compression are produced by threaded support rods on either side of the halo ring. ■ Flexion and extension are accommodated by a serrated split articulation coupling attached to the halo ring, which can be adjusted in 4-degree increments.	■ Simplifies application while promoting patient comfort ■ Eliminates shoulder pressure and discomfort by using a flexible padded strap instead of the vest's solid plastic shoulder ■ Accommodates the tall patient with modified hardware and shorter uprights and allows unobstructed access for medial and lateral X-rays
Trippi-Wells tongs 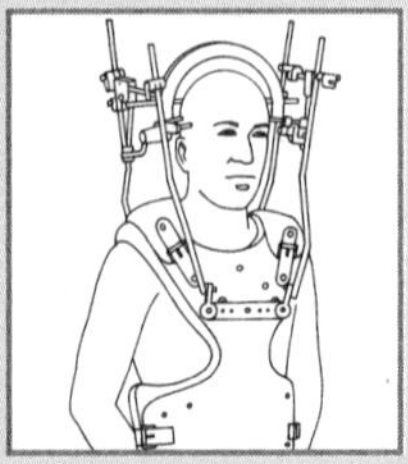	■ Traction is produced by four pins that compress the skull. ■ Flexion and extension are obtained by adjusting the midline vertical plate.	■ Applies tensile force to the neck or spine while allowing patient mobility ■ Makes it possible to change from mobile to stationary traction without interrupting traction ■ Adjusts to three planes for mobile and stationary traction ■ Allows unobstructed access for medial and lateral X-rays

■ Remove the headboard and any furniture at the head of the bed to provide ample working space.

ALERT

Never put the patient's head on a pillow before applying the halo to avoid further injury to the spinal cord.

■ Elevate the bed to a working level that gives the physician easy access to the front and back of the halo unit.
■ Stand at the head of the bed, and see if the patient's chin lines up with his midsternum, indicating proper alignment. If ordered, support the patient's head in your hands and gently rotate the neck into alignment without flexing or extending it.

Assisting with halo application

■ Ask another nurse to help you with the procedure.
■ Explain the procedure to the patient, wash your hands, and provide privacy.
■ Have the assisting nurse hold the patient's head and neck stable while the physician removes the cervical collar or sandbags. Maintain this support until the halo is secure, while you assist with pin insertion.
■ The physician measures the patient's head with a tape measure and refers to the halo-ring conversion chart to determine the correct ring size. (The ring should clear the head by $^{2}/_{3}''$ [1.5 cm] and fit $^{1}/_{3}''$ [1 cm] above the bridge of the nose.)
■ The physician selects four pin sites: $^{1}/_{2}''$ above the lateral one-third of each eyebrow and $^{1}/_{2}''$ above the top of each ear in the occipital area. He also takes into account the degree and type of correction needed to provide proper cervical alignment.
■ Trim the hair at the pin sites with scissors to facilitate subsequent care and help prevent infection. Then use 4″ × 4″ gauze pads soaked in antiseptic cleaning solution to clean the sites.
■ Open the halo-vest unit using sterile technique to avoid contamination. The physician puts on the sterile gloves and removes the halo and the Allen wrench. He then places the halo over the patient's head and inserts the four positioning pins to hold the halo in place temporarily.
■ Help the physician prepare the anesthetic. First, clean the injection port of the multiple-dose vial of lidocaine with the alcohol pad. Then, invert the vial so the physician can insert a 25G needle attached to the 3-ml syringe and withdraw the anesthetic.
■ The physician injects the anesthetic at the four pin sites. He may change needles on the syringe after each injection.
■ The physician removes four of the five skull pins from the sterile setup and firmly screws in each pin at a 90-degree angle to the skull. When the pins are in place, he removes the positioning pins. He then tightens the skull pins with the torque screwdriver.

Applying the vest

■ After the physician measures the patient's chest and abdomen, he selects a vest of appropriate size.
■ Place the sheepskin liners inside the front and back of the vest to make it more comfortable to wear and to help prevent pressure ulcers.
■ Help the physician carefully raise the patient while the other nurse supports the head and neck. Slide the back of the vest under the patient and gently lay him down. The physician then fastens the front of the vest on the patient's chest using Velcro straps.
■ The physician attaches the metal bars to the halo and vest and tightens each bolt in turn to avoid tightening any single bolt completely, causing maladjusted tension. When halo-vest traction is in place, X-rays should be taken immediately to check the depth of the skull pins and verify proper alignment.

Caring for the patient

■ Take routine and neurologic vital signs at least every 2 hours for 24 hours (preferably every hour for 48 hours) and then every 4 hours until stable.

ACTION STAT!

Notify the physician immediately if you observe any loss of motor function or any decreased sensation from baseline because these findings could indicate spinal cord trauma.

- Put on gloves. Gently clean the pin sites every 4 hours with cotton-tipped applicators. Rinse the sites with normal saline solution to remove any excess cleaning solution. Then clean the pin sites with antiseptic cleaning solution. Meticulous pin-site care prevents infection and removes debris that might block drainage and lead to abscess formation. Watch for signs of infection—a loose pin, swelling or redness, purulent drainage, pain at the site—and notify the physician if these signs develop.
- The physician retightens the skull pins with the torque screwdriver 24 and 48 hours after the halo is applied. If the patient complains of a headache after the pins are tightened, obtain an order for an analgesic.

ACTION STAT!

If pain occurs with jaw movement or any movement of the head or neck, notify the physician immediately because this may indicate that the pins have slipped onto the thin temporal plate.

- Examine the halo-vest unit every shift to make sure that it's secure and that the patient's head is centered within the halo. If the vest fits correctly, you should be able to insert one or two fingers under the jacket at the shoulder and chest when the patient is lying supine.
- Wash the patient's chest and back daily. First, place the patient on his back. Loosen the bottom Velcro straps so you can get to the chest and back. Then, reaching under the vest, wash and dry the skin. Check for tender, reddened areas or pressure spots that may develop into ulcers. If necessary, use a hair dryer to dry damp sheepskin because moisture predisposes the skin to pressure ulcer formation. Lightly dust the skin with medicated powder or cornstarch to prevent itching. If itching persists, check to see if the patient is allergic to sheepskin and if any drug he's taking might cause a skin rash. If your facility's policy allows, change the vest lining as necessary.
- Turn the patient on his side (less than 45 degrees) to wash his back. Then close the vest.
- Be careful not to put any stress on the apparatus, which could knock it out of alignment and lead to subluxation of the cervical spine.

Special considerations

ALERT

Keep two conventional wrenches available at all times; they may be taped to the patient's halo-vest on the chest area. In case of cardiac arrest, use them to remove the distal anterior bolts. Pull the two upright bars outward. Unfasten the Velcro straps, and remove the front of the vest. Use the sturdy back of the vest as a board for cardiopulmonary resuscitation (CPR). Some vests have a hinged front to raise the breast plate for CPR. Know the type of vest your patient has. To prevent subluxating the cervical injury, start CPR with the jaw thrust maneuver, which avoids hyperextension of the neck. Pull the patient's mandible forward while maintaining proper head and neck alignment. This maneuver pulls the tongue forward to open the airway.

- Never lift the patient up by the vertical bars. This could strain or tear the skin at the pin sites or misalign the traction.
- To prevent falls, walk with the ambulatory patient. Remember, he'll have difficulty seeing objects at or near his feet, and the weight of the halo-vest unit (about 10 lb [4.5 kg]) may throw him off balance. If the patient is in a wheelchair, lower the leg rests to prevent the chair from tipping backward.
- Because the vest limits chest expansion, routinely assess pulmonary function, especially in the patient with pulmonary disease.

- Teach the patient to turn slowly—in small increments—to avoid losing his balance.
- Remind him to avoid bending forward because the extra weight of the halo apparatus could cause him to fall. Teach him to bend at the knees rather than the waist.
- Have a physical therapist teach the patient how to use assistive devices to extend his reach and to help him put on socks and shoes.
- Suggest that he wear shirts that button in front and that are larger than usual to accommodate the halo-vest.
- Most important, teach the patient about pin-site care and about shampooing and hair care.

Complications

- Paralysis below the break caused by compression of the cord due to manipulation of the patient's neck during application of halo-vest traction causing subluxation of the spinal cord, or possible pushing of a bone fragment into the spinal cord
- Puncture of the skull and dura mater causing a loss of cerebrospinal fluid and a serious central nervous system infection due to inaccurate positioning of the skull pins
- Infection at the pin sites due to nonsterile technique during application of the halo or inadequate pin-site care
- Pressure ulcers developing if the vest fits poorly or chafes the skin

Patient teaching

- Teach the patient how to perform pin-site care and about shampooing and hair care.
- Make sure the patient understands activity restrictions before discharge.

Documentation

Record the date and time that the halo-vest traction was applied. Also note the length of the procedure and the patient's response. After application, record routine and neurologic vital signs. Document pin-site care and note any signs of infection.

Hand hygiene

The success of infection control in the United States has been due in a large part to recognizing the individual as a primary source of health care-associated infections (HAIs). The hands are the conduits for almost every transfer of potential pathogens from one patient to another, from a contaminated object to the patient, or from a staff member to the patient. To protect patients from HAIs, hand hygiene must be performed routinely and thoroughly.

The Centers for Disease Control and Prevention guidelines define hand hygiene as hand washing, antiseptic hand washing, antiseptic hand rub, or surgical hand antisepsis. Plain soap, detergents, or antimicrobial-containing products may be used to wash the hands. Hand hygiene can be broken down into two processes. Mechanical removal of microorganisms occurs when the hands are washed with plain soap or detergent; in this process, microorganisms are removed from the hands, which are then rinsed. Chemical removal of microorganisms occurs when the hands are washed with an antimicrobial agent; this process kills or inhibits the growth of microorganisms. The decision as to when hand hygiene should occur depends on four factors:

- intensity of contact with patients or fomites
- degree of contamination that's likely to occur with contact
- susceptibility of patients to infection
- procedure to be performed.

Equipment

Hand washing

Antibacterial or antimicrobial soap or detergent ♦ warm running water ♦ paper towels ♦ optional: antiseptic cleaning agent, fingernail brush, disposable sponge brush or plastic cuticle stick

Hand sanitizing

Alcohol-based hand rub

Proper hand hygiene technique

To minimize the spread of infection, follow these basic hand-washing instructions. With your hands angled downward under the faucet, adjust the water temperature until it's comfortably warm.

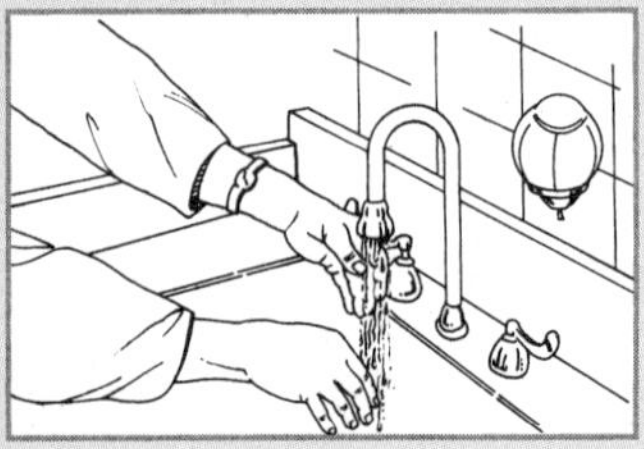

Work up a generous lather by scrubbing vigorously for 10 seconds. Be sure you clean beneath your fingernails, around your knuckles, and along the sides of your fingers and hands.

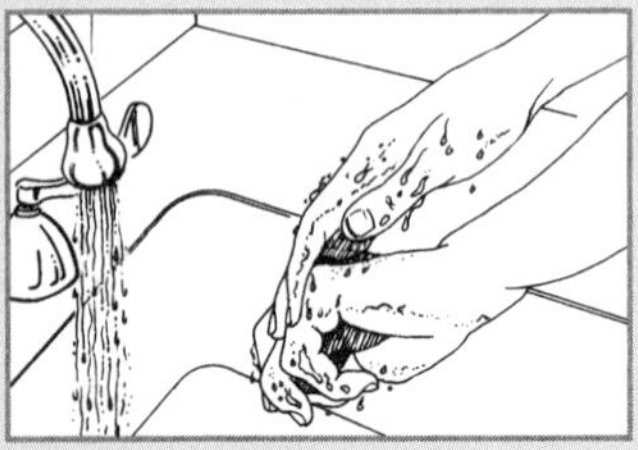

Rinse your hands completely to wash away suds and microorganisms. Pat dry with a paper towel. To prevent recontaminating your hands on the faucet handles, cover each one with a dry paper towel before turning off the water.

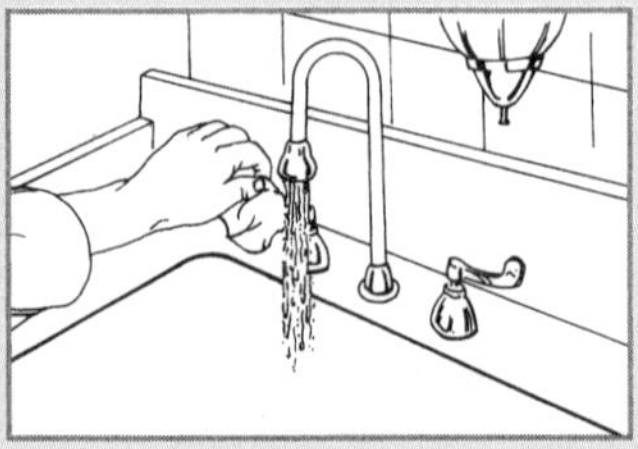

Key steps

Hand washing

- Remove rings as your facility policy dictates because they harbor dirt and skin microorganisms. Remove your watch or wear it well above the wrist.
- Wet your hands and wrists with warm water and apply soap from a dispenser. Don't use bar soap because it allows cross-contamination. Hold your hands below elbow level to prevent water from running up your arms and back down, thus contaminating clean areas. (See *Proper hand hygiene technique*.)
- Work up a generous lather by rubbing your hands together vigorously for about 10 seconds. Soap and warm water reduce surface tension and this, aided by friction, loosens surface microorganisms, which wash away in the lather.
- Pay special attention to the area under the fingernails and around the cuticles and to the thumbs, knuckles, and sides of the fingers and hands because microorganisms thrive in these protected or overlooked areas. If you don't remove your rings, move them up and down your fingers to clean beneath them.
- Avoid splashing water on yourself or the floor because microorganisms spread more easily on wet surfaces and because slippery floors are dangerous. Also avoid touching the sink or faucets because they're considered contaminated.
- Rinse hands and wrists well because running water flushes suds, soil, and microorganisms away.
- Pat hands and wrists dry with a paper towel. Avoid rubbing, which can cause abrasion and chapping.
- If the sink isn't equipped with knee or foot controls, turn off the faucets by gripping them with a dry paper towel to avoid recontaminating your hands.

Hand sanitizing

- Apply a small amount of the alcohol-based hand rub to all surfaces of the hands.
- Rub hands together until all of the product has dried (usually 30 seconds).

Special considerations

- Wash your forearms as well as your hands thoroughly before participating in a sterile procedure, or whenever your hands are grossly contaminated. Clean under the fingernails as well and in and around the cuticles with a fingernail brush, disposable sponge brush, or plastic cuticle stick. Use these softer implements because brushes, metal files, or other hard objects may injure your skin and, if reused, may be a source of contamination.
- Artificial nails may serve as a reservoir for microorganisms; therefore, they shouldn't be worn in health care facilities. Naturally long nails may also harbor more microorganisms; keep nails trimmed short, no more than 1/4" beyond the edge of the finger.
- Follow your facility's policy concerning when to wash with soap and when to use an antiseptic cleaning agent. Typically, you'll wash with soap before coming on duty, before and after direct or indirect patient contact, before preparing or serving food, before preparing or administering medications, before and after performing any bodily functions (such as blowing your nose or using the bathroom), after direct or indirect contact with a patient's excretions, secretions, or blood, and after completing your shift.
- Use an antiseptic cleaning agent before performing invasive procedures, wound care, and dressing changes, and after contamination. Antiseptics are also recommended for hand hygiene in isolation rooms, neonate nurseries, and before caring for a highly susceptible patient.
- If your hands aren't visibly soiled, an alcohol-based hand rub is preferred for routine decontamination. Always wash your hands after removing gloves.
- If you're providing care in the patient's home, bring your own supply of soap and disposable paper towels. If there's no running water, use an alcohol-based hand sanitizer.
- Don't use an alcohol-based hand sanitizer if you contact items contaminated with *Clostridium difficile* or *Bacillus anthracis* (Anthrax). These organisms can form spores and alcohol won't kill them. Wash your hands with soap and water or antiseptic soap and water if either of these organisms is known or suspected to be present.
- It's important to keep hands soft and use lotion between washings because microorganisms are more difficult to remove from rough or chapped hands.

Complications

- Dryness, cracking, and irritation due to frequent hand hygiene that strips the skin of its natural oils (especially in those with sensitive skin)

Patient teaching

- Teach the patient proper hand hygiene when he'll be providing self-care.

Documentation

Document proper hand hygiene as it pertains to specific patient care.

Hemodialysis

Hemodialysis is performed to remove toxic wastes from the blood of patients in renal failure. This potentially life-saving procedure removes blood from the body, circulates it through a purifying dialyzer, and then returns it to the body. Various access sites can be used for this procedure. (See *Hemodialysis access sites,* page 232.) The most common access device for long-term treatment is an arteriovenous (AV) fistula. (See "Arteriovenous fistula care," page 15.)

Differential diffusion across a semipermeable membrane (the underlying mechanism in hemodialysis) extracts by-products of protein metabolism, such as urea and uric acid, as well as creatinine and excess body water. This process restores or maintains the balance of the body's buffer system and electrolyte level. Hemodialysis thus promotes a rapid return to normal serum values and helps prevent complications associated with uremia.

Hemodialysis provides temporary support for patients with acute reversible renal failure. It's also used for regular long-term treatment of patients with chronic end-stage renal disease. A less common indication for hemodialysis is acute poisoning,

Hemodialysis access sites

Hemodialysis requires vascular access. The site and type of access may vary, depending on the expected duration of dialysis, the surgeon's preference, and the patient's condition.

Subclavian vein catheterization

Using the Seldinger technique, the physician or surgeon inserts an introducer needle into the subclavian vein. He then inserts a guide wire through the introducer needle and removes the needle. Using the guide wire, he next threads a 5" to 12" (12.5 to 30.5 cm) plastic or Teflon catheter (with a Y-hub) into the patient's vein.

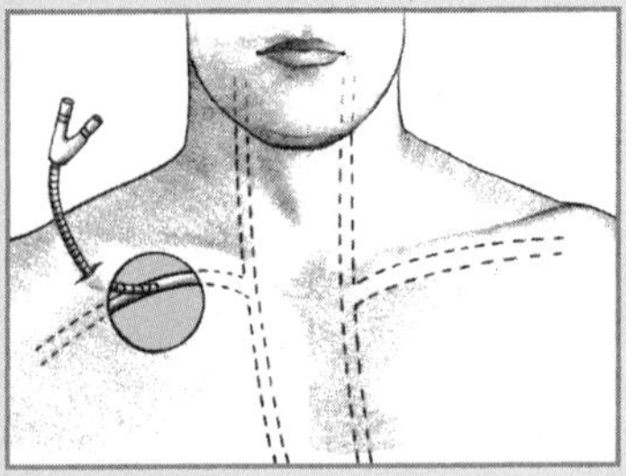

Femoral vein catheterization

Using the Seldinger technique, the physician or surgeon inserts an introducer needle into the left or right femoral vein. He then inserts a guide wire through the introducer needle and removes the needle.

Using the guide wire, he next threads a 5" to 12" plastic or Teflon catheter with a Y-hub or two catheters, one for inflow and another placed about ½" (1 cm) distal to the first for outflow.

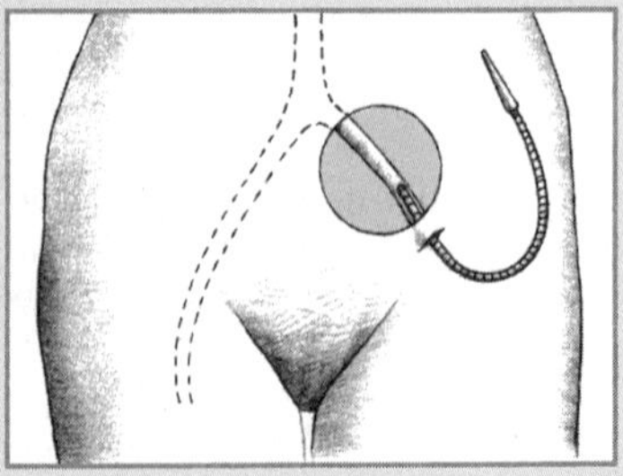

Arteriovenous fistula

To create a fistula, the surgeon makes an incision into the patient's wrist or lower forearm, then a small incision in the side of an artery and another in the side of a vein. He sutures the edges of the incisions together to make a common opening 3 to 7 mm long.

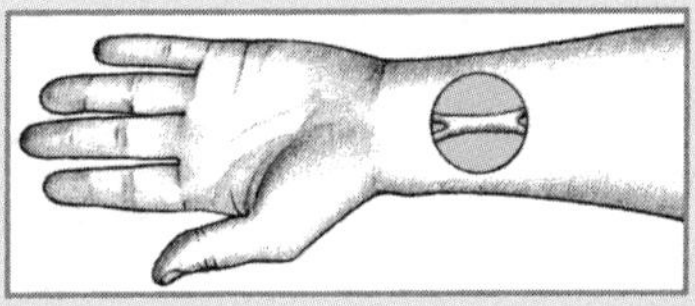

Arteriovenous shunt

To create a shunt, the surgeon makes an incision in the patient's wrist, lower forearm, or (rarely) an ankle. He then inserts a 6" to 10" (15 to 25.5 cm) transparent Silastic cannula into an artery and another into a vein. Finally, he tunnels the cannulas out through stab wounds and joins them with a piece of Teflon tubing.

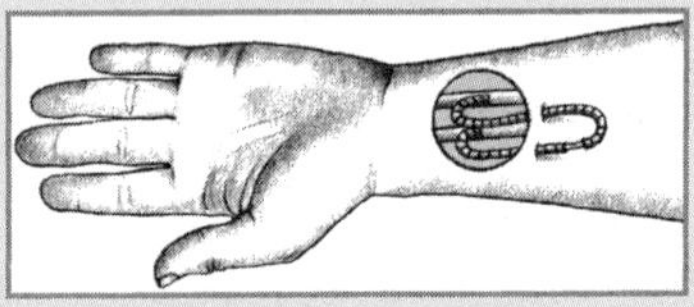

Arteriovenous graft

To create a graft, the surgeon makes an incision in the patient's forearm, upper arm, or thigh. He then tunnels a natural or synthetic graft under the skin and sutures the distal end to an artery and the proximal end to a vein.

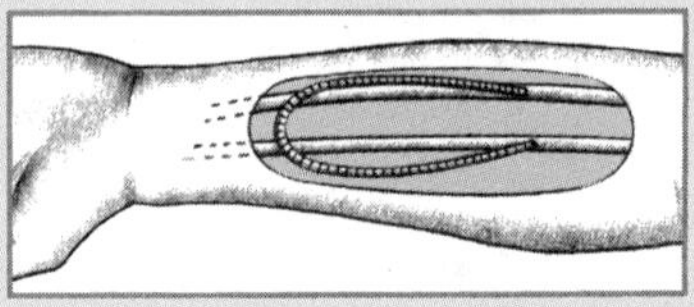

such as barbiturate or analgesic overdose. The patient's condition (rate of creatinine accumulation, weight gain) determines the number and duration of hemodialysis treatments.

Specially trained personnel usually perform this procedure in a hemodialysis unit. However, if the patient is acutely ill and unstable, hemodialysis can be done at the bedside in the intensive care unit.

Equipment

Preparing the hemodialysis machine

Hemodialysis machine with appropriate dialyzer ♦ I.V. solution, administration sets, lines, and related equipment ♦ dialysate ♦ optional: heparin, 3-ml syringe with needle, medication label, hemostats

Hemodialysis with a double-lumen catheter

Antiseptic pads ♦ two sterile 4″ × 4″ gauze pads ♦ two 3-ml and two 5-ml syringes ♦ tape ♦ heparin bolus syringe ♦ clean gloves ♦ sterile labels ♦ sterile marker

Hemodialysis with an AV fistula

Two winged fistula needles (each attached to a 10-ml syringe filled with heparin flush solution) ♦ linen-saver pad ♦ antiseptic pads ♦ sterile 4″ × 4″ gauze pads ♦ tourniquet ♦ clean gloves ♦ adhesive tape ♦ sterile labels ♦ sterile marker ♦ antiseptic cleaning solution

Hemodialysis with an AV shunt

Alcohol pads ♦ antiseptic pads ♦ sterile gloves ♦ two sterile shunt adapters ♦ sterile Teflon connector ♦ two bulldog clamps ♦ two 10-ml syringes ♦ normal saline solution ♦ four short strips of adhesive tape ♦ optional: sterile shunt spreader, sterile labels, sterile marker

Discontinuing hemodialysis with a double-lumen catheter

Sterile 4″× 4″ gauze pads ♦ antiseptic pads ♦ precut gauze dressing ♦ clean and sterile gloves ♦ normal saline solution ♦ alcohol pads ♦ heparin flush solution ♦ luer-lock injection caps ♦ optional: transparent occlusive dressing, skin barrier preparation, tape, materials for culturing drainage, sterile labels, sterile marker

Discontinuing hemodialysis with an AV fistula

Clean gloves ♦ sterile 4″ × 4″ gauze pads ♦ two adhesive bandages ♦ hemostats ♦ optional: sterile absorbable gelatin sponges (Gelfoam)

Discontinuing hemodialysis with an AV shunt

Sterile gloves ♦ two bulldog clamps ♦ two hemostats ♦ antiseptic cleaning solution ♦ sterile 4″ × 4″ gauze pads ♦ alcohol pads ♦ elastic gauze bandages ♦ plasticized or hypoallergenic tape

Preparation

- Prepare the hemodialysis equipment following the manufacturer's instructions and your facility's protocol.
- Maintain strict sterile technique to prevent introducing pathogens into the patient's bloodstream during dialysis.
- Make sure to test the dialyzer and dialysis machine for residual disinfectant after rinsing, and to test all the alarms.

Key steps

- Confirm the patient's identity using two patient identifiers according to your facility's policy.
- Weigh the patient. To determine ultrafiltration requirements, compare his present weight to his weight after the last dialysis and his target weight. Record his baseline vital signs, taking his blood pressure while he's sitting and standing. Auscultate his heart for rate, rhythm, and abnormalities. Observe respiratory rate, rhythm, and quality. Assess for edema. Check his mental status and the condition and patency of the access site. Check for problems since the last dialysis, and evaluate previous laboratory data.
- Help the patient into a comfortable position (supine or sitting in recliner chair with feet elevated). Make sure that the access site is well supported and resting on a clean drape.

■ If the patient is undergoing hemodialysis for the first time, explain the procedure in detail.
■ Use standard precautions in all cases to prevent transmission of infection. Wash your hands before beginning.
■ Label all medications, medication containers, and other solutions on and off the sterile field.

Beginning hemodialysis with a double-lumen catheter

■ Prepare venous access. If the extension tubing isn't already clamped, clamp it to prevent air from entering the catheter. Clean each catheter extension tube, clamp, and luer-lock injection cap with antiseptic pads to remove contaminants. Next, place a sterile 4″ × 4″ gauze pad under the extension tubing, and place two 5-ml syringes and two sterile gauze pads on the drape.
■ Prepare the anticoagulant regimen as ordered.
■ Identify arterial and venous blood lines, and place them near the drape.
■ To remove clots and ensure catheter patency, remove catheter caps, attach syringes to each catheter port, open one clamp, and aspirate 1.5 to 3 ml of blood. Close the clamp and repeat the procedure with the other port. Flush each port with 5 ml of heparin flush solution.
■ Attach blood lines to patient access. First, remove the syringe from the arterial port, and attach the line to the arterial port. Administer the heparin according to protocol. This prevents clotting in the extracorporeal circuit.
■ Grasp the venous blood line and attach it to the venous port. Open the clamps on the extension tubing, and secure the tubing to the patient's extremity with tape to reduce tension on the tube and minimize trauma to the insertion site.
■ Begin hemodialysis according to your facility's policy.

Beginning hemodialysis with an AV fistula

■ Flush the fistula needles, using attached syringes containing heparinized normal saline solution, and set them aside.
■ Place a linen-saver pad under the patient's arm.
■ Using sterile technique, clean a 3″ × 10″ (7.5 × 25 cm) area of skin over the fistula with antiseptic pads. Discard each pad after one wipe.
■ Apply a tourniquet above the fistula to distend the veins and facilitate venipuncture. Be sure to avoid occluding the fistula.
■ Put on clean gloves. Perform the venipuncture with a fistula needle. Remove the needle guard and squeeze the wing tips firmly together. Insert the arterial needle at least 1″ (2.5 cm) above the anastomosis, being careful not to puncture the fistula.
■ Release the tourniquet and flush the needle with heparin flush solution to prevent clotting. Clamp the arterial needle tubing with a hemostat, and secure the wing tips of the needle to the skin with adhesive tape to prevent it from dislodging within the vein.
■ Perform another venipuncture with the venous needle a few inches above the arterial needle. Flush the needle with heparin flush solution. Clamp the venous needle tubing, and secure the wing tips of the venous needle as you did the arterial needle.
■ Remove the syringe from the end of the arterial tubing, uncap the arterial line from the hemodialysis machine, and connect the two lines. Tape the connection securely to prevent it from separating during the procedure. Repeat these two steps for the venous line.
■ Release the hemostats and start hemodialysis.

Beginning hemodialysis with an AV shunt

■ Remove the bulldog clamps and place them within easy reach of the sterile field. Remove the shunt dressing, and clean the shunt, using sterile technique, as you would for daily care. (See "Arteriovenous fistula care," page 15.) Clean the bulldog clamps with an alcohol pad.
■ Assemble the shunt adapters according to the manufacturer's directions.
■ Clean the arterial and venous shunt connection with antiseptic pads to remove contaminants. Use a separate pad for each

tube, and wipe in one direction only, from the insertion site to the connection sites. Allow the tubing to air-dry.

- Put on sterile gloves.
- Clamp the arterial side of the shunt with a bulldog clamp to prevent blood from flowing through it. Clamp the venous side to prevent leakage when the shunt is opened.
- Open the shunt by separating its sides with your fingers or with a sterile shunt spreader, if available. Both sides of the shunt should be exposed. Always inspect the Teflon connector on one side of the shunt to see if it's damaged or bent. If necessary, replace it before proceeding. Note which side contains the connector so you can use the new one to close the shunt after treatment.
- To adapt the shunt to the lines of the machine, attach a shunt adapter and 10-ml syringe filled with about 8 ml of normal saline solution to the side of the shunt containing the Teflon connector. Attach the new Teflon connector to the other side of the shunt with the second adapter. Attach the second 10-ml syringe filled with about 8 ml of normal saline solution to the same side.
- Flush the shunt's arterial tubing by releasing its clamp and gently aspirating it with the normal saline solution-filled syringe. Flush the tubing slowly, observing it for signs of fibrin buildup. Repeat the procedure on the venous side of the shunt.
- Secure the shunt to the adapter connection with adhesive tape to prevent separation during treatment.
- Connect the arterial and venous lines to the adapters and secure the connections with tape. Tape each line to the patient's arm to prevent unnecessary strain on the shunt during treatment.
- Begin hemodialysis according to your facility's policy.

Discontinuing hemodialysis with a double-lumen catheter

- Wash your hands.
- Clamp the extension tubing to prevent air from entering the catheter. Clean all connection points on the catheter and blood lines as well as the clamps to reduce the risk of systemic or local infection.
- Place a clean drape under the catheter, and place two sterile 4″ × 4″ gauze pads on the drape beneath the catheter lines. Soak the pads with antiseptic cleaning solution. Prepare the catheter flush solution with normal saline or heparin flush solution as ordered.
- Put on clean gloves. Grasp each blood line with a gauze pad and disconnect each line from the catheter.
- Flush each port with normal saline solution to clean the extension tubing and catheter of blood. Administer additional heparin flush solution as ordered to ensure catheter patency. Attach luer-lock injection caps to prevent air entry or blood loss. Clamp the extension tubing.
- When hemodialysis is complete, re-dress the catheter insertion site; also re-dress it if it's occluded, soiled, or wet. Position the patient supine with his face turned away from the insertion site so that he doesn't contaminate the site by breathing on it.
- Wash your hands and remove the outer occlusive dressing. Put on sterile gloves, remove the old inner dressing, and discard the gloves and the inner dressing.
- Set up a sterile field, and observe the site for drainage. Obtain a drainage sample for culture if necessary. Notify the practitioner if the suture is missing.
- Put on sterile gloves and clean the insertion site with an alcohol pad to remove skin oils. Clean the site with an antiseptic pad and allow it to air-dry.
- Place a precut gauze dressing under the catheter, and place another gauze dressing over the catheter.
- Apply a skin barrier preparation to the skin surrounding the gauze dressing. Cover the gauze and catheter with a transparent occlusive dressing.
- Apply a 4″ to 5″ (10 to 12.5 cm) piece of 2″ tape over the cut edge of the dressing to reinforce the lower edge.

Discontinuing hemodialysis with an AV fistula

- Wash your hands. Turn the blood pump on the hemodialysis machine to 50 to 100 ml/minute.

- Put on clean gloves and remove the tape from the connection site of the arterial lines. Clamp the needle tubing with the hemostat and disconnect the lines. The blood in the machine's arterial line will continue to flow toward the dialyzer, followed by a column of air. Just before the blood reaches the point where the normal saline solution enters the line, clamp the blood line with another hemostat.
- Unclamp the normal saline solution to allow a small amount to flow through the line. Unclamp the hemostat on the machine line. This allows all blood to flow into the dialyzer where it passes through the filter and back to the patient through the venous line.
- After blood is retransfused, clamp the venous needle tubing and the machine's venous line with hemostats. Turn off the blood pump.
- Remove the tape from the connection site of the venous lines and disconnect the lines.
- Remove the venipuncture needle and apply pressure to the site with a folded 4″ × 4″ gauze pad until all bleeding stops, usually within 10 minutes. Apply an adhesive bandage. Repeat the procedure on the arterial line.
- When hemodialysis is complete, assess the patient's weight, vital signs (including standing blood pressure), and mental status. Compare your findings with your predialysis assessment data. Document your findings.
- Disinfect and rinse the delivery system according to the manufacturer's instructions.

Discontinuing hemodialysis with an AV shunt

- Wash your hands. Turn the blood pump on the hemodialysis machine to 50 to 100 ml/minute.
- Put on the sterile gloves and remove the tape from the connection site of the arterial lines. Clamp the arterial cannula with a bulldog clamp, and then disconnect the lines. The blood in the machine's arterial line will continue to flow toward the dialyzer, followed by a column of air. Just before the blood reaches the point where the normal saline solution enters the line, clamp the blood line with a hemostat.
- Unclamp the normal saline solution to allow a small amount to flow through the line. Reclamp the normal saline solution line and unclamp the hemostat on the machine line. This allows all blood to flow into the dialyzer where it's circulated through the filter and back to the patient through the venous line.
- Just before the last volume of blood enters the patient, clamp the venous cannula with a bulldog clamp and the machine's venous line with a hemostat.
- Remove the tape from the connection site of the venous lines. Turn off the blood pump and disconnect the lines.
- Reconnect the shunt cannula. Remove the older of the two Teflon connectors and discard it. Connect the shunt, taking care to position the Teflon connector equally between the two cannulas. Remove the bulldog clamps.
- Secure the shunt connection with plasticized or hypoallergenic tape to prevent accidental disconnection.
- Clean the shunt and its site with the gauze pads soaked with antiseptic cleaning solution. When the cleaning procedure is finished, remove the antiseptic solution with alcohol pads.
- Make sure that blood flows through the shunt adequately.
- Apply a dressing to the shunt site and wrap it securely (but not too tightly) with elastic gauze bandages. Attach the bulldog clamps to the outside dressing.
- When hemodialysis is complete, assess the patient's weight, vital signs, and mental status. Compare your findings with your predialysis assessment data. Document your findings.
- Disinfect and rinse the delivery system according to the manufacturer's instructions.

Special considerations

- Obtain blood samples from the patient as ordered. Samples are usually drawn before beginning hemodialysis.

ALERT

To avoid pyrogenic reactions and bacteremia with septicemia resulting from contamination, use strict sterile technique during preparation of the machine. Discard equipment that has fallen on the floor or that has been disconnected and exposed to the air.

DEVICE SAFETY

Immediately report a machine malfunction or equipment defect.

- Avoid unnecessary handling of shunt tubing. However, be sure to inspect the shunt carefully for patency by observing its color. Look for clots and serum and cell separation, and check the temperature of the Silastic tubing. Assess the shunt insertion site for signs of infection, such as purulent drainage, inflammation, and tenderness, which may indicate the body's rejection of the shunt. Check to see if the shunt insertion tips are exposed.

DO'S & DON'TS

Make sure that you complete each step in this procedure correctly. Overlooking a single step or performing it incorrectly can cause unnecessary blood loss or inefficient treatment from poor clearances or inadequate fluid removal. For example, never allow a normal saline solution bag to run dry while priming and soaking the dialyzer. This can cause air to enter the patient portion of the dialysate system. Ultimately, failure to perform accurate hemodialysis therapy can lead to patient injury and even death.

- If bleeding continues after you remove an AV fistula needle, apply pressure with a sterile, absorbable gelatin sponge. If bleeding persists, apply a similar sponge soaked in topical thrombin solution.
- Throughout hemodialysis, carefully monitor the patient's vital signs. Read blood pressure at least hourly or as often as every 15 minutes, if necessary. Monitor the patient's weight before and after the procedure to ensure adequate ultrafiltration during treatment. (Many dialysis units are now equipped with bed scales.)
- Perform periodic tests for clotting time on the patient's blood samples and samples from the dialyzer. If the patient receives meals during treatment, make sure that they're light.
- Continue necessary drug administration during dialysis unless the drug would be removed in the dialysate; if so, administer the drug after dialysis.

Complications

- Fever caused by bacterial endotoxins in the dialysate
- Early dialysis disequilibrium syndrome caused by rapid fluid removal and electrolyte changes during hemodialysis; signs and symptoms including headache, nausea, vomiting, restlessness, hypertension, muscle cramps, backache, and seizures
- Hypovolemia and hypotension caused by excessive removal of fluid during ultrafiltration; hyperglycemia and hypernatremia caused by diffusion of the sugar and sodium content of the dialysate solution into the blood; these conditions, in turn, causing hyperosmolarity
- Cardiac arrhythmias occurring during hemodialysis resulting from electrolyte and pH changes in the blood; also developing in patients taking antiarrhythmic drugs because the dialysate removes these drugs during treatment
- Angina developing in patients with anemia or preexisting arteriosclerotic cardiovascular disease because of the physiologic stress on the blood during purification and ultrafiltration (Reduced oxygen levels resulting from extracorporeal blood flow or membrane sensitivity may require increasing oxygen administration during hemodialysis.)
- Fatal air embolism resulting if the dialyzer retains air, if tubing connections become loose, or if the normal saline solution container empties; symptoms including chest pain, dyspnea, coughing, and cyanosis
- Hemolysis resulting from obstructed flow of the dialysate concentrate or from incorrect setting of the conductivity alarm limits; symptoms including chest pain,

dyspnea, cherry red blood, arrhythmias, acute decrease in hematocrit, and hyperkalemia

- Hyperthermia (fatal) resulting if the dialysate becomes overheated
- Exsanguination resulting from separations of the blood lines or from rupture of the blood lines or dialyzer membrane

Patient teaching

- Before the patient leaves the health care facility, teach him how to care for his vascular access site. Instruct him to keep the incision clean and dry to prevent infection, and to clean it daily until it heals completely and the sutures are removed (usually 10 to 14 days after surgery). He should notify the practitioner of pain, swelling, redness, or drainage in the affected arm. Teach him how to use a stethoscope to auscultate for bruits and how to palpate a thrill.
- Explain that after the access site heals, he may use the arm freely. In fact, exercise is beneficial because it helps stimulate vein enlargement.
- Remind him not to allow any treatments or procedures on the accessed arm, including blood pressure monitoring or needle punctures.
- Tell him to avoid putting excessive pressure on the arm. He shouldn't sleep on it, wear constricting clothing on it, or lift heavy objects or strain with it. He also should avoid getting wet for several hours after dialysis.
- Teach the patient exercises for the affected arm to promote vascular dilation and enhance blood flow. He may start by squeezing a small rubber ball or other soft object for 15 minutes, when advised by the practitioner.
- If the patient will be performing hemodialysis at home, thoroughly review all aspects of the procedure with the patient and his family. Give them the phone number of the dialysis center. Emphasize that training for home hemodialysis is a complex process requiring 2 to 3 months to ensure that the patient or family member performs it safely and competently. Keep in mind that this procedure is stressful.

Documentation

Record the time treatment began and any problems with it. Note the patient's vital signs and weight before and during treatment. Note the time blood samples were taken for testing, the test results, and treatment for complications. Record the time the treatment was completed and the patient's response to it.

Hydrotherapy

Treating diseases or injuries by immersing part or all of the patient's body in water is known as hydrotherapy. Commonly used to debride serious burns and to hasten healing, hydrotherapy also promotes circulation and comfort in patients with peripheral vascular disease and musculoskeletal disorders such as arthritis. Although hydrotherapy usually involves immersing the patient in a tub of water ("tubbing"), showers or other water-spray techniques may replace tubbing in some health care facilities and burn centers. (See *Positioning the patient for hydrotherapy*.) The nurse or physical therapist usually assists the patient into the tub or shower area if he's ambulatory. If he isn't ambulatory, he can enter the water using a stretcher or hoist device.

Hydrotherapy is contraindicated in the presence of sudden changes: fever, electrolyte or fluid imbalance, or unstable vital signs. Always follow the standard precautions guidelines.

Equipment

Water tank or tub or shower table ♦ chemical additives as ordered ♦ padded table for patient to sit or lie on while performing exercises ♦ stretcher ♦ headrest ♦ hydraulic hoist ♦ gown ♦ surgical cap ♦ mask ♦ gloves (for removing dressings) ♦ shoulder-length gloves (for tubbing) ♦ apron ♦ debridement instruments ♦ razor, shaving cream, mild soap, shampoo, and washcloth (for general cleaning) ♦ fluffed gauze pads ♦ cotton-tipped applicators ♦ sterile sheets ♦ warm, sterile bath blankets

Barriers, sheets, and bath blankets may be sterile or clean, depending on the patient's condition and your facility's infection-control policies.

Preparation

- Thoroughly clean and disinfect the tub or shower, its equipment, and the tub or shower room before each treatment to prevent cross-contamination. After cleaning, place the tub liner in the tub and fill the tub with warm water (98° to 104° F [36.6° to 40° C]).
- Attach the headrest to the sides of the tub. Add prescribed chemicals (such as sodium chloride) to the water to maintain the normal isotonic level (usually 0.9%) and to prevent dialysis and tissue irritation. Also add potassium chloride to prevent potassium loss and calcium hypochlorite detergent as ordered.
- Get bath blankets from the blanket warmer, and ensure that the room is warm enough to avoid chilling the patient.

Key steps

- If this is the patient's first treatment, explain the procedure to him to allay his fears and promote cooperation. As necessary (before debridement, for example), administer an analgesic about 20 minutes before the procedure.
- Check the patient's vital signs.
- If the patient is receiving an I.V. infusion, make sure he has enough I.V. solution to last through the procedure. Be sure that the I.V. site is covered and kept dry.
- Transfer the patient to a stretcher, and transport him to the therapy room. If he's ambulatory, he may walk unassisted, provided that the therapy room is nearby.
- Wash your hands, and put on your gown, gloves, mask, and surgical cap.
- Remove the outer dressings and dispose of them properly before immersing the patient. Leave the inner gauze layer on the wound unless it can be easily removed.
- If the patient is ambulatory, position him on the padded table for transfer to the tub, or assist him into the tub and situate him on the already lowered padded table.
- If the patient isn't ambulatory, attach the stretcher to the overhead hydraulic hoist. Ensure that the hoist hooks are fastened securely. Use the hoist to transfer the patient to and from the tub.

Positioning the patient for hydrotherapy

Immerse the patient in a tub or Hubbard tank (as shown). Alternatively, you may spray his wounds with water as he lies on a special shower table. Hydrotherapy is traumatic and painful for the burn patient. Provide continual support and encouragement.

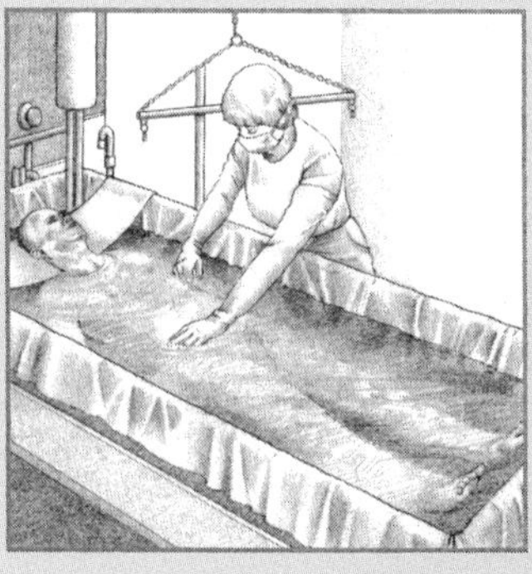

- Lower the patient into the tub. Position him so that the headrest supports his head. Allow him to soak for 3 to 5 minutes.
- Remove your gloves, wash your hands, and put on the shoulder-length tubbing gloves and apron.
- Remove remaining gauze dressings, if any, from the patient's wounds.
- If ordered, place the tub's agitator into the water and turn it on. The motor may burn out if it's turned on out of the water. Some tubs have aerators to agitate the water.
- Clean all unburned areas first (encourage the patient to do this if he can). Wash unburned skin, and clip or shave hair near the wound. Shave facial hair, shampoo the scalp, and give mouth care, as appropriate. Provide perineal care, and clean inside the patient's nose and the folds of the ears and eyes with cotton-tipped applicators.
- Gently scrub burned areas with fluffed gauze pads to remove topical agents, exudates, necrotic tissue, and other debris.

Debride the wound after turning off the agitator.

- Exercise the patient's extremities with active or passive range of motion, depending on his condition and exercise tolerance. Alternatively, you may have the physical therapist exercise the patient.
- After you've completed the treatment, use the hoist to raise the patient above the water.
- With the patient still suspended over the water, spray-rinse his body to remove debris from shaving, cleaning, and debridement.
- Transfer the patient to a stretcher covered with a clean sheet and bath blanket, and cover him with a warm sterile sheet (a blanket may be added for warmth). Pat unburned areas dry to prevent chilling.
- Remove the wet or damp linens, and cover the patient with dry linens. Remove your gown, gloves, and mask before transporting the patient to the dressing area for further debridement, if needed, and new sterile dressings.
- Have the tub drained, cleaned, and disinfected according to your facility's policy.

Special considerations

- Remain with the patient at all times to prevent accidents in the tub. Limit hydrotherapy to 20 or 30 minutes. Watch the patient closely for adverse reactions.
- Patients with an endotracheal tube may receive hydrotherapy. Spray their wounds while they're suspended over the tub on a padded table. Immerse patients with long-standing tracheostomies only with a practitioner's order.
- If necessary, weigh the patient during hydrotherapy to assess nutritional status and fluid shift. Use a hoist that has a table scale.
- Whirlpool treatments should be discontinued when the wounds are assessed as clean because the whirlpool's agitating water may result in trauma to the regenerating tissue.

Complications

- Infection caused by incomplete disinfection of tub, drains, and faucets, or cross-contamination from members of the tubbing team
- Patient chilling easily from decreased resistance to temperature changes
- Fluid or electrolyte imbalance (or both) resulting from a chemical imbalance between the patient and the tub solution

Documentation

Record the date, time, and patient's reaction. Note the patient's condition (vital signs and wound appearance). Document any wound infection or bleeding. Note treatments given, such as debridement, and dressing changes. Record any special treatments in the nursing care plan.

Hyperthermia-hypothermia blanket

A blanket-sized aquathermia pad, the hyperthermia-hypothermia blanket raises, lowers, or maintains body temperature through conductive heat or cold transfer between the blanket and the patient. It can be operated manually or automatically.

In manual operation, the nurse or practitioner sets the temperature on the unit. The blanket reaches and maintains this temperature regardless of the patient's temperature. The temperature control must be adjusted manually to reach a different setting. The nurse monitors the patient's body temperature with a conventional thermometer.

In automatic operation, the unit directly and continually monitors the patient's temperature by means of a thermistor probe (rectal, skin, or esophageal) and alternates heating and cooling cycles as necessary to achieve and maintain the desired body temperature. The thermistor probe may also be used in conjunction with manual operation but isn't essential. The unit is equipped with an alarm to warn of abnormal temperature fluctuations and a circuit breaker that protects against current overload.

The blanket is most commonly used to reduce high fever when more conservative measures—such as baths, ice packs, and antipyretics—are unsuccessful. Its other uses include maintaining normal temperature during surgery or shock; inducing hypothermia during surgery to decrease metabolic activity and thereby reduce oxygen requirements; reducing intracranial pressure; controlling bleeding and intractable pain in patients with amputations, burns, or cancer; and providing warmth in cases of severe hypothermia.

Equipment

Hyperthermia-hypothermia control unit ♦ fluid for the control unit (distilled water or distilled water and 20% ethyl alcohol) ♦ thermistor probe (rectal, skin, or esophageal) ♦ patient thermometer ♦ one or two hyperthermia-hypothermia blankets ♦ one or two disposable blanket covers (or one or two sheets or bath blankets) ♦ lanolin or a mixture of lanolin and cold cream ♦ adhesive tape ♦ towel ♦ sphygmomanometer ♦ gloves, if necessary ♦ patient gown ♦ optional: protective wraps for the patient's hands and feet

Disposable hyperthermia-hypothermia blankets are available for single-patient use.

Preparation

DEVICE SAFETY

Inspect the control unit and each blanket for leaks and the plugs and connecting wires for broken prongs, kinks, and fraying. If you detect or suspect malfunction, don't use the equipment.

- Review the practitioner's order, and prepare one or two blankets by covering them with disposable covers (or use a sheet or bath blanket when positioning the blanket on the patient). The cover absorbs perspiration and condensation, which could cause tissue breakdown if left on the skin.
- Connect the blanket to the control unit, and set the controls for manual or automatic operation and for the desired blanket or body temperature. Make sure the machine is properly grounded before plugging it in.
- Turn on the machine and add liquid to the unit reservoir, if necessary, as fluid fills the blanket. Allow the blanket to preheat or precool so that the patient receives immediate thermal benefit. Place the control unit at the foot of the bed.

Key steps

- Assess the patient's condition, and explain the reason for the procedure and what to expect. Provide privacy, and make sure the room is warm and free of drafts. Check your facility's policy and, if necessary, make sure the patient or a responsible family member has signed a consent form.
- Explain to the patient the need for frequent monitoring and position changes.
- Wash your hands thoroughly. If the patient isn't already wearing a patient gown, ask him to put one on. Use a gown with cloth ties rather than metal snaps or pins to prevent heat or cold injury.
- Take the patient's temperature, pulse, respirations, and blood pressure to serve as a baseline, and assess his level of consciousness, pupil reaction, limb strength, and skin condition.
- Keeping the bottom sheet in place and the patient recumbent, roll the patient to one side and slide the rolled blanket halfway underneath him, so that its top edge aligns with his neck. Then roll the patient back, and pull and flatten the blanket across the bed. Place a pillow under the patient's head. Make sure his head doesn't lie directly on the blanket because the blanket's rigid surface may be uncomfortable and the heat or cold may lead to tissue breakdown. Use a sheet or bath blanket as insulation between the patient and the blanket.
- Apply lanolin or a mixture of lanolin and cold cream to the patient's skin where it touches the blanket to help protect the skin from heat or cold sensation.
- In automatic operation, insert the thermistor probe in the patient's rectum and tape it in place to prevent accidental dislodgment. If rectal insertion is contraindicated, tuck a skin probe deep into the axilla, and secure it with tape. If the patient is comatose or anesthetized, insert an esophageal probe. Plug the other end of the probe into the correct jack on the unit's control panel.

Using a warming system

Shivering, the compensatory response to falling body temperature, may use more oxygen than the body can supply—especially in a surgical patient. In the past, patients were covered with blankets to warm their bodies. Now, health care facilities may supply a warming system, such as the Bair Hugger patient-warming system (shown below).

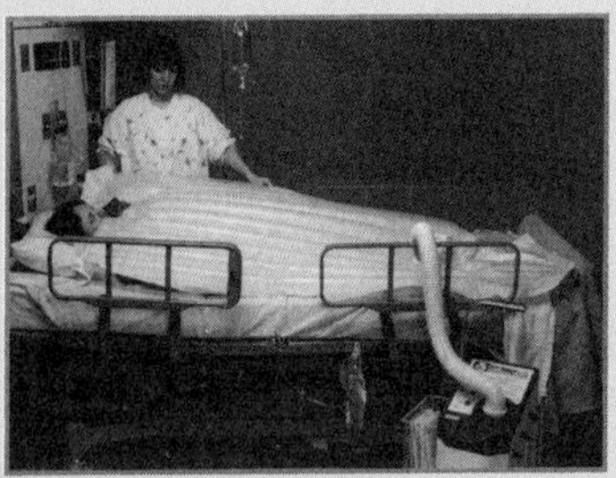

This system helps to gradually increase body temperature by drawing air through a filter, warming the air to the desired temperature, and circulating it through a hose to a warming blanket placed over the patient.

When using the warming system, follow these guidelines:

- Use a bath blanket in a single layer over the warming blanket to minimize heat loss.
- Place the warming blanket directly over the patient with the paper side facing down and the clear tubular side facing up.
- Make sure the connection hose is at the foot of the bed.
- Take the patient's temperature during the first 15 to 30 minutes and at least every 30 minutes while the warming blanket is in use.
- Obtain guidelines from the patient's practitioner for discontinuing use of the warming blanket.

- Place a sheet or, if ordered, the second hyperthermia-hypothermia blanket over the patient. This increases the thermal benefit by trapping cooled or heated air.
- Wrap the patient's hands and feet if he wishes to minimize chilling and promote comfort. Monitor vital signs and perform a neurologic assessment every 5 minutes until the desired body temperature is reached and then every 15 minutes until temperature is stable or as ordered.
- Check fluid intake and output hourly or as ordered. Observe the patient regularly for color changes in skin, lips, and nail beds and for edema, induration, inflammation, pain, and sensory impairment. If they occur, discontinue the procedure and notify the practitioner.
- Reposition the patient every 30 minutes to 1 hour, unless contraindicated, to prevent skin breakdown. Keep the patient's skin, bedclothes, and blanket cover free of perspiration and condensation, and reapply cream to exposed body parts as needed.
- After turning off the machine, follow the manufacturer's directions. Some units must remain plugged in for at least 30 minutes to allow the condenser fan to remove water vapor from the mechanism. Continue to monitor the patient's temperature until it stabilizes because body temperature can fall as much as 5° F (2.8° C) after this procedure.
- Remove all equipment from the bed. Dry the patient and make him comfortable. Supply a fresh patient gown, if necessary. Cover him lightly.
- Continue to perform neurologic checks and monitor vital signs, fluid intake and output, and general condition every 30 minutes for 2 hours and then hourly or as ordered.
- Return the equipment to the central supply department for cleaning, servicing, and storage.

Special considerations

- If the patient shivers excessively during hypothermia treatment, discontinue the procedure and notify the practitioner immediately. By increasing metabolism, shivering elevates body temperature.

- Avoid lowering the temperature more than 1 degree every 15 minutes to prevent premature ventricular contractions.
- Don't use pins to secure catheters, tubes, or blanket covers because an accidental puncture can result in fluid leakage and burns.
- With hyperthermia or hypothermia therapy, the patient may experience a secondary defense reaction (vasoconstriction or vasodilation, respectively) that causes body temperature to rebound and thus defeat the treatment's purpose.
- If the patient requires isolation, place the blanket, blanket cover, and probe in a plastic bag clearly marked with the type of isolation so that the central supply department can give it special handling. If the blanket is disposable, discard it, using appropriate precautions.
- To avoid bacterial growth in the reservoir or blankets, always use sterile distilled water and change it monthly. Check to see if facility policy calls for adding a bacteriostatic agent to the water. Avoid using deionized water because it may corrode the system.
- To gradually increase body temperature, especially in postoperative patients, the practitioner may order a disposable warming system. (See *Using a warming system*.)
- Tell the patient the signs and symptoms to report.

Complications

- Shivering, marked changes in vital signs, increased intracranial pressure, respiratory distress or arrest, cardiac arrest, oliguria, and anuria

Documentation

Record the patient's pulse, respirations, blood pressure, neurologic signs, fluid intake and output, skin condition, and position change. Record the patient's temperature and that of the blanket every 30 minutes while the blanket is in use. Also document the type of hyperthermia-hypothermia unit used; control settings (manual or automatic and temperature settings); date, time, duration, and the patient's tolerance of treatment; and signs of complications.

IJK

Incentive spirometry

Incentive spirometry involves using a breathing device to help the patient achieve maximum ventilation. The device measures respiratory flow or respiratory volume and induces the patient to take a deep breath and hold it for several seconds. This deep breath increases lung volume, boosts alveolar inflation, and promotes venous return. This exercise also establishes alveolar hyperinflation for a longer time than is possible with a normal deep breath, thus preventing and reversing the alveolar collapse that causes atelectasis and pneumonitis.

Devices used for incentive spirometry provide a visual incentive to breathe deeply. Some are activated when the patient inhales a certain volume of air; the device then estimates the amount of air inhaled. Others contain plastic floats, which rise according to the amount of air the patient pulls through the device when he inhales.

Patients at low risk for developing atelectasis may use a flow incentive spirometer. Patients at high risk may need a volume incentive spirometer, which measures lung inflation more precisely.

Incentive spirometry benefits the patient on prolonged bed rest, especially the postoperative patient who may regain his normal respiratory pattern slowly due to such predisposing factors as abdominal or thoracic surgery, advanced age, inactivity, obesity, smoking, and decreased ability to cough effectively and expel lung secretions.

Equipment

Flow or volume incentive spirometer, as indicated, with sterile disposable flow tube and mouthpiece (the tube and mouthpiece are sterile on first use and clean on subsequent uses) ♦ stethoscope ♦ watch ♦ pencil and paper

Preparation

- Assemble the ordered equipment at the patient's bedside.
- Read the manufacturer's instructions for spirometer setup and operation.
- Remove the sterile flow tube and mouthpiece from the package, and attach them to the device.
- Set the flow rate or volume goal as determined by the practitioner or respiratory therapist and based on the patient's preoperative performance.
- Turn on the machine, if necessary.

Key steps

- Confirm the patient's identity using two patient identifiers according to your facility's policy.
- Assess the patient's condition.
- Explain the procedure to the patient, making sure that he understands the importance of performing this exercise regularly to maintain alveolar inflation.
- Wash your hands.
- Help the patient into a comfortable sitting or semi-Fowler's position to promote optimal lung expansion. If you're using a flow incentive spirometer and the patient can't assume or maintain this position, he can perform the procedure in any position as long as the device remains upright. Tilt-

ing a flow incentive spirometer decreases the required patient effort and reduces the exercise's effectiveness.

- Auscultate the patient's lungs to provide a baseline for comparison with posttreatment auscultation.
- Instruct the patient to insert the mouthpiece and close his lips tightly around it because a weak seal may alter flow or volume readings.
- Instruct the patient to exhale normally and then inhale as slowly and as deeply as possible. If he has difficulty with this step, tell him to suck as he would through a straw but more slowly. Ask the patient to retain the entire volume of air he inhaled for 3 seconds or, if you're using a device with a light indicator, until the light turns off. This deep breath creates sustained transpulmonary pressure near the end of inspiration and is sometimes called a sustained maximal inspiration.
- Tell the patient to remove the mouthpiece and exhale normally. Allow him to relax and take several normal breaths before attempting another breath with the spirometer. Repeat this sequence 5 to 10 times during every waking hour. Note tidal volumes.
- Evaluate the patient's ability to cough effectively, and encourage him to cough after each effort because deep lung inflation may loosen secretions and facilitate their removal. Observe any expectorated secretions.
- Auscultate the patient's lungs, and compare findings with the first auscultation.
- Instruct the patient to remove the mouthpiece. Wash the device in warm water and shake it dry. Avoid immersing the spirometer itself because this enhances bacterial growth and impairs the internal filter's effectiveness in preventing inhalation of extraneous material.
- Place the mouthpiece in a plastic storage bag between exercises, and label it and the spirometer, if applicable, with the patient's name to avoid inadvertent use by another patient.

Special considerations

- If the patient is scheduled for surgery, make a preoperative assessment of his respiratory pattern and capability to ensure the development of appropriate postoperative goals. Teach the patient how to use the spirometer before surgery so that he can concentrate on your instructions and practice the exercise. A preoperative evaluation will also help in establishing a postoperative therapeutic goal.
- Avoid exercising at mealtime to prevent nausea. Provide paper and pencil so the patient can note exercise times. Exercise frequency varies with the patient's condition and ability.
- Immediately after surgery, monitor the exercise frequently to ensure compliance and assess achievement.

Complications

- Hyperventilation, increased surgical pain, nausea, barotrauma, fatigue, and possible exacerbation of bronchospasm

Patient teaching

- Explain the importance of continuing incentive spirometry after discharge, as directed.

Documentation

Record any preoperative teaching you provided. Document the preoperative flow or volume levels, date and time of the procedure, type of spirometer, flow or volume levels achieved, and number of breaths taken. Also record the patient's condition before and after the procedure, his tolerance of the procedure, and the results of both auscultations.

Incontinence management

Urinary incontinence (UI) afflicts approximately 10 million adults, including 1.5 million nursing home residents, in the United States. Studies have found that fecal incontinence affects up to 47% of the patients in such facilities. Because of the social stigma of UI, many patients never report the problem to their practitioner. UI is neither a disease nor a part of normal aging but may be caused by confusion, dehydration, fecal impaction, or restricted mobility. It's also a sign of various disorders, such as prostatic hyperplasia, bladder calculus, bladder cancer, urinary tract infection (UTI), stroke, diabetic neuropathy, Guillain-Barré syndrome, multiple sclerosis (MS), prostate cancer, prostatitis, spinal cord injury, and urethral stricture. It may also result from urethral sphincter damage after prostatectomy. In addition, certain drugs, including diuretics, hypnotics, sedatives, anticholinergics, antihypertensives, and alpha antagonists, may trigger UI.

According to the National Institute on Aging, UI has four distinct types:

- Urge incontinence—the involuntary loss of urine associated with a strong desire to void (urgency). It can occur in healthy people, but also in people with diabetes, Alzheimer's disease, Parkinson's disease, stroke, and MS. It can also be a sign of bladder cancer.
- Stress incontinence—usually presents clinically as the involuntary loss of urine from sudden physical strain, such as a sneeze, cough, quick movement, or during exercise. It's the most common type that occurs in younger and middle-aged women.
- Overflow incontinence—results in the involuntary loss of urine due to overdistention of the bladder, which causes dribbling because the distended bladder can't contract strongly enough to force a urine stream. This can occur in men with enlarged prostates or patients with diabetes or spinal cord injuries.
- Functional incontinence—results in urine leakage even though the bladder and urethra function normally. This condition is usually related to cognitive or environmental factors, such as mental impairment or the inability to get to the toilet in time because of arthritis or other disorders.

Care of persons with UI should include attention to toileting schedules, monitoring of fluid and dietary intake, strategies to decrease urine loss at night, use of protective garments, and prevention and early treatment of skin breakdown. Pharmacologic treatment includes medications that prevent bladder contractions, relax muscles to help the bladder fully empty, or contract muscles to cut down on leakage. Surgical treatment includes transurethral resection of the prostate in men, repair of the anterior vaginal wall or retropelvic suspension of the bladder in women, urethral sling, and bladder augmentation.

Fecal incontinence, the involuntary passage of feces, may occur gradually (as in dementia) or suddenly (as in spinal cord injury), but most commonly occurs as a result of diarrhea or constipation. It can also result from many factors, such as fecal stasis and impaction secondary to reduced activity; inappropriate diet; untreated painful anal conditions; chronic laxative use; reduced fluid intake; neurologic deficit; pelvic, prostatic, or rectal surgery; or the use of certain medications, including antihistamines, psychotropics, and iron preparations. Not usually a sign of serious illness, fecal incontinence can seriously impair an individual's physical and psychological well-being.

Management of fecal incontinence includes managing the patient's diet, bowel retraining, and biofeedback to improve sensation and control. Surgery, such as a sphincteroplasty to repair the anal sphincter muscles or to transpose muscle from another part of the body, can also be done if appropriate.

Patients with urinary or fecal incontinence should be carefully assessed for underlying disorders. Most can be treated; some can even be cured.

Equipment

Bladder retraining record sheet ♦ gloves ♦ stethoscope (to assess bowel sounds) ♦ lubricant ♦ moisture barrier cream ♦ incontinence pads ♦ bedpan ♦ specimen container ♦ laboratory request form ♦ optional: stool collection kit, urinary catheter

Key steps

- Whether the patient reports urinary or fecal incontinence or both, you'll need to perform initial and continuing assessments to plan effective interventions.

Urinary incontinence

- Ask the patient when he first noticed urine leakage and whether it began suddenly or gradually. Have him describe his typical urinary pattern: Does incontinence usually occur during the day or at night? Ask him to rate his urinary control: Does he have moderate control, or is he completely incontinent? If he sometimes urinates with control, ask him to identify when and how much he usually urinates.

- Evaluate related problems, such as urinary hesitancy, frequency, urgency, nocturia, and decreased force or an interrupted urine stream. Ask the patient to describe previous treatment he has had for incontinence or measures he has performed by himself. Ask about medications, including nonprescription drugs.
- Assess the patient's environment. Is a toilet or commode readily available, and how long does the patient take to reach it? After the patient is in the bathroom, assess his manual dexterity; for example, how easily does he manipulate his clothes?
- Evaluate the patient's mental status and cognitive function.
- Quantify the patient's normal daily fluid intake.
- Review the patient's medication and diet history for drugs and foods that affect digestion and elimination.
- Review or obtain the patient's medical history, noting especially the number and route of births (in women) and incidence of UTIs, prostate disorders, spinal injury or tumor, stroke, and bladder, prostate, or pelvic surgery. Assess for such disorders as delirium, dehydration, urine retention, restricted mobility, fecal impaction, infection, inflammation, or polyuria.
- Inspect the urethral meatus for obvious inflammation or anatomic defects. Have the female patient bear down while you note any urine leakage. Gently palpate the abdomen for bladder distention, which signals urine retention. If possible, have the patient examined by a urologist.
- Obtain specimens for appropriate laboratory tests as ordered. Label each specimen container and send it to the laboratory with a request form.
- Begin incontinence management by implementing an appropriate bladder retraining program. (See *Bladder retraining,* page 248.)
- To manage stress incontinence, begin an exercise program to help strengthen the pelvic floor muscles. (See *Strengthening pelvic floor muscles,* page 249.)
- To manage functional incontinence, frequently assess the patient's mental and functional status. Regularly remind him to void. Respond to his calls promptly, and help him get to the bathroom quickly. Provide positive reinforcement.
- To ensure healthful hydration and to prevent a UTI, make sure that the patient maintains adequate daily fluid intake (six to eight 8-oz glasses of fluid). Restrict fluid intake after 6 p.m.

Fecal incontinence

- Ask the patient with fecal incontinence to identify its onset, duration, severity, and pattern (for instance, determine whether it occurs at night or with diarrhea). Focus the history on GI, neurologic, and psychological disorders.
- Note the frequency, consistency, and volume of stool passed in the previous 24 hours. Obtain a stool specimen, if ordered. Protect the patient's bed with an incontinence pad.
- Assess for chronic constipation, GI and neurologic disorders, and laxative abuse. Inspect the abdomen for distention, and auscultate for bowel sounds. If not contraindicated, put on gloves, apply lubricant, and check for fecal impaction (a factor in overflow incontinence). Remove gloves when finished. Checking for fecal impaction may stimulate a bowel movement, so keep a bedpan readily available.
- Assess the patient's medication regimen. Check for drugs that affect bowel activity, such as aspirin, anticholinergics, anti-Parkinson drugs, aluminum hydroxide, calcium carbonate antacids, diuretics, iron preparations, opiates, tranquilizers, tricyclic antidepressants, and phenothiazines.
- For the neurologically capable patient with chronic incontinence, provide bowel retraining.
- Advise the patient to consume a fiber-rich diet, with raw, leafy vegetables (such as carrots and lettuce), unpeeled fruits (such as apples), and whole grains (such as wheat or rye breads and cereals). If the pa-

Bladder retraining

The incontinent patient typically feels frustrated, embarrassed, and hopeless. Fortunately, his problem can usually be corrected by bladder retraining—a program that aims to establish a regular voiding pattern. Follow these guidelines.

Assess elimination patterns

First, assess the patient's intake and voiding patterns and reason for each accidental voiding (such as a coughing spell). Use an incontinence monitoring record.

Establish a voiding schedule

Encourage the patient to void regularly, for example, every 2 hours. When he can stay dry for 2 hours, increase the interval by 30 minutes every day until he achieves a 3- to 4-hour voiding schedule. Teach the patient to practice relaxation techniques such as deep breathing, which help decrease the sense of urgency.

Record results and remain positive

Keep a record of continence and incontinence for about 5 days. Remember, both your own and your patient's positive attitudes are crucial to his successful bladder retraining.

Take steps for success

Here are some tips to boost the patient's success:

- Situate the patient's bed near a bathroom or portable toilet. Leave a light on at night. If the patient needs assistance getting out of bed or a chair, promptly answer the call for help.
- Teach the patient measures to prevent urinary tract infections, such as adequate fluid intake (at least 2 qt [2 L]/day unless contraindicated), drinking cranberry juice, wearing cotton underpants, and bathing with nonirritating soaps.
- Encourage the patient to empty his bladder completely before and after meals and at bedtime.
- Advise him to urinate whenever the urge arises and never to ignore it.
- Instruct the patient to take prescribed diuretics upon rising in the morning.
- Advise him to limit the use of sleeping aids, sedatives, and alcohol; they decrease the urge to urinate and can increase incontinence, especially at night.
- If the patient is overweight, encourage weight loss.
- Suggest exercises to strengthen pelvic muscles.
- Instruct the patient to increase dietary fiber.
- Monitor the patient for signs of anxiety and depression.
- Reassure the patient that periodic incontinent episodes don't mean that the program has failed. Encourage persistence, tolerance, and a positive attitude.

tient has a lactose deficiency, suggest calcium supplements to replace calcium lost by eliminating dairy products from the diet.

- Encourage adequate fluid intake.
- Teach the elderly patient to gradually eliminate laxative use. Point out that using laxative agents to promote regular bowel movement may have the opposite effect, producing either constipation or incontinence over time. Suggest natural laxatives, such as prunes and prune juice, instead.
- Promote regular exercise by explaining how it helps to regulate bowel motility. Even a nonambulatory patient can perform some exercises while sitting or lying in bed.

Special considerations

- To rid the bladder of residual urine, teach the patient to perform Valsalva's or Credé's maneuver, or institute clean intermittent catheterization. Use an indwelling urinary catheter only as a last resort because of the risk of UTI.
- For fecal incontinence, maintain effective hygienic care to increase the patient's com-

Strengthening pelvic floor muscles

Stress incontinence, the most common kind of urinary incontinence in women, usually results from weakening of the urethral sphincter. In men, it may sometimes occur after a radical prostatectomy.

You can help a patient prevent or minimize stress incontinence by teaching her pelvic floor (Kegel) exercises to strengthen the pubococcygeal muscles. Here's how.

Learning Kegel exercises

First, explain how to locate the muscles of the pelvic floor. Instruct the patient to tense the muscles around the anus, as if to retain stool.

Next, teach the patient to tighten the muscles of the pelvic floor to stop the flow of urine while urinating and then to release the muscles to restart the flow. Once learned, these exercises can be done anywhere at any time.

Establishing a regimen

Explain to the patient that contraction and relaxation exercises are essential to muscle retraining. Suggest that she start out by contracting the pelvic floor muscles for 10 seconds, then relax for 10 seconds before slowly tightening the muscles and then releasing them.

Typically, the patient starts with 15 contractions in the morning and afternoon and 20 at night. Or she may exercise for 10 minutes three times per day, working up to 25 contractions at a time as strength improves.

Advise the patient not to use stomach, leg, or buttock muscles. Also discourage leg crossing or breath holding during these exercises.

fort and prevent skin breakdown and infection. Clean the perineal area frequently, and apply a moisture barrier cream. Control foul odors as well.

- Schedule extra time to provide encouragement and support for the patient, who may feel shame, embarrassment, and powerlessness from loss of control.

Complications

- Skin breakdown and infection
- Psychological problems including social isolation, loss of independence, lowered self-esteem, and depression

Patient teaching

- Advise the patient to consume a fiber-rich diet with raw, leafy vegetables, unpeeled fruits, and whole grains.
- Encourage adequate fluid intake
- Encourage exercise, explaining to the patient about how it helps regulate bowel motility.
- Suggest the use of natural laxatives, such as prunes and prune juice. Encourage the patient to gradually eliminate over-the-counter laxative use.

Documentation

Record all bladder and bowel retraining efforts, noting scheduled bathroom times, food and fluid intake, elimination amounts, and the patient's response to training efforts, as appropriate. Record the duration of continent periods.

Intermittent infusion device, drug administration

Intermittent infusion devices allow drugs to be given intermittently by infusion, I.V. bolus, or I.V. push injection methods. It eliminates the need for multiple venipunctures or for maintaining venous access with a continuous I.V. infusion (saline lock).

Equipment

Gloves ♦ alcohol pads ♦ three 3-ml syringes with needleless adapter ♦ normal saline solution ♦ extra intermittent infusion device ♦ prescribed drug in an I.V. container with administration set and needle (for infusion) or in a syringe with needle (for I.V. bolus or push) ♦ tourniquet ♦ optional: T-connector, sterile bacteriostatic water

Preparation

- Check the order on the patient's drug record against the prescriber's order.
- Wash your hands, and then wipe the tops of the normal saline solution, heparin flush solution, and drug containers with alcohol pads.
- Fill two of the 3-ml syringes (bearing 22G needles) with normal saline solution; draw 1 ml of heparin flush solution into the third syringe, according to your facility's policy.
- If you'll be infusing the drug, insert the administration set spike into the I.V. container, attach the needleless adapter, and prime the line.
- If you'll be injecting the drug I.V., fill a syringe with the prescribed drug.

Key steps

- Confirm the patient's identity by asking his name and checking the name, room number, and bed number on his wristband.
- If your facility uses a bar-code scanning system, scan your ID badge, the patient's ID bracelet, and the medication's bar code.
- Explain the procedure to the patient.
- Put on gloves.
- Wipe the injection port of the intermittent infusion device with an alcohol pad, and insert the needleless adapter of a saline-filled syringe.
- Aspirate the syringe to verify the patency of the device. If no blood appears during aspiration, apply a tourniquet slightly above the site, keep it in place for about 1 minute, and then aspirate again. If blood still doesn't appear, remove the tourniquet and inject normal saline solution slowly.

ACTION STAT!

Stop the injection immediately if you feel any resistance because this may mean the device is occluded. If you feel resistance, insert a new saline lock.

- If you feel no resistance, watch for signs of infiltration (puffiness or pain at the site) as you slowly inject the saline solution. If these signs occur, insert a new intermittent infusion device.
- If blood is aspirated, slowly inject the saline solution and observe for signs of infiltration.
- Withdraw the saline syringe and needleless adapter.
- Flush with dilute normal saline solution to prevent clotting in the device.

Giving I.V. bolus or push injections

- Insert the needleless adapter and syringe with the drug for the I.V. bolus or push injection into the injection port of the device.
- Inject the drug at the required rate.
- Remove the needleless adapter and syringe from the injection port.
- Insert the needleless adapter of the remaining saline-filled syringe into the injection port, and slowly inject the normal saline solution to flush all drug through the device.
- Remove the needleless adapter and syringe, and insert and inject the heparin (or saline) flush solution to prevent clotting in the device.

Giving an infusion

- Insert and secure the needleless adapter attached to the administration set.
- Open the infusion line and adjust the flow rate as needed.
- To give fluids and drugs simultaneously or to give a drug incompatible with the primary I.V. solution, use a T-connector or needleless adapter.
- Infuse drug for the prescribed length of time; then flush the device with normal saline solution to prevent clotting in the device.

Special considerations

- In the last step, to avoid clotting in the device, flush with bacteriostatic water if the drug you're injecting (such as diazepam) is incompatible with normal saline solution.

- Change intermittent infusion devices every 48 to 72 hours, according to universal precautions guidelines and your facility's policy.

Complications

- Infiltration
- Specific reaction to infused drug

Documentation

Record the type, amount, and times of drug given. Document I.V. solutions used to dilute the drug and flush the line on the intake record. If you can't rotate injection sites because the patient has fragile veins, document this fact. Note the use of normal saline solution.

Intermittent infusion device insertion

Also called a *saline lock,* an intermittent infusion device consists of a cannula with an attached injection cap. Filled with saline solution to prevent blood clot formation, the device maintains venous access in patients who are receiving I.V. medication regularly or intermittently but who don't require continuous infusion.

A saline lock should be inserted using sterile technique and maintaining standard precautions. If contamination occurs or is suspected, or the integrity of the product is compromised, it should be removed immediately.

Considerations when choosing the size of an I.V. catheter include size and condition of the vein, the viscosity of the fluid to be infused, the patient's age, and the type and duration of I.V. therapy. (See *Choosing the right I.V. catheter size.*)

An intermittent infusion device is superior to an I.V. line that's maintained at a moderately slow infusion rate because it minimizes the risk of fluid overload and electrolyte imbalance. It also cuts costs, reduces the risk of contamination by eliminating I.V. solution containers and administration sets, increases patient comfort and mobility, reduces patient anxiety and, if inserted in a large vein, allows collection of multiple blood samples without repeated venipuncture.

Choosing the right I.V. catheter size

Catheters come in various sizes (gauges). Choose the shortest catheter with the largest gauge appropriate for the type and duration of the infusion. The larger the gauge number, the smaller the catheter's bore.

- 24 gauge—used mostly in neonates, pediatric patients, and elderly patients
- 22 gauge—used especially in children and elderly patients
- 18 gauge—best used for blood, blood products, and viscous medications
- 16 gauge—(largest catheter) used in major surgeries, obstetric emergencies, and traumas

Equipment

Intermittent infusion device ♦ needleless system device ♦ normal saline solution ♦ tourniquet ♦ alcohol pad or other approved antimicrobial solution ♦ venipuncture equipment ♦ transparent semipermeable dressing ♦ tape

Prefilled saline cartridges are available for use in a syringe cartridge holder.

Key steps

- Confirm the patient's identity using two patient identifiers according to your facility's policy.
- Wash your hands thoroughly to prevent contamination of the venipuncture site.
- Explain the procedure to the patient, and describe the purpose of the intermittent infusion device.
- Remove the set from its packaging, wipe the port with an alcohol pad, and inject normal saline solution to fill the tubing and needleless system. This removes air from the system, preventing formation of an air embolus.

- Select a venipuncture site. Put on gloves. Apply a tourniquet 2″ (5.1 cm) proximal to the chosen area.
- Clean the venipuncture site with alcohol or other approved antimicrobial solution according to your facility's policy and manufacturer's directions.
- Perform the venipuncture and ensure correct needle placement in the vein. Then release the tourniquet.
- Tape the set in place. Loop the tubing, if applicable, so the injection port is free and easily accessible.
- Flush the catheter with saline solution.
- Apply a transparent semipermeable dressing. On the dressing label, write the time, date, and your initials, and place the label on the dressing.
- Remove and discard gloves.
- Inject normal saline solution every 8 to 24 hours or according to your facility's policy to maintain the patency of the intermittent infusion device. Inject the saline slowly to prevent stinging.

Special considerations

- When accessing an intermittent infusion device, be sure to stabilize the device to prevent dislodging it from the vein.
- If the patient feels a burning sensation during the injection of saline, stop the injection and check the cannula placement. If the cannula is in the vein, inject the saline at a slower rate to minimize irritation. If the needle isn't in the vein, remove and discard it. Then select a new venipuncture site and, using fresh equipment, restart the procedure.
- Change the intermittent infusion device every 48 to 72 hours, according to your facility's policy, using a new venipuncture site. Some facilities use a transparent semipermeable dressing. This allows more patient freedom and better observation of the injection site.
- If the practitioner orders an I.V. infusion discontinued and an intermittent infusion device inserted in its place, convert the existing line by disconnecting the I.V. tubing and inserting a male adapter plug into the device.
- Most health care facilities require the use of luer-lock systems on all infusion cannulas and lines.

Complications

- Same as for the use of a peripheral I.V. line (see *Risks of peripheral I.V. therapy*, pages 380 to 387)

Patient teaching

- If you're caring for a patient who will be going home with a peripheral line, teach him how to care for the I.V. site and how to identify complications.
- If he must observe movement restrictions, make sure that he understands which movements to avoid.
- Because the patient may have special drug delivery equipment that differs from the type used in the facility, be sure to demonstrate the equipment and have the patient give a return demonstration.
- Tell the patient to report problems with the I.V. line—for instance, if the solution stops infusing or if an alarm goes off on the infusion pump. Explain that the I.V. site will be changed at established intervals by a home care nurse.
- Teach the patient or caregiver how and when to flush the device.
- Finally, teach the patient to document daily whether the I.V. site is free from pain, swelling, and redness.

Documentation

Record the date and time of insertion; type, brand, and gauge of the needle and length of the cannula; anatomic location of the insertion site; the patient's tolerance of the procedure; and the date and time of each saline flush.

Internal fixation

Open reduction is a surgical procedure to realign a fracture; internal fixation is the addition of devices to stabilize the fracture. Internal fixation devices include nails, screws, pins, wires, and rods. They can be used individually or in combination with metal plates to attain stabilization. (See *Internal fixation devices.*)

Internal fixation devices

Choice of a specific internal fixation device depends on the location, type, and configuration of the fracture.

In trochanteric or subtrochanteric fractures, the surgeon may use a hip pin or nail, with or without a screw plate. A pin or plate with extra nails stabilizes the fracture by impacting the bone ends at the fracture site.

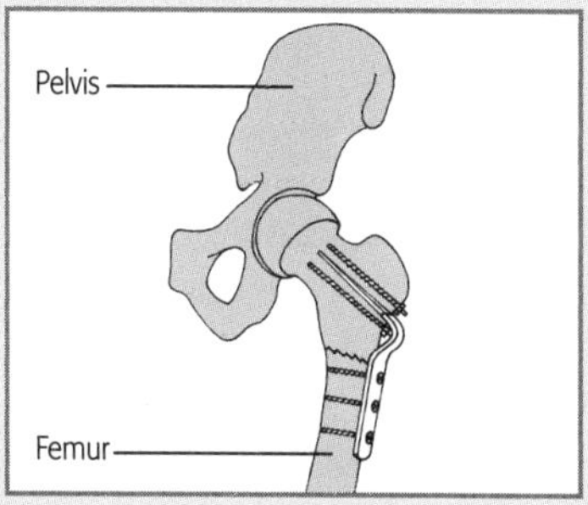

In an uncomplicated fracture of the femoral shaft, the surgeon may use an intramedullary rod. This device permits early ambulation with partial weight bearing.

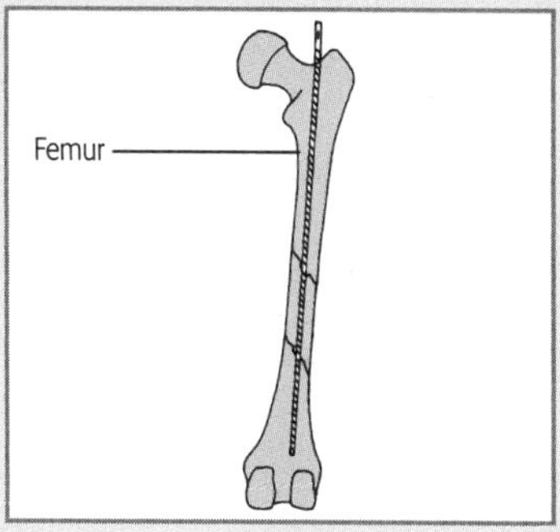

Another choice for fixation of a long-bone fracture is a screw plate, shown below on the tibia.

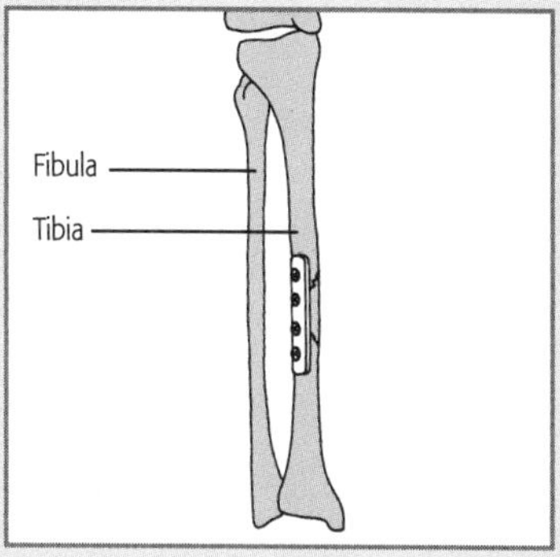

In an arm fracture, the surgeon may fix the involved bones with a plate, rod, or nail. Most radial and ulnar fractures may be fixed with plates, whereas humeral fractures are commonly fixed with rods.

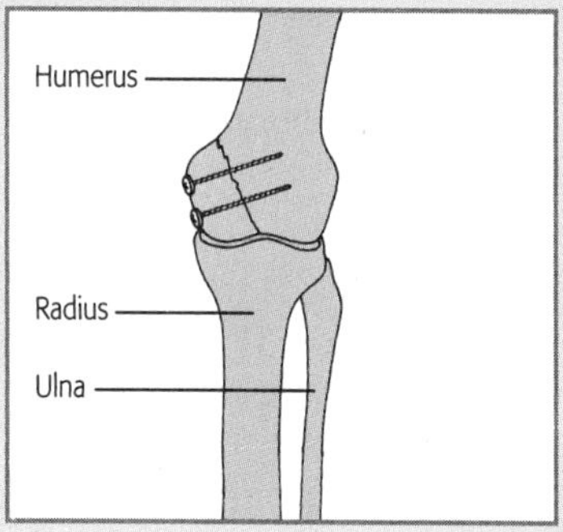

Typically, internal fixation is used to treat fractures of the face and jaw, spine, bones of the arms and legs, and fractures involving a joint (most commonly, the hip). Internal fixation permits earlier mobilization and can shorten hospitalization, particularly in elderly patients with hip fractures.

Equipment

Ice bag ♦ pain medication (analgesic or opioid) ♦ incentive spirometer ♦ compression stockings

Patients with leg fractures

Overhead frame with trapeze ♦ pressure-relief mattress ♦ crutches or walker ♦ pillow (hip fractures may require abductor pillows)

Preparation

- Equipment is collected and prepared in the operating room.

Key steps

- Explain the procedure to the patient to alleviate his fears. Tell him what to expect during postoperative assessment and monitoring, teach him how to use an incentive spirometer, and prepare him for proposed exercise and progressive ambulation regimens if necessary.
- After the procedure, monitor the patient's vital signs every 2 to 4 hours for 24 hours, then every 4 to 8 hours, according to your facility's protocol. Changes in the patient's vital signs may indicate hemorrhage or infection.
- Monitor fluid intake and output every 4 to 8 hours.
- Perform neurovascular checks every 2 to 4 hours for 24 hours, then every 4 to 8 hours as appropriate. Assess color, warmth, sensation, movement, edema, capillary refill, and pulses of the affected area. Compare findings with the unaffected side.
- Apply an ice bag to the operative site, as ordered, to reduce swelling, relieve pain, and lessen bleeding.
- Administer opioids, as ordered, before exercising or mobilizing the affected area to promote comfort. If the patient is using patient-controlled analgesia, instruct him to administer a dose before exercising or mobilizing.
- Monitor the patient for pain unrelieved by opioids and for burning, tingling, or numbness, which may indicate infection, impaired circulation, or compartment syndrome.
- Elevate the affected limb on a pillow, if appropriate, to minimize edema.
- Check surgical dressings for excessive drainage or bleeding. Check the incision site for signs of infection, such as erythema, drainage, edema, and unusual pain.
- Assist and encourage the patient to perform range-of-motion and other muscle-strengthening exercises, as ordered, to promote circulation, improve muscle tone, and maintain joint function.
- Teach the patient to perform progressive ambulation and mobilization using an overhead frame with trapeze, or crutches or a walker, as appropriate.
- Continue anticoagulation therapy as ordered by the practitioner.
- Teach the patient signs and symptoms of venous thromboembolism.

Special considerations

- To avoid the complications of immobility after surgery, have the patient use an incentive spirometer. Apply compression stockings and a sequential compression device, as appropriate. The patient may also require a pressure-relief mattress.

Complications

- Wound infection and, more critically, infection involving metal fixation devices requiring reopening of the incision, draining the suture line, (possibly removing the fixation device), and administering wound dressings and antibiotic therapy
- Malunion, nonunion, fat or pulmonary embolism, neurovascular impairment, and chronic pain

Patient teaching

- Before discharge, instruct the patient and his family how to care for the incisional site and recognize signs and symptoms of infection.
- Teach the patient and his family about administering pain medication, practicing an exercise regimen (if any), and using assistive ambulation devices (such as crutches or a walker), if appropriate.

Documentation

In the patient record, document perioperative findings on cardiovascular, respiratory, and neurovascular status. Name pain-management techniques used. Describe incision appearance and alignment of the affected bone. Document the patient's response to teaching about appropriate exercise, care of the incision site, use of assistive devices (if appropriate), and symptoms that should be reported to the practitioner.

Intra-aortic balloon counterpulsation

Providing temporary support for the heart's left ventricle, intra-aortic balloon counterpulsation (IABC) mechanically displaces blood within the aorta by means of an intra-aortic balloon attached to an external pump console. The balloon is usually inserted through the common femoral artery and positioned with its tip just distal to the left subclavian artery. It monitors myocardial perfusion and the effects of drugs on myocardial function and perfusion. When used correctly, IABC improves two key aspects of myocardial physiology: It increases the supply of oxygen-rich blood to the myocardium, and it decreases myocardial oxygen demand.

IABC is recommended for patients with a wide range of low-cardiac-output disorders or cardiac instability, including refractory anginas, ventricular arrhythmias associated with ischemia, and pump failure caused by cardiogenic shock, intraoperative myocardial infarction (MI), or low cardiac output after bypass surgery. IABC is also indicated for patients with low cardiac output secondary to acute mechanical defects after MI (such as ventricular septal defect, papillary muscle rupture, or left ventricular aneurysm).

Perioperatively, the technique is used to support and stabilize patients with a suspected high-grade lesion who are undergoing such procedures as angioplasty, thrombolytic therapy, cardiac surgery, and cardiac catheterization.

IABC is contraindicated in patients with severe aortic regurgitation, aortic aneurysm, or severe peripheral vascular disease.

Equipment

IABC console and balloon catheters ♦ dacron graft (for surgically inserted balloon) ♦ electrocardiogram (ECG) monitor and electrodes ♦ I.V. solution and infusion set ♦ sedative ♦ pain medication ♦ arterial line catheter ♦ heparin flush solution, transducer, and flush setup ♦ pulmonary artery (PA) catheter setup ♦ temporary pacemaker setup ♦ #18G angiography needle ♦ sterile drape ♦ sterile gloves ♦ gown ♦ mask ♦ sutures ♦ antiseptic and saline solution or sterile water for irrigation and suction setup ♦ oxygen setup and respirator, if necessary ♦ defibrillator and emergency medications ♦ fluoroscope ♦ indwelling urinary catheter ♦ urinometer ♦ arterial blood gas (ABG) kits and tubes for laboratory studies ♦ antiseptic swabs and ointment ♦ dressing materials ♦ 4″ × 4″ gauze pads ♦ clippers ♦ optional: defibrillator, atropine, I.V. heparin, low-molecular-weight dextran

Preparation

- Depending on your facility's policy, you or a perfusionist must balance the pressure transducer in the external pump console and calibrate the oscilloscope monitor to ensure accuracy.

Key steps

- Explain to the patient that the physician will place a special balloon catheter in his aorta to help his heart pump more easily. Briefly explain the insertion procedure, and mention that the catheter will be connected to a large console next to his bed. Tell him that the balloon will temporarily reduce his heart's workload to promote rapid healing of the ventricular muscle. Let him know that it will be removed after his heart can resume an adequate workload. (See *How the intra-aortic balloon pump works*, page 256.)

Preparing for intra-aortic balloon insertion

- Make sure the patient or a family member understands and signs a consent form. Verify that the form is attached to his chart.
- Obtain the patient's baseline vital signs, including pulmonary artery pressure (PAP). (A PA line should already be in place.) Attach the patient to an ECG machine for continuous monitoring. Be sure to apply chest electrodes in a standard lead II position—or in whatever position produces the largest R wave—because the R wave triggers balloon inflation and deflation. Obtain a baseline ECG.

How the intra-aortic balloon pump works

Made of polyurethane, the intra-aortic balloon is attached to an external pump console by means of a large-lumen catheter. The illustrations here show the direction of blood flow when the pump inflates and deflates the balloon.

Balloon inflation

The balloon inflates as the aortic valve closes and diastole begins. Diastole increases perfusion to the coronary arteries.

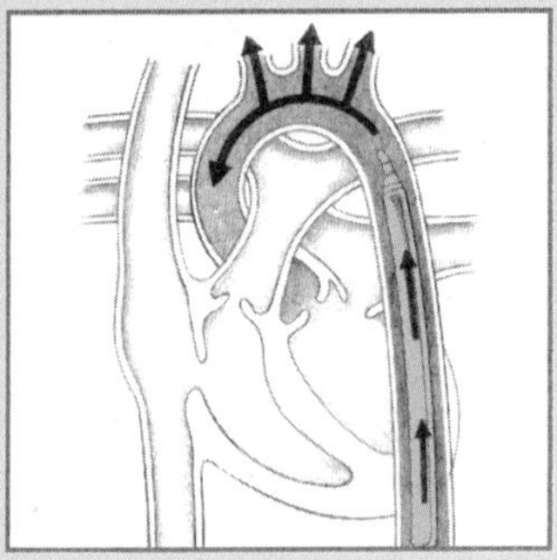

Balloon deflation

The balloon deflates before ventricular ejection, when the aortic valve opens. This permits ejection of blood from the left ventricle against a lowered resistance. As a result, aortic end-diastolic pressure and afterload decrease and cardiac output rises.

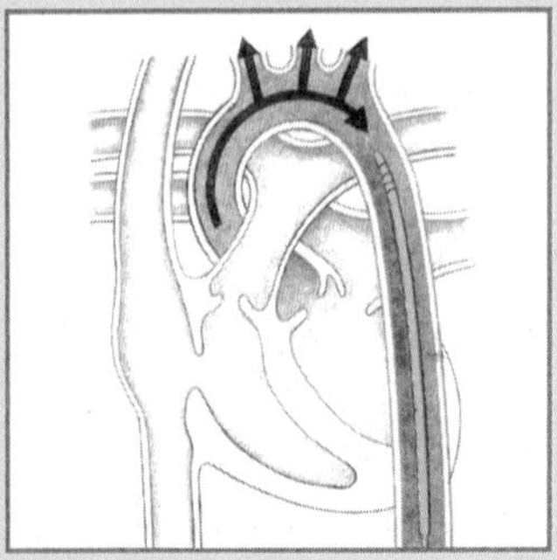

- Attach another set of ECG electrodes to the patient unless the ECG pattern is being transmitted from the patient's bedside monitor to the balloon pump monitor through a phone cable. Administer oxygen as ordered and as necessary.
- Make sure the patient has an arterial line, a PA line, and a peripheral I.V. line in place. The arterial line is used for withdrawing blood samples, monitoring blood pressure, and assessing the timing and effectiveness of therapy. The PA line allows measurement of PAP, aspiration of blood samples, and cardiac output studies. Increased PAP indicates increased myocardial workload and ineffective balloon pumping. Cardiac output studies are usually performed with and without the balloon to check the patient's progress. The central lumen of the intra-aortic balloon, used to monitor central aortic pressure, produces an augmented pressure waveform that allows you to check for proper timing of the inflation-deflation cycle and demonstrates the effects of counterpulsation, elevated diastolic pressure, and reduced end-diastolic and systolic pressures. (See *Interpreting intra-aortic balloon waveforms.*)
- Insert an indwelling catheter so you can measure the patient's urine output and assess his fluid balance and renal function. To reduce the risk of infection, clip hair bilaterally from the lower abdomen to the lower thigh, including the pubic area.
- Observe and record the patient's peripheral leg pulse and document sensation, movement, color, and temperature of the legs.
- Administer a sedative as ordered.

Inserting the intra-aortic balloon percutaneously

- The physician may insert the balloon percutaneously through the femoral artery into the descending thoracic aorta, using a modified Seldinger technique. First, he accesses the vessel with an 18G angiography needle and removes the inner stylet.
- Then he passes the guide wire through the needle and removes the needle.
- After passing a #8 French vessel dilator over the guide wire into the vessel, he re-

Interpreting intra-aortic balloon waveforms

During intra-aortic balloon counterpulsation, you can use electrocardiogram and arterial pressure waveforms to determine whether the balloon pump is functioning properly.

Normal inflation-deflation timing

Balloon inflation occurs after aortic valve closure; deflation, during isovolumetric contraction, just before the aortic valve opens. In a properly timed waveform, like the one shown at right, the inflation point lies at or slightly above the dicrotic notch. Both inflation and deflation cause a sharp V. Peak diastolic pressure exceeds peak systolic pressure; peak systolic pressure exceeds assisted peak systolic pressure.

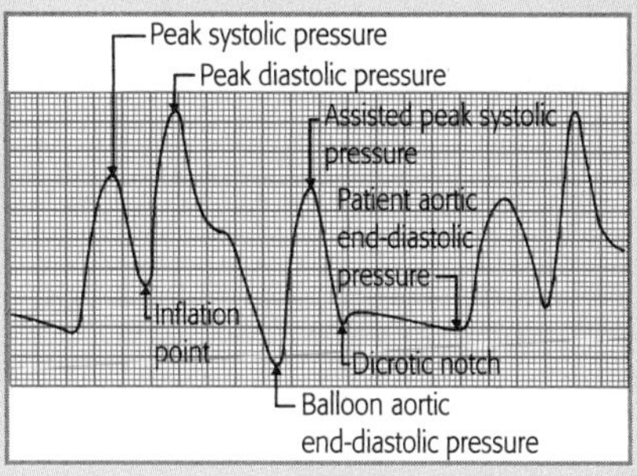

Early inflation

With *early inflation,* the inflation point lies before the dicrotic notch. Early inflation dangerously increases myocardial stress and decreases cardiac output.

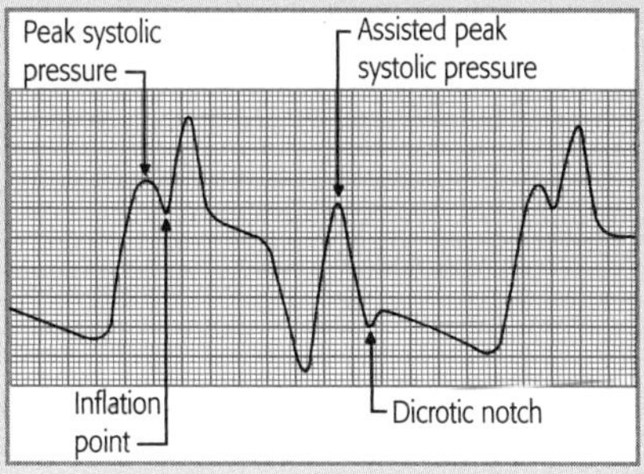

Early deflation

With *early deflation,* a U shape appears and peak systolic pressure is less than or equal to assisted peak systolic pressure. This won't decrease afterload or myocardial oxygen consumption.

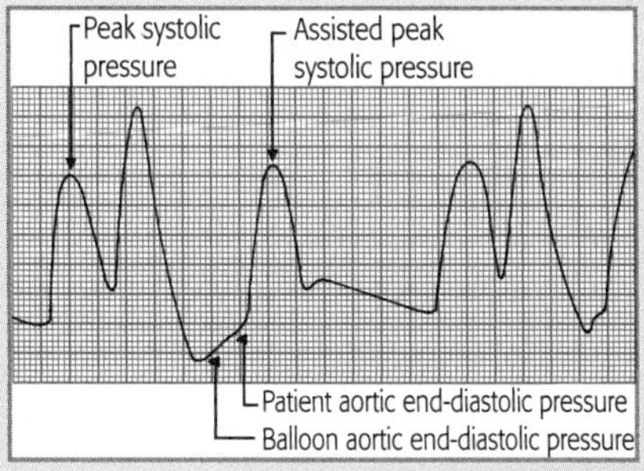

(continued)

Interpreting intra-aortic balloon waveforms *(continued)*

Late inflation

With *late inflation,* the dicrotic notch precedes the inflation point, and the notch and the inflation point create a W shape. This can lead to a reduction in peak diastolic pressure, coronary and systemic perfusion augmentation time, and augmented coronary perfusion pressure.

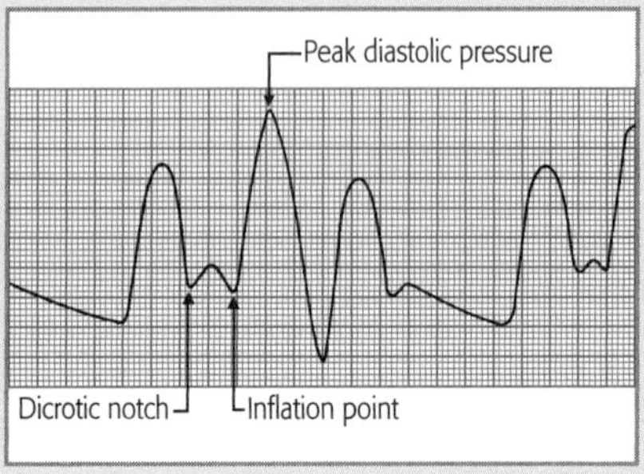

Late deflation

With *late deflation,* peak systolic pressure exceeds assisted peak systolic pressure. This threatens the patient by increasing afterload, myocardial oxygen consumption, cardiac workload, and preload. It occurs when the balloon has been inflated for too long.

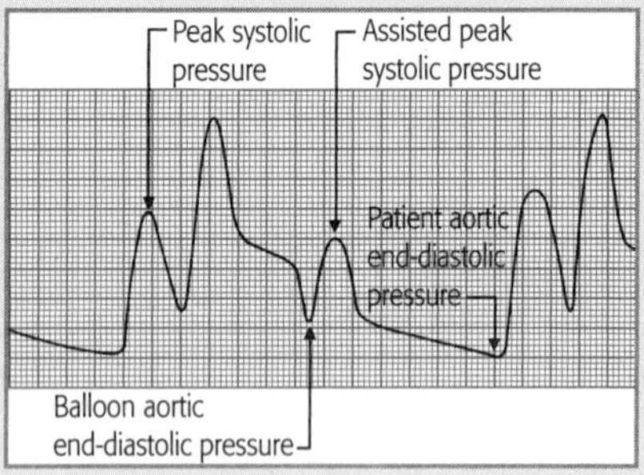

moves the vessel dilator, leaving the guide wire in place.

- Next, the physician passes an introducer (dilator and sheath assembly) over the guide wire into the vessel until about 1″ (2.5 cm) remains above the insertion site. He then removes the inner dilator, leaving the introducer sheath and guide wire in place.
- After passing the balloon over the guide wire into the introducer sheath, the physician advances the catheter into position, ⅜″ to ¾″ (1 to 2 cm) distal to the left subclavian artery under fluoroscopic guidance.
- The physician attaches the balloon to the control system to initiate counterpulsation. The balloon catheter then unfurls.

Inserting the intra-aortic balloon surgically

- If the physician chooses not to insert the catheter percutaneously, he usually inserts it by femoral arteriotomy.
- After making an incision and isolating the femoral artery, the physician attaches a Dacron graft to a small opening in the arterial wall.
- He then passes the catheter through this graft. Using fluoroscopic guidance as necessary, he advances the catheter up the descending thoracic aorta and places the catheter tip between the left subclavian artery and the renal arteries.
- The physician sews the Dacron graft around the catheter at the insertion point and connects the other end of the catheter to the pump console.
- If the balloon can't be inserted through the femoral artery, the physician inserts it in an antegrade direction through the ante-

rior wall of the ascending aorta. He positions it $\frac{3}{8}''$ to $\frac{3}{4}''$ (1 to 2 cm) beyond the left subclavian artery and brings the catheter out through the chest wall.

Monitoring the patient after balloon insertion

ALERT

If the control system malfunctions or becomes inoperable, don't let the balloon catheter remain dormant for more than 30 minutes. Get another control system and attach it to the balloon; then resume pumping. In the meantime, inflate the balloon manually, using a 60-ml syringe and room air a minimum of once every 5 minutes, to prevent thrombus formation in the catheter.

- Obtain a chest X-ray to verify correct balloon placement.
- Assess and record pedal and posterior tibial pulses as well as color, sensation, and temperature in the affected limb every 15 minutes for 1 hour, then hourly.

ACTION STAT!

Notify the physician immediately if you detect circulatory changes; the balloon may need to be removed.

- Observe and record the patient's baseline arm pulses, arm sensation and movement, and arm color and temperature every 15 minutes for 1 hour after balloon insertion, then every 2 hours while the balloon is in place. Loss of left arm pulses may indicate upward balloon displacement. Notify the physician of any changes.
- Monitor the patient's urine output every hour. Note baseline blood urea nitrogen (BUN) and serum creatinine levels, and monitor these levels daily. Changes in urine output, BUN, and serum creatinine levels may signal reduced renal perfusion from downward balloon displacement.
- Auscultate and record bowel sounds every 4 hours. Check for abdominal distention and tenderness as well as changes in the patient's elimination patterns.
- Measure the patient's temperature every 1 to 4 hours. If it's elevated, obtain blood samples for a culture, send them to the laboratory immediately, and notify the physician. Culture any drainage at the insertion site.
- Monitor the patient's hematologic status. Observe for bleeding gums, blood in the urine or stools, petechiae, and bleeding at the insertion site. Monitor his platelet count, hemoglobin levels, and hematocrit daily. Expect to administer blood products to maintain hematocrit at 30%. If the platelet count drops, expect to administer platelets.
- Monitor partial thromboplastin time (PTT) every 6 hours while the heparin dose is adjusted to maintain PTT at $1\frac{1}{2}$ to 2 times the normal value, then every 12 to 24 hours while the balloon remains in place.
- Measure PAP and pulmonary artery wedge pressure (PAWP) every 1 to 2 hours, as ordered. A rising PAWP reflects preload, signaling increased ventricular pressure and workload; notify the physician if this occurs. Some patients require I.V. nitroprusside during IABC to reduce preload and afterload.
- Obtain samples for ABG analysis, as ordered.
- Monitor serum electrolyte levels—especially sodium and potassium—to assess the patient's fluid and electrolyte balance and help prevent arrhythmias.
- Watch for signs and symptoms of a dissecting aortic aneurysm: a blood pressure differential between the left and right arms, elevated blood pressure, syncope, pallor, diaphoresis, dyspnea, a throbbing abdominal mass, a reduced red blood cell count with an elevated white blood cell count, and pain in the chest, abdomen, or back. Notify the physician immediately if you detect any of these complications.

Weaning the patient from IABC

- Assess the cardiac index, systemic blood pressure, and PAWP to help the physician evaluate the patient's readiness for weaning—usually about 24 hours after balloon insertion. The patient's hemodynamic status should be stable on minimal doses of inotropic agents, such as dopamine (Intropin) or dobutamine (Dobutrex).

- To begin weaning, gradually decrease the frequency of balloon augmentation to 1:2 and 1:4, as ordered. Although your facility has its own weaning protocol, be aware that assist frequency is usually maintained for an hour or longer. If the patient's hemodynamic indices remain stable during this time, weaning may continue.
- Avoid leaving the patient on a low augmentation setting for more than 2 hours to prevent embolus formation.
- Assess the patient's tolerance of weaning.

ACTION STAT!

Signs and symptoms of poor tolerance include confusion and disorientation, urine output below 30 ml/hour, cold and clammy skin, chest pain, arrhythmias, ischemic ECG changes, and elevated PAP. If the patient develops any of these problems, notify the physician at once.

Removing the intra-aortic balloon

- The balloon is removed when the patient's hemodynamic status remains stable after the frequency of balloon augmentation is decreased. The control system is turned off and the connective tubing is disconnected from the catheter to ensure balloon deflation.
- The physician withdraws the balloon until the proximal end of the catheter contacts the distal end of the introducer sheath.
- The physician then applies pressure below the puncture site and removes the balloon and introducer sheath as a unit, allowing a few seconds of free bleeding to prevent thrombus formation.
- To promote distal bleedback, the physician applies pressure above the puncture site.
- Apply direct pressure to the site for 30 minutes or until bleeding stops. (In some facilities, this is the physician's responsibility.)
- If the balloon was inserted surgically, the physician will close the Dacron graft and suture the insertion site. The cardiologist usually removes a percutaneous catheter.
- After balloon removal, provide wound care according to your facility's policy. Record the patient's pedal and posterior tibial pulses, and the color, temperature, and sensation of the affected limb. Enforce bed rest as appropriate (usually for 24 hours).

Special considerations

- Before using the IABC control system, make sure you know what the alarms and messages mean and how to respond to them.

ACTION STAT!

You must respond immediately to alarms and messages.

- Change the dressing at the balloon insertion site every 24 hours or as needed, using strict sterile technique. Don't let povidone-iodine solution come in contact with the catheter.
- Make sure the head of the bed is elevated no more than 30 degrees.
- Watch for pump interruptions, which may result from loose ECG electrodes or leadwires, static or 60-cycle interference, catheter kinking, or improper body alignment.
- Make sure the PTT is within normal limits before the balloon is removed to prevent bleeding.

Complications

- Arterial embolism stemming from clot formation on the balloon surface
- Extension or rupture of an aortic aneurysm, femoral or iliac artery perforation, femoral artery occlusion, and sepsis
- Bleeding at the insertion site aggravated by pump-induced thrombocytopenia caused by platelet aggregation around the balloon

Documentation

Document all aspects of patient assessment and management, including the patient's response to therapy. If you're responsible for the IABC device, document all routine checks, problems, and troubleshooting measures. If a technician is responsible for the IABC device, record only when and why the technician was notified as well as the result of his actions on the patient, if any. Also document any teaching of the patient, family, or close friends as well as their responses.

Intracranial pressure monitoring

Intracranial pressure (ICP) monitoring measures pressure exerted by the brain, blood, and cerebrospinal fluid (CSF) against the inside of the skull. Normal ICP is 0 to 15 mm Hg, with the ICP threshold of 20 to 25 mm Hg as the highest acceptable limit before instituting treatment. Indications for monitoring ICP include head trauma with bleeding or edema, overproduction or insufficient absorption of CSF, cerebral hemorrhage, and space-occupying brain lesions. ICP monitoring can detect elevated ICP early, before clinical danger signs develop. Prompt intervention can then help avert or diminish neurologic damage caused by cerebral hypoxia and shifts of brain mass.

The four basic ICP monitoring systems are intraventricular catheter, subarachnoid bolt, epidural sensor, and intraparenchymal pressure monitoring. (See *Understanding ICP monitoring,* pages 262 and 263.)

Regardless of which system is used, the procedure is typically performed by a neurosurgeon in the operating room, emergency department, or intensive care unit. Insertion of an ICP monitoring device requires sterile technique to reduce the risk of central nervous system (CNS) infection. Setting up equipment for the monitoring systems also requires strict asepsis.

Equipment

Monitoring unit and transducers as ordered ♦ 16 to 20 sterile 4″ × 4″ gauze pads ♦ linen-saver pads ♦ electric clippers or hair scissors ♦ sterile drapes ♦ sterile gown ♦ surgical mask ♦ sterile gloves ♦ head dressing supplies (two rolls of 4″ elastic gauze dressing, one roll of 4″ roller gauze, adhesive tape) ♦ antiseptic solution ♦ sterile marker ♦ sterile labels ♦ optional: suction apparatus, I.V. pole, and yardstick

Preparation

- Monitoring units and setup protocols are varied and complex and differ among health care facilities. Check your facility's guidelines for your particular unit.
- Various types of preassembled ICP monitoring units are available, each with its own setup protocols. These units are designed to reduce the risk of infection by eliminating the need for multiple stopcocks, manometers, and transducer dome assemblies. Some facilities use units that have miniaturized transducers rather than transducer domes.

Key steps

- Confirm the patient's identity using two patient identifiers according to facility policy.
- Explain the procedure to the patient or his family. Make sure the patient or a responsible family member has signed a consent form.
- Determine whether the patient is allergic to iodine preparations.
- Provide privacy if the procedure is being done in an open emergency department or intensive care unit.
- Wash your hands.
- Obtain baseline routine and neurologic vital signs to aid in prompt detection of decompensation during the procedure.
- Place the patient in the supine position, and elevate the head of the bed 30 degrees (or as ordered).
- Place linen-saver pads under the patient's head. Clip his hair at the insertion site, as indicated by the physician, to decrease the risk of infection. Carefully fold and remove the linen-saver pads to avoid spilling loose hair onto the bed. Drape the patient with sterile drapes. Scrub the insertion site for 2 minutes with chlorhexidine solution.
- The physician puts on the sterile gown, mask, and sterile gloves. He then opens the interior wrap of the sterile supply tray and proceeds with insertion of the catheter or bolt. Label all medications, medication

Understanding ICP monitoring

Intracranial pressure (ICP) can be monitored using one of four systems.

Intraventricular catheter monitoring

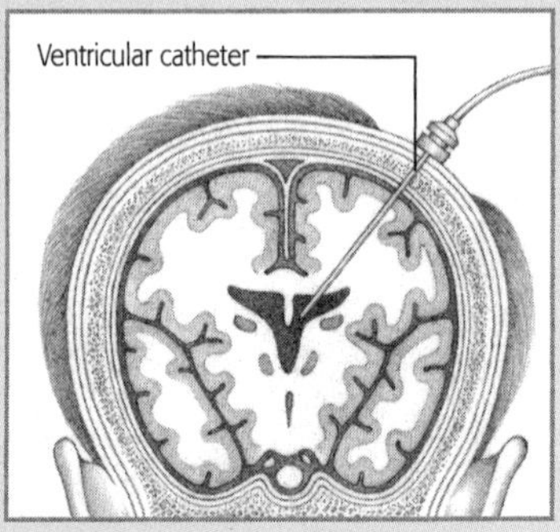

In this procedure, which monitors ICP directly, the physician inserts a small polyethylene or silicone rubber catheter into the lateral ventricle through a burr hole.

Although this method measures ICP most accurately, it carries the greatest risk of infection. This is the only type of ICP monitoring that allows evaluation of brain compliance and drainage of significant amounts of cerebrospinal fluid (CSF).

Contraindications usually include stenotic cerebral ventricles, cerebral aneurysms in the path of catheter placement, and suspected vascular lesions.

Subarachnoid bolt monitoring

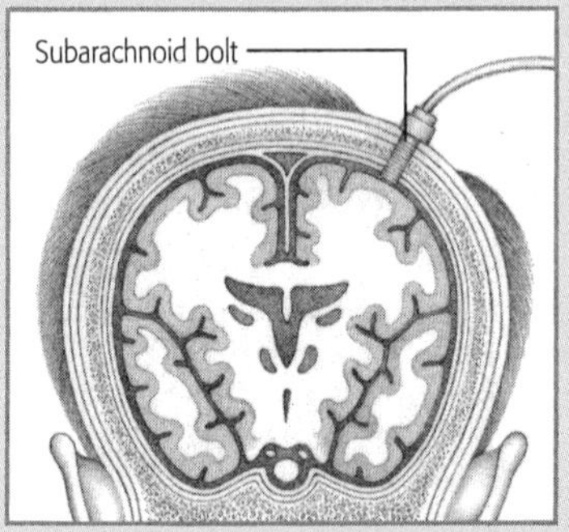

This procedure involves insertion of a special bolt into the subarachnoid space through a twist-drill burr hole that's positioned in the front of the skull behind the hairline.

Placing the bolt is easier than placing an intraventricular catheter, especially if a computed tomography scan reveals that the cerebrum has shifted or the ventricles have collapsed. This type of ICP monitoring also carries less risk of infection and parenchymal damage because the bolt doesn't penetrate the cerebrum.

containers, and other solutions on and off the sterile field.

- To facilitate placement of the device, hold the patient's head in your hands or attach a long strip of 4″ roller gauze to one side rail, and bring it across the patient's forehead to the opposite rail. Reassure the conscious patient to help ease his anxiety. Talk to him frequently to assess his level of consciousness (LOC) and detect signs of deterioration. Watch for cardiac arrhythmias and abnormal respiratory patterns.
- After insertion, put on sterile gloves and apply antiseptic solution and a sterile dressing to the site. If not done by the physician, connect the catheter to the appropriate monitoring device, depending on the system used. (See *Setting up an ICP monitoring system,* page 264.)
- If the physician has set up a ventriculostomy drainage system, attach the drip chamber to the headboard or bedside I.V. pole as ordered.
- Inspect the insertion site at least every 24 hours (or according to your facility's policy) for redness, swelling, and drainage. Clean the site, reapply antiseptic solution, and apply a fresh sterile dressing.
- Assess the patient's clinical status, and take routine and neurologic vital signs every hour, or as ordered. Make sure

Epidural or subdural sensor monitoring

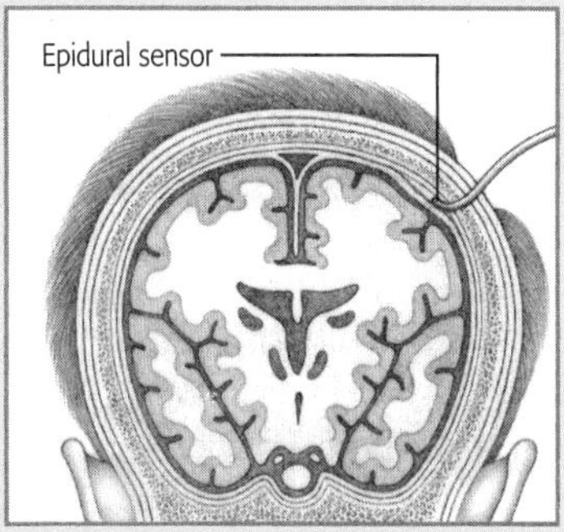

ICP can also be monitored from the epidural or subdural space. For epidural monitoring, a fiber-optic sensor is inserted into the epidural space through a burr hole. This system's main drawback is its questionable accuracy because ICP isn't being measured directly from a CSF-filled space.

For subdural monitoring, a fiber-optic transducer-tipped catheter is tunneled through a burr hole, and its tip is placed on brain tissue under the dura mater. The main drawback to this method is its inability to drain CSF.

Intraparenchymal monitoring

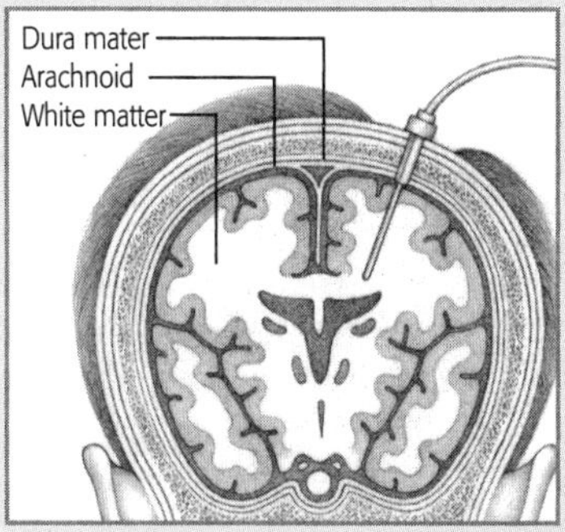

In this procedure, the physician inserts a catheter through a small subarachnoid bolt and, after puncturing the dura, advances the catheter a few centimeters into the brain's white matter. There's no need to balance or calibrate the equipment after insertion.

Although this method doesn't provide direct access to CSF, measurements are accurate because brain tissue pressure correlate well with ventricular pressures. Intraparenchymal monitoring may be used to obtain ICP measurements in patients with compressed or dislocated ventricles.

you've obtained orders for waveforms and pressure parameters from the physician.

- Calculate cerebral perfusion pressure (CPP) hourly; use the equation: CPP − MAP = ICP (MAP refers to mean arterial pressure).
- Observe digital ICP readings and waves. Remember, the pattern of readings is more significant than any single reading. (See *Interpreting ICP waveforms*, pages 265 and 266.)

ACTION STAT!

If you observe continually elevated ICP readings, note how long they're sustained. If they last several minutes, notify the physician immediately.

- Finally, record and describe any CSF drainage.

Special considerations

ALERT

In infants, ICP monitoring can be performed without penetrating the scalp. In this external method, a photoelectric transducer with a pressure-sensitive membrane is taped to the anterior fontanel. The transducer responds to pressure at the site and transmits readings to a bedside monitor and

(Text continues on page 266.)

Setting up an ICP monitoring system

To set up an intracranial pressure (ICP) monitoring system, follow these steps, using strict aseptic technique.

- Begin by opening a sterile towel. On the sterile field, place a 20-ml luer-lock syringe, an 18G needle, a 250-ml bag filled with normal saline solution (with outer wrapper removed), and a disposable transducer.
- Put on sterile gloves and gown, and fill the 20-ml syringe with normal saline solution from the I.V. bag.
- Remove the injection cap from the patient line and attach the syringe. Turn the system stopcock off to the short end of the patient line, and flush through to the drip chamber (as shown below). Allow a few drops to flow through the flow chamber (the manometer), the tubing, and the one-way valve into the drainage bag. (Fill the tubing and the manometer slowly to minimize air bubbles. If any air bubbles surface, be sure to force them from the system.)

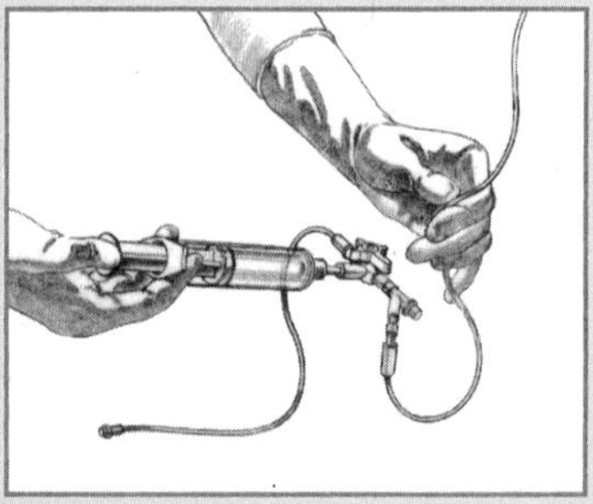

- Attach the manometer to the I.V. pole at the head of the bed.
- Slide the drip chamber onto the manometer, and align the chamber to the zero point (as shown top of next column).
- Next, connect the transducer to the monitor.
- Put on a clean pair of sterile gloves.
- Keeping one hand sterile, turn the patient stopcock off to the patient.

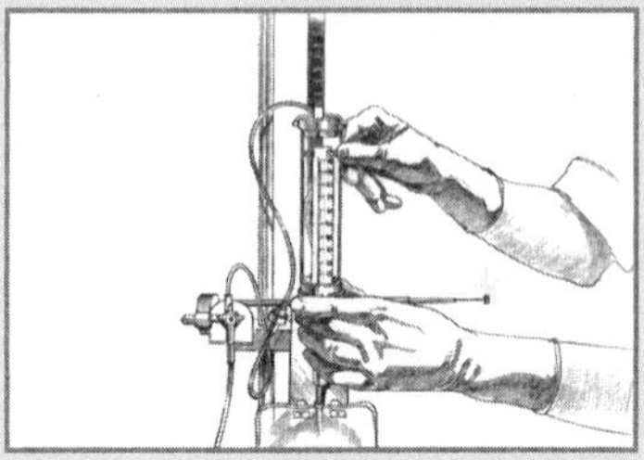

- Align the zero point with the center line of the patient's head, level with the middle of the ear (as shown below).
- Lower the flow chamber to zero, and turn the stopcock off to the dead-end cap. With a clean hand, balance the system according to monitor guidelines.

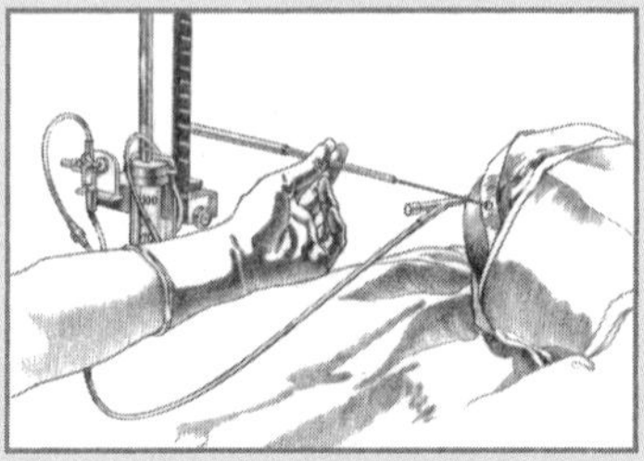

- Turn the system stopcock off to drainage, and raise the flow chamber to the ordered height (as shown below).
- Return the stopcock to the ordered position, and observe the monitor for the return of ICP patterns.

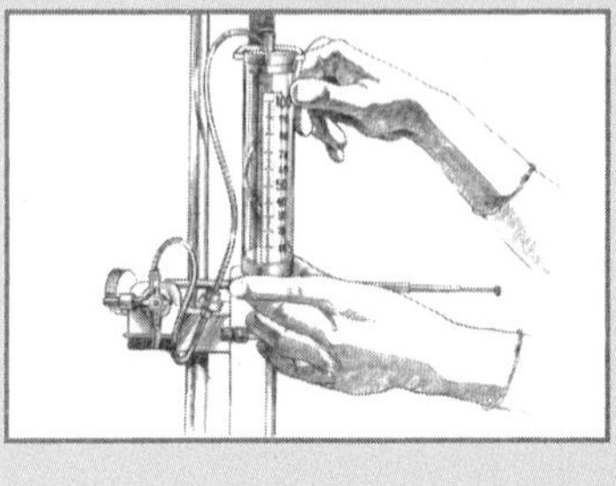

Interpreting ICP waveforms

Three waveforms—A, B, and C—are used to monitor intracranial pressure (ICP). A (plateau) waves are an ominous sign of intracranial decompensation and poor compliance. B waves correlate with changes in respiration, and C waves correlate with changes in arterial pressure.

Normal waveform

A normal ICP waveform typically shows a steep upward systolic slope followed by a downward diastolic slope with a dicrotic notch. In most cases, this waveform occurs continuously and indicates an ICP between 0 and 15 mm Hg—normal pressure.

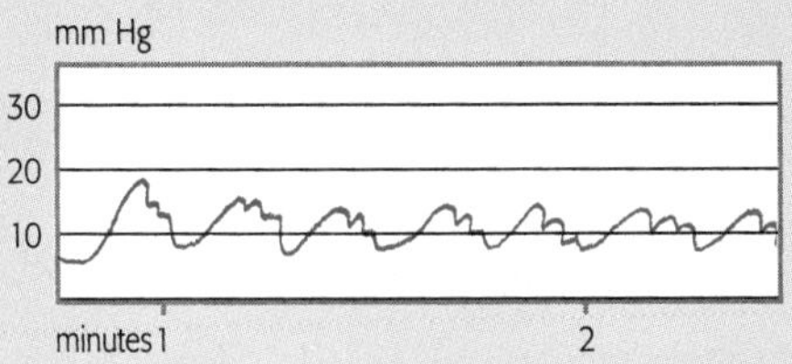

A waves

The most clinically significant ICP waveforms are A waves (shown at right), which may reach elevations of 50 to 100 mm Hg, persist for 5 to 20 minutes, then drop sharply—signaling exhaustion of the brain's compliance mechanisms. A waves may come and go, spiking from temporary rises in thoracic pressure or from any condition that increases ICP beyond the brain's compliance limits. Activities, such as sustained coughing or straining during defecation, can cause temporary elevations in thoracic pressure.

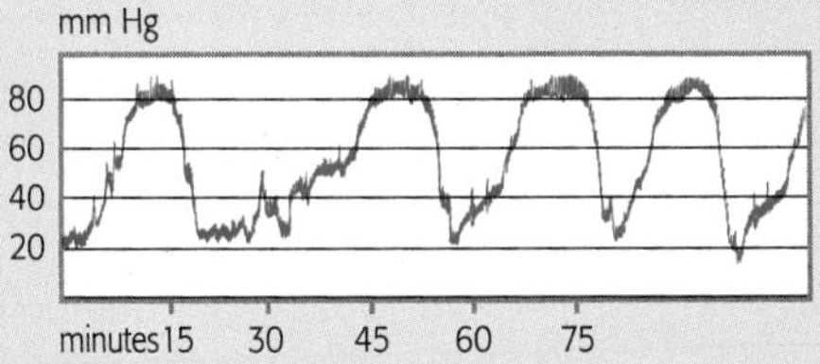

B waves

B waves, which appear sharp and rhythmic with a sawtooth pattern, occur every 1½ to 2 minutes and may reach elevations of 50 mm Hg. The clinical significance of B waves isn't clear, but the waves correlate with respiratory changes and may occur more frequently with decreasing compensation. Because B waves sometimes precede A waves, notify the physician if B waves occur frequently.

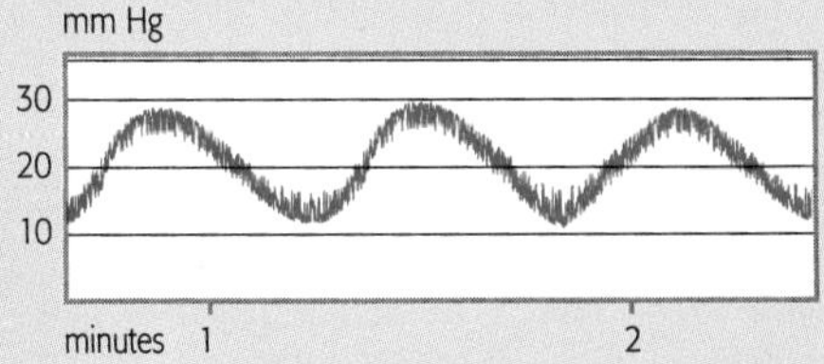

(continued)

Interpreting ICP waveforms *(continued)*

C waves

Like B waves, C waves are rapid and rhythmic, but they aren't as sharp. Clinically insignificant, they may fluctuate with respirations or systemic blood pressure changes.

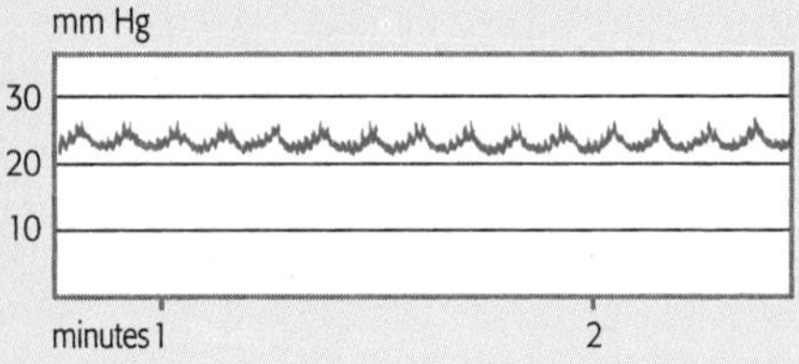

Waveform showing equipment problem

A waveform that looks like the one shown at right signals a problem with the transducer or monitor. Check for line obstruction, and determine if the transducer needs rebalancing.

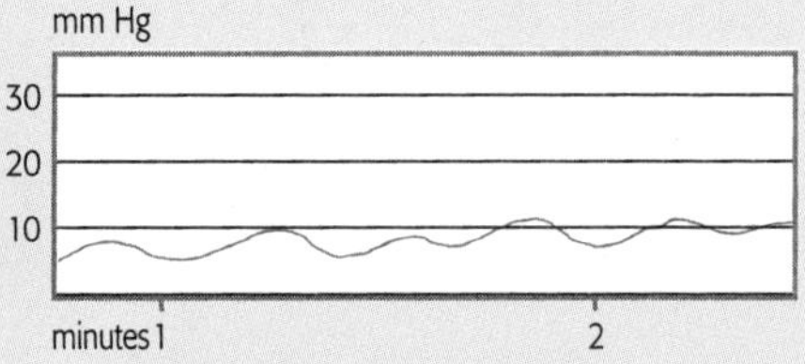

recording system. The external method is restricted to infants because pressure readings can be obtained only at fontanels, the incompletely ossified areas of the skull.

- Osmotic diuretic agents such as mannitol (Osmitrol) reduce cerebral edema by shrinking intracranial contents. Given by I.V. drip or bolus, mannitol draws water from tissues into plasma; it doesn't cross the blood-brain barrier. Monitor serum electrolyte levels and osmolality readings closely because the patient may become dehydrated very quickly. Be aware that a rebound increase in ICP may occur. (See *Managing increased ICP*.)
- To avoid rebound increased ICP, 50 ml of albumin may be given with the mannitol bolus. Note, however, that you'll see a residual rise in ICP before it decreases. If your patient has heart failure or severe renal dysfunction, monitor for problems in adapting to the increased intravascular volumes.
- Fluid restriction, usually 1,200 to 1,500 ml/day, prevents cerebral edema from developing or worsening.
- Barbiturate-induced coma depresses the reticular activating system and reduces the brain's metabolic demand. Reduced demand for oxygen and energy reduces cerebral blood flow, thereby lowering ICP.
- Hyperventilation with oxygen from a handheld resuscitation bag or ventilator helps rid the patient of excess carbon dioxide, thereby constricting cerebral vessels and reducing cerebral blood volume and ICP. However, only normal brain tissues respond because blood vessels in damaged areas have reduced vasoconstrictive ability.

ALERT

Hyperventilation with a handheld resuscitation bag or a ventilator should be performed with care because hyperventilation can cause ischemia.

- Before tracheal suctioning, hyperventilate the patient with 100% oxygen as ordered. Apply suction for a maximum of 10 seconds. Avoid inducing hypoxia because this condition greatly increases cerebral blood flow.

Managing increased ICP

By performing nursing care gently, slowly, and cautiously, you can best help manage—or even significantly reduce—increased intracranial pressure (ICP). If possible, urge your patient to participate in his own care. Here are some steps you can take to manage increased ICP:

- Plan your care to include rest periods between activities. This allows the patient's ICP to return to baseline, thus avoiding lengthy and cumulative pressure elevations.
- Speak to the patient before attempting any procedures, even if he appears comatose. Touch him on an arm or leg first before touching him in a more personal area, such as the face or chest. This is especially important if the patient doesn't know you or if he's confused or sedated.
- Suction the patient 10 seconds or less and only when needed to remove secretions and maintain airway patency. Avoid depriving him of oxygen for long periods while suctioning; always hyperventilate the patient with oxygen before and after the procedure. Monitor his heart rate while suctioning. If multiple catheter passes are needed to clear secretions, hyperventilate the patient between them to bring ICP as close to baseline as possible.
- To promote venous drainage, keep the patient's head in the midline position, even when he's positioned on his side. Avoid flexing the neck or hip more than 90 degrees, and keep the head of the bed elevated 30 to 45 degrees.
- To avoid increasing intrathoracic pressure, which raises ICP, discourage Valsalva's maneuver and isometric muscle contractions. To avoid isometric contractions, distract the patient when giving him painful injections (by asking him to wiggle his toes and by massaging the area before injection to relax the muscle) and have him concentrate on breathing through difficult procedures such as bed-to-stretcher transfers. To keep the patient from holding his breath when moving around in bed, tell him to relax as much as possible during position changes. If necessary, administer a stool softener to help prevent constipation and unnecessary straining during defecation.
- If the patient is heavily sedated, monitor his respiratory rate and blood gas levels. Depressed respirations will compromise ventilations and oxygen exchange. Maintaining adequate respiratory rate and volume helps reduce ICP.
- If you're in a specialty unit, you may be able to routinely hyperventilate the patient to counter sustained ICP elevations. This procedure is one of the best ways to reduce high ICP at bedside for short periods. Consult your facility's protocol.

- Because fever raises brain metabolism, which increases cerebral blood flow, fever reduction (achieved by administering acetaminophen [Tylenol], sponge baths, or a hypothermia blanket) also helps to reduce ICP. However, rebound increases in ICP and brain edema may occur if rapid rewarming takes place after hypothermia or if cooling measures induce shivering.
- Withdrawal of CSF through the drainage system reduces CSF volume and thus reduces ICP. Although less commonly used, surgical removal of a skull-bone flap provides room for the swollen brain to expand. If this procedure is performed, keep the site clean and dry to prevent infection and maintain sterile technique when changing the dressing.

Complications

- CNS infection (most common) resulting from contamination of the equipment setup or of the insertion site

ALERT

Be especially cautious when positioning the ventriculostomy; if the drip chamber is too high, it may raise ICP; if it's too low, it may cause excessive CSF drainage. Such loss can rapidly decompress the cranial contents and damage bridging cortical veins, leading to hematoma formation. Decompression can also lead to rupture of existing hematomas or aneurysms, causing hemorrhage.

ALERT

Watch for signs of impending or overt decompensation: pupillary dilation (unilateral or bilateral), decreased pupillary response to light, decreasing LOC, rising systolic blood pressure and widening pulse pressure, bradycardia, slowed, irregular respirations and, in late decompensation, decerebrate posturing.

Documentation

Record the time and date of the insertion procedure and the patient's response. Note the insertion site and the type of monitoring system used. Record ICP digital readings and waveforms and CPP hourly in your notes, on a flowchart, or directly on readout strips, depending on your facility's policy. Document any factors that may affect ICP (for example, drug therapy, stressful procedures, or sleep).

Record routine and neurologic vital signs hourly, and describe the patient's clinical status. Note the amount, character, and frequency of any CSF drainage (for example, "between 6 p.m. and 7 p.m., 15 ml of blood-tinged CSF"). Record the ICP reading in response to drainage.

Intradermal injections

Because little systemic absorption of intradermally injected agents takes place, this type of injection is used primarily to produce a local effect, as in allergy or tuberculin testing. Intradermal injections are administered in small volumes (usually 0.5 ml or less) into the outer layers of the skin.

The ventral forearm is the most commonly used site for intradermal injection because of its easy accessibility and lack of hair. In extensive allergy testing, the outer aspect of the upper arms may be used as well as the area of the back located between the scapulae. (See *Intradermal injection sites.*)

Equipment

Patient's medication record and chart ♦ tuberculin syringe with a 26G or 27G $^{1}/_{2}''$ to $^{3}/_{8}''$ needle ♦ prescribed medication ♦ gloves ♦ alcohol pads

Preparation

- Verify the order on the patient's medication record by checking it against the prescriber's orders.
- Inspect the medication to make sure it isn't abnormally discolored or cloudy and doesn't contain precipitates.
- Wash your hands.
- Choose equipment appropriate to the prescribed medication and injection site, and make sure it works properly.
- Check the medication label against the patient's medication record.
- Read the label again as you draw up the medication for injection.

Key steps

- Confirm the patient's identity using two patient identifiers according to your facility's policy.
- If your facility uses a bar code scanning system, be sure to scan your ID badge, the patient's ID bracelet, and the medication's bar code.
- Tell him where you'll be giving the injection.
- Instruct the patient to sit up and to extend his arm and support it on a flat surface, with the ventral forearm exposed.
- Put on gloves.
- With an alcohol pad, clean the surface of the ventral forearm about two or three fingerbreadths distal to the antecubital space.

DO'S & DON'TS

Make sure the test site you have chosen is free from hair or blemishes.

- Allow the skin to dry completely before administering the injection.

Intradermal injection sites

The most common intradermal injection site is the ventral forearm. Other sites (indicated by dotted areas) include the upper chest, upper arm, and shoulder blades. Skin in these areas is usually lightly pigmented, thinly keratinized, and relatively hairless, facilitating detection of adverse reactions.

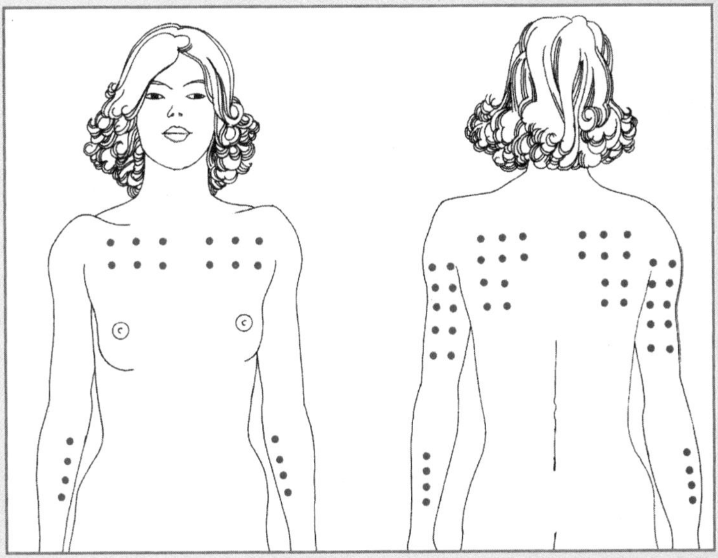

■ While holding the patient's forearm in your hand, stretch the skin taut with your thumb.
■ With your free hand, hold the needle at a 10- to 15-degree angle to the patient's arm, with its bevel up.
■ Insert the needle about 1/8″ (0.3 cm) below the epidermis at sites 2″ (5 cm) apart. Stop when the needle's bevel tip is under the skin, and inject the antigen slowly. You should feel some resistance as you do this, and a wheal should form as you inject the antigen. (See *Giving an intradermal injection*.) If no wheal forms, you have injected the antigen too deeply; withdraw the needle, and administer another test dose at least 2″ from the first site.
■ Withdraw the needle at the same angle at which it was inserted. Don't rub the site. This could irritate the underlying tissue, which may affect test results.

Giving an intradermal injection

Secure the patient's forearm. Insert the needle at a 10- to 15-degree angle so that it just punctures the skin's surface. The antigen should raise a small wheal as it's injected.

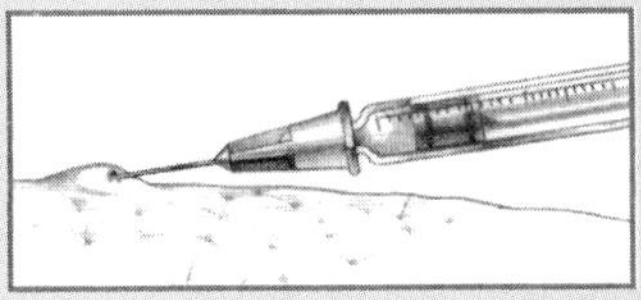

■ Circle each test site with a marking pen, and label each site according to the recall antigen given. Instruct the patient to refrain from washing off the circles until the test is completed.

- Dispose of needles and syringes according to your facility's policy.
- Remove and discard your gloves.
- Assess the patient's response to the skin testing in 24 to 48 hours.

Special considerations

ACTION STAT!

In patients who are hypersensitive to the test antigens, a severe anaphylactic response can result. This requires immediate epinephrine injection and other emergency resuscitation procedures. Be especially alert after giving a test dose of penicillin or tetanus antitoxin.

Complications

- None known

Patient teaching

- Tell the patient not to wash the CIRCLED injection site until after the results are determined.

Documentation

On the patient's medication record, document the type and amount of medication given, the time it was given, and the injection site. Note skin reactions and other adverse reactions.

Intramuscular injections

I.M. injections deposit medication deep into muscle tissue. This route of administration provides rapid systemic action and absorption of relatively large doses (up to 5 ml in appropriate sites). I.M. injections are recommended for patients who are uncooperative or can't take medication orally and for drugs that are altered by digestive juices. Because muscle tissue has few sensory nerves, I.M. injection allows less painful administration of irritating drugs.

The site for an I.M. injection must be chosen carefully, taking into account the patient's general physical status and the purpose of the injection. I.M. injections shouldn't be administered at inflamed, edematous, or irritated sites or at sites that contain moles, birthmarks, scar tissue, or other lesions. They may also be contraindicated in patients with impaired coagulation mechanisms, occlusive peripheral vascular disease, edema, and shock; after thrombolytic therapy; and during an acute myocardial infarction because these conditions impair peripheral absorption. I.M. injections require sterile technique to maintain the integrity of muscle tissue.

Oral or I.V. routes are preferred for administration of drugs that are poorly absorbed by muscle tissue, such as phenytoin, digoxin, chlordiazepoxide, and diazepam.

Equipment

Patient's medication record and chart ♦ prescribed medication ♦ diluent or filter needle, if needed ♦ 3- or 5-ml syringe ♦ 20G to 25G 1″ to 3″ needle ♦ gloves ♦ alcohol pads ♦ 2″ × 2″ gauze pad

The prescribed medication must be sterile. The needle may be packaged separately or already attached to the syringe. Needles used for I.M. injections are longer than subcutaneous needles because they must reach deep into the muscle. Needle length also depends on the injection site, patient's size, and amount of subcutaneous fat covering the muscle. The needle gauge for I.M. injections should be larger to accommodate viscous solutions and suspensions.

Preparation

- Verify the order on the patient's medication record by checking it against the prescriber's order. Also note whether the patient has any allergies, especially before the first dose.
- Check the prescribed medication for color and clarity. Also note the expiration date. Never use medication that's cloudy or discolored or contains a precipitate unless the manufacturer's instructions allow it. Remember that for some drugs (such as suspensions), the presence of drug particles is normal. Observe for abnormal

changes. If in doubt, check with the pharmacist.

- Choose equipment appropriate to the prescribed medication and injection site, and make sure it works properly. The needle should be straight, smooth, and free of burrs.
- Gather all necessary equipment and proceed to the patient's room.

Single-dose ampules

- Wrap an alcohol pad around the ampule's neck and snap off the top, directing the force away from your body.
- Attach a filter needle to the needle and withdraw the medication, keeping the needle's bevel tip below the level of the solution.
- Tap the syringe to clear air from it. Cover the needle with the needle sheath.
- Before discarding the ampule, check the medication label against the patient's medication record.
- Discard the filter needle and the ampule.
- Attach the appropriate needle to the syringe.

Single-dose or multidose vials

- Reconstitute powdered drugs according to instructions. Make sure all crystals have dissolved in the solution. Warm the vial by rolling it between your palms to help the drug dissolve faster.
- Wipe the stopper of the medication vial with an alcohol pad, and then draw up the prescribed amount of medication.
- Read the medication label as you select the medication, as you draw it up, and after you've drawn it up to verify the correct dosage.
- Don't use an air bubble in the syringe. A holdover from the days of reusable syringes, air bubbles can affect the medication dosage by 5% to 100%. Modern disposable syringes are calibrated to administer the correct dose without an air bubble.

Key steps

- Confirm the patient's identity using two patient identifiers according to your facility's policy.
- If your facility uses a bar code scanning system, be sure to scan your ID badge, the patient's ID bracelet, and the medication's bar code.
- Provide privacy, explain the procedure to the patient, and wash your hands.
- Select an appropriate injection site. The gluteal muscles (gluteus medius and minimus and the upper outer corner of the gluteus maximus) are used most commonly for healthy adults, although the deltoid muscle may be used for a small-volume injection (2 ml or less). Remember to rotate injection sites for patients who require repeated injections.
- For infants and children, the vastus lateralis muscle of the thigh is used most often because it's usually the best developed and contains no large nerves or blood vessels, minimizing the risk of serious injury. The rectus femoris muscle may also be used in infants but is usually contraindicated in adults.
- Position and drape the patient, making sure the injection site is accessible.
- Loosen the protective needle sheath, but don't remove it.
- After selecting the injection site, gently tap it to stimulate the nerve endings and minimize pain when the needle is inserted. (See *Locating I.M. injection sites,* page 272.) Clean the skin at the site with an alcohol pad. Move the pad outward in a circular motion to a circumference of about 2" (5 cm) from the injection site, and allow the skin to dry. Keep the alcohol pad for later use.
- Put on gloves. With the thumb and index finger of your nondominant hand, gently stretch the skin of the injection site taut.
- While you hold the syringe in your dominant hand, remove the needle sheath by slipping it between the free fingers of your nondominant hand and then drawing back the syringe.
- Position the syringe at a 90-degree angle to the skin surface, with the needle a couple of inches from the skin. Tell the patient that he'll feel a prick as you insert the needle. Then quickly and firmly thrust the needle through the skin and subcutaneous tissue, deep into the muscle.
- Support the syringe with your nondominant hand, if desired. Pull back slightly on

Locating I.M. injection sites

The illustrations below show the most common sites for administering an I.M. injection.

Deltoid

Find the lower edge of the acromial process and the point on the lateral arm in line with the axilla. Insert the needle 1" to 2" (2.5 to 5 cm) below the acromial process, usually two or three fingerbreadths, at a 90-degree angle or angled slightly toward the process. Typical injection: 0.5 ml (range: 0.5 to 2.0 ml).

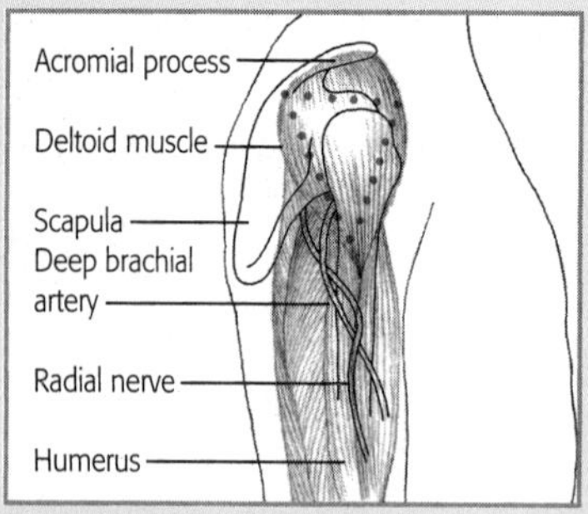

Dorsogluteal

Inject above and outside a line drawn from the posterior superior iliac spine to the greater trochanter of the femur. Or, divide the buttock into quadrants and inject in the upper outer quadrant, about 2" to 3" (5 to 7.5 cm) below the iliac crest. Insert the needle at a 90-degree angle. Typical injection: 1 to 4 ml (range: 1 to 5 ml).

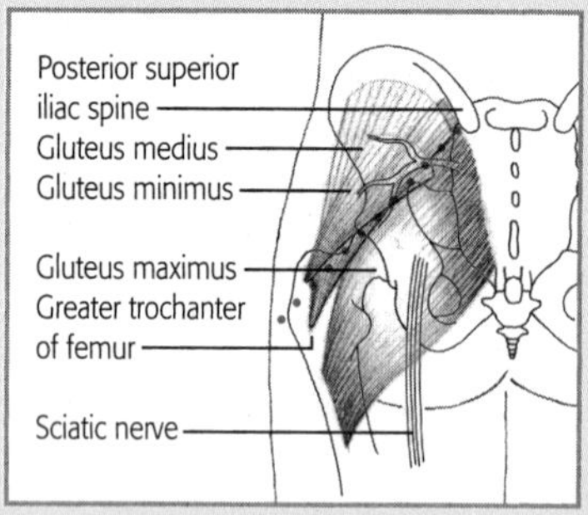

Ventrogluteal

Locate the greater trochanter of the femur with the heel of your hand. Then, spread your index and middle fingers from the anterior superior iliac spine to as far along the iliac crest as you can reach. Insert the needle between the two fingers at a 90-degree angle to the muscle. (Remove your fingers before inserting the needle.) Typical injection: 1 to 4 ml (range: 1 to 5 ml).

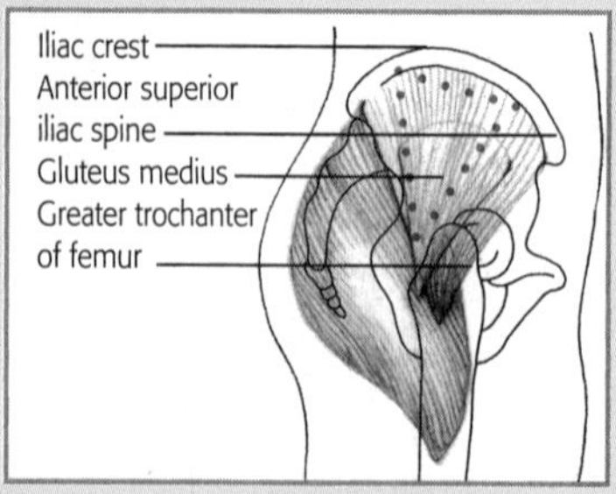

Vastus lateralis

Use the lateral muscle of the quadriceps group, from a handbreadth below the greater trochanter to a handbreadth above the knee. Insert the needle into the middle third of the muscle parallel to the surface on which the patient is lying. You may have to bunch the muscle before insertion. Typical injection: 1 to 4 ml (range: 1 to 5 ml; 1 to 3 ml for infants).

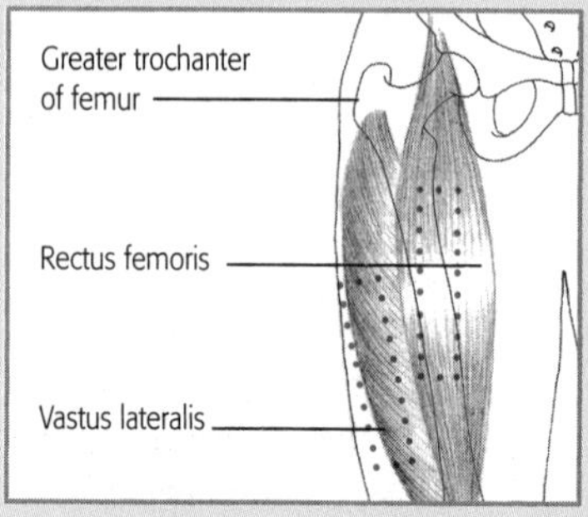

the plunger with your dominant hand to aspirate for blood. If no blood appears, slowly inject the medication into the muscle. A slow, steady injection rate allows the muscle to distend gradually and accept the medication under minimal pressure. You should feel little or no resistance against the force of the injection.

ALERT

If blood appears in the syringe on aspiration, the needle is in a blood vessel. If this occurs, stop the injection, withdraw the needle, prepare another injection with new equipment, and inject another site. Don't inject the bloody solution.

- After the injection, gently but quickly remove the needle at a 90-degree angle.
- Using a gloved hand, cover the injection site immediately with the used alcohol pad or 2″ × 2″ gauze pad, apply gentle pressure, and unless contraindicated, massage the relaxed muscle to help distribute the drug.
- Remove the alcohol pad, and inspect the injection site for signs of active bleeding or bruising. If bleeding continues, apply pressure to the site; if bruising occurs, you may apply ice.
- Watch for adverse reactions at the site for 10 to 30 minutes after the injection.
- An older patient will probably bleed or ooze from the site after the injection because of decreased tissue elasticity. Applying a small pressure bandage may be helpful.
- Discard all equipment according to standard precautions and your facility's policy.

DO'S & DON'TS

Don't recap needles; dispose of them in an appropriate sharps container to avoid needle-stick injuries.

Special considerations

- To slow their absorption, some drugs for I.M. administration are dissolved in oil or other special solutions. Mix these preparations well before drawing them into the syringe.
- The gluteal muscles can be used as the injection site only after a toddler has been walking for about 1 year.
- Never inject into sensitive muscles, especially those that twitch or tremble when you assess site landmarks and tissue depth. Injections into these trigger areas may cause sharp or referred pain, such as the pain caused by nerve trauma.
- Keep a rotation record that lists all available injection sites, divided into various body areas, for patients who require repeated injections. Rotate from a site in the first area to a site in each of the other areas. Then return to a site in the first area that is at least 1″ (2.5 cm) away from the previous injection site in that area.
- If the patient has experienced pain or emotional trauma from repeated injections, consider numbing the area before cleaning it by holding ice on it for several seconds or consider the use of an eutectic mixture of local anesthetics cream applied 60 to 90 minutes prior to the procedure. If you must inject more than 5 ml of solution, divide the solution and inject it at two separate sites.
- Always encourage the patient to relax the muscle you'll be injecting because injections into tense muscles are more painful than usual and may bleed more readily.
- I.M. injections can damage local muscle cells, causing elevations in serum enzyme levels (creatine kinase [CK]) that can be confused with elevations resulting from cardiac muscle damage, as in myocardial infarction. To distinguish between skeletal and cardiac muscle damage, diagnostic tests for suspected myocardial infarction must identify the isoenzyme of CK specific to cardiac muscle and include tests to determine lactate dehydrogenase and aspartate aminotransferase levels. If it's important to measure these enzyme levels, suggest that the physician switch to I.V. administration and adjust dosages accordingly.
- Dosage adjustments are usually necessary when changing from the I.M. route to the oral route.

Complications

- Sterile abscesses developing due to accidental injection of concentrated or irritating medications into subcutaneous tissue or other areas where they can't be fully ab-

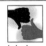

sorbed (Such abscesses result from the body's natural immune response in which phagocytes attempt to remove the foreign matter.)
- Deposits of unabsorbed medications due to failure to rotate sites in patients who require repeated injections (Such deposits can reduce the desired pharmacologic effect and may lead to abscess formation or tissue fibrosis.)
- Quick absorption of I.M. medications in older patients due to decreased muscle mass

Documentation
Chart the drug administered, dose, date, time, route of administration, and injection site. Also, note the patient's tolerance of the injection and the injection's effects, including any adverse effects.

Isolation equipment use

Use of isolation equipment prevents spread of infection from patient to patient, patient to health care worker, or health care worker to patient. Its use reduces risk of infection in immunocompromised patients. Proper equipment must be selected and those who use it must be adequately trained. There are different types of isolation precautions, including droplet, airborne, and contact. They each require different equipment and are instituted in varying circumstances.

Equipment
Door card announcing isolation precautions ♦ gowns ♦ gloves ♦ goggles ♦ masks ♦ specially marked laundry bags ♦ plastic trash bags ♦ optional: isolation cart, water-soluble laundry bags

Preparation
- An isolation cart may be used when the patient's room has no anteroom. It should include a work area (such as a pull-out shelf), drawers or a cabinet area for holding isolation supplies and, possibly, a pole on which to hang coats or jackets.
- Remove the cover from the isolation cart, if needed, and set up the work area.
- Check the cart or anteroom to ensure that correct and sufficient supplies are in place for the designated isolation category.

Key steps
- Remove your watch (or push it well up your arm) and any rings, according to your facility's policy, to prevent the growth of microorganisms under jewelry.
- Wash your hands with an antiseptic cleaning agent to prevent the growth of microorganisms under gloves.
- Explain to the patient the need for isolation precautions.
- Explain that anyone entering the room must wear a gown, gloves, and a mask.

Putting on isolation garb
- Put on the gown and wrap it around the back of your uniform.
- Tie the strings or fasten the snaps or pressure-sensitive tabs at the neck.
- Make sure your uniform is completely covered, and secure the gown at the waist.
- Place the mask snugly over your nose and mouth.
- Secure ear loops around your ears or tie the strings behind your head high enough so the mask won't slip off.
- If the mask has a metal strip, squeeze it to fit your nose firmly but comfortably.
- If you wear glasses, tuck the mask under their lower edge.
- Put on the gloves.
- Pull the gloves over the gown cuffs to cover the edges of the sleeves.

Removing isolation garb
ALERT

The outside surfaces of your barrier clothes are contaminated.

- Wearing gloves, untie the gown's waist strings.
- With your gloved left hand, remove the right glove by pulling on the cuff, turning the glove inside out as you pull. Don't touch any skin with the outside of either glove. (See *Removing contaminated gloves*.)

Removing contaminated gloves

Proper removal techniques are essential for preventing the spread of pathogens from gloves to your skin surface. Follow these steps:

1. Using your left hand, pinch the right glove near the top. Avoid allowing the glove's outer surface to buckle inward against your wrist.

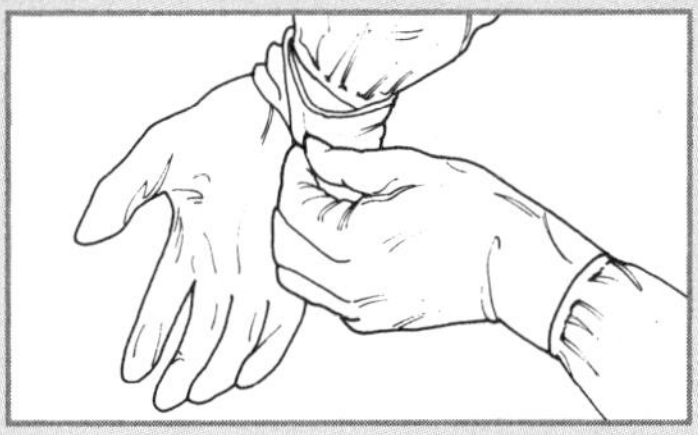

2. Pull downward, allowing the glove to turn inside out as it comes off. Keep the right glove in your left hand after removing it.

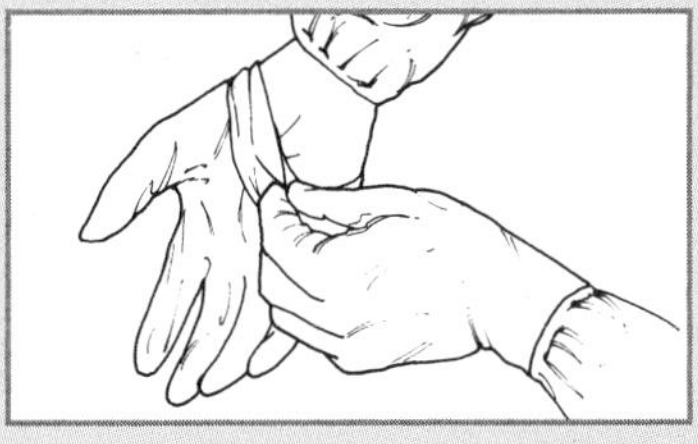

3. Now insert the first two fingers of your ungloved right hand under the edge of the left glove. Avoid touching the glove's outer surface or folding it against your left wrist.

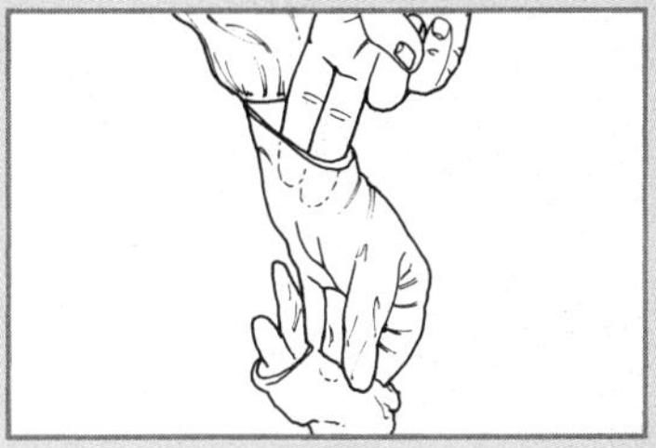

4. Pull downward so the glove turns inside out as it comes off. Continue pulling until the left glove completely encloses the right and its uncontaminated inner surface is facing out.

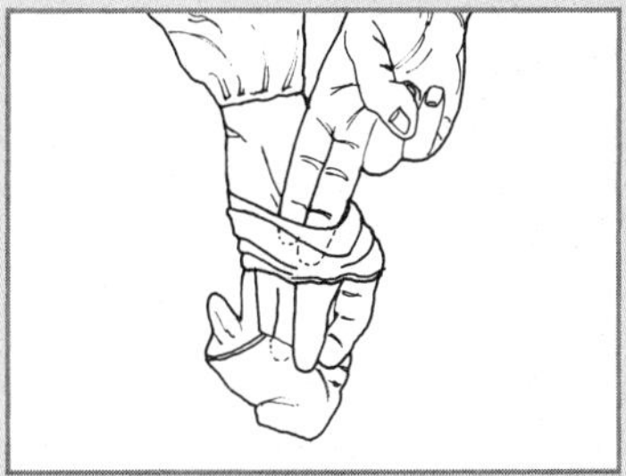

- Remove the left glove by wedging one or two fingers of your right hand inside the glove and pulling it off, turning it inside out as you remove it.
- Discard the gloves in the trash container that contains a plastic trash bag.
- Untie your mask, holding it only by the strings.
- Discard the mask in the trash container.
- If the patient has a disease spread by airborne pathogens, remove the mask last.
- Untie the neck straps of your gown.
- Grasp the outside of the gown at the back of the shoulders and pull the gown down over your arms, turning it inside out as you remove it to contain the pathogens.
- Holding the gown well away from your uniform, fold it inside out.
- Discard it in the specially marked laundry bags or trash container, as needed.
- If the sink is inside the patient's room, wash your hands and forearms with soap or antiseptic before leaving the room.
- Turn off the faucet using a paper towel, and discard the towel in the room.
- Grasp the door handle with a clean paper towel to open it; discard the towel in a trash container inside the room.
- Close the door from the outside with your bare hand.
- If the sink is in an anteroom, wash your hands and forearms with soap or antiseptic after leaving the room.

Using I.V. clamps

With a roller clamp, you can increase or decrease the flow through the I.V. line by turning a wheel.

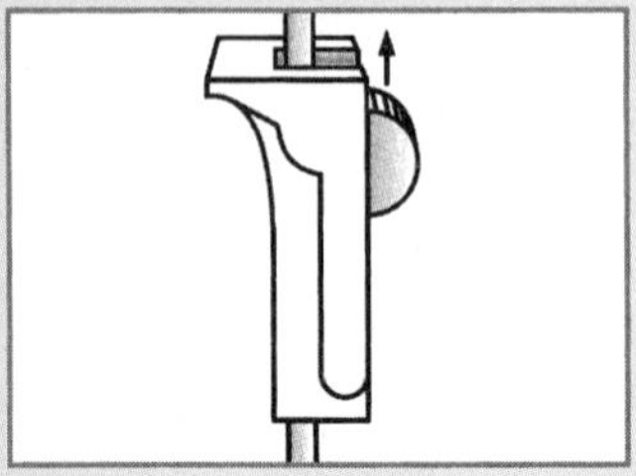

With a slide clamp, you can open or close the line by moving the clamp horizontally. However, you can't make fine adjustments to the flow rate.

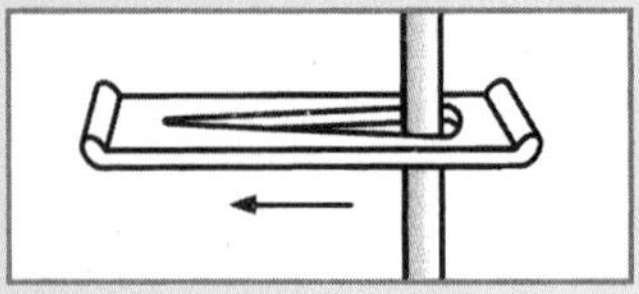

Special considerations

- Use gown, gloves, goggles, and mask only once; discard in the appropriate container before leaving a contaminated area.
- If your mask is reusable, undamaged, and not damp, keep it for future use.

ALERT

Isolation garb loses its effectiveness when wet because moisture lets organisms seep through the material. Change masks and gowns as soon as moisture is noticeable or according to the manufacturer's recommendations or your facility's policy.

- At the end of your shift, restock used items for the next person.
- After patient transfer or discharge, return the isolation cart to the appropriate area for cleaning and restocking of supplies.
- An isolation room or other room prepared for isolation purposes must be thoroughly cleaned and disinfected before use by another patient.

Complications

- None known

Documentation

Document that isolation precautions were initiated.

I.V. infusion rates and manual control

Infusion rates are vital to the safe administration of I.V. fluids and medications. Information necessary to calculate infusion rates includes:

- volume of fluid to be infused
- total infusion time
- calibration of the administration set—number of drops per milliliter (found on I.V. tubing package).

Many devices can regulate the infusion of I.V. solution, including clamps, the flow regulator (or rate minder), and the volumetric pump. (See *Using I.V. clamps*.)

When regulated by a clamp, the infusion rate is usually measured in drops per minute; by a volumetric pump, in milliliters per hour. The infusion regulator can be set to deliver the desired amount of solution, also in milliliters per hour. Less accurate than infusion pumps, infusion regulators are most reliable when used with inactive adult patients. With any device, the infusion rate can be easily monitored by using a time tape, which indicates the prescribed solution level at hourly intervals.

Equipment

I.V. administration set with clamp ♦ 1" paper or adhesive tape (or premarked time tape) ♦ infusion pump (if infusing medication) ♦ watch with second hand ♦ drip rate chart, as necessary ♦ pen

Standard macrodrip sets deliver from 10 to 20 drops/ml, depending on the manufacturer; microdrip sets, 60 drops/ml; and blood transfusion sets, 10 drops/ml. A commercially available adapter can convert a macrodrip set to a microdrip system.

Key steps

- The infusion rate requires close monitoring and correction because such factors as

Calculating infusion rates

When calculating the infusion rate of I.V. solutions, remember that the number of drops required to deliver 1 ml varies with the type and manufacturer of the administration set used. The illustration on the left shows a standard (macrodrip) set, which delivers from 10 to 20 drops/ml. The illustration in the center shows a pediatric (microdrip) set, which delivers about 60 drops/ml. The illustration on the right shows a blood transfusion set, which delivers about 10 drops/ml.

To calculate the infusion rate, you must know the calibration of the drip rate for each manufacturer's product. Use this formula to calculate specific drip rates:

$$\frac{\text{volume of infusion (in ml)}}{\text{time of infusion (in minutes)}} \times \text{drip factor (in drops/ml)} = \text{drops/minute}$$

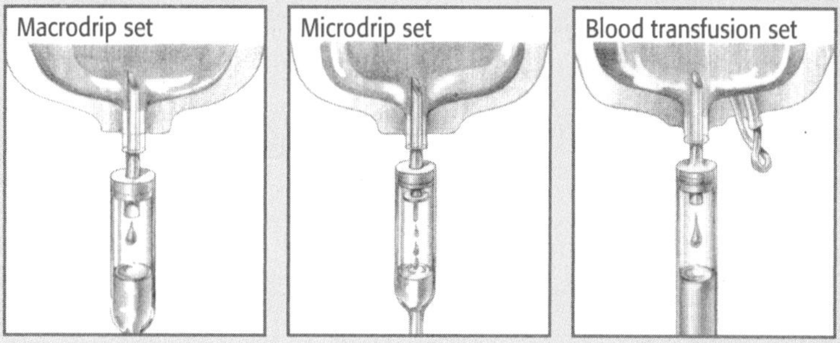

venous spasm, venous pressure changes, patient movement or manipulation of the clamp, and bent or kinked tubing can cause the infusion rate to vary markedly.

Calculating and setting the drip rate

- Follow the steps in *Calculating infusion rates*, to determine the proper drip rate, or use your unit's drip rate chart.
- After calculating the desired drip rate, remove your watch and hold it next to the drip chamber of the I.V. administration set to allow simultaneous observation of the watch and the drops.
- Release the clamp to the approximate drip rate. Then count drops for 1 minute to account for flow irregularities.
- Adjust the clamp, as necessary, and count drops for 1 minute. Continue to adjust the clamp and count drops until the correct rate is achieved.

Making a time tape

- Calculate the number of milliliters to be infused per hour. Place a piece of tape vertically on the container alongside the volume-increment markers.
- Starting at the current solution level, move down the number of milliliters to be infused in 1 hour, and mark the appropriate time and a horizontal line on the tape at this level. Then continue to mark 1-hour intervals until you reach the bottom of the container.
- Check the infusion rate every 15 minutes until stable. Then recheck it every hour or according to your facility's policy and adjust as necessary.
- With each check, inspect the I.V. site for complications, and assess the patient's response to therapy.

Special considerations

- If the infusion rate slows significantly, a slight rate increase may be necessary.
- If the rate must be increased by more than 30%, consult the practitioner.
- When infusing drugs, use an I.V. pump, if possible, to avoid infusion rate inaccuracies.

Managing I.V. flow-rate deviations

Problem	Cause	Intervention
Flow rate too fast	▪ Patient or visitor manipulates the clamp	▪ Instruct the patient not to touch the clamp, and place tape over it. Restrain the patient or administer the I.V. solution with an infusion pump if necessary.
	▪ Tubing disconnected from the catheter	▪ Wipe the distal end of the tubing with alcohol, reinsert firmly into the catheter hub, and tape at the connection site. Consider using tubing with luer-lock connections.
	▪ Change in patient position	▪ Administer the I.V. solution with an infusion pump.
	▪ Bevel against vein wall (positional cannulation)	▪ Manipulate cannula, and place a 2" x 2" gauze pad over or under the catheter hub to change angle. Reset flow clamp at desired rate. If necessary, remove cannula and reinsert.
	▪ Flow clamp drifting as a result of patient movement	▪ Place tape below the clamp.
Flow rate too slow	▪ Venous spasm after insertion	▪ Apply warm soaks over site.
	▪ Venous obstruction from bending arm	▪ Secure with an arm board, if necessary.
	▪ Pressure change (decreasing fluid in bottle causes solution to run slower due to decreasing pressure)	▪ Readjust the flow rate.
	▪ Elevated blood pressure	▪ Readjust the flow rate. Use an infusion pump.
	▪ Cold solution	▪ Allow the solution to warm to room temperature before hanging.
	▪ Change in solution viscosity from medication added	▪ Readjust the flow rate.

Managing I.V. flow-rate deviations *(continued)*

Problem	Cause	Intervention
Flow rate too slow *(continued)*	▪ I.V. container too low or patient's arm or leg too high	▪ Hang the container higher or remind the patient to keep his arm below heart level.
	▪ Bevel against vein wall (positional cannulation)	▪ Withdraw the needle slightly, or place a folded 2" x 2" gauze pad over or under the catheter hub to change the angle.
	▪ Excess tubing dangling below insertion site	▪ Replace the tubing with a shorter piece, or tape the excess tubing to the I.V. pole, below the flow clamp (make sure the tubing is not kinked).
	▪ Cannula too small	▪ Remove the cannula in use and insert a larger-bore cannula, or use an infusion pump.
	▪ Infiltration or clotted cannula	▪ Remove the cannula in use and insert a new cannula.
	▪ Kinked tubing	▪ Check the tubing over its entire length and unkink it.
	▪ Clogged filter	▪ Remove the filter and replace it with a new one.
	▪ Tubing memory (tubing compressed at area clamped)	▪ Massage or milk the tubing by pinching and wrapping it around a pencil four or five times. Quickly pull the pencil out of the coiled tubing.

▪ Always use a pump when infusing solutions by way of a central line.
▪ Large-volume solution containers have about 10% more fluid than the amount indicated on the bag to allow for tubing purges. Thus, a 1,000-ml bag or bottle contains an additional 100 ml; similarly, a 500-ml container holds an extra 50 ml; and a 250-ml container, 25 ml.

Complications

▪ Insufficient intake of fluids, drugs, and nutrients caused by an excessively slow infusion rate
▪ Circulatory overload—possibly leading to heart failure and pulmonary edema as well as adverse effects—due to an excessively rapid rate of fluid or drug infusion (see *Managing I.V. flow-rate deviations*)

Documentation

Record the original flow rate when setting up a peripheral line. If you adjust the rate, record the change, the date and time, and your initials.

I.V. pumps

Various types of I.V. pumps electronically regulate the flow of I.V. solutions or drugs with great accuracy.

Volumetric pumps, used for high-pressure infusion of drugs or for the accurate delivery of fluids or drugs, have mechanisms to propel the solution at the desired rate under pressure. The peristaltic pump applies pressure to the I.V. tubing to force the solution through it. (Not all peristaltic pumps are volumetric; some count drops.) These pumps are also indicated for use with arterial lines. Most volumetric pumps operate at high pressures (up to 45 psi), delivering from 1 to 999 ml/hour with about 98% accuracy.

For the administration of vesicants, a low-pressure pump—one that operates at 10 to 25 psi—is the instrument of choice. The portable syringe pump, another type of volumetric pump, delivers small amounts of fluid over a long period. It's used for administering fluids to infants and for delivering intra-arterial drugs. Other specialized devices include the controlled-release infusion system, secondary syringe converter, and patient-controlled analgesia device.

Equipment

Peristaltic pump ♦ I.V. pole ♦ I.V. solution ♦ sterile administration set ♦ sterile peristaltic tubing or cassette, if needed ♦ alcohol pads ♦ adhesive tape

Tubing and cassettes vary with each manufacturer.

Preparation

To set up a volumetric pump

- Attach the pump to the I.V. pole.
- Swab the port on the I.V. container with alcohol, insert the administration set spike, and fill the drip chamber to prevent air bubbles from entering the tubing.
- Prime the tubing and close the clamp. Follow the manufacturer's instructions for tubing placement.

Key steps

- Position the pump on the same side of the bed as the I.V. or anticipated venipuncture site to avoid crisscrossing I.V. lines over the patient. If necessary, perform the venipuncture.
- Plug in the machine and attach its tubing to the needle or catheter hub.
- Depending on the machine, turn it on and press the START button. Set the appropriate dials on the front panel to the desired infusion rate and volume. Always set the volume dial at 50 ml less than the prescribed volume or 50 ml less than the volume in the container so that you can hang a new container before the old one empties.
- Check the patency of the I.V. line and watch for infiltration.
- Tape all connections.
- Turn on the alarm switches. Then explain the alarm system to the patient to prevent anxiety when a change in the infusion activates the alarm.

Special considerations

- Monitor the pump and the patient frequently to ensure the device's correct operation and flow rate and to detect infiltration and such complications as infection and air embolism.
- If electrical power fails, the pump will automatically switch to battery power.

DEVICE SAFETY

Check the manufacturer's recommendations before administering opaque fluids, such as blood, because some pumps fail to detect opaque fluids and others may cause hemolysis of infused blood.

- Remove I.V. solutions from the refrigerator 1 hour before infusing them to help release small gas bubbles from the solutions. Small bubbles in the solution can join to form larger bubbles, which can activate the pump's air-in-line alarm.

Complications

- See "Peripheral I.V. line insertion," page 373, for complications associated with I.V. pumps

■ Infiltration developing rapidly with infusion by a volumetric pump because the increased subcutaneous pressure won't slow the infusion rate until significant edema occurs

Patient teaching

■ Schedule a teaching session with the patient or his family so you can answer questions they may have about the procedure before the patient's discharge.
■ Make sure that the patient and his family understand the purpose of using the pump. If necessary, demonstrate how it works. Also demonstrate how to maintain the system (tubing, solution, and site assessment and care) until you're confident that the patient and family can proceed safely.
■ As time permits, have the patient repeat the demonstration.
■ Discuss what complications to watch for, such as infiltration, and review the measures to take if complications occur.

Documentation

In addition to routine documentation of the I.V. infusion, record the use of a pump on the I.V. record and in your notes.

I.V. therapy preparation

Selection and preparation of equipment are essential for accurate delivery of an I.V. solution. Selection of an I.V. administration set depends on the rate and type of infusion and the type of I.V. solution container. There are two types of drip sets available, the macrodrip and the microdrip. The macrodrip set can deliver a solution in large quantities and at rapid rates because it delivers a larger amount of solution with each drop than the microdrip set. The microdrip set, used for pediatric patients and certain adult patients requiring small or closely regulated amounts of I.V. solution, delivers a smaller quantity of solution with each drop.

Administration tubing with a secondary injection port permits separate or simultaneous infusion of two solutions; tubing with a piggyback port and a backcheck valve permits intermittent infusion of a secondary solution and, on its completion, a return to infusion of the primary solution. Vented I.V. tubing is selected for solutions in nonvented bottles; nonvented tubing is selected for solutions in bags or vented bottles. Assembly of I.V. equipment requires sterile technique to prevent contamination, which can cause local or systemic infection.

Equipment

I.V. solution ♦ alcohol pads ♦ I.V. administration set ♦ in-line (0.2 micron containing a membrane that's bacterial/particulate-retentive and also air-eliminating) filter, if needed ♦ I.V. pole ♦ medication and label, if necessary

Preparation

■ Verify the type, volume, and expiration date of the I.V. solution. Discard outdated solution.
■ If the solution is contained in a glass bottle, inspect the bottle for chips and cracks; if it's in a plastic bag, squeeze the bag to detect leaks.
■ Examine the I.V. solution for particles, abnormal discoloration, and cloudiness. If present, discard the solution and notify the pharmacy or dispensing department.
■ If ordered, add medication to the solution, and place a completed medication-added label on the container.
■ Remove the administration set from its box, and check for cracks, holes, and missing clamps.

Key steps

■ Tell the patient that a plastic catheter or needle will be placed in his vein and about how long the catheter or needle will stay in place.
■ Explain to the patient that the practitioner will decide what fluids he needs.
■ Tell the patient that I.V. fluid may feel cold at first but the feeling will subside and to report any discomfort.
■ Wash your hands thoroughly to prevent introducing contaminants during preparation.

DO'S & DON'TS

Indications for in-line filters

An in-line filter removes pathogens and particles from I.V. solutions. Because an in-line filter is expensive and its installation is awkward and time-consuming, these filters aren't used routinely. Many facilities require that a filter be used only when administering an admixture. If you're unsure of whether to use a filter, check your facility's policy or follow this list of do's & don'ts.

Do's

Use an in-line filter:

- when administering solutions to an immunodeficient patient
- when administering total parenteral nutrition
- when using additives comprising many separate particles, such as antibiotics requiring reconstitution, or when administering several additives
- when using rubber injection ports or plastic diaphragms repeatedly
- when phlebitis is likely to occur.

Change the in-line filter according to the manufacturer's recommendations (and with administration set change).

Use an add-on filter of larger pore size (1.2 microns) when infusing lipid emulsions or total nutrient admixtures that require filtration.

If a positive-pressure electronic infusion device is used, consider the pound per square inch (psi) rating of the filter. If the psi from the infusion device exceeds that of the filter, the filter will crack or break under the pressure.

Don'ts

Don't use an in-line filter:

- when administering solutions with large particles, such as blood and its components, suspensions, lipid emulsions, and high-molecular-volume plasma expanders
- when administering a drug dose of 5 mg or less.

- Slide the flow clamp of the administration set tubing down to the drip chamber or injection port, and close the clamp.

Setting up a bag

- Place the bag on a flat, stable surface or hang it on an I.V. pole.
- Remove the protective cap or tear the tab from the tubing insertion port.
- Remove the protective cap from the administration set spike.
- Holding the port firmly with one hand, insert the spike with your other hand.
- Hang the bag on the I.V. pole, if you haven't already, and squeeze the drip chamber until it's half full.

Setting up a nonvented bottle

- Remove the bottle's metal cap and inner disk, if present.
- Place the bottle on a stable surface and wipe the rubber stopper with an alcohol pad.
- Remove the protective cap from the administration set spike, and push the spike through the center of the bottle's rubber stopper. Avoid twisting or angling the spike to prevent pieces of the stopper from breaking off and falling into the solution.
- Invert the bottle. If its vacuum is intact, you'll hear a hissing sound and see air bubbles rise (this may not occur if you've already added medication). If the vacuum isn't intact, discard the bottle and begin again.
- Hang the bottle on the I.V. pole, and squeeze the drip chamber until it's half full.

Setting up a vented bottle

- Remove the bottle's metal cap and latex diaphragm to release the vacuum. If the vacuum isn't intact (except after medication has been added), discard the bottle and begin again.

- Place the bottle on a stable surface and wipe the rubber stopper with an alcohol pad.
- Remove the protective cap from the administration set spike, and push the spike through the insertion port next to the air vent tube opening.
- Hang the bottle on the I.V. pole, and squeeze the drip chamber until it's half full.

Priming the I.V. tubing

- If necessary, attach a filter to the opposite end of the I.V. tubing, and follow the manufacturer's instructions for filling and priming it. Purge the tubing before attaching the filter to avoid forcing air into the filter and, possibly, clogging some filter channels. Most filters are positioned with the distal end of the tubing facing upward so that the solution will completely wet the filter membrane and all air bubbles will be eliminated from the line. (See *Indications for in-line filters.*)
- If you aren't using a filter, aim the distal end of the tubing over a wastebasket or sink and slowly open the flow clamp. (Most distal tube coverings allow the solution to flow without having to remove the protective cover.)
- Leave the clamp open until the I.V. solution flows through the entire length of the tubing to release trapped air bubbles and force out all the air.
- Invert all Y-ports and backcheck valves and tap them, if necessary, to fill them with solution.
- After priming the tubing, close the clamp. Then loop the tubing over the I.V. pole.
- Label the container with the patient's name and room number, date and time, the container number, ordered rate and duration of infusion, and your initials.

Special considerations

- Before initiation of I.V. therapy, the patient should be told what to expect.
- Always use sterile technique when preparing I.V. solutions. If you contaminate the administration set or container, replace it with a new one to prevent introducing contaminants into the system.

Documenting insertion of a venipuncture device

After you establish an I.V. route, remember to document the date, time, and venipuncture site together with the equipment used, such as the type and gauge of catheter or needle. Record how the patient tolerated the procedure and any patient teaching that you performed with the patient and his family, such as explaining the purpose of I.V. therapy, describing the procedure itself, and discussing possible complications.

You'll need to update your records each time you change the insertion site and change the venipuncture device or the I.V. tubing. Also document any reason for changing the I.V. site, such as extravasation, phlebitis, occlusion, patient removal, or routine change, according to your facility's policy.

- If necessary, you can use vented tubing with a vented bottle. To do this, don't remove the latex diaphragm. Instead, insert the spike into the larger indentation in the diaphragm.
- Change I.V. tubing every 48 or 72 hours according to your facility's policy or more frequently if you suspect contamination. Change the filter according to the manufacturer's recommendations or sooner if it becomes clogged.

Complications

- None known

Documentation

Document the type of solution used and any additives to the solution. (See *Documenting insertion of a venipuncture device.*)

L

Latex allergy protocol

Latex—a natural product of the rubber tree—is used in many products in the health care field as well as other areas. With the increased use of latex in barrier protection and medical equipment, many more nurses and patients are becoming hypersensitive to it. Certain groups of people, such as those who have had or will have multiple surgical procedures (especially those with a history of spina bifida), health care workers (especially those in the emergency department and operating room), and workers who manufacture latex and latex-containing products, are at an increased risk for developing latex allergy. Still others may have a genetic predisposition to latex allergy.

People who are allergic to certain "cross-reactive" foods—including apricots, cherries, grapes, kiwis, passion fruit, bananas, avocados, chestnuts, tomatoes, and peaches—may also be allergic to latex. Exposure to latex elicits an allergic response similar to the one elicited by these foods.

For people with latex allergy, latex becomes a hazard when its protein comes in direct contact with mucous membranes or is inhaled, which happens when powdered latex surgical gloves are used. People with asthma are at a greater risk for developing worsening symptoms from airborne latex.

The diagnosis of latex allergy is based on the patient's history and physical examination. Laboratory testing should be performed to confirm or eliminate the diagnosis. Skin testing can be done, but the Ala-STAT test, Hycor assay, and the Pharmacia CAP test are the only U.S. Food and Drug Administration–approved blood tests available. Some laboratories may also choose to perform an enzyme-linked immunosorbent assay.

Latex allergy can produce myriad symptoms, including a rash, hives, generalized itching (on the hands and arms, for example); sneezing and coughing (hay fever-type signs); bronchial asthma, scratchy throat, or difficulty breathing; itchy, watery, or burning eyes; edema of the face, hands, or neck; and anaphylaxis.

To help identify the patient at risk for latex allergy, ask latex allergy-specific questions during the health history. If the patient's history reveals a latex sensitivity, he's assigned to one of three categories based on the extent of his sensitization. Group 1 includes patients who have a history of anaphylaxis or a systemic reaction when exposed to a natural latex product. Group 2 patients have a clear history of an allergic reaction of a nonsystemic type. Group 3 patients don't have a previous history of latex hypersensitivity but are designated as "high risk" because of an associated medical condition, occupation, or "crossover" allergy.

If you determine that the patient has a latex sensitivity, make sure that he doesn't come in contact with latex because such contact could result in a life-threatening hypersensitivity reaction. Also, be sure to record the patient's allergies in his permanent medical record. Creating a latex-free environment is the only way to safeguard him. (See *Creating a latex-free environment*.) Hypoallergenic latex gloves contain signifi-

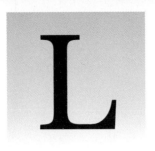

Creating a latex-free environment

- Ask all patients about latex sensitivity. Use a screening questionnaire to determine whether your patient has latex sensitivity.
- Include information about latex allergy on the patient's identification bracelet. Make sure the information is also noted on the front of the patient's chart and in your facility's database.
- Post a latex allergy sign in the patient's room.
- Implement and disseminate latex allergy protocols and lists of nonlatex substitutes that can be used to care for the patient.
- Remove all latex-containing products that may come in contact with the patient.
- Use tubing made of polyvinyl chloride.
- Check adhesives and tapes, including electrocardiogram electrodes and dressing supplies, for latex content.
- Have a special latex-free crash cart outside the patient's room at all times during the patient's hospitalization.
- Notify central supply and the pharmacy that the patient has a latex allergy so that latex contact is eliminated from drugs and other materials prepared for the patient.
- Notify dietary staff of relevant food allergies and instruct them to avoid handling the patient's food with powdered latex gloves.

cant amounts of latex allergens and shouldn't be worn in the vicinity of someone who's allergic to latex. Many health care facilities now designate "latex-free" equipment, which is usually kept on a cart that can be moved into the patient's room.

Equipment

Latex allergy patient identification bracelet ♦ latex-free equipment cart with necessary supplies, including room contents ♦ anaphylaxis kit ♦ optional: latex allergy sign

Preparation

- After you've determined that the patient has a latex allergy or is sensitive to latex, arrange for him to be placed in a private room. If that isn't possible, make the room latex-free, even if the roommate hasn't been designated as hypersensitive to latex. This prevents the spread of airborne particles from latex products used on the other patient.

Key steps

- Assess all patients being admitted to the delivery room or short-procedure unit or having a surgical procedure for possible latex allergy.
- If the patient has a confirmed latex allergy, bring a cart with latex-free supplies into his room.
- Document in the patient's chart (according to your facility's policy) that the patient has a latex allergy. If policy requires that the patient wear a latex allergy patient identification bracelet, place it on the patient.
- If the patient will be receiving anesthesia, make sure that "latex allergy" is clearly visible on the front of his chart. Notify the circulating nurse in the surgical unit, the postanesthesia care unit nurses, and other team members that the patient has a latex allergy. (See *Anesthesia induction and latex allergy,* page 286.)
- If the patient must be transported to another area of the facility, make certain the latex-free cart accompanies him and that all health care workers who come in contact with him are wearing nonlatex gloves. The patient should wear a mask with cloth ties when leaving his room to protect him from inhaling airborne latex particles.
- If the patient will have an I.V. line, make sure that I.V. access is accomplished using all latex-free products. Post a latex allergy sign on the I.V. tubing to prevent access of the line using latex products.

Anesthesia induction and latex allergy

Latex allergy can cause signs and symptoms in both conscious and anesthetized patients.

Causes of intraoperative reaction
- Latex contact with mucous membrane
- Latex contact with intraperitoneal serosal lining
- Inhalation of airborne latex particles during anesthesia
- Injection of antibiotics and anesthetic agents through latex ports

Signs and symptoms in a conscious patient
- Abdominal cramping
- Anxiety
- Bronchoconstriction
- Diarrhea
- Feeling of faintness
- Generalized pruritus
- Itchy eyes
- Nausea
- Shortness of breath
- Swelling of soft tissue (hands, face, tongue)
- Vomiting
- Wheezing

Signs and symptoms in an anesthetized patient
- Bronchospasm
- Cardiopulmonary arrest
- Facial edema
- Flushing
- Hypotension
- Laryngeal edema
- Tachycardia
- Urticaria
- Wheezing

- Flush I.V. tubing with 50 ml of I.V. solution to rinse the tubing out because of latex ports in the I.V. tubing.
- Place a warning label on I.V. bags that says, "Don't use latex injection ports."
- Use a nonlatex tourniquet. If none is available, use a latex tourniquet over clothing.
- Remove the vial stopper to mix and draw up medications.
- Use latex-free oxygen administration equipment. Remove the elastic, and tie equipment on with gauze.
- Wrap your stethoscope with a nonlatex product to protect the patient from latex contact.
- Wrap Tegaderm over the patient's finger before using pulse oximetry.
- Use latex-free syringes when administering medication through a syringe.
- Make sure that an anaphylaxis kit is readily available. If the patient has an allergic reaction to latex, you must act immediately. (See *Managing a latex allergy reaction*.)

Special considerations

- Remember that signs and symptoms of latex allergy usually occur within 30 minutes of anesthesia induction. However, the time of onset can range from 10 minutes to 5 hours.

DO'S & DON'TS

Don't forget that, as a health care worker, you're in a position to develop a latex hypersensitivity. If you suspect that you're sensitive to latex, contact the employee health services department concerning facility protocol for latex-sensitive employees. Use latex-free products as often as possible to help reduce your exposure to latex.

- Don't assume that if something doesn't look like rubber it isn't latex. Latex can be found in a wide variety of equipment, including electrocardiograph leads, oral and nasal airway tubing, tourniquets, nerve stimulation pads, temperature strips, and blood pressure cuffs.

Complications

- None known

Patient teaching

- Inform the patient about the importance of wearing latex allergy identification.
- Explain the importance of informing all health care providers of the latex allergy.

ACTION STAT!

Managing a latex allergy reaction

If you determine that your patient is having an allergic reaction to a latex product, act immediately. Make sure that you perform emergency interventions using latex-free equipment. If the latex product that caused the reaction is known, remove it and perform these measures.

- If the allergic reaction develops during medication administration or a procedure, stop the medication or procedure immediately.
- Assess airway, breathing, and circulation.
- Administer 100% oxygen with continuous pulse oximetry.
- Start I.V. volume expanders with lactated Ringer's solution or normal saline solution.
- Administer epinephrine according to the patient's symptoms.
- Administer famotidine, as ordered.
- If bronchospasm is evident, treat it with nebulized albuterol, as ordered.
- Secondary treatment for latex allergy reaction is aimed at treating the swelling and tissue reaction to the latex as well as breaking the chain of events associated with the allergic reaction. It includes:
  - diphenhydramine
  - methylprednisolone
  - famotidine.
- Document the event and the exact cause (if known). If latex particles have entered the I.V. line, insert a new I.V. line with a new catheter, new tubing, and new infusion attachments as soon as possible.

Documentation

Document initiation of latex allergy precautions. Document any allergic reaction that the patient may have, along with what precipitated the reaction, treatment, and the patient's response.

Lipid emulsion administration

Typically given as separate solutions in conjunction with parenteral nutrition, lipid emulsions are a source of calories and essential fatty acids. A deficiency in essential fatty acids can hinder wound healing, adversely affect the production of red blood cells, and impair prostaglandin synthesis.

Lipid emulsions may also be given alone. They can be administered through either a peripheral or a central venous line.

Lipid emulsions are contraindicated in patients who have a condition that disrupts normal fat metabolism, such as pathologic hyperlipidemia, lipid nephrosis, or acute pancreatitis. They must be used cautiously in patients who have liver disease, pulmonary disease, anemia, or coagulation disorders and in those who are at risk for developing a fat embolism.

Equipment

Lipid emulsion ♦ I.V. administration set with vented spike (a separate adapter may be used if an administration set with vented spike isn't available) ♦ access pin with reflux valve ♦ tape ♦ time tape ♦ alcohol pads

If administering the lipid emulsion as part of a 3-in-1 solution, also obtain a filter that's 1.2 microns or greater because lipids will clog a smaller filter.

Preparation

- Inspect the lipid emulsion for opacity and consistency of color and texture. If the emulsion looks frothy or oily or contains particles or if you think its stability or sterility is questionable, return the bottle to the pharmacy.
- To prevent aggregation of fat globules, don't shake the lipid container excessively.
- Protect the emulsion from freezing, and never add anything to it.

- Make sure you have the correct lipid emulsion, and verify the prescriber's order and the patient's name.

Key steps

- Explain the procedure to the patient to promote his cooperation.

Connecting the tubing

- First, connect the I.V. tubing to the access pin. Access pins with reflux valves take the place of needles when connecting piggyback tubing to primary tubing.
- Close the flow clamp on the I.V. tubing. If the tubing doesn't contain luer-lock connections, tape all connections securely to prevent accidental separation, which can lead to air embolism, exsanguination, and sepsis.
- Using sterile technique, remove the protective cap from the lipid emulsion bottle, and wipe the rubber stopper with an alcohol pad.
- Hold the bottle upright and, using strict sterile technique, insert the vented spike through the inner circle of the rubber stopper.
- Invert the bottle, and squeeze the drip chamber until it fills to the level indicated in the tubing package instructions.
- Open the flow clamp and prime the tubing. Gently tap the tubing to dislodge air bubbles trapped in the Y-ports. If necessary, attach a time tape to the lipid emulsion container to allow accurate measurement of fluid intake.
- Label the tubing, noting the date and time the tubing was hung.

Starting the infusion

- If this is the patient's first lipid infusion, administer a test dose at the rate of 1 ml/minute for 30 minutes.
- Monitor the patient's vital signs, and watch for signs and symptoms of an adverse reaction, such as fever; flushing, sweating, or chills; a pressure sensation over the eyes; nausea; vomiting; headache; chest and back pain; tachycardia; dyspnea; and cyanosis. An allergic reaction is usually due either to the source of lipids or to eggs, which occur in the emulsion as egg phospholipids, an emulsifying agent.
- If the patient has no adverse reactions to the test dose, begin the infusion at the prescribed rate. Use an infusion pump if you'll be infusing the lipids at less than 20 ml/hour. The maximum infusion rate is 125 ml/hour for a 10% lipid emulsion and 60 ml/hour for a 20% lipid emulsion.

Special considerations

- Always maintain strict sterile technique while preparing and handling equipment.
- Observe the patient's reaction to the lipid emulsion. Most patients report a feeling of satiety; some complain of an unpleasant metallic taste.
- Change the I.V. tubing and the lipid emulsion container every 24 hours.
- Monitor the patient for hair and skin changes. Also, closely monitor his lipid tolerance rate. Cloudy plasma in a centrifuged sample of citrated blood indicates that the lipids haven't been cleared from the patient's bloodstream.
- A lipid emulsion may clear from the blood at an accelerated rate in patients with full-thickness burns, multiple traumatic injuries, or a metabolic imbalance. This is because catecholamines, adrenocortical hormones, thyroxine, and growth hormone enhance lipolysis and embolization of fatty acids.
- Obtain weekly laboratory tests, as ordered. The usual tests include liver function studies, prothrombin time, platelet count, and serum triglyceride levels. Whenever possible, draw blood for triglyceride levels at least 6 hours after the completion of the lipid emulsion infusion to avoid falsely elevated results.
- A lipid emulsion is an excellent medium for bacterial growth. Therefore, never rehang a partially empty bottle of emulsion.
- Report any adverse reactions to the patient's physician so that he can change the parenteral nutrition regimen as needed.

Complications

- Fever, dyspnea, cyanosis, nausea, vomiting, headache, flushing, diaphoresis, lethargy, syncope, chest and back pain, slight pressure over the eyes, irritation at the infusion site, hyperlipidemia, hypercoagulability, and thrombocytopenia occurring immediately or early in fewer than 1% of patients

- Thrombocytopenia in infants receiving a 20% I.V. lipid emulsion
- Hepatomegaly, splenomegaly, jaundice secondary to central lobular cholestasis, and blood dyscrasias (such as thrombocytopenia, leukopenia, and transient increases in liver function studies) occurring as delayed but uncommon and associated with prolonged administration
- Deficiency of essential fatty acids indicated by dry or scaly skin, thinning hair, abnormal liver function studies, and thrombocytopenia
- Brown pigmentation in the reticuloendothelial system (unknown reasons)
- Lipid accumulation of peripheral parenteral nutrition in the lungs of premature or low-birth-weight neonates

Documentation

Record the times of all dressing changes and solution changes, the condition of the catheter insertion site, your observations of the patient's condition, and any complications and resulting treatments.

Lumbar puncture

Lumbar puncture involves the insertion of a sterile needle into the subarachnoid space of the spinal canal, usually between the third and fourth lumbar vertebrae. This procedure is used to determine the presence of blood in cerebrospinal fluid (CSF), to obtain CSF specimens for laboratory analysis, and to inject dyes for contrast in radiologic studies. It's also used to administer drugs or anesthetics and to relieve intracranial pressure (ICP) by removing CSF.

Performed by a physician or advanced practice nurse, lumbar puncture requires sterile technique and careful patient positioning. This procedure is contraindicated in patients with ICP, lumbar deformity, or infection at the puncture site. It isn't recommended in patients with increased ICP because the rapid reduction in pressure that follows withdrawal of CSF can cause tonsillar herniation and medullary compression.

Equipment

Overbed table ♦ one or two pairs of sterile gloves for the practitioner ♦ sterile gloves for the nurse ♦ antiseptic solution ♦ sterile gauze pads ♦ alcohol pads ♦ sterile fenestrated drape ♦ 3-ml syringe for local anesthetic ♦ 25G 3/4" sterile needle for injecting anesthetic ♦ local anesthetic (usually 1% lidocaine) ♦ 18G or 20G 3½" spinal needle with stylet (22G needle for children) ♦ three-way stopcock ♦ manometer ♦ small adhesive bandage ♦ three sterile collection tubes with stoppers ♦ laboratory request forms and laboratory biohazard transport bag ♦ sterile marker ♦ sterile labels ♦ light source such as a gooseneck lamp ♦ optional: patient-care reminder

Disposable lumbar puncture trays contain most of the needed sterile equipment.

Preparation

- Gather the equipment and take it to the patient's bedside.

Key steps

- Confirm the patient's identity using two patient identifiers according to your facility's policy.
- Explain the procedure to the patient to ease his anxiety and ensure his cooperation. Make sure a consent form has been signed.
- Inform the patient that he may experience headache after lumbar puncture, but reassure him that his cooperation during the procedure minimizes such an effect. (*Note:* Sedatives and analgesics are usually withheld before this test if there's evidence of a central nervous system disorder because they may mask important symptoms.)
- Immediately before the procedure, provide privacy and instruct the patient to void.
- Wash your hands thoroughly.
- Label all tubes and medications on and off the sterile field.
- Open the equipment tray on an overbed table, being careful not to contaminate the sterile field when you open the wrapper. Label all medications, medication contain-

Positioning for lumbar puncture

Have the patient lie on his side at the edge of the bed, with his chin tucked to his chest and his knees drawn up to his abdomen. Make sure the patient's spine is curved and his back is at the edge of the bed (as shown below). This position widens the spaces between the vertebrae, easing insertion of the needle.

To help the patient maintain this position, place one of your hands behind his neck and the other hand behind his knees, and pull gently. Hold the patient firmly in this position throughout the procedure to prevent accidental needle displacement.

Patient positioning

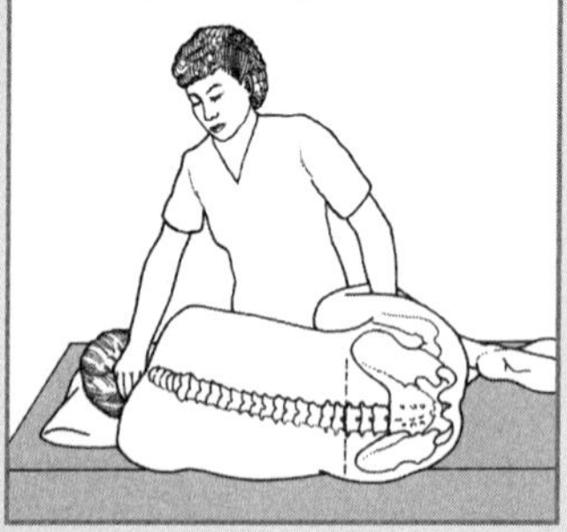

Typically, the practitioner inserts the needle between the third and fourth lumbar vertebrae (as shown below).

Needle insertion

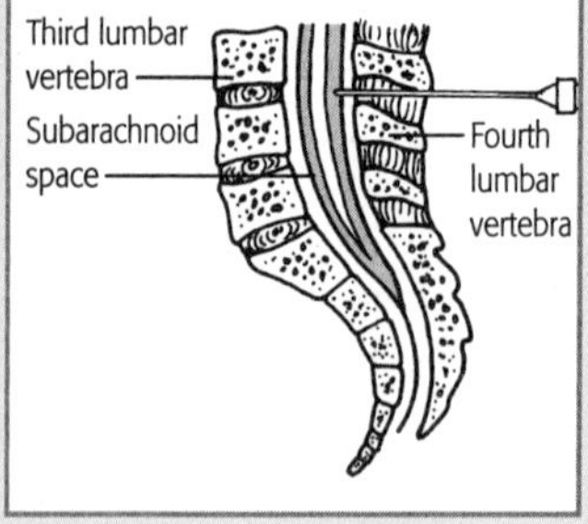

ers, and other solutions on and off the sterile field.

- Provide adequate lighting at the puncture site, and adjust the height of the patient's bed to allow the practitioner to perform the procedure comfortably.
- Position the patient and reemphasize the importance of remaining as still as possible to minimize discomfort and trauma. (See *Positioning for lumbar puncture.*)
- The practitioner cleans the puncture site with sterile gauze pads soaked in antiseptic solution, wiping in a circular motion away from the puncture site; he uses three different pads to prevent contamination of spinal tissues by the body's normal skin flora. Next, he drapes the area with the fenestrated drape to provide a sterile field. (If the practitioner uses povidone-iodine pads instead of sterile gauze pads, he may remove his sterile gloves and put on another pair to avoid introducing povidone-iodine into the subarachnoid space with the lumbar puncture needle.)
- If no ampule of anesthetic is included on the equipment tray, clean the injection port of a multidose vial of anesthetic with an alcohol pad. Then invert the vial 45 degrees so that the practitioner can insert a 25G needle and syringe and withdraw the anesthetic for injection.
- Before the practitioner injects the anesthetic, tell the patient he'll experience a transient burning sensation and local pain. Ask him to report any other persistent pain or sensations because they may indicate irritation or puncture of a nerve root, requiring repositioning of the needle.
- When the practitioner inserts the sterile spinal needle into the subarachnoid space between the third and fourth lumbar vertebrae, instruct the patient to remain still and breathe normally. If necessary, hold the patient firmly in position to prevent sudden movement that may displace the needle.
- If the lumbar puncture is being performed to administer contrast media for radiologic studies or spinal anesthetic, the practitioner injects the dye or anesthetic at this time.
- When the needle is in place, the practitioner attaches a manometer with a three-

way stopcock to the needle hub to read CSF pressure. If ordered, help the patient extend his legs to provide a more accurate pressure reading.

- The practitioner then detaches the manometer and allows CSF to drain from the needle hub into the collection tubes. When he has collected 2 to 3 ml in each tube, mark the tubes in sequence, insert a stopper to secure them, and label them.
- If the practitioner suspects an obstruction in the spinal subarachnoid space, he may check for Queckenstedt's sign. After he takes an initial CSF pressure reading, compress the patient's neck vein for 10 seconds as ordered. This increases ICP and—if no subarachnoid block exists—causes CSF pressure to rise as well. The practitioner then takes pressure readings every 10 seconds until the pressure stabilizes.
- After the practitioner collects the specimens and removes the spinal needle, clean the puncture site with povidone-iodine and apply a small adhesive bandage.
- Send the CSF specimens to the laboratory immediately, with completed laboratory request forms in a laboratory biohazard transport bag.

Special considerations

ACTION STAT!

During lumbar puncture, watch closely for signs of adverse reaction, including elevated pulse rate, pallor, and clammy skin. Alert the practitioner immediately to any significant changes.

- The patient may be ordered to lie flat for 8 to 12 hours after the procedure. If necessary, place a patient-care reminder on his bed to this effect.
- Collected CSF specimens must be sent to the laboratory immediately; they can't be refrigerated for later transport.

Complications

- Headache (common)
- Reaction to the anesthetic, meningitis, epidural or subdural abscess, bleeding into the spinal canal, CSF leakage through the dural defect remaining after needle withdrawal, local pain caused by nerve root irritation, edema or hematoma at the puncture site, transient difficulty voiding, and fever
- Tonsillar herniation and medullary compression (serious yet rare)

Documentation

Record the initiation and completion times of the procedure, the patient's response, administration of drugs, number of specimen tubes collected, time of transport to the laboratory, and color, consistency, and any other characteristics of the collected specimens.

M

Male incontinence device

Many patients don't require an indwelling urinary catheter to manage their incontinence. For male patients, a male incontinence device reduces the risk of urinary tract infection from catheterization, promotes bladder retraining when possible, helps prevent skin breakdown, and improves the patient's self-image. The device consists of a condom catheter secured to the shaft of the penis and connected to a leg bag or drainage bag. It has no contraindications but can cause skin irritation and edema.

Equipment

Condom catheter ♦ drainage bag ♦ extension tubing ♦ hypoallergenic tape or incontinence sheath holder ♦ commercial adhesive strip or skin-bond cement ♦ elastic adhesive or Velcro, if needed ♦ gloves ♦ electric clippers, if needed ♦ basin ♦ soap ♦ washcloth ♦ towel

Preparation

- Fill the basin with lukewarm water.
- Bring the basin and the remaining equipment to the patient's bedside.

Key steps

- Confirm the patient's identity using two patient identifiers according to facility policy.
- Explain the procedure to the patient, wash your hands thoroughly, put on gloves, and provide privacy.

Applying the device

- If the patient is circumcised, wash the penis with soap and water, rinse well, and pat dry with a towel. If the patient is uncircumcised, gently retract the foreskin and clean beneath it. Rinse well but don't dry because moisture provides lubrication and prevents friction during foreskin replacement. Replace the foreskin to avoid penile constriction. Then, if necessary, clip the hair at the base and shaft of the penis to prevent the adhesive strip or skin-bond cement from pulling it out.
- If you're using a precut commercial adhesive strip, insert the glans penis through its opening, and position the strip 1" (2.5 cm) from the scrotal area. If you're using uncut adhesive, cut a strip to fit around the shaft of the penis. Remove the protective covering from one side of the adhesive strip and press this side firmly to the penis to enhance adhesion. Then remove the covering from the other side of the strip. If a commercial adhesive strip isn't available, apply skin-bond cement and let it dry for a few minutes.
- Position the rolled condom catheter at the tip of the penis, with its drainage opening at the urinary meatus.
- Unroll the catheter upward, past the adhesive strip on the shaft of the penis. Then gently press the sheath against the strip until it adheres. (See *How to apply a condom catheter*.)
- After the condom catheter is in place, secure it with hypoallergenic tape or an incontinence sheath holder.
- Using extension tubing, connect the condom catheter to the leg bag or drainage bag. Remove and discard your gloves.

Removing the device

- Put on gloves and simultaneously roll the condom catheter and adhesive strip off the penis and discard them. If you've used skin-bond cement rather than an adhesive strip, remove it with solvent. Also remove and discard the hypoallergenic tape or incontinence sheath holder.
- Clean the penis with lukewarm water, rinse thoroughly, and dry. Check for swelling or signs of skin breakdown.
- Remove the leg bag by closing the drain clamp, unlatching the leg straps, and disconnecting the extension tubing at the top of the bag. Discard your gloves.

Special considerations

- If hypoallergenic tape or an incontinence sheath holder isn't available, secure the condom with a strip of elastic adhesive or Velcro. Apply the strip snugly—but not too tightly—to prevent circulatory constriction.
- Inspect the condom catheter for twists and the extension tubing for kinks to prevent obstruction of urine flow, which could cause the condom to balloon, eventually dislodging it.

Complications

- Circulatory constriction
- Obstruction of urine flow
- Skin irritation and edema

Patient teaching

- Teach the patient how to apply the catheter.
- Instruct the patient about the signs and symptoms of infection.
- Teach the patient to check his penis for signs of irritation.

Documentation

Record the date and time of application and removal of the incontinence device. Also note skin condition and the patient's response to the device, including voiding pattern, to assist with bladder retraining.

How to apply a condom catheter

Apply an adhesive strip to the shaft of the penis about 1" (2.5 cm) from the scrotal area.

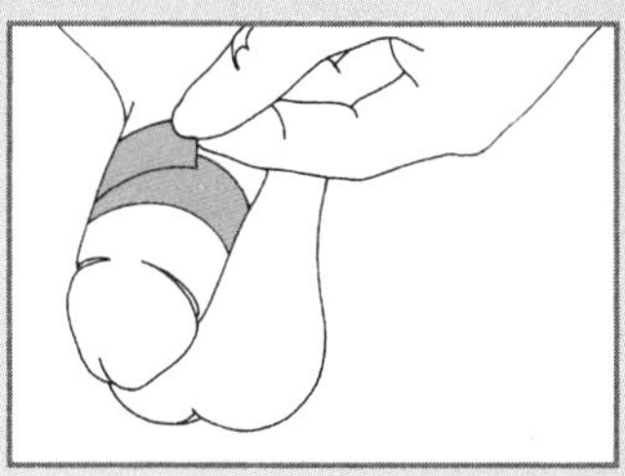

Then roll the condom catheter on to the penis past the adhesive strip, leaving about 1" clearance at the end. Press the sheath gently against the strip until it adheres.

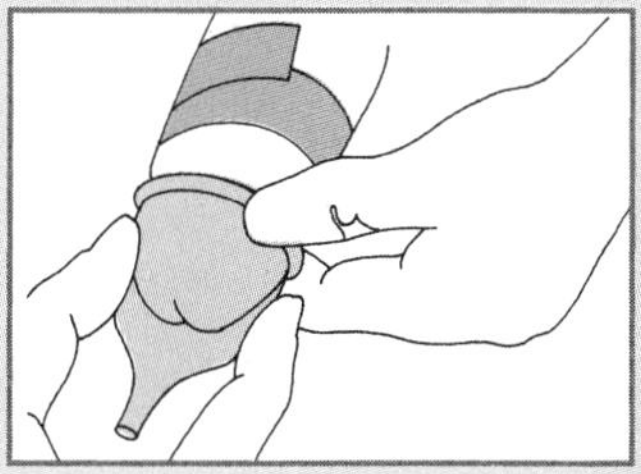

Manual ventilation

A handheld resuscitation bag is an inflatable device that can be attached to a face mask or directly to an endotracheal (ET) or tracheostomy tube to allow manual delivery of oxygen or room air to the lungs of a patient who can't breathe by himself or has inadequate ventilation. Typically used in an emergency, manual ventilation can also be performed while the patient is disconnected temporarily from a mechanical ventilator, such as during a tubing change, during transport, or before suctioning. In such instances, the use of a handheld resuscitation bag maintains ventilation. Oxygen administration with a resuscitation bag can help improve a compromised cardiorespiratory system.

Equipment

Handheld resuscitation bag (1 to 2 L) ♦ mask ♦ oxygen source (wall unit or tank)

Using a PEEP valve

Add positive end-expiratory pressure (PEEP) to manual ventilation by attaching a PEEP valve to the resuscitation bag. This may improve oxygenation if the patient hasn't responded to increased fraction of inspired oxygen levels. Always use a PEEP valve to manually ventilate a patient who has been receiving PEEP on the ventilator.

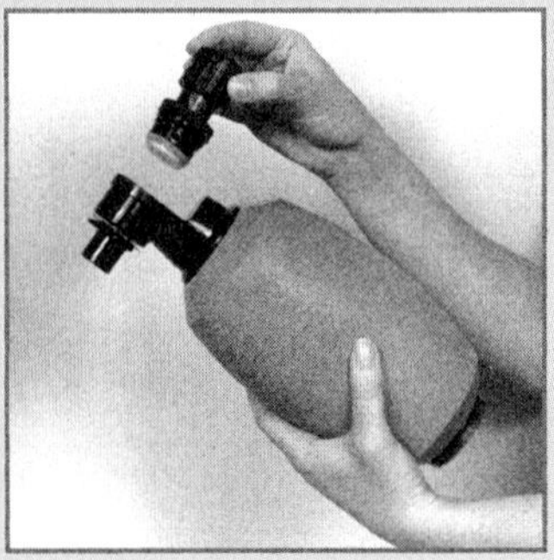

♦ oxygen tubing ♦ nipple adapter attached to oxygen flowmeter ♦ oxygen reservoir, positive end-expiratory pressure (PEEP) valve (see *Using a PEEP valve*)

Preparation

- The typical bag-mask device used for positive-pressure ventilation has a self-inflating bag with a nonrebreathing valve connected to the face mask. Unless the patient is intubated or has a tracheostomy, select a mask that fits snugly over the mouth and nose. Attach the mask to the resuscitation bag.
- If oxygen is readily available, connect the handheld resuscitation bag to the oxygen.
- Attach one end of the tubing to the bottom of the bag and the other end to the nipple adapter on the flowmeter of the oxygen source.
- Adjust the oxygen to a minimal flow rate of 10 to 12 L/minute, oxygen greater than 40%. Ideally, an oxygen reservoir should be used. This device attaches to an adapter on the bottom of the bag and delivers 100% oxygen.

Key steps

- Before using the handheld resuscitation bag, check the patient's upper airway for foreign matter. If present, remove it because this alone may restore spontaneous respirations. Suction the patient to remove secretions that may obstruct the airway. If necessary, insert an oropharyngeal or nasopharyngeal airway to maintain airway patency. If the patient has a tracheostomy or ET tube in place, suction the tube.
- If appropriate, remove the bed's headboard and stand at the head of the bed to help keep the patient's neck extended and to free space at the side of the bed for other activities such as cardiopulmonary resuscitation.
- Use the head-tilt, chin-lift maneuver to move the tongue away from the base of the pharynx and prevent airway obstruction. If trauma is present, use the jaw-thrust method. (See *Using a handheld resuscitation bag and mask.*)
- Keeping your nondominant hand on the patient's mask, exert downward pressure to seal the mask against his face. For the adult patient, use your dominant hand to compress the bag to give 8 to 10 breaths/minute.
- Depress the 1-L bag by one-half to two-thirds of its volume or a 2-L bag about one-third its volume to deliver a tidal volume sufficient to achieve a visible chest rise.
- Deliver each breath over 1 second. Allow the patient to exhale before giving another ventilation.

ALERT

For infants and children, use a pediatric handheld resuscitation bag with a volume of at least 450 to 500 ml. Deliver 20 breaths/-minute, or one compression of the bag every 3 to 5 seconds.

DO'S & DON'TS

Deliver breaths with the patient's inspiratory effort, if present. Don't attempt to deliver a breath as the patient exhales.

Using a handheld resuscitation bag and mask

Bag-mask resuscitation by one rescuer

1. Circle the edges of the mask with the index and first finger of one hand while lifting the jaw with the other fingers. Make sure there's a tight seal. Use the other hand to compress the bag.

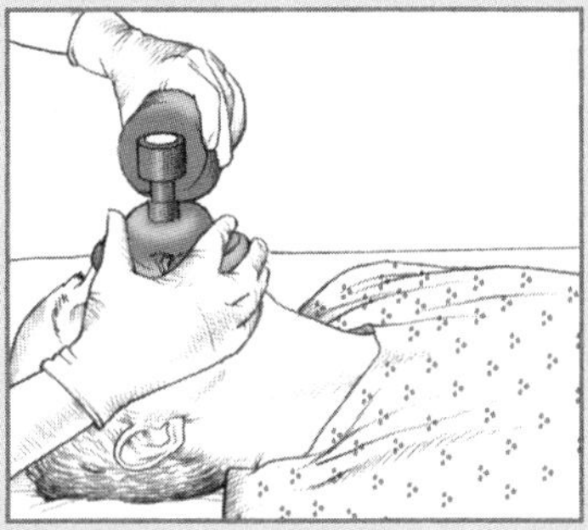

2. Make sure the patient's mouth remains open underneath the mask. Attach the bag to the mask and to the tubing leading to the oxygen source.

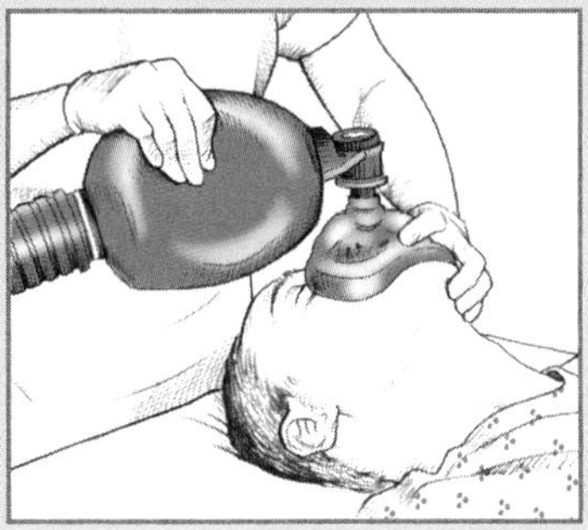

3. Alternatively, if the patient has a tracheostomy or endotracheal tube in place, remove the mask from the bag and attach the handheld resuscitation bag directly to the tube.

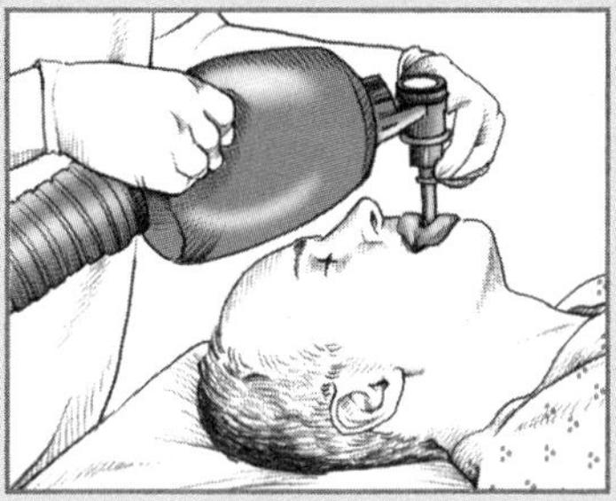

Bag-mask resuscitation by two rescuers

One rescuer stands at the victim's head and uses the thumb and the first finger of both hands to completely seal the edges of the mask. The other fingers lift the jaw and extend the victim's neck. The second rescuer squeezes the bag over 2 seconds until the chest rises.

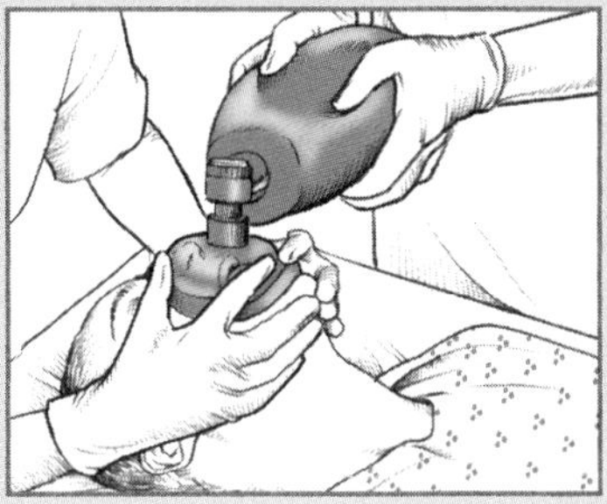

- Observe the patient's chest to make sure that it rises and falls with each compression. If ventilation fails to occur, check the fit of the mask and the patency of the patient's airway; if necessary, reposition his head and ensure patency with an oral airway.

Special considerations

- Avoid neck hyperextension if the patient has a possible cervical injury; instead, use the jaw-thrust technique to open the airway.
- If you need both hands to keep the patient's mask in place and maintain hyperextension, use the lower part of your arm to compress the bag against your side.

- Observe for vomiting through the clear part of the mask. If vomiting occurs, stop the procedure immediately, lift the mask, turn the patient to his side, wipe and suction vomitus, and resume resuscitation.
- Underventilation occurs because the handheld resuscitation bag is difficult to keep positioned tightly on the patient's face while ensuring an open airway. Furthermore, the volume of air delivered to the patient varies with the type of bag used and the hand size of the person compressing the bag. An adult with a small or medium-sized hand may not consistently deliver sufficient air. For these reasons, have someone assist with the procedure, if possible.
- Aspiration of vomitus can result in pneumonia, and gastric distention may result from air forced into the patient's stomach.

Complications

- None known

Documentation

In an emergency, record the date and time you started and stopped the procedure, manual ventilation efforts, oxygen flow rate, any complications and interventions taken, and the patient's response to treatment, according to your facility's policy for respiratory arrest.

In a nonemergency situation, record the date and time of the procedure, reason and length of time the patient was disconnected from mechanical ventilation and received manual ventilation, any complications and interventions taken, and the patient's tolerance of the procedure.

Mechanical traction

Mechanical traction is used to reduce fractures, treat dislocations, correct or prevent deformities, improve or correct contractures, or decrease muscle spasms. It works by exerting a pulling force on an injured or diseased part of the body—usually the spine, pelvis, or bones of the arms or legs, while countertraction pulls in the opposite direction.

The three types of traction are manual, skin, and skeletal. Manual traction involves placing hands on the affected body part and applying a steady pull, usually during a procedure such as cast application, fracture reduction, or halo application.

Skin traction is ordered when a light, temporary, or noncontinuous pulling force is required. Contraindications for skin traction include a severe injury with open wounds, an allergy to tape or other skin traction equipment, circulatory disturbances, dermatitis, and varicose veins.

In skeletal traction, an orthopedist inserts a pin or wire through the bone and attaches the traction equipment to the pin or wire to exert a direct, constant, longitudinal pulling force. Indications for skeletal traction include fractures of the tibia, femur, and humerus. Infections, such as osteomyelitis, contraindicate skeletal traction.

Nursing responsibilities for this procedure include supervising the setup of the traction frame. (See *Traction frames*.) The design of the patient's bed usually dictates whether to use a claw clamp or I.V.-post-type frame. (However, the claw-type Balkan frame is rarely used.) A nurse with special skills, an orthopedic technician, or the practitioner can set up the specific traction. Instructions for setting up these traction units usually accompany the equipment.

After the patient is placed in the specific type of traction ordered by the orthopedist, the nurse is responsible for preventing complications from immobility; for routinely inspecting the equipment; for adding traction weights as ordered; and, in patients with skeletal traction, for monitoring the pin insertion sites for signs of infection. (See *Comparing types of traction,* page 298.)

Equipment

Claw-type basic frame

102″ (259-cm) plain bar ♦ two 66″ (167.6-cm) swivel-clamp bars ♦ two upper-panel clamps ♦ two lower-panel clamps

Traction frames

You may encounter three types of traction frames, as described below.

Claw-type basic frame

With a claw-type basic frame, claw attachments secure the uprights to the footboard and headboard.

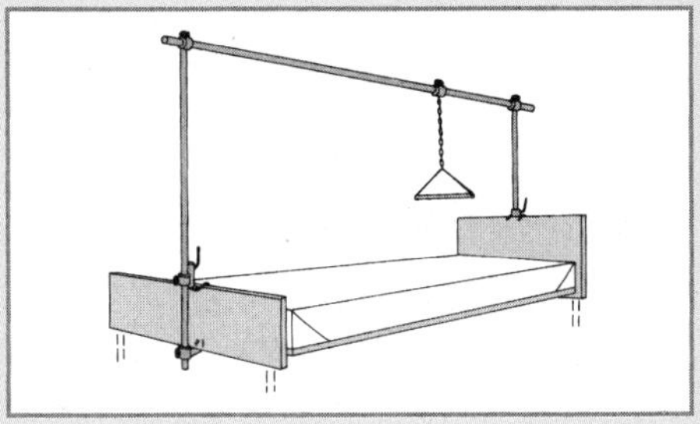

I.V.-type basic frame

With an I.V.-type basic frame, I.V. posts, placed in I.V. holders, support the horizontal bars across the foot and head of the bed. These horizontal bars then support the two uprights.

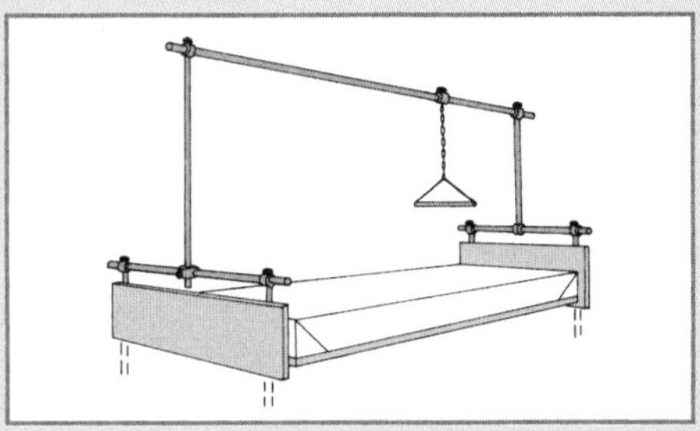

I.V.-type Balkan frame

An I.V.-type Balkan frame features I.V. posts and horizontal bars (secured in the same manner as those for the I.V.-type basic frame) that support four uprights.

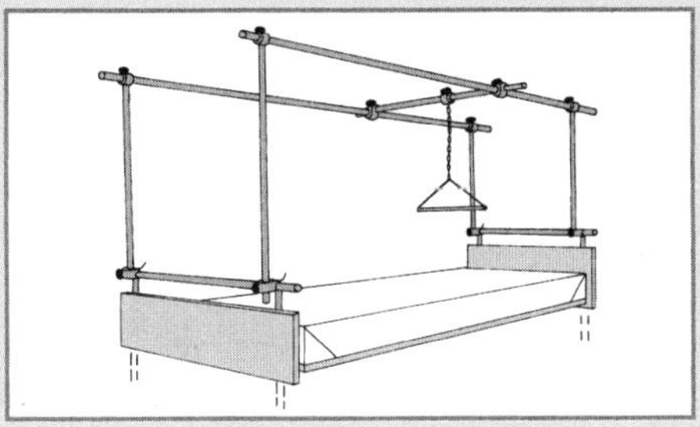

I.V.-type basic frame

102″ plain bar ♦ 27″ (68.6-cm) double-clamp bar ♦ 48″ (122-cm) swivel-clamp bar ♦ two 36″ (91.5-cm) plain bars ♦ four 4″ (10-cm) I.V. posts with clamps ♦ cross clamp

I.V.-type Balkan frame

Two 102″ plain bars ♦ two 27″ double-clamp bars ♦ two 48″ swivel-clamp bars ♦ five 36″ plain bars ♦ four 4″ I.V. posts with clamps ♦ eight cross clamps

All frame types

Trapeze with clamp ♦ wall bumper or roller

Skeletal traction care

Sterile cotton-tipped applicators ♦ prescribed antiseptic solution ♦ sterile gauze pads ♦ optional: antimicrobial ointment

Comparing types of traction

Traction therapy applies a pulling force to an injured or diseased limb. For traction to be effective, it must be combined with an equal mix of countertraction. Weights provide the pulling force. Countertraction is produced by positioning the patient's body weight against the traction pull.

Skin traction

Skin traction immobilizes a body part intermittently over an extended period through direct application of a pulling force on the patient's skin. The force may be applied using adhesive or nonadhesive traction tape or other skin traction devices, such as a boot, belt, or halter.

This traction exerts a light pull and uses up to 8 lb (3.6 kg) per extremity for an adult.

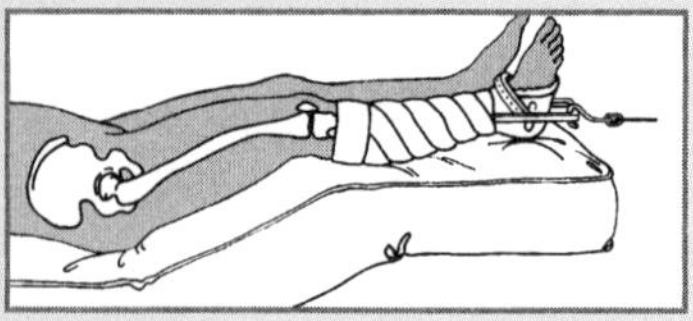

Skeletal traction

Skeletal traction immobilizes a body part for prolonged periods by attaching weighted equipment directly to the patient's bones. This may be accomplished with pins, screws, wires, or tongs. The amount of weight applied is determined by body size and extent of injury.

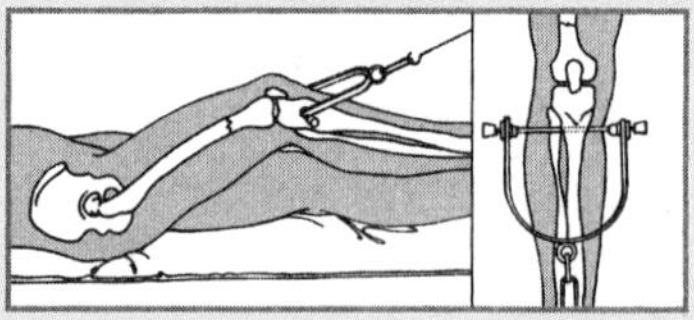

Preparation

- Arrange with central supply or the appropriate department to have the traction equipment transported to the patient's room on a traction cart.
- If appropriate, gather the equipment for pin-site care at the patient's bedside. Pin-site care protocols may vary with each facility or practitioner.

Key steps

- Confirm the patient's identity using two patient identifiers according to facility policy.
- Explain the purpose of traction to the patient. Emphasize the importance of maintaining proper body alignment after the traction equipment is set up.

Setting up a claw-type basic frame

- Attach one lower-panel and one upper-panel clamp to each 66″ swivel-clamp bar.
- Fasten one bar to the footboard and one to the headboard by turning the clamp knobs clockwise until they're tight and then pulling back on the upper clamp's rubberized bar until it's tight.
- Secure the 102″ horizontal plain bar atop the two vertical bars, making sure that the clamp knobs point up.
- Using the appropriate clamp, attach the trapeze to the horizontal bar about 2′ (61 cm) from the head of the bed.

Setting up an I.V.-type basic frame

- Attach one 4″ I.V. post with clamp to each end of both 36″ horizontal plain bars.
- Secure an I.V. post in each I.V. holder at the bed corners. Using a cross clamp, fasten the 48″ vertical swivel-clamp bar to the middle of the horizontal plain bar at the foot of the bed.
- Fasten the 27″ vertical double-clamp bar to the middle of the horizontal plain bar at the head of the bed.
- Attach the 102″ horizontal plain bar to the tops of the two vertical bars, making sure that the clamp knobs point up.

- Using the appropriate clamp, attach the trapeze to the horizontal bar about 2′ from the head of the bed.

Setting up an I.V.-type Balkan frame

- Attach one 4″ I.V. post with clamp to each end of two 36″ horizontal plain bars.
- Secure an I.V. post in each I.V. holder at the bed corners.
- Attach a 48″ vertical swivel-clamp bar, using a cross clamp, to each I.V. post clamp on the horizontal plain bar at the foot of the bed.
- Fasten one 36″ horizontal plain bar across the midpoints of the two 48″ swivel-clamp bars, using two cross clamps.
- Attach a 27″ vertical double-clamp bar to each I.V. post clamp on the horizontal bar at the head of the bed.
- Using two cross clamps, fasten a 36″ horizontal plain bar across the midpoints of two 27″ double-clamp bars.
- Clamp a 102″ horizontal plain bar onto the vertical bars on each side of the bed, making sure that the clamp knobs point up.
- Use two cross clamps to attach a 36″ horizontal plain bar across the two overhead bars, about 2′ from the head of the bed.
- Attach the trapeze to this 36″ horizontal bar.

After setting up any frame

- Attach a wall bumper or roller to the vertical bar or bars at the head of the bed. This protects the walls from damage caused by the bed or equipment.

Caring for the traction patient

- Show the patient how much movement he's allowed and instruct him not to readjust the equipment. Tell him to report pain or pressure from the traction equipment.
- At least once per shift, make sure that the traction equipment connections are tight. Check for impingements such as ropes rubbing on the footboard or getting caught between pulleys. Friction and impingement reduce the effectiveness of traction.
- Inspect the traction equipment to ensure the correct alignment.
- Inspect the ropes for fraying, which can eventually cause a rope to break.
- Make sure that the ropes are positioned properly in the pulley track. An improperly positioned rope changes the degree of traction.
- To prevent tampering and aid stability and security, make sure that all rope ends are taped above the knot.
- Inspect the equipment regularly to make sure that the traction weights hang freely. Weights that touch the floor, bed, or each other reduce the amount of traction.
- About every 2 hours, check the patient for proper body alignment, and reposition the patient as necessary. Misalignment causes ineffective traction and may keep the fracture from healing properly.
- To prevent complications from immobility, assess the patient's neurovascular integrity routinely. His condition, the hospital routine, and the practitioner's orders determine the frequency of neurovascular assessments.
- Provide skin care, encourage coughing and deep-breathing exercises, and assist with ordered range-of-motion exercises for unaffected extremities. Typically, an order for compression stockings is written. Check elimination patterns and provide laxatives as ordered.
- For the patient with skeletal traction, make sure that the protruding pin or wire ends are covered with cork to prevent them from tearing the bedding or injuring the patient and staff.
- Check the pin site and surrounding skin regularly for signs of infection.
- If ordered, clean the pin site and surrounding skin. Pin-site care varies. Check your facility's policy, or follow orders prescribed by the practitioner.

Special considerations

- When using skin traction, apply ordered weights slowly and carefully to avoid jerking the affected extremity. To avoid injury in case the ropes break, arrange the weights so they don't hang over the patient.

- When applying Buck's traction, make sure that the line of pull is always parallel to the bed and not angled downward to prevent pressure on the heel. Placing a flat pillow under the extremity may be helpful as long as it doesn't alter the line of pull.

Complications

- Pressure ulcers; muscle atrophy, weakness, or contractures; and osteoporosis
- GI disturbances, such as constipation; urinary problems, including stasis and calculi; respiratory problems, such as stasis of secretions and hypostatic pneumonia; and circulatory disturbances, including stasis and thrombophlebitis
- Depression or other emotional disturbances
- Osteomyelitis originating at the pin or wire sites

Documentation

In the patient record, document the amount of traction weight used daily, noting the application of additional weights and the patient's tolerance. Document equipment inspections and patient care, including routine checks of neurovascular integrity, skin condition, respiratory status, and elimination patterns. If applicable, note the condition of the pin site and any care given.

Mechanical ventilation

A mechanical ventilator moves air in and out of a patient's lungs. Although the equipment serves to ventilate a patient, it doesn't ensure adequate gas exchange. Mechanical ventilators may use either positive or negative pressure to ventilate the patient.

Positive-pressure ventilators exert a positive pressure on the airway, which causes inspiration while increasing tidal volume (V_T). The inspiratory cycles of these ventilators may vary in volume, pressure, or time. For example, a volume-cycled ventilator—the type used most commonly—delivers a preset volume of air each time, regardless of the amount of lung resistance. A pressure-cycled ventilator generates flow until the machine reaches a preset pressure regardless of the volume delivered or the time required to achieve the pressure. A time-cycled ventilator generates flow for a preset period. A high-frequency ventilator uses high respiratory rates and low V_T to maintain alveolar ventilation.

Negative-pressure ventilators act by creating negative pressure, which pulls the thorax outward and allows air to flow into the lungs. Examples of such ventilators are the iron lung, cuirass (chest shell), and body wrap. Negative-pressure ventilators are used mainly to treat neuromuscular disorders, such as Guillain-Barré syndrome, myasthenia gravis, and poliomyelitis.

Other indications for ventilator use include central nervous system disorders, such as cerebral hemorrhage and spinal cord transsection, acute respiratory distress syndrome, pulmonary edema, chronic obstructive pulmonary disease, flail chest, and acute hypoventilation.

Equipment

Oxygen source ♦ air source that can supply 50 psi ♦ mechanical ventilator ♦ humidifier ♦ ventilator circuit tubing, connectors, and adapters ♦ condensation collection trap ♦ in-line thermometer ♦ gloves ♦ handheld resuscitation bag with reservoir ♦ suction equipment ♦ sterile distilled water ♦ equipment for arterial blood gas (ABG) analysis ♦ optional: oximeter, capnography device

Preparation

DEVICE SAFETY

In most health care facilities, respiratory therapists assume responsibility for setting up the ventilator. If necessary, check the manufacturer's instructions for setting it up.

- In most cases, you'll need to add sterile distilled water to the humidifier and connect the ventilator to the appropriate gas source.

Key steps

- Verify the practitioner's order for ventilator support. If the patient isn't already intubated, prepare him for intubation. (See "Endotracheal intubation," page 161.)
- When possible, explain the procedure to the patient and his family to help reduce anxiety and fear. Assure them that staff members are nearby to provide care.
- Perform a complete physical assessment and draw blood for ABG analysis to establish a baseline.
- Suction the patient, if necessary, using a closed suction catheter.
- Plug the ventilator into the electrical outlet and turn it on. Adjust the settings on the ventilator as ordered. Make sure that the ventilator's alarms are set, as ordered, and the humidifier is filled with sterile distilled water. Attach a capnographic device to measure carbon dioxide levels to confirm placement of the endotracheal (ET) tube, detect disconnection from the ventilator, and for early detection of complications.
- Put on gloves if you haven't already. Connect the ET tube to the ventilator. Observe for chest expansion, and auscultate for bilateral breath sounds to verify that the patient is being ventilated.
- Monitor the patient's ABG values after the initial ventilator setup (usually 20 to 30 minutes), after changes in ventilator settings, and as the patient's clinical condition indicates to determine whether the patient is being adequately ventilated and to avoid oxygen toxicity. Be prepared to adjust ventilator settings depending on ABG values.
- Check the ventilator tubing frequently for condensation, which can cause resistance to airflow and which may also be aspirated by the patient. As needed, drain the condensate into a collection trap or briefly disconnect the patient from the ventilator (ventilating him with a handheld resuscitation bag, if necessary), and empty the water into an appropriate receptacle.

DO'S & DON'TS

Don't drain the condensate into the humidifier because the condensation may be contaminated with the patient's secretions and is considered infectious. Also, avoid accidental drainage of condensation into the patient's airway.

- Inspect the humidification device regularly and remove condensate as needed. Inspect heat and moisture exchangers, and replace if secretions contaminate the insert or filter. Note humidifier settings. The heated humidifier should be set to deliver an inspired gas temperature of 91.4° F (33° C) plus or minus 3.6° F (2° C) and should provide a minimum of 30 mg/L of water vapor with routine use to an intubated patient.
- If you're using a heated humidifier, monitor the inspired air temperature as close to the patient's airway as possible. The inspiratory gas shouldn't be greater than 98.6° F (37° C) at the opening of the airway. Check that the high temperature alarm is set no higher than 98.6° F and no lower than 86° F (30° C). Observe the amount and consistency of the patient's secretions. If the secretions are copious or increasingly tenacious when a heat and moisture exchanger is used, a heated humidifier should be used instead.
- Check the in-line thermometer to make sure that the temperature of the air delivered to the patient is close to body temperature.
- When monitoring the patient's vital signs, count spontaneous breaths as well as ventilator-delivered breaths.
- Change, clean, or dispose of the ventilator tubing and equipment according to your facility's policy.
- When ordered, begin to wean the patient from the ventilator. (See *Weaning from the ventilator,* page 302.)

Special considerations

- Make sure the ventilator alarms are on at all times. These alarms alert the nursing staff to potentially hazardous conditions and changes in the patient's status. If an alarm sounds and the problem can't be identified easily, disconnect the patient from the ventilator and use a handheld resuscitation bag to ventilate him. (See *Responding to ventilator alarms,* pages 303 and 304.)

Weaning from the ventilator

Successful weaning from the ventilator depends on the patient's ability to breathe on his own. This means that he must have a spontaneous respiratory effort that can keep him ventilated, a stable cardiovascular system, and sufficient respiratory muscle strength and level of consciousness to sustain spontaneous breathing. The patient should meet some or all of the following criteria.

Readiness criteria

- Arterial oxygen saturation ($Sa{O_2}$) greater than 92% on fraction of inspired oxygen less than or equal to 40%, positive end-expiratory pressure less than or equal to 5 cm H_2O
- Hemodynamically stable, adequately resuscitated and doesn't require vasoactive support
- Serum electrolyte levels and pH within normal range
- Hematocrit greater than 25%
- Core body temperature greater than 96.8° F (36° C) and less than 102.2° F (39° C)
- Pain is adequately managed
- Successful withdrawal of a neuromuscular blocker
- Arterial blood gas values within normal limits or at patient's baseline

Weaning intervention (long term—more than 72 hours)

- Transfer to pressure-support ventilation (PSV) mode and adjust support level to maintain patient's respiratory rate at less than 35 breaths/minute.
- Observe for 30 minutes for signs of early failure, such as:
  - sustained respiratory rate greater than 35 breaths/minute
  - $Sa{O_2}$ less than 89%
  - tidal volume less than or equal to 5 ml/kg
  - sustained minute ventilation greater than 200 ml/kg/minute
  - evidence of respiratory or hemodynamic distress: labored respiratory pattern, increased diaphoresis or anxiety or both, sustained heart rate greater than 20% higher or lower than baseline, systolic blood pressure greater than 180 mm Hg or less than 90 mm Hg higher.
- If tolerated, continue trial for 2 hours, then return patient to "rest" settings by adding ventilator breaths or increasing PSV to achieve a total respiratory rate of less than 20 breaths/minute.
- After 2 hours of rest, repeat trial for 2 to 4 hours at same PSV level as previous trial. If the patient exceeds the tolerance criteria, stop the trial and return to "rest" settings. In this case, the next trial should be performed at a higher support level than the failed trial.
- Record the results after each weaning episode, including specific parameters and the time frame if failure was observed.
- The goal is to increase trial lengths and reduce the PSV level needed in increments.
- With each successful trial, the PSV level may be decreased by 2 to 4 cm H_2O, the time interval may be increased by 1 to 2 hours, or both while keeping the patient within tolerable parameters.
- Ensure nocturnal ventilation at "rest" settings (with a respiratory rate of less than 20 breaths/minute) for at least 6 hours each night until the patient's weaning trials demonstrate readiness to discontinue support.

- Provide emotional support to the patient during all phases of mechanical ventilation to reduce anxiety and promote successful treatment. Even if the patient is unresponsive, continue to explain all procedures and treatment to him.
- Unless contraindicated, turn the patient from side to side every 1 to 2 hours to facilitate lung expansion and removal of secretions. Perform active or passive range-of-motion exercises for all extremities to reduce the hazards of immobility. If the pa-

Responding to ventilator alarms

Signal	Possible cause	Interventions
Low-pressure alarm	■ Tube disconnected from ventilator	■ Reconnect the tube to the ventilator.
	■ Endotracheal (ET) tube displaced above vocal cords or tracheostomy tube extubated	■ Check tube placement and reposition, if needed. If extubation or displacement has occurred, ventilate the patient manually and call the practitioner immediately.
	■ Leaking tidal volume from low cuff pressure (from an underinflated or ruptured cuff or a leak in the cuff or one-way valve)	■ Listen for a whooshing sound around the tube, indicating an air leak. If you hear one, check cuff pressure. If you can't maintain pressure, call the practitioner; he may need to insert a new tube.
	■ Ventilator malfunction	■ Disconnect the patient from the ventilator and ventilate him manually, if necessary. Obtain other ventilator.
	■ Leak in ventilator circuitry (from loose connection or hole in tubing, loss of temperature-sensitive device, or cracked humidification jar)	■ Make sure all connections are intact. Check for holes or leaks in the tubing and replace, if necessary. Check the humidification jar and replace if cracked.
High-pressure alarm	■ Increased airway pressure or decreased lung compliance caused by worsening disease	■ Auscultate the lungs for evidence of increasing lung consolidation, barotrauma, or wheezing. Call the practitioner, if indicated.
	■ Patient biting on oral ET tube	■ Insert a bite-block, if needed.
	■ Secretions in airway	■ Listen for secretions in the airway. To remove them, suction the patient or have him cough.
	■ Condensate in large-bore tubing	■ Check tubing for condensate, and remove any fluid.
	■ Intubation of right mainstem bronchus	■ Check tube position. If it has slipped, call the practitioner; he may need to reposition it.
	■ Patient coughing, gagging, or attempting to talk	■ If the patient fights the ventilator, provide explanations and use a communication board. If these fail, the practitioner may order a sedative or neuromuscular blocking agent.
	■ Chest wall resistance	■ Reposition the patient to see if doing so improves chest expansion. If repositioning doesn't help, administer the prescribed analgesic.

(continued)

Responding to ventilator alarms *(continued)*

Signal	Possible cause	Interventions
High-pressure alarm *(continued)*	■ Failure of high-pressure relief valve	■ Have the faulty equipment replaced.
	■ Bronchospasm	■ Assess the patient for the cause. Report to the practitioner and treat as ordered.

tient's condition permits, position him upright at regular intervals to increase lung expansion. When moving the patient or the ventilator tubing, be careful to prevent condensation in the tubing from flowing into the lungs because aspiration of this contaminated moisture can cause infection. Provide care for the patient's artificial airway as needed.

■ Assess the patient's peripheral circulation, and monitor his urine output for signs of decreased cardiac output. Watch for signs and symptoms of fluid volume excess or dehydration.

■ Place the call bell within the patient's reach, and establish a method of communication, such as a communication board, because intubation and mechanical ventilation impair the patient's ability to speak. An artificial airway, such as a tracheostomy, may help the patient to speak by allowing air to pass through his vocal cords.

■ Administer a sedative or neuromuscular blocking agent, as ordered, to relax the patient or eliminate spontaneous breathing efforts that can interfere with the ventilator's action. Remember that the patient receiving a neuromuscular blocking medication requires close observation because of his inability to breathe or communicate.

■ If the patient is receiving a neuromuscular blocking agent, make sure that he also receives a sedative. Neuromuscular blocking agents cause paralysis without altering the patient's level of consciousness (LOC). Reassure the patient and his family that the paralysis is temporary. Also make sure that emergency equipment is readily available in case the ventilator malfunctions or the patient is accidentally extubated. Continue to explain all procedures to the patient, and take extra steps to ensure his safety, such as raising the side rails during turning and covering and lubricating his eyes.

■ Make sure that the patient gets adequate rest and sleep because fatigue can delay weaning from the ventilator. Provide subdued lighting, safely muffle equipment noises, and restrict staff access to the area to promote quiet during rest periods.

■ When weaning the patient, continue to observe for signs of hypoxia. Schedule weaning to fit comfortably and realistically within the patient's daily regimen. Avoid scheduling sessions after meals, baths, or lengthy therapeutic or diagnostic procedures. Have the patient help you set up the schedule to give him some sense of control over a frightening procedure. As the patient's tolerance for weaning increases, help him sit up out of bed to improve his breathing and sense of well-being. Suggest diversionary activities to take his mind off breathing.

Complications

■ Tension pneumothorax, decreased cardiac output, oxygen toxicity, fluid volume excess caused by humidification, infection, and such GI complications as distention or bleeding from stress ulcers

Patient teaching

■ If the patient will be discharged on a ventilator, evaluate the family's or the caregiver's ability and motivation to provide such care.

■ Well before discharge, develop a teaching plan that will address the patient's needs. For example, teaching should include information about ventilator care and settings, artificial airway care, suctioning, respiratory therapy, communication, nutrition, therapeutic exercise, the signs and symptoms of infection, and ways to troubleshoot minor equipment malfunctions.

- Also evaluate the patient's need for adaptive equipment, such as a hospital bed, wheelchair or walker with a ventilator tray, patient lift, and bedside commode. Determine whether the patient needs to travel; if so, select appropriate portable and backup equipment.
- Before discharge, have the patient's caregiver demonstrate her ability to use the equipment. At discharge, contact a durable medical equipment vendor and a home health nurse to follow up with the patient. Also refer the patient to community resources, if available.

Documentation

Document the date and time of initiation of mechanical ventilation. Name the type of ventilator used for the patient, and note its settings. Include ET tube or tracheostomy size, position, and pressure. Describe the patient's subjective and objective response to mechanical ventilation, including his vital signs, breath sounds, accessory muscle use, skin color, chest motion, intake and output, and weight. Note any spontaneous respirations. List any complications and interventions taken. Record all pertinent laboratory data, including ABG analysis results, end-tidal carbon dioxide values, and oxygen saturation levels.

During weaning, record the date and time of each session, the weaning method used, and baseline and subsequent vital signs, oxygen saturation levels, and ABG values. Describe the patient's subjective and objective responses, including LOC, respiratory effort, arrhythmias, skin color, and need for suctioning.

List all complications and interventions taken. If the patient was receiving pressure support ventilation (PSV) or using a T-piece or tracheostomy collar, note the duration of spontaneous breathing and the patient's ability to maintain the weaning schedule. If using intermittent mandatory ventilation, with or without PSV, record the control breath rate, the time of each breath reduction, and the rate of spontaneous respirations.

Mixed venous oxygen saturation

Mixed venous oxygen saturation monitoring uses a fiber-optic thermodilution pulmonary artery (PA) catheter to continuously monitor oxygen delivery to tissues and oxygen consumption by tissues. This process allows rapid detection of impaired oxygen delivery. It's used to evaluate a patient's response to drug therapy, endotracheal tube suctioning, ventilator setting changes, positive end-expiratory pressure, and fraction of inspired oxygen. Mixed venous oxygen saturation ($S\bar{v}O_2$) usually ranges from 60% to 80%; normal value is 75%.

Equipment

Fiber-optic PA catheter ♦ co-oximeter (monitor) ♦ optical module and cable ♦ gloves

Preparation

- Review the manufacturer's instructions for assembly and use of the fiber-optic PA catheter.
- Connect the optical module and cable to the monitor.
- Peel back catheter wrapping just enough to uncover the fiber-optic connector and attach the fiber-optic connector to the optical module; don't remove the rest of the catheter.
- Calibrate the fiber-optic catheter per manufacturer instructions.
- Assist with pulmonary catheter insertion if necessary.

Key steps

- Wash your hands and put on gloves.
- Explain the procedure to the patient.
- Assist with insertion of the fiber-optic catheter.
- After insertion, ensure correct positioning and function.
- Observe digital readout and record the $S\bar{v}O_2$ on graph paper. (See *$S\bar{v}O_2$ waveforms*, page 306.)

$S\bar{v}O_2$ waveforms

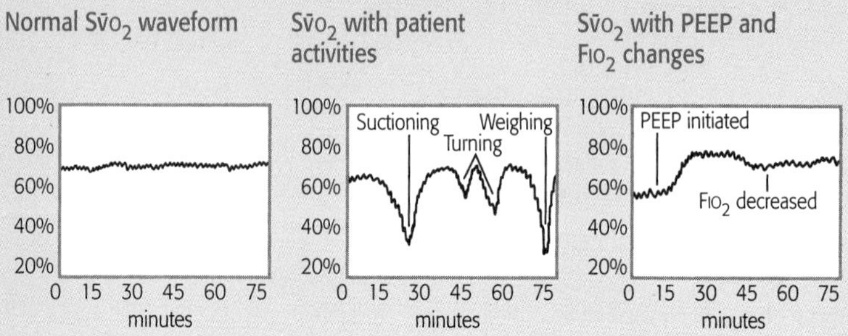

- Repeat readings at least hourly to monitor and document trends.
- Set alarms 10% above and 10% below patient's current $S\bar{v}O_2$ reading.

Recalibrating the monitor

- Draw a blood sample from the distal port of the PA catheter and send it for laboratory analysis.
- Compare the laboratory's $S\bar{v}O_2$ reading with that of the fiber-optic catheter.
- If the catheter values and monitor values differ by more than 4%, follow the manufacturer's instructions to enter the $S\bar{v}O_2$ value obtained by the laboratory into the oximeter.
- Recalibrate the monitor every 24 hours or whenever the catheter has been disconnected from the optical module.

Special considerations

ACTION STAT!

If the patient's $S\bar{v}O_2$ drops below 60% or varies by more than 10% for 3 minutes or longer, reassess the patient. If the $S\bar{v}O_2$ doesn't return to the baseline value after nursing interventions, notify the practitioner. This could indicate hemorrhage, hypoxia, shock, or arrhythmias.

- $S\bar{v}O_2$ may also decrease as a result of increased oxygen demand from hyperthermia, shivering, or seizures.
- If the intensity of the tracing is low, make sure that all connections are secure and the catheter is patent and not kinked.
- If the tracing is damped or erratic, aspirate blood from the catheter to check for patency.
- If aspiration is unsuccessful, anticipate catheter replacement and notify the practitioner.
- Determine if the catheter is wedged by checking the PA waveform.
- If the catheter has wedged, turn the patient from side to side and instruct him to cough.

ACTION STAT!

If the catheter remains wedged, notify the practitioner immediately.

- Monitor for signs and symptoms of infection, such as redness or drainage at the catheter site.

Complications

- Thrombosis
- Thromboembolism
- Infection

Documentation

Record the $S\bar{v}O_2$ value on a flowchart and attach a tracing. Note significant changes in the patient's status. For comparison, note the $S\bar{v}O_2$ as measured by the fiber-optic catheter whenever a blood sample is obtained for laboratory analysis of $S\bar{v}O_2$.

N

Nasal packing

In the highly vascular nasal mucosa, even seemingly minor injuries can cause major bleeding and blood loss. When routine therapeutic measures, such as direct pressure, cautery, and vasoconstrictive drugs, fail to control epistaxis (nosebleed), the patient's nose may have to be packed to stop anterior bleeding (which runs out of the nose) or posterior bleeding (which runs down the throat). If blood drains into the nasopharyngeal area or lacrimal ducts, the patient may also appear to bleed from the mouth and eyes.

Most nasal bleeding originates at a plexus of arterioles and venules in the anteroinferior septum. Only about 1 in 10 nosebleeds occurs in the posterior nose, which usually bleeds more heavily than the anterior location.

A nurse typically assists the physician with anterior or posterior nasal packing. (See *Types of nasal packing,* page 308.) She may also assist with nasal balloon catheterization, a procedure that applies pressure to a posterior bleeding site. (See *Nasal balloon catheters,* page 309.)

Whichever procedure the patient undergoes, you should provide ongoing encouragement and support to reduce his discomfort and anxiety. You should also perform ongoing assessment to determine the procedure's success and to detect possible complications.

Equipment

Anterior and posterior packing

Gowns ♦ goggles ♦ masks ♦ sterile gloves ♦ emesis basin ♦ facial tissues ♦ patient drape (towels, incontinence pads, or gown) ♦ nasal speculum and tongue blades (may be in preassembled head and neck examination kit) ♦ directed illumination source (such as headlamp or strong flashlight) or fiber-optic nasal endoscope, light cables, and light source ♦ suction apparatus with sterile suction-connecting tubing and sterile nasal aspirator tip ♦ sterile bowl and sterile saline solution for flushing out suction apparatus ♦ sterile tray or sterile towels ♦ sterile cotton-tipped applicators ♦ local anesthetic spray (topical 4% lidocaine [Xylocaine]) or vial of local anesthetic solution (such as 2% lidocaine or 1% to 2% lidocaine with epinephrine 1:100,000) ♦ sterile cotton balls or cotton pledgets ♦ 10-ml syringe with 22G 1½" needle ♦ silver nitrate sticks ♦ electrocautery device with grounding plate and small tip ♦ topical nasal decongestant ♦ absorbable hemostatic (such as Gelfoam, Avitene, Surgicel, or thrombin) ♦ sterile normal saline solution (1-g container and 60-ml syringe with luer-lock tip, or 5-ml bullets for moistening nasal tampons) ♦ hypoallergenic tape ♦ antibiotic ointment ♦ equipment for measuring vital signs ♦ equipment for drawing blood

Anterior packing

Two packages of 1½" (3.8-cm) petroleum strip gauze (3′ to 4′ [0.9 to 1.2 m]) ♦ bayonet forceps or two nasal tampons

(*Text continues on page 310.*)

Types of nasal packing

Nosebleeds may be controlled with anterior or posterior nasal packing.

Anterior nasal packing

The physician may treat an anterior nosebleed by packing the anterior nasal cavity with a 3′ to 4′ (0.9- to 1.2 m) strip of antibiotic-impregnated petroleum gauze (shown below) or with a nasal tampon.

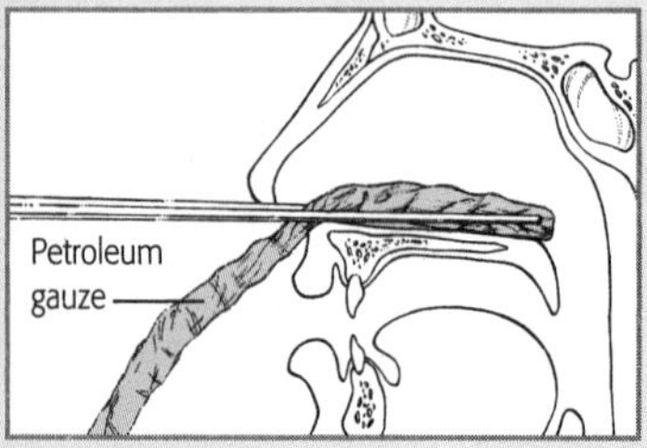

A nasal tampon is made of tightly compressed absorbent material with or without a central breathing tube. The physician inserts a lubricated tampon along the floor of the nose and, with the patient's head tilted backward, instills 5 to 10 ml of antibiotic or normal saline solution. This causes the tampon to expand, stopping the bleeding. The tampon should be moistened periodically, and the central breathing tube should be suctioned regularly.

In a child or a patient with blood dyscrasias, the physician may fashion an absorbable pack by moistening a gauze-like, regenerated cellulose material with a vasoconstrictor. Applied to a visible bleeding point, this substance will swell to form a clot. The packing is absorbable and doesn't need removal.

Posterior nasal packing

Posterior packing consists of a gauze roll shaped and secured by three sutures (one suture at each end and one in the middle) or a balloon-type catheter. To insert the packing, the physician advances one or two soft catheters into the patient's nostrils (shown below). When the catheter tips appear in the nasopharynx, the physician grasps them with a Kelly clamp or bayonet forceps and pulls them forward through the mouth. He secures the two end sutures to the catheter tip and draws the catheter back through the nostrils.

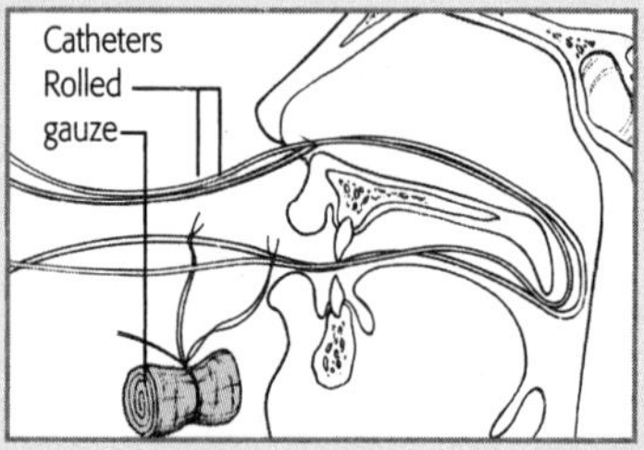

This step brings the packing into place with the end sutures hanging from the patient's nostril. (The middle suture emerges from the patient's mouth to free the packing, when needed.)

The physician may weigh the nose sutures with a clamp. Then he will pull the packing securely into place behind the soft palate and against the posterior end of the septum (nasal choana).

After he examines the patient's throat (to ensure that the uvula hasn't been forced under the packing), he inserts anterior packing and secures the whole apparatus by tying the posterior pack strings around rolled gauze or a dental roll at the nostrils (shown below).

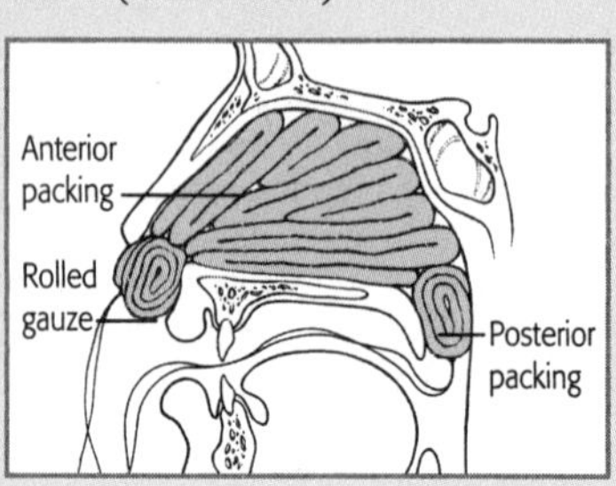

Nasal balloon catheters

To control epistaxis, the physician may use a balloon catheter instead of nasal packing. Self-retaining and disposable, the catheter may have a single or double balloon to apply pressure to bleeding nasal tissues. If bleeding is still uncontrolled, the physician may choose to use arterial ligation, cryotherapy, or arterial embolization.

When inserted and inflated, the single-balloon catheter (shown below) compresses the blood vessels while a soft, collapsible external bulb prevents the catheter from dislodging posteriorly.

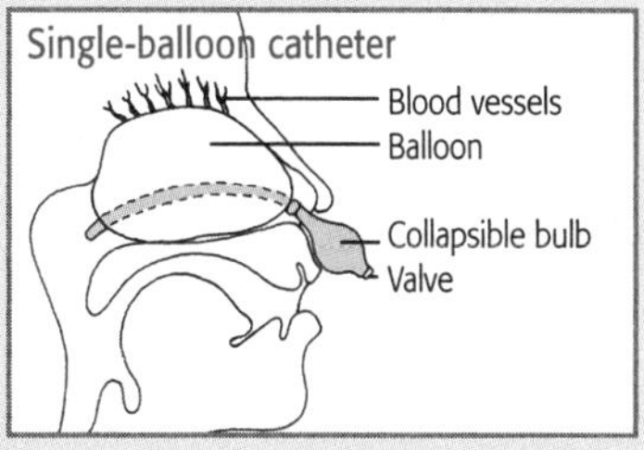

The double-balloon catheter (shown below) is used for simultaneous anterior and posterior nasal packing. The posterior balloon compresses the posterior vessels serving the nose, including the bleeding vessels; the anterior balloon compresses bleeding intranasal vessels. This catheter contains a central airway for breathing comfort.

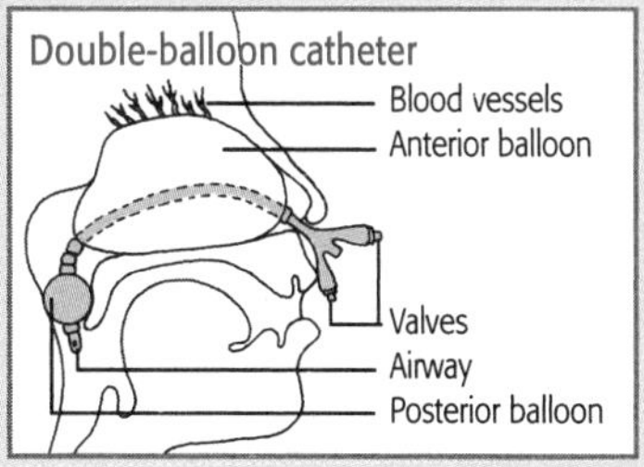

Assisting with insertion

To assist with inserting a single- or double-balloon catheter, prepare the patient as you would for nasal packing. Be sure to discuss the procedure thoroughly to alleviate the patient's anxiety and promote his cooperation.

Explain that the catheter tip will be lubricated with an antibiotic or a water-soluble lubricant to ease passage and prevent infection.

Providing routine care

The tip of the single-balloon catheter will be inserted in the nostrils until it reaches the posterior pharynx. Then the balloon will be inflated with normal saline solution, pulled gently into the posterior nasopharynx, and secured at the nostrils with the collapsible bulb. With a double-balloon catheter, the posterior balloon is inflated with normal saline solution; then the anterior balloon is inflated.

To check catheter placement, mark the catheter at the nasal vestibule; then inspect for that mark and observe the oropharynx for the posteriorly placed balloon. Assess the nostrils for irritation or erosion. Remove secretions by gently suctioning the airway of a double-balloon catheter or by dabbing away crusted external secretions if the patient has a catheter with no airway.

To prevent damage to nasal tissue, the physician may order the balloon be deflated for 10 minutes every 24 hours. If bleeding recurs or remains uncontrolled, reinflate the balloon and contact the physician, who may add packing.

Recognizing complications

The patient may report difficulty breathing, swallowing, or eating, and the nasal mucosa may sustain damage from pressure. Balloon deflation may dislodge clots and nasal debris into the oropharynx, which could prompt coughing, gagging, or vomiting.

Posterior packing

Two #14 or #16 French catheters with 30-cc balloon or two single- or double-chamber nasal balloon catheters ♦ marking pen

Assessment and bedside use

Tongue blades ♦ flashlight ♦ long hemostats or sponge forceps ♦ 60-ml syringe for deflating balloons (if applicable) ♦ if nasal tampons are in place: saline bullets for applying moisture and small flexible catheters for suctioning central breathing tube ♦ drip pad or moustache dressing supplies ♦ mouth care supplies ♦ water or artificial saliva ♦ external humidification

Preparation

- Wash your hands.
- Assemble all equipment at the patient's bedside.
- Label all medication on and off the sterile field.
- Make sure the headlamp works.
- Plug in the suction apparatus, and connect the tubing from the collection bottle to the suction source.
- Test the suction equipment to make sure it works properly.
- At the bedside, create a sterile field. (Use the sterile towels or the sterile tray.)
- Using sterile technique, place all sterile equipment on the sterile field.
- If the physician will inject a local anesthetic rather than spray it into the nose, place the 22G 1½" needle attached to the 10-ml syringe on the sterile field.
- When the physician readies the syringe, clean the stopper on the anesthetic vial, and hold the vial so he can withdraw the anesthetic. This practice allows the physician to avoid touching his sterile gloves to the nonsterile vial.
- Open the packages containing the sterile suction-connecting tubing and aspirating tip, and place them on the sterile field.
- Fill the sterile bowl with normal saline solution so that the suction tubing can be flushed as necessary.
- Thoroughly lubricate the anterior or posterior packing with antibiotic ointment.
- If the patient needs a nasal balloon catheter, test the balloon for leaks by inflating the catheter with normal saline solution. Remove the solution before insertion.

Key steps

- Make sure that all people caring for the patient wear gowns, gloves, and goggles during insertion of packing to prevent possible contamination from splattered blood.
- Check the patient's vital signs, and observe for hypotension with postural changes. Hypotension suggests significant blood loss. Also monitor airway patency because the patient will be at risk for aspirating or vomiting swallowed blood.
- Explain the procedure to the patient, and offer reassurance to reduce his anxiety and promote cooperation.
- If ordered, administer a sedative or tranquilizer to reduce the patient's anxiety and decrease sympathetic stimulation, which can exacerbate a nosebleed.
- Help the patient sit with his head tilted forward to minimize blood drainage into the throat and prevent aspiration.
- Turn on the suction apparatus and attach the connecting tubing so the physician can aspirate the nasal cavity to remove clots before locating the bleeding source.
- To inspect the nasal cavity, the physician will use a nasal speculum and an external light source or a fiber-optic nasal endoscope. To remove collected blood and help visualize the bleeding vessel, he will use suction or cotton-tipped applicators. The nose may be treated early with a topical vasoconstrictor such as phenylephrine (Neo-Synephrine) to slow bleeding and aid visualization.

Anterior nasal packing

- Help the physician apply topical vasoconstricting agents to control bleeding or to use chemical cautery with silver nitrate sticks.
- To enhance the vasoconstrictor's action, apply manual pressure to the nose for about 10 minutes.
- If bleeding persists, you may help insert an absorbable nasal pack directly on the bleeding site. The pack swells to form an artificial clot.

- If these methods fail, prepare to assist with electrocautery or insertion of anterior nasal packing. (Even if only one side is bleeding, both sides may require packing to control bleeding.)
- While the anterior pack is in place, use the cotton-tipped applicators to apply petroleum jelly to the patient's lips and nostrils to prevent drying and cracking.

Posterior nasal packing

- Wash your hands, and put on sterile gloves.
- If the physician identifies the bleeding source in the posterior nasal cavity, lubricate the soft catheters to ease insertion.
- Instruct the patient to open his mouth and to breathe normally through his mouth during catheter insertion to minimize gagging as the catheters pass through the nostril.
- Help the physician insert the packing as directed.
- Help the patient assume a comfortable position with his head elevated 45 to 90 degrees. Assess him for airway obstruction or any respiratory changes.
- Monitor the patient's vital signs regularly to detect changes that may indicate hypovolemia or hypoxemia.

Special considerations

- Patients with posterior packing are usually hospitalized for monitoring. If mucosal oozing persists, apply a moustache dressing by securing a folded gauze pad over the nasal vestibules with tape or a commercial nasal dressing holder. Change the pad when soiled.
- Test the patient's call bell to make sure he can summon help if needed.

ACTION STAT!

Keep emergency equipment (flashlight, tongue blade, syringe, and hemostats) at the patient's bedside to speed packing removal if it becomes displaced and occludes the airway.

- Once the packing is in place, compile assessment data carefully to help detect the underlying cause of nosebleeds. Mechanical factors include a deviated septum, injury, and a foreign body. Environmental factors include drying and erosion of the nasal mucosa. Other possible causes are upper respiratory tract infection, anticoagulant or salicylate therapy, blood dyscrasias, cardiovascular or hepatic disorders, tumors of the nasal cavity or paranasal sinuses, chronic nephritis, and familial hemorrhagic telangiectasia.
- If significant blood loss occurs or if the underlying cause remains unknown, expect the physician to order a complete blood count and coagulation profile as soon as possible. Blood transfusion may be necessary. After the procedure, the physician may order arterial blood gas analysis to detect any pulmonary complications and arterial oxygen saturation monitoring to assess for hypoxemia. If necessary, prepare to administer supplemental humidified oxygen with a face mask and to give antibiotics and decongestants as ordered.
- Because a patient with nasal packing must breathe through his mouth, provide thorough mouth care often. Artificial saliva, room humidification, and ample fluid intake also relieve dryness caused by mouth breathing.
- Until the pack is removed, the patient should be on modified bed rest. As ordered, administer moderate doses of nonaspirin analgesics, decongestants, and sedatives along with prophylactic antibiotics to prevent sinusitis or related infections.
- Nasal packing is usually removed in 2 to 5 days. After an anterior pack is removed, instruct the patient to avoid rubbing or picking his nose, inserting any object into his nose, and blowing his nose forcefully for 48 hours or as ordered.

Complications

- Hypoxemia
- Aspiration of blood in patients with posterior packing
- Exacerbation of underlying pulmonary conditions
- Airway obstruction
- Otitis media
- Hematotympanum and pressure necrosis of nasal structures, especially the septum

- Hypotension in the patient with significant blood loss, increasing the risk of aspiration and hypoxemia, caused by sedation

Patient teaching

- Tell the patient to expect reduced ability to detect smell and taste. Make sure he has a working smoke detector at home.
- Advise him to eat soft foods because his eating and swallowing abilities will be impaired.
- Instruct him to drink fluids often or to use artificial saliva to cope with dry mouth.
- Teach him measures to prevent nosebleeds, and instruct him to seek medical help if these measures fail to stop bleeding.

Documentation

Record the type of pack used to ensure its removal at the appropriate time. On the intake and output record, document the estimated blood loss and all fluid administered. Note the patient's vital signs, his response to sedation or position changes, the results of any laboratory tests, and any drugs administered, including topical agents. Record any complications. Document discharge instructions and clinical follow-up plans.

Nasoenteric-decompression tube care

The patient with a nasoenteric-decompression tube needs special care and continuous monitoring to ensure tube patency, to maintain suction and bowel decompression, and to detect such complications as fluid-electrolyte imbalances related to aspiration of intestinal contents. Precise intake and output records are an integral part of the patient's care. Frequent mouth and nose care is also essential to provide comfort and to prevent skin breakdown. Finally, a patient with a nasoenteric-decompression tube will need encouragement and support during insertion and removal of the tube and while the tube is in place.

Equipment

Suction apparatus with intermittent suction capability (stationary or portable unit) ♦ container of water ♦ intake and output record sheets ♦ mouthwash and water mixture ♦ petroleum jelly or water-soluble lubricant ♦ cotton-tipped applicators ♦ safety pin ♦ tape or rubber band ♦ disposable irrigation set ♦ irrigant ♦ labels for tube lumens ♦ optional: throat comfort measures, such as gargle, viscous lidocaine, throat lozenges, ice collar, sour hard candy, or gum

Preparation

- Assemble the suction apparatus and set up the suction unit.
- If indicated, test the unit by turning it on and placing the end of the suction tubing in a container of water. If the tubing draws in water, the unit works.

Key steps

- Explain to the patient and his family the purpose of the procedure. Answer questions clearly and thoroughly to ease anxiety and enhance cooperation.
- After tube insertion, have the patient lie quietly on his right side for about 2 hours to promote the tube's passage. After the tube advances past the pylorus, his activity level may increase, as ordered.
- After the tube advances to the desired position, coil the excess external tubing and secure it to the patient's gown or bed linens with a safety pin attached to tape or a rubber band looped around it. This prevents kinks in the tubing, which would interrupt suction. Once in the desired location, the tube may be taped to the patient's face.
- Maintain slack in the tubing so the patient can move comfortably and safely in bed. Show him how far he can move without dislodging the tube.
- After securing the tube, connect it to the tubing on the suction machine to begin decompression.

DEVICE SAFETY

Check the suction machine at least every 2 hours to confirm proper functioning and to ensure tube patency and bowel decompression. Excessive negative pressure may draw the mucosa into the tube openings, impair the suction's effectiveness, and injure the mucosa. By using intermittent suction, you may avoid these problems. To check functioning in an intermittent suction unit, look for drainage in the connecting tube and dripping into the collecting container.

- Empty the container every 8 hours and measure the contents.
- After decompression and before extubation, as ordered, provide a clear-to-full liquid diet to assess bowel function.
- Record intake and output accurately to monitor fluid balance. If you irrigate the tube, its length may prohibit aspiration of the irrigant, so record the amount of instilled irrigant as "intake." Typically, normal saline solution supersedes water as the preferred irrigant because water, which is hypotonic, may increase electrolyte loss through osmotic action, especially if you irrigate the tube often.
- Observe the patient for signs and symptoms of disorders related to suctioning and intubation. Signs and symptoms of dehydration, a fluid-volume deficit, or a fluid-electrolyte imbalance include dry skin and mucous membranes, decreased urine output, lethargy, exhaustion, and fever.
- Watch for signs and symptoms of pneumonia related to the patient's inability to clear his pharynx or cough effectively with a tube in place. Be alert for fever, chest pain, tachypnea or labored breathing, and diminished breath sounds over the affected area.
- Observe drainage characteristics: color, amount, consistency, odor, and any unusual changes.
- Provide mouth care frequently (at least every 4 hours) to increase the patient's comfort and promote a healthy oral cavity. If the tube remains in place for several days, mouth-breathing will leave the lips, tongue, and other tissues dry and cracked.
- Encourage the patient to brush his teeth or rinse his mouth with the mouthwash and water mixture.
- Lubricate the patient's lips with petroleum jelly applied with a cotton-tipped applicator.
- At least every 4 hours, gently clean and lubricate the patient's external nostrils with either petroleum jelly or water-soluble lubricant on a cotton-tipped applicator to prevent skin breakdown.
- Watch for peristalsis to resume, signaled by bowel sounds, passage of flatus, decreased abdominal distention, and possibly, a spontaneous bowel movement. These signs may require tube removal.

Special considerations

- If the suction machine works improperly, replace it immediately. If the machine works properly but no drainage accumulates in the collection container, suspect an obstruction in the tube.
- As ordered, irrigate the tube with the irrigation set to clear the obstruction. (See *Clearing a nasoenteric-decompression tube obstruction,* page 314.)
- If your patient is ambulatory and his tube connects to a portable suction unit, he may move short distances while connected to the unit. Or, if feasible and ordered, the tube can be disconnected and clamped briefly while he moves around.
- If the tubing irritates the patient's throat or makes him hoarse, offer relief with mouthwash, gargles, viscous lidocaine, throat lozenges, an ice collar, sour hard candy, or gum, as appropriate.
- Make sure the tube isn't pressing on the nostril to prevent skin breakdown.
- If the tip of the balloon falls below the ileocecal valve (confirmed by X-ray), the tube can't be removed nasally. Rather, it has to be advanced and removed through the anus.
- If the balloon at the end of the tube protrudes from the anus, notify the practitioner. Most likely, the tube can be disconnected from suction, the proximal end severed, and the remaining tube removed gradually through the anus either manually or by peristalsis.

DO'S & DON'TS

Clearing a nasoenteric-decompression tube obstruction

If your patient's nasoenteric-decompression tube appears to be obstructed, notify the practitioner right away. He may order the following measures to restore patency quickly and efficiently:

- First, disconnect the tube from the suction source and irrigate with normal saline solution. Use gravity flow to help clear the obstruction unless ordered otherwise.
- If irrigation doesn't reestablish patency, the tube may be obstructed by its position against the gastric mucosa. To rectify this, tug slightly on the tube to move it away from the mucosa.
- If gentle tugging doesn't restore patency, the tube may be kinked and may need additional manipulation. Before proceeding, though, take these precautions:
  - Never reposition or irrigate a nasoenteric-decompression tube (without a practitioner's order) in the patient who has had GI surgery.
  - Avoid manipulating a tube in a patient who had the tube inserted during surgery. To do so may disturb new sutures.
  - Don't try to reposition a tube in a patient who was difficult to intubate (because of an esophageal stricture, for example).

Complications

- Fluid volume deficit, electrolyte imbalance, and pneumonia

Documentation

Record the frequency and type of mouth and nose care provided. Describe the therapeutic effect, if any. Document in your notes the amount, color, consistency, and odor of the drainage obtained each time you empty the collection container.

Record the amount of drainage on the intake and output sheet. Always document the amount of any irrigant or other fluid introduced through the tube or taken orally by the patient.

If the suction machine malfunctions, note the length of time it wasn't functioning and the nursing action taken. Document the amount and character of any vomitus. Also note the patient's tolerance of the tube's insertion and removal.

Nasoenteric-decompression tube insertion and removal

The nasoenteric-decompression tube is inserted nasally and advanced beyond the stomach into the intestinal tract. It's used to aspirate intestinal contents for analysis and to treat intestinal obstruction. The tube may also help to prevent nausea, vomiting, and abdominal distention after GI surgery. A physician will usually insert or remove a nasoenteric-decompression tube, but sometimes a nurse will remove it.

The nasoenteric-decompression tube may have a preweighted tip and a balloon at one end of the tube that holds air or water to stimulate peristalsis and facilitate the tube's passage through the pylorus and into the intestinal tract. (See *Common types of nasoenteric-decompression tubes.*)

Equipment

Sterile 10-ml syringe ♦ 21G needle ♦ nasoenteric-decompression tube ♦ container of water ♦ 5 to 10 ml of water, as ordered ♦ suction-decompression equipment ♦ gloves ♦ towel or linen-saver pad ♦ water-soluble lubricant ♦ 4″ × 4″ gauze pad ♦ ½″ hypoallergenic tape ♦ bulb syringe or 60-ml catheter-tip syringe ♦ rubber band ♦ safety pin ♦ clamp ♦ specimen container ♦ basin of ice or warm water ♦ penlight ♦ waterproof marking pen ♦ glass of water with straw ♦ optional: ice chips, local anesthetic

Common types of nasoenteric-decompression tubes

The type of nasoenteric-decompression tube chosen for your patient will depend on the size of the patient and his nostrils, the estimated duration of intubation, and the reason for the procedure. For example, to remove viscous material from the patient's intestinal tract, the practitioner may select a tube with a wide bore and a single lumen.

Whichever tube you use, you'll need to provide good mouth care and check the patient's nostrils often for signs of irritation. If you see any signs of irritation, retape the tube so that it doesn't cause tension, and then lubricate the nostril. Or check with the practitioner to see if the tube can be inserted through the other nostril.

Most tubes are impregnated with a radiopaque mark so that placement can easily be confirmed by X-ray or other imaging technique. Tubes, such as the preweighted Andersen Miller-Abbot type intestinal tube (shown below), have a tungsten-weighted inflatable latex balloon tip designed for temporary management of mechanical obstruction in the small or large intestines.

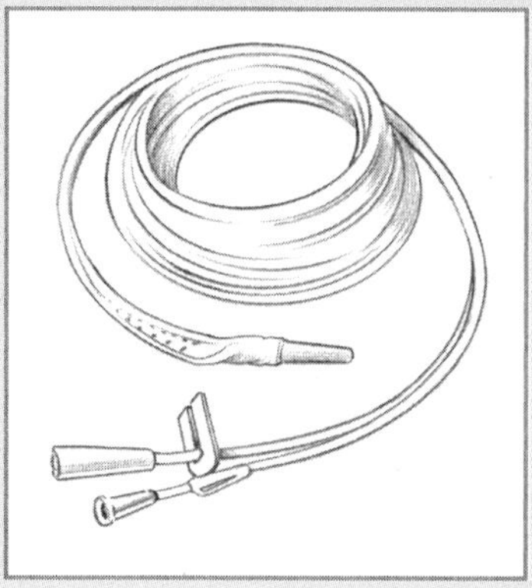

Preparation

- Stiffen a flaccid tube by chilling it in a basin of ice to facilitate insertion. To make a stiff tube flexible, dip it into warm water.
- Air or water is added to the balloon either before or after insertion of the tube, depending on the type of tube used. Follow the manufacturer's recommendations.
- Set up suction-decompression equipment, if ordered, and make sure it works properly.

Key steps

- Confirm the patient's identity using two patient identifiers according to facility policy.
- Explain the procedure to the patient, forewarning him that he may experience some discomfort. Provide privacy and adequate lighting. Wash your hands and put on gloves.
- Position the patient as the physician specifies, usually in semi-Fowler's or high Fowler's position. You may also need to help the patient hold his neck in a hyperextended position.
- Protect the patient's chest with a linen-saver pad or towel.
- Agree with the patient on a signal that can be used to stop the insertion briefly if necessary.

Assisting with insertion

- The physician assesses the patency of the patient's nostrils. To evaluate which nostril has better airflow in a conscious patient, he holds one nostril closed and then the other as the patient breathes. In an unconscious patient, he examines each nostril with a penlight to check for polyps, a deviated septum, or other obstruction.
- To decide how far the tube must be inserted to reach the stomach, the physician places the tube's distal end at the tip of the patient's nose and then extends the tube to the earlobe and down to the xiphoid process. He either marks the tube with a waterproof marking pen or holds it at this point.
- The physician applies water-soluble lubricant to the first few inches of the tube

to reduce friction and tissue trauma and to facilitate insertion.

- If the balloon already contains water, the physician holds it so the fluid runs to the bottom. Then he pinches the balloon closed to retain the fluid as the insertion begins.
- Tell the patient to breathe through his mouth or to pant as the balloon enters his nostril. After the balloon begins its descent, the physician releases his grip on it, allowing the weight of the fluid or the preweighted tip to pull the tube into the nasopharynx. When the tube reaches the nasopharynx, the physician instructs the patient to lower his chin and to swallow. In some cases, the patient may sip water through a straw to facilitate swallowing as the tube advances, but not after the tube reaches the trachea. This prevents injury from aspiration. The physician continues to advance the tube slowly to prevent it from curling or kinking in the stomach.
- To confirm the tube's passage into the stomach, the physician aspirates stomach contents with a bulb syringe.
- To keep the tube out of the patient's eyes and to help avoid undue skin irritation, fold a 4″ × 4″ gauze pad in half and tape it to the patient's forehead with the fold directed toward the patient's nose. The physician can slide the tube through this sling, leaving enough slack for the tube to advance.
- Position the patient as directed to help advance the tube. He'll typically lie on his right side until the tube clears the pylorus (about 2 hours). The physician will confirm passage by X-ray.
- After the tube clears the pylorus, the physician may direct you to advance it 2″ to 3″ (5 to 7.5 cm) every hour and to reposition the patient until the premeasured mark reaches the patient's nostril. Gravity and peristalsis will help advance the tube. (Notify the physician if you can't advance the tube.)
- Keep the remaining premeasured length of tube well lubricated to ease passage and prevent irritation.

DO'S & DON'TS

Don't tape the tube while it advances to the premeasured mark unless the physician asks you to do so.

- After the tube progresses the necessary distance, the physician will order an X-ray to confirm tube positioning. When the tube is in place, secure the external tubing with tape to help prevent further progression.
- Loop a rubber band around the tube and pin the rubber band to the patient's gown with a safety pin.
- If ordered, attach the tube to intermittent suction.

Removing the tube

- Assist the patient into semi-Fowler's or high Fowler's position. Drape a linen-saver pad or towel across the patient's chest.
- Wash your hands and put on gloves.
- Clamp the tube and disconnect it from the suction. This prevents the patient from aspirating any gastric contents that leak from the tube during withdrawal.
- If your patient has a tube with an inflated balloon tip, attach a 10-ml syringe to the balloon port and withdraw the air or water.
- Slowly withdraw between 6″ and 8″ (15 and 20 cm) of the tube. Wait 10 minutes and withdraw another 6″ to 8″. Wait another 10 minutes. Continue this procedure until the tube reaches the patient's esophagus (with 18″ [46 cm] of the tube remaining inside the patient). At this point, you can gently withdraw the tube completely.

Special considerations

- For a double- or triple-lumen tube, note which lumen accommodates balloon inflation and which accommodates drainage.
- Apply a local anesthetic, if ordered, to the nostril or the back of the throat to dull sensations and the gag reflex for intubation. Letting the patient gargle with a liquid anesthetic or holding ice chips in his mouth for a few minutes serves the same purpose.

Complications

- Reflux esophagitis, nasal or oral inflammation, and nasal, laryngeal, or esophageal ulceration

Documentation

Record the date and time the nasoenteric-decompression tube was inserted and by whom. Note the patient's tolerance of the procedure; the type of tube used; the suction type and amount; and the color, amount, and consistency of drainage. Also note the date, time, and name of the person removing the tube and the patient's tolerance of the removal procedure.

Nasogastric tube care

A nasogastric (NG) tube is indicated for feeding or administering drugs and other oral agents. Providing effective NG tube care requires meticulous monitoring of the patient and the equipment. Monitoring the patient involves checking drainage from the NG tube and assessing GI function. Monitoring the equipment involves verifying correct tube placement and irrigating the tube to ensure patency and to prevent mucosal damage.

Specific care varies only slightly for the most commonly used NG tubes: the single-lumen Levin tube and the double-lumen Salem sump tube.

Equipment

Irrigant (usually normal saline solution) ♦ irrigant container ♦ 60-ml catheter-tip syringe ♦ bulb syringe ♦ suction equipment ♦ sponge-tipped swabs, or toothbrush and toothpaste ♦ petroleum jelly ♦ ½″ or 1″ hypoallergenic tape ♦ water-soluble lubricant ♦ gloves ♦ pH test strip ♦ linen-saver pad ♦ optional: emesis basin

Preparation

- Make sure the suction equipment works properly.
- When using a Salem sump tube with suction, connect the larger, primary lumen (for drainage and suction) to the suction equipment and select the appropriate setting, as ordered (usually low, constant suction).
- If the practitioner doesn't specify the setting, follow the manufacturer's directions.
- A Levin tube usually calls for intermittent low suction.

Key steps

- Confirm the patient's identity using two patient identifiers according to facility policy.
- Explain the procedure to the patient and provide privacy.
- Wash your hands, and put on gloves.

Irrigating an NG tube

- Review the irrigation schedule (usually every 4 hours), if the practitioner orders this procedure.
- Assess tube placement by looking for discrepancies in tube markings or by measuring the external tube length and comparing it with the length documented in the chart. Have the patient open his mouth so that you can check to see if the tube is coiled.
- Aspirate stomach contents to check correct positioning in the stomach and to prevent the patient from aspirating the irrigant.
- Examine the aspirate and place a small amount on the pH test strip. The probability of gastric placement is increased if the aspirate has a typical gastric fluid appearance (grassy-green, clear and colorless with mucus shreds, or brown with a pH of less than or equal to 5.0).
- If the tube is used for gastric suction, the aspirate will be green or clear and colorless with off-white or tan mucus.
- Measure the amount of irrigant in the bulb syringe or in the 60-ml catheter-tip syringe (usually 10 to 20 ml) to maintain an accurate intake and output record.
- When using suction with a Salem sump tube or a Levin tube, unclamp and disconnect the tube from the suction equipment while holding it over a linen-saver pad or an emesis basin to collect any drainage.
- Slowly instill the irrigant into the NG tube. (When irrigating the Salem sump tube, you may instill small amounts of solution into the vent lumen without interrupting suction; however, you should in-

still greater amounts into the larger, primary lumen.)

- Gently aspirate the solution with the bulb syringe or 60-ml catheter-tip syringe or connect the tube to the suction equipment, as ordered. Gentle aspiration prevents excessive pressure on a suture line and on delicate gastric mucosa. Report any bleeding.
- Reconnect the tube to suction after completing irrigation.

Instilling solution through an NG tube

DO'S & DON'TS

If the practitioner orders instillation, inject the solution, and don't aspirate it.

- Note the amount of instilled solution as "intake" on the intake and output record.
- Reattach the tube to suction as ordered.
- After attaching the Salem sump tube's primary lumen to suction, instill 10 to 20 cc of air into the vent lumen to verify patency. Listen for a soft hiss in the vent. If you don't hear this sound, suspect a clogged tube; recheck patency by instilling 10 ml of normal saline solution and 10 to 20 cc of air in the vent.

Monitoring patient comfort and condition

- Provide mouth care once per shift or as needed. Depending on the patient's condition, use sponge-tipped swabs to clean his teeth or help him to brush them with toothbrush and toothpaste. Coat the patient's lips with petroleum jelly to prevent dryness caused by mouth breathing.
- Change the tape securing the tube as needed or at least daily. Clean the skin, apply fresh tape, and dab water-soluble lubricant on the nostrils as needed.
- Regularly check the tape that secures the tube because sweat and nasal secretions may loosen the tape.
- Assess bowel sounds regularly (every 4 to 8 hours) to verify GI function.
- Measure the drainage amount and update the intake and output record every 8 hours. Be alert for electrolyte imbalances with excessive gastric output.
- Inspect gastric drainage and note its color, consistency, odor, and amount. Normal gastric secretions have no color or appear yellow-green from bile and have a mucoid consistency. Immediately report any drainage with a coffee-bean color because it may indicate bleeding. If you suspect that the drainage contains blood, use a screening test (such as Hematest) for occult blood according to facility policy.

Special considerations

- Irrigate the NG tube with 30 ml of irrigant before and after instilling medication. Wait about 30 minutes, or as ordered, after instillation before reconnecting the suction equipment to allow sufficient time for the medication to be absorbed.
- When no drainage appears, check the suction equipment for proper function. Then, holding the NG tube over a linen-saver pad or an emesis basin, separate the tube and the suction source. Check the suction equipment by placing the suction tubing in an irrigant container. If the apparatus draws the water, check the NG tube for proper function. Be sure to note the amount of water drawn into the suction container on the intake and output record.
- A dysfunctional NG tube may be clogged or incorrectly positioned. Attempt to irrigate the tube, reposition the patient, or rotate and reposition the tube. However, if the tube was inserted during surgery, avoid this maneuver to ensure that the movement doesn't interfere with gastric or esophageal sutures. Notify the practitioner.
- If you can ambulate the patient and interrupt suction, disconnect the NG tube from the suction equipment. Clamp the tube to prevent stomach contents from draining out of the tube.
- If the patient has a Salem sump tube, watch for gastric reflux in the vent lumen when pressure in the stomach exceeds atmospheric pressure. This problem may result from a clogged primary lumen or from a suction system that's set up improperly. Assess the suction equipment for proper functioning. Then irrigate the NG tube and instill 30 cc of air into the vent tube to maintain patency. Don't attempt to stop reflux by clamping the vent tube. Unless

contraindicated, elevate the patient's torso more than 30 degrees, and keep the vent tube above his midline to prevent a siphoning effect.

Complications

- Epigastric pain and vomiting
- Hemorrhage
- Perforation
- Dehydration and electrolyte imbalances
- Pain, swelling, and salivary dysfunction signaling parotitis
- Nasal skin breakdown and discomfort and increased mucus secretions
- Aspiration pneumonia
- Gastric mucosa damage

Patient teaching

- If possible, teach the patient who requires long-term treatment how to administer feedings himself through the NG tube. Have him observe the procedure several times before trying it himself.
- Remain with the patient when he performs the procedure for the first few times so that you can provide assistance and answer any questions. Encourage him and correct any errors in technique, as necessary.

Documentation

Regularly record tube placement confirmation (usually every 4 to 8 hours). Keep a precise record of fluid intake and output, including the instilled irrigant in fluid input. Track the irrigation schedule and note the actual time of each irrigation. Describe drainage color, consistency, odor, and amount. Note tape change times and condition of the nares.

Nasogastric tube drug instillation

Besides providing an alternate means of nourishment, a nasogastric (NG) tube or gastrostomy tube allows direct instillation of medication into the GI system of patients who can't ingest the drug orally. Before instillation, the patency and positioning of the tube must be carefully checked because the procedure is contraindicated if the tube is obstructed or improperly positioned; if the patient is vomiting around the tube; or if his bowel sounds are absent.

Oily medications and enteric-coated or sustained-release tablets or capsules are contraindicated for instillation through an NG tube. Oily medications cling to the sides of the tube and resist mixing with the irrigating solution, and crushing enteric-coated or sustained-release tablets to facilitate transport through the tube destroys their intended properties.

Equipment

Patient's medication record and chart ♦ prescribed medication ♦ towel or linen-saver pad ♦ 50- or 60-ml piston-type catheter-tip syringe ♦ feeding tubing ♦ two 4″ × 4″ gauze pads ♦ pH test strip ♦ gloves ♦ diluent ♦ cup for mixing medication and fluid ♦ spoon ♦ 50 ml of water ♦ rubber band ♦ gastrostomy tube and funnel, if needed ♦ optional: mortar and pestle, clamp

For maximum control of suction, use a piston syringe instead of a bulb syringe. The liquid for diluting the medication can be juice, water, or a nutritional supplement.

Preparation

- Gather equipment for use at the bedside.
- Liquids should be at room temperature. Administering cold liquids through an NG tube can cause abdominal cramping.
- Although this isn't a sterile procedure, make sure the cup, syringe, spoon, and gauze are clean.

Key steps

- Confirm the patient's identity using two patient identifiers according to facility policy.
- Verify the order on the patient's medication record by checking it against the practitioner's order.
- Wash your hands and put on gloves.
- Check the label on the medication three times before preparing it for administration to make sure you'll be giving the medication correctly.
- If your facility utilizes a bar code scanning system, be sure to scan your ID

Giving medications through an NG tube

Holding the nasogastric (NG) tube at a level somewhat above the patient's nose, pour up to 30 ml of diluted medication into the syringe barrel. To prevent air from entering the patient's stomach, hold the tube at a slight angle and add more medication before the syringe empties. If necessary, raise the tube slightly higher to increase the flow rate.

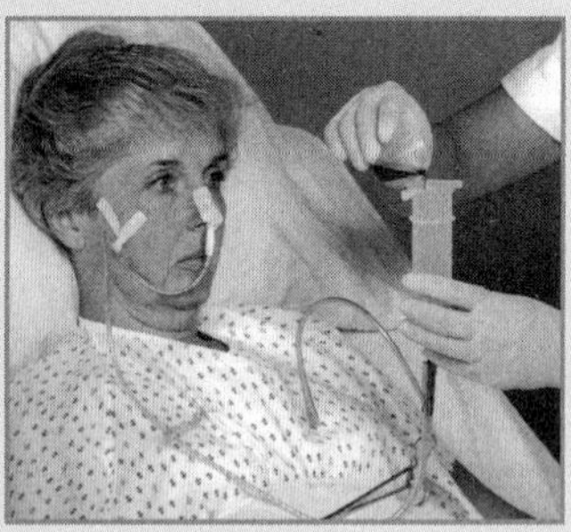

After you've delivered the whole dose, position the patient on her right side, head slightly elevated, to minimize esophageal reflux.

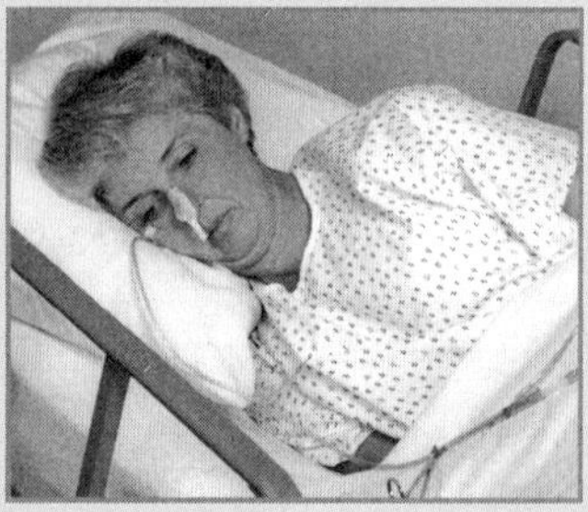

badge, the patient's ID bracelet, and the medication's bar code.

- If the prescribed medication is in tablet form, crush the tablets to ready them for mixing in a cup with the diluting liquid. Request liquid forms of medications, if available. Bring the medication and equipment to the patient's bedside.
- Explain the procedure to the patient; provide privacy.
- Unpin the tube from the patient's gown. To avoid soiling the sheets, fold back the bed linens to the patient's waist and drape his chest with a towel or linen-saver pad.
- Elevate the head of the bed so that the patient is in Fowler's position, as tolerated.
- After unclamping the tube, take the 50- or 60-ml syringe and attach it to the end of the tube.
- Aspirate stomach contents and place a small amount on a pH test strip. Probability of gastric placement is increased if aspirate has a typical gastric fluid appearance (grassy-green, clear and colorless with mucus shreds, or brown) and pH is ≤ 5.0. If no gastric contents appear when you draw back on the syringe, the tube may have risen into the esophagus, and you'll have to advance it before proceeding.
- If you meet resistance when aspirating for gastric contents, stop the procedure. Resistance may indicate a nonpatent tube or improper tube placement. (Keep in mind that some smaller NG tubes may collapse when aspiration is attempted.) If the tube seems to be in the stomach, resistance probably means that the tube is lying against the stomach wall. To relieve resistance, withdraw the tube slightly or turn the patient.
- After you have established that the tube is patent and in the correct position, clamp the tube, detach the syringe, and lay the end of the tube on the 4″ × 4″ gauze pad.
- Mix the crushed tablets or liquid medication with the diluent. If the medication is in capsule form, open the capsules and empty their contents into the liquid. Pour liquid medications directly into the diluent. Stir well. (If the medication was in tablet form, make sure the particles are small enough to pass through the eyes at the distal end of the tube.)
- Reattach the syringe, without the piston, to the end of the tube and open the clamp.
- Deliver the medication slowly and steadily. (See *Giving medications through an NG tube*.)
- If the medication flows smoothly, slowly add more until the entire dose has been given.

Giving medications through a gastrostomy tube

Surgically inserted into the stomach, a gastrostomy tube reduces the risk of fluid aspiration, a constant danger with a nasogastric (NG) tube. To administer medication by this route, prepare the patient and medication as for an NG tube. Then gently lift the dressing around the tube to assess the skin for irritation. Report any irritation to the practitioner. If none appears, follow these steps:

- Remove the dressing that covers the tube. Then remove the dressing or plug at the tip of the tube, and attach the syringe or funnel to the tip.
- Release the clamp and instill about 10 ml of water into the tube through the syringe. If the water flows in easily, the tube is patent. If it flows in slowly, raise the funnel to increase pressure. If the water still doesn't flow properly, stop the procedure and notify the practitioner.

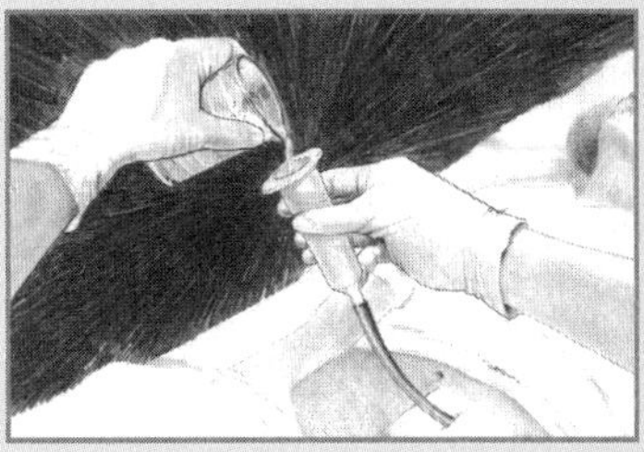

- Pour up to 30 ml of medication into the syringe or funnel. Tilt the tube to allow air to escape as the fluid flows downward. Just before the syringe empties, add medication as needed.
- After giving the medication, pour in about 30 ml of water to irrigate the tube.
- Tighten the clamp, place a 4" × 4" gauze pad on the end of the tube, and secure it with a rubber band.
- Cover the tube with two more 4" × 4" gauze pads, and secure them firmly with tape.
- Keep the head of the bed elevated for at least 30 minutes after the procedure to aid digestion.

Do's & don'ts

If the medication doesn't flow properly, don't force it. If it's too thick, dilute it with water. If you suspect that tube placement is inhibiting the flow, stop the procedure and reevaluate tube placement.

- Watch the patient's reaction throughout the instillation. If he shows any sign of discomfort, stop the procedure immediately.
- As the last of the medication flows out of the syringe, start to irrigate the tube by adding 30 to 50 ml of water. Irrigation clears medication from the sides of the tube and from the distal end, reducing the risk of clogging.
- For a child, irrigate the tube using only 15 to 30 ml of water.
- When the water stops flowing, quickly clamp the tube. Detach the syringe and dispose of it.
- Fasten the NG tube to the patient's gown.
- Remove the towel or linen-saver pad and replace bed linens.
- Leave the patient in Fowler's position, or have him lie on his right side with the head of the bed partially elevated. Tell him to maintain this position for at least 30 minutes after the procedure. This position facilitates the downward flow of medication into his stomach and prevents esophageal reflux.
- You may be asked to deliver medications through a gastrostomy tube. (See *Giving medications through a gastrostomy tube.*)
- If medication is prescribed for a patient with a gastrostomy feeding button, ask the practitioner to order the liquid form of the drug if possible. If not, you may give a

tablet or capsule dissolved in 30 to 50 ml of warm water (15 to 30 ml for children). To administer medication this way, use the same procedure as for feeding the patient through the button. (See "Gastrostomy feeding button care," page 221.) Then draw up the dissolved medication into a syringe and inject it into the feeding tube.

- Withdraw the medication syringe, and flush the tube with 50 ml of warm water.
- Flush the tube with 30 ml of water for a child.
- Then replace the safety plug, and keep the patient upright at a 30-degree angle for 30 minutes after giving the medication.

Special considerations

DO'S & DON'TS

To prevent instillation of too much fluid (for an adult, more than 400 ml of liquid at one time), don't schedule the drug instillation with the patient's regular tube feeding, if possible.

- If you must schedule a tube feeding and medication instillation simultaneously, give the medication first to ensure that the patient receives the prescribed drug therapy even if he can't tolerate an entire feeding. Remember to avoid giving foods that interact adversely with the drug. Tube feedings of Osmolite or Isocal must be held 2 hours before and 2 hours after phenytoin administration.
- If the patient receives continuous tube feedings, stop the feeding and check the quantity of residual stomach contents. If it's more than 50% of the previous hour's intake, withhold the medication and feeding and notify the practitioner. An excessive amount of residual contents may indicate intestinal obstruction or paralytic ileus.
- If the NG tube is attached to suction, be sure to turn off the suction for 20 to 30 minutes after administering medication.

Complications

- None known

Patient teaching

- If possible, teach the patient who requires long-term treatment to instill his medication himself through the NG tube. Have him observe the procedure several times before trying it himself.
- Remain with the patient when he performs the procedure for the first few times so that you can provide assistance and answer any questions. Encourage him and correct any errors in technique, as necessary.

Documentation

Record the instillation of medication, date and time of instillation, dose, and patient's tolerance of the procedure. On his intake and output sheet, note the amount of fluid instilled. Document patient teaching that was done.

Nasogastric tube insertion and removal

Usually inserted to decompress the stomach, a nasogastric (NG) tube can prevent vomiting after major surgery. An NG tube is typically in place for 48 to 72 hours after surgery, by which time peristalsis usually resumes. It may remain in place for shorter or longer periods, however, depending on its use.

The NG tube has other diagnostic and therapeutic applications, especially in assessing and treating upper GI bleeding, collecting gastric contents for analysis, performing gastric lavage, aspirating gastric secretions, and administering medications and nutrients.

Inserting an NG tube requires close observation of the patient and verification of proper placement. Removing the tube requires careful handling to prevent injury or aspiration. The tube must be inserted with extra care in a pregnant patient and in one with an increased risk of complications. For example, the practitioner will order an NG tube for a patient with aortic aneurysm, myocardial infarction, gastric hemorrhage, or esophageal varices only if he believes that the benefits outweigh the risks of intubation.

Types of NG tubes

The practitioner will choose the type and diameter of nasogastric (NG) tube that best suits the patient's needs, including lavage, aspiration, enteral therapy, or stomach decompression. Choices may include the Levin, Salem sump, and Moss tubes.

Levin tube

The Levin tube is a rubber or plastic tube that has a single lumen, a length of 42″ to 50″ (107 to 127 cm), and holes at the tip and along the side.

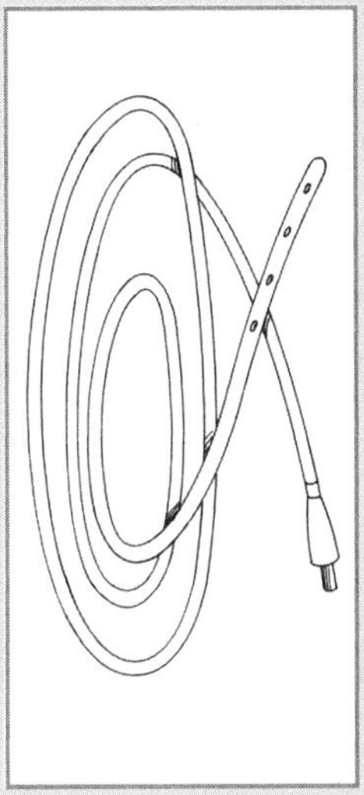

Salem sump tube

The Salem sump tube is a double-lumen tube made of clear plastic and has a blue sump port (pigtail) that allows atmospheric air to enter the patient's stomach. Thus, the tube floats freely and doesn't adhere to or damage gastric mucosa. The larger port of this 48″ (122-cm) tube serves as the main suction conduit. The tube has openings at 17.7″ (45 cm), 21.7″ (55 cm), 25.6″ (65 cm), and 29.5″ (75 cm) as well as a radiopaque line to verify placement.

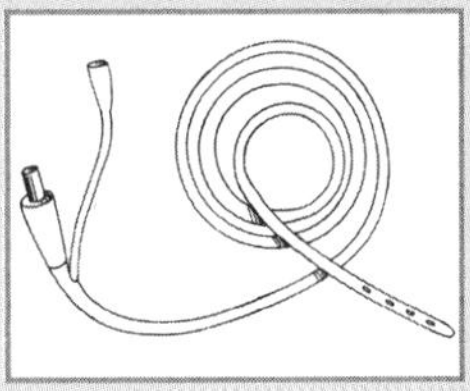

Moss tube

The Moss tube has a radiopaque tip and three lumens. The first, positioned and inflated in the cardia, serves as a balloon inflation port. The second is an esophageal aspiration port. The third is a duodenal feeding port.

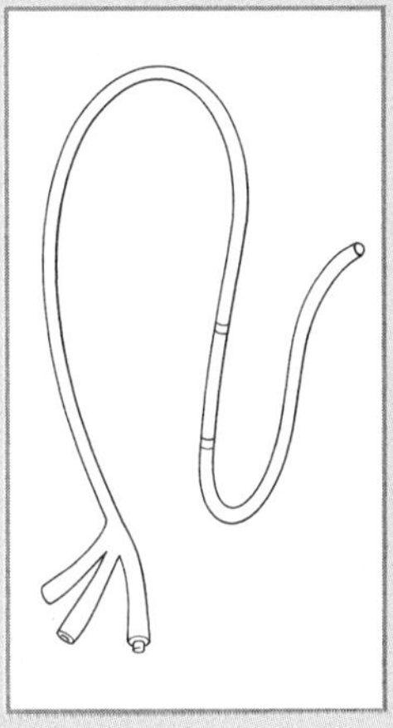

Most NG tubes have a radiopaque marker or strip at the distal end so that tube position can be verified by X-ray. If the position can't be confirmed, the practitioner may order fluoroscopy to verify placement.

The most common NG tubes are the Levin tube, which has one lumen, and the Salem sump tube, which has two lumens, one for suction and drainage and a smaller one for ventilation. Air flows through the vent lumen continuously. This protects the delicate gastric mucosa by preventing a vacuum from forming should the tube adhere to the stomach lining. The Moss tube, which has a triple lumen, is usually inserted during surgery. (See *Types of NG tubes*.)

Equipment

Insertion of NG tube

Tube (usually #12, #14, #16, or #18 French for a normal adult) ♦ towel or linen-saver pad ♦ facial tissues ♦ emesis basin ♦ penlight ♦ 1″ or 2″ hypoallergenic tape ♦ gloves ♦ water-soluble lubricant ♦ cup or glass of water with straw (if appropriate) ♦ pH test strip ♦ tongue blade ♦ catheter-tip or bulb syringe or irrigation set ♦ safety pin ♦ ordered suction equipment ♦ optional: metal clamp, alcohol pad, warm water, large basin or plastic container, rubber band

Removal of NG tube

Gloves ♦ catheter-tip syringe ♦ normal saline solution ♦ towel or linen-saver pad ♦ adhesive remover ♦ facial tissues ♦ optional: clamp

Preparation

- Inspect the NG tube for defects, such as rough edges or partially closed lumens.
- Then check the tube's patency by flushing it with water.
- To ease insertion, increase a stiff tube's flexibility by coiling it around your gloved fingers for a few seconds or by dipping it into warm water. Stiffen a limp rubber tube by briefly chilling it in ice.

Key steps

- Whether you're inserting or removing an NG tube, be sure to provide privacy, wash your hands, and put on gloves before inserting the tube. Check the practitioner's order to determine the type of tube that should be inserted.

Inserting an NG tube

- Confirm the patient's identity using two patient identifiers according to facility policy.
- Explain the procedure to the patient to ease anxiety and promote cooperation. Inform her that she may experience some nasal discomfort, that she may gag, and that her eyes may water. Emphasize that swallowing will ease the tube's advancement.
- Agree on a signal that the patient can use if she wants you to stop briefly during the procedure.
- Gather and prepare all necessary equipment.
- Help the patient into high Fowler's position unless contraindicated.
- Stand at the patient's right side if you're right-handed or at her left side if you're left-handed to ease insertion.
- Drape the towel or linen-saver pad over the patient's chest to protect her gown and bed linens from spills.
- Have the patient gently blow her nose to clear her nostrils.
- Place the facial tissues and emesis basin well within the patient's reach.
- Help the patient face forward with her neck in a neutral position.
- To determine how long the NG tube must be to reach the stomach, hold the end of the tube at the tip of the patient's nose. Extend the tube to the patient's earlobe and then down to the xiphoid process (as shown below).

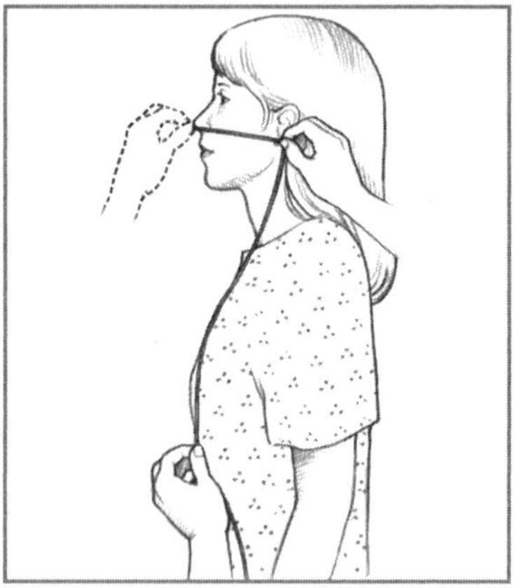

- Mark this distance on the tubing with tape, or note the marking already on the tube. (Average measurements for an adult range from 22″ to 26″ [56 to 66 cm].) It may be necessary to add 2″ (5.1 cm) to this measurement in tall individuals to ensure entry into the stomach.
- To determine which nostril will allow easier access, use a penlight and inspect for a deviated septum or other abnormalities. Ask the patient if she ever had nasal surgery or a nasal injury. Assess airflow in both nostrils by occluding one nostril at a time while the patient breathes through her nose. Choose the nostril with the better airflow.
- Lubricate the first 3″ (7.6 cm) of the tube with a water-soluble gel to minimize injury to the nasal passages. Using a water-soluble lubricant prevents lipoid pneumonia, which may result from aspiration of an oil-based lubricant or from accidental slippage of the tube into the trachea.
- Instruct the patient to hold her head straight and upright.
- Grasp the tube with the end pointing downward, curve it if necessary, and care-

fully insert it into the more patent nostril (as shown below).

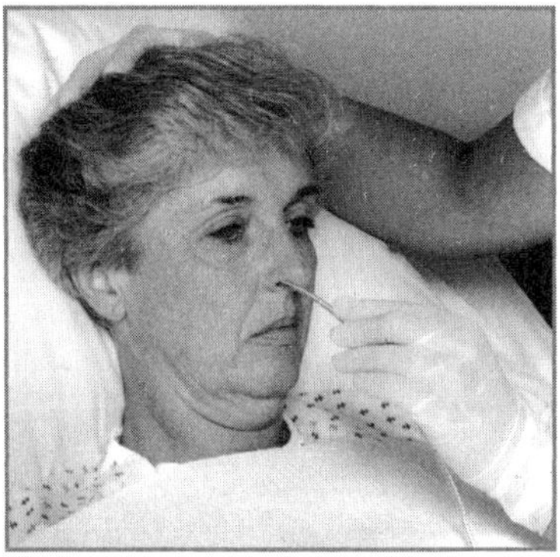

- Aim the tube downward and toward the ear closer to the chosen nostril. Advance it slowly to avoid pressure on the turbinates and resultant pain and bleeding.
- When the tube reaches the nasopharynx, you'll feel resistance. Instruct the patient to lower her head slightly to close the trachea and open the esophagus. Then rotate the tube 180 degrees toward the opposite nostril to redirect it so that the tube won't enter the patient's mouth.
- Unless contraindicated, offer the patient a cup or glass of water with a straw. Direct her to sip and swallow as you slowly advance the tube (as shown below). This helps the tube pass to the esophagus. (If you aren't using water, ask the patient to swallow.)

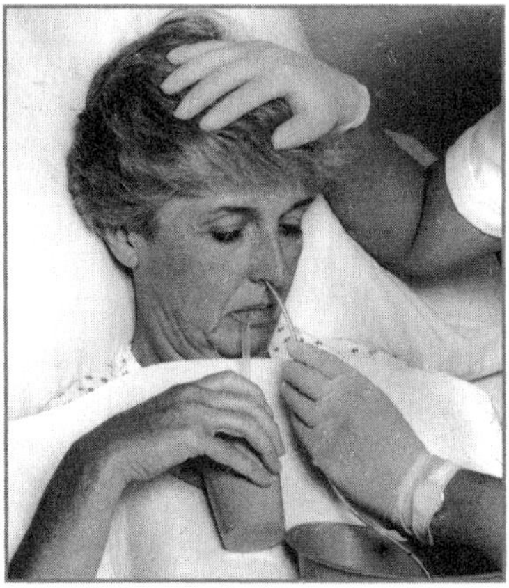

Ensuring proper tube placement

- Use a tongue blade and penlight to examine the patient's mouth and throat for signs of a coiled section of tubing (especially in an unconscious patient). Coiling indicates an obstruction.
- Keep an emesis basin and facial tissues readily available for the patient.
- As you carefully advance the tube and the patient swallows, watch for respiratory distress signs, which may mean the tube is in the bronchus and must be removed immediately.
- Stop advancing the tube when the tape mark or the tube marking reaches the patient's nostril.
- Attach a catheter-tip or bulb syringe to the tube and try to aspirate stomach contents (as shown below). If you don't obtain stomach contents, position the patient on her left side to move the contents into the stomach's greater curvature, and aspirate again. When confirming tube placement, never place the tube's end in a container of water. If the tube is positioned incorrectly in the trachea, the patient may aspirate water. Gently aspirate stomach contents. Examine the aspirate and place a small amount on the pH test strip. Probability of gastric placement is increased if the aspirate has a typical gastric fluid appearance (grassy-green, clear and colorless with mucus shreds, or brown) and the pH is ≤ 5.0.

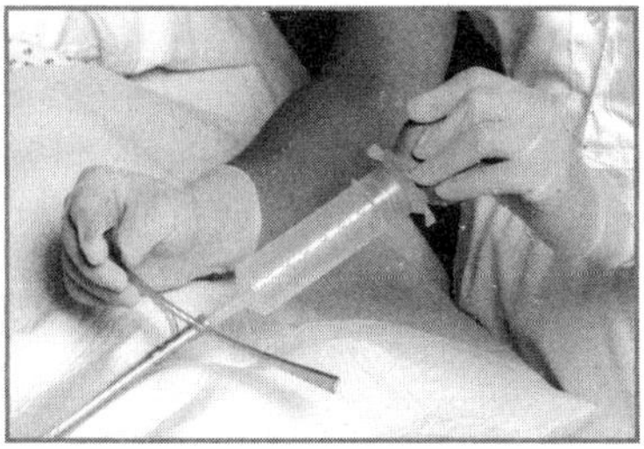

- Ideally, proper tube placement should be confirmed by X-ray.
- Secure the NG tube to the patient's nose with hypoallergenic tape (or other designated tube holder). If the patient's skin is oily, wipe the bridge of the nose with an alcohol pad and allow it to dry. You'll need

about 4″ (10 cm) of 1″ tape. Split one end of the tape up the center about 1½″ (4 cm). Make tabs on the split ends (by folding sticky sides together). Stick the uncut tape end on the patient's nose so that the split in the tape starts about ½″ (1.3 cm) to 1½″ from the tip of her nose. Crisscross the tabbed ends around the tube (as shown below). Then apply another piece of tape over the bridge of the nose to secure the tube.

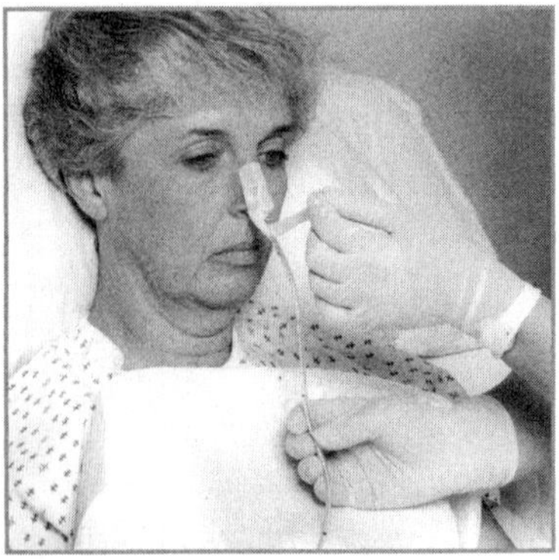

- Alternatively, stabilize the tube with a prepackaged product that secures and cushions it at the nose (as shown below).

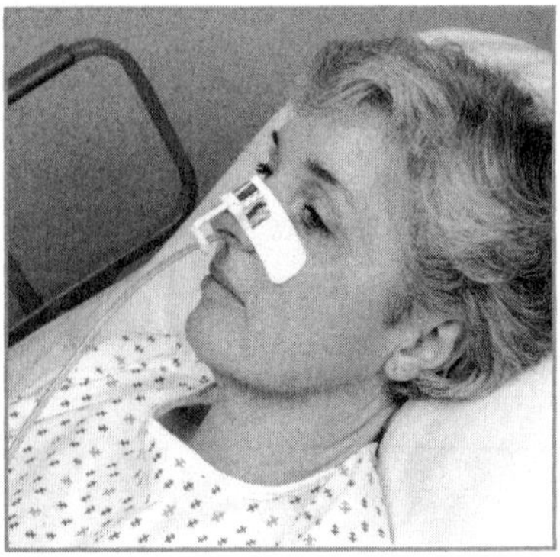

- To reduce discomfort from the weight of the tube, tie a slipknot around the tube with a rubber band, and then secure the rubber band to the patient's gown with a safety pin, or wrap another piece of tape around the end of the tube and leave a tab. Then fasten the tape tab to the patient's gown.
- Attach the tube to suction equipment, if ordered, and set the designated suction pressure.
- Provide frequent nose and mouth care while the tube is in place.

Removing an NG tube

- Confirm the patient's identity using two patient identifiers according to facility policy.
- Explain the procedure to the patient, informing her that it may cause some nasal discomfort and sneezing or gagging.
- Assess bowel function by auscultating for peristalsis or flatus.
- Help the patient into semi-Fowler's position. Then drape a towel or linen-saver pad across her chest to protect her gown and bed linens from spills.
- Wash your hands, and put on gloves.
- Using a catheter-tip syringe, flush the tube with 10 ml of normal saline solution to ensure that the tube doesn't contain stomach contents that could irritate tissues during tube removal.
- Untape the tube from the patient's nose, and then unpin it from her gown.
- Clamp the tube by folding it in your hand.
- Ask the patient to hold her breath to close the epiglottis. Then withdraw the tube gently and steadily. (When the distal end of the tube reaches the nasopharynx, you can pull it quickly.)
- When possible, immediately cover and remove the tube because its sight and odor may nauseate the patient.
- Assist the patient with thorough mouth care, and clean the tape residue from her nose with adhesive remover.
- For the next 48 hours, monitor the patient for signs of GI dysfunction, including nausea, vomiting, abdominal distention, and food intolerance. GI dysfunction may necessitate reinsertion of the tube.

Special considerations

- Ross-Hanson tape is a helpful device for calculating the correct tube length. Place the narrow end of this measuring tape at the tip of the patient's nose. Extend the tape to the patient's earlobe and down to the tip of the xiphoid process. Mark this distance on the edge of the tape labeled "nose to ear to xiphoid." The corresponding measurement on the opposite edge of the tape is the proper insertion length.

- If the patient has a deviated septum or other nasal condition that prevents nasal insertion, pass the tube orally after removing any dentures, if necessary. Sliding the tube over the tongue, proceed as you would for nasal insertion.
- When using the oral route, remember to coil the end of the tube around your hand. This helps curve and direct the tube downward at the pharynx.
- If your patient is unconscious, tilt her chin toward her chest to close the trachea. Then advance the tube between respirations to ensure that it doesn't enter the trachea.
- While advancing the tube in an unconscious patient (or in a patient who can't swallow), stroke the patient's neck to encourage the swallowing reflex and to facilitate passage down the esophagus.

ACTION STAT!

While advancing the tube, observe for signs that it has entered the trachea, such as choking or breathing difficulties in a conscious patient and cyanosis in an unconscious patient or a patient without a cough reflex. If these signs occur, remove the tube immediately. Allow the patient time to rest; then try to reinsert the tube.

- After tube placement, vomiting suggests tubal obstruction or incorrect position. Assess immediately to determine the cause.

Complications

- Skin erosion at the nostril, sinusitis, esophagitis, esophagotracheal fistula, gastric ulceration, and pulmonary and oral infection
- Electrolyte imbalances and dehydration

Patient teaching

- An NG tube may be inserted or removed at home. Indications for insertion include gastric decompression and short-term feeding.
- A home care nurse or the patient may insert the tube, deliver the feeding, and remove the tube.

Documentation

Record the type and size of the NG tube and the date, time, and route of insertion. Note the type and amount of suction, if used, and describe the drainage, including the amount, color, character, consistency, and odor. Note the patient's tolerance of the procedure, especially any signs or symptoms that signal complications, such as nausea, vomiting, or abdominal distention. Document any subsequent irrigation procedures and continuing problems after irrigation. When you remove the tube, be sure to record the date and time. Describe the color, consistency, and amount of gastric drainage. Note the patient's tolerance of the procedure, especially any unusual events such as nausea, vomiting, abdominal distention, or food intolerance.

Nasopharyngeal airway insertion and care

Insertion of a nasopharyngeal airway—a soft rubber or latex uncuffed catheter—establishes or maintains a patent airway. This airway is the typical choice for patients who have had recent oral surgery or facial trauma and for patients with loose, cracked, or avulsed teeth. It's also used to protect the nasal mucosa from injury when the patient needs frequent nasotracheal suctioning. This type of airway may also be tolerated better than an oropharyngeal airway by a patient who isn't deeply unconscious.

The airway follows the curvature of the nasopharynx, passing through the nose and extending from the nostril to the posterior pharynx. The bevel-shaped pharyngeal end of the airway facilitates insertion, and its funnel-shaped nasal end helps prevent slippage.

Insertion of a nasopharyngeal airway is preferred when an oropharyngeal airway is contraindicated or fails to maintain a patent airway. A nasopharyngeal airway is contraindicated if the patient is receiving anticoagulant therapy or has a hemorrhagic disorder, sepsis, or pathologic nasopharyngeal deformity. It's been found that airway bleeding can occur in up to 30% of patients after insertion.

Equipment

Nasopharyngeal airway insertion

Nasopharyngeal airway of proper size ♦ tongue blade ♦ water-soluble lubricant ♦ gloves ♦ optional: suction equipment

Nasopharyngeal airway cleaning

Hydrogen peroxide ♦ water ♦ basin ♦ optional: pipe cleaner

Preparation

- Measure the diameter of the patient's nostril and the distance from the tip of his nose to his earlobe.
- Select an airway that's a slightly smaller diameter than the nostril and about 1″ (2.5 cm) longer than measured. The sizes for this type of airway are labeled according to their internal diameter. The recommended size for a large adult is 8 to 9 mm; for a medium adult, 7 to 8 mm; for a small adult, 6 to 7 mm.
- Lubricate the distal half of the airway's surface with a water-soluble lubricant to prevent traumatic injury during insertion.

Key steps

- Put on gloves.
- In a nonemergency situation, explain the procedure to the patient.
- Properly insert the airway. (See *Inserting a nasopharyngeal airway.*)
- After the airway is inserted, check it regularly to detect dislodgment or obstruction.
- When the patient's natural airway is patent, remove the airway in one smooth motion. If the airway sticks, apply lubricant around the nasal end of the tube and around the nostril, and then gently rotate the airway until it's free.

Special considerations

- When you insert the airway, remember to use a chin-lift or jaw-thrust technique to anteriorly displace the patient's mandible.

ACTION STAT!

Immediately after insertion, assess the patient's respirations. If absent or inadequate, initiate ar-

Inserting a nasopharyngeal airway

First, hold the airway beside the patient's face to make sure it's the proper size (as shown below). It should be slightly smaller than the patient's nostril diameter and slightly longer than the distance from the tip of his nose to his earlobe.

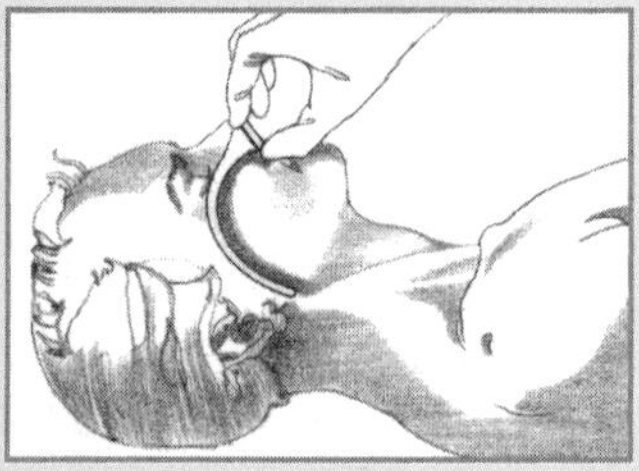

To insert the airway, hyperextend the patient's neck (unless contraindicated). Then push up the tip of his nose and pass the airway into his nostril (as shown below). Avoid pushing against any resistance to prevent tissue trauma and airway kinking.

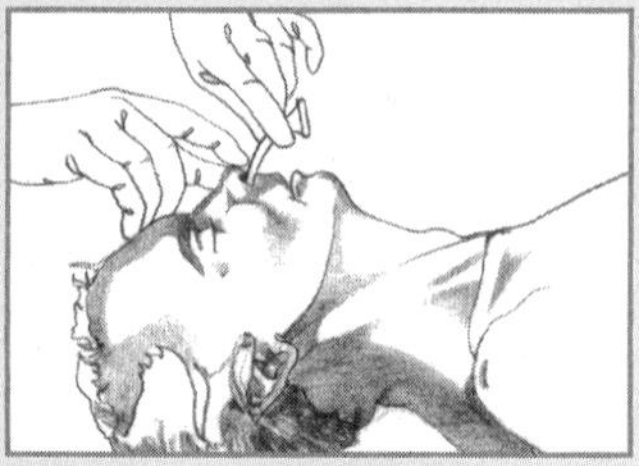

To check for correct airway placement, first close the patient's mouth. Then place your finger over the tube's opening to detect air exchange. Depress the patient's tongue with a tongue blade, and look for the airway tip behind the uvula.

tificial positive-pressure ventilation with a mouth-to-mask technique, a handheld resuscitation bag, or an oxygen-powered breathing device.

- If the patient coughs or gags, the tube may be too long. If so, remove the airway and insert a shorter one.
- At least once every 8 hours, remove the airway to check nasal mucous membranes for irritation or ulceration.
- Clean the airway by placing it in a basin and rinsing it with hydrogen peroxide and then with water. If secretions remain, use a pipe cleaner to remove them. Reinsert the clean airway into the other nostril (if it's patent) to avoid skin breakdown.

Complications

- Sinus infection
- Injury to the nasal mucosa
- Gastric distention and hypoventilation
- Laryngospasm, retching, or vomiting

Documentation

Record the date and time of the airway's insertion, size of the airway, removal and cleaning of the airway, shifts from one nostril to the other, condition of the mucous membranes, suctioning, any complications and interventions taken, and the patient's tolerance of the procedure.

Nephrostomy and cystostomy tube care

Two urinary diversion techniques—nephrostomy and cystostomy—ensure adequate drainage from the kidneys or bladder and help prevent urinary tract infection or kidney failure. (See *Urinary diversion techniques,* page 330.)

A nephrostomy tube drains urine directly from a kidney when a disorder inhibits the normal flow of urine. The tube is usually placed percutaneously, though sometimes it's surgically inserted through the renal cortex and medulla into the renal pelvis from a lateral incision in the flank. The usual indication is obstructive disease, such as calculi in the ureter or ureteropelvic junction, or an obstructing tumor. Draining urine with a nephrostomy tube also allows kidney tissue damaged by obstructive disease to heal.

A cystostomy tube drains urine from the bladder, diverting it from the urethra. This type of tube is used after certain gynecologic procedures, bladder surgery, prostatectomy, and for severe urethral strictures or traumatic injury. Inserted about 2" (5 cm) above the symphysis pubis, a cystostomy tube may be used alone or with an indwelling urethral catheter.

Equipment

Dressing changes

Antiseptic solution and pads ♦ 4" × 4" gauze pads ♦ sterile cup or emesis basin ♦ waterproof, disposable plastic bag ♦ linen-saver pad ♦ clean gloves (for dressing removal) ♦ sterile gloves (for new dressing) ♦ forceps ♦ precut 4" × 4" drain dressings or transparent semipermeable dressings ♦ adhesive tape (preferably hypoallergenic)

Nephrostomy-tube irrigation

3-ml syringe ♦ alcohol pad or antiseptic pad ♦ normal saline solution ♦ optional: hemostat

Commercially prepared sterile dressing kits may be available.

Preparation

- Wash your hands and assemble all equipment at the patient's bedside.
- Open several packages of gauze pads, place them in the sterile cup or emesis basin, and pour the antiseptic solution over them. Or, if available, open several packages of antiseptic pads.
- If you're using a commercially packaged dressing kit, open it using sterile technique.
- Fill the cup with antiseptic solution.
- Open the plastic bag and place it away from the other equipment to avoid contaminating the sterile field.

Key steps

- Wash your hands, provide privacy, and explain the procedure to the patient.

Urinary diversion techniques

A cystostomy or a nephrostomy can be used to create a permanent diversion, to relieve obstruction from an inoperable tumor, or to provide an outlet for urine after cystectomy. A temporary diversion can relieve obstruction from a calculus or ureteral edema.

In a *cystostomy,* a catheter is inserted percutaneously through the suprapubic area into the bladder. In a *nephrostomy,* a catheter is inserted percutaneously through the flank into the renal pelvis.

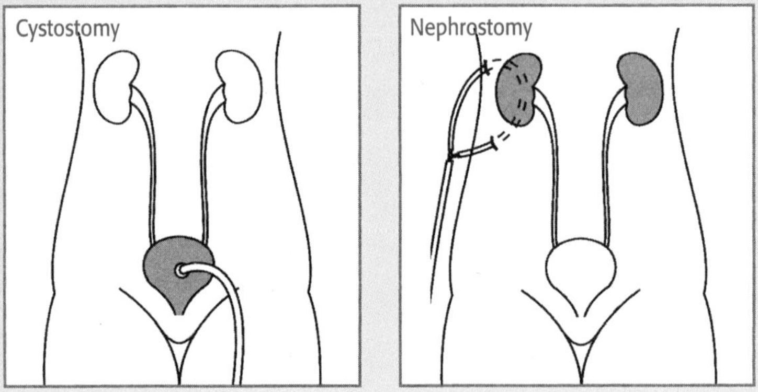

Changing a dressing

- Help the patient to lie on his back (for a cystostomy tube) or on the side opposite the tube (for a nephrostomy tube) so that you can see the tube clearly and change the dressing more easily.
- Place the linen-saver pad under the patient to absorb excess drainage and keep him dry.
- Put on the clean gloves. Carefully remove the tape around the tube, and then remove the wet or soiled dressing. Discard the tape and dressing in the plastic bag. Remove the gloves and discard them in the bag.
- Put on the sterile gloves. Pick up a saturated pad or dip a dry one into the cup of antiseptic solution.
- To clean the wound, wipe only once with each pad, moving from the insertion site outward. Discard the used pad in the plastic bag. Don't touch the bag to avoid contaminating your gloves.
- Pick up a sterile 4″ × 4″ drain dressing and place it around the tube. If necessary, overlap two drain dressings to provide maximum absorption. Or, depending on facility policy, apply a transparent semipermeable dressing over the site and tubing to allow observation of the site without removing the dressing.
- Secure the dressing with hypoallergenic tape. Then tape the tube to the patient's lateral abdomen to prevent tension on the tube. (See *Taping a nephrostomy tube*.)
- Dispose of all equipment appropriately. Clean the patient as necessary.

Irrigating a nephrostomy tube

- Fill the 3-ml syringe with the normal saline solution.
- Clean the junction of the nephrostomy tube and drainage tube with the alcohol pad or antiseptic pad, and disconnect the tubes.
- Insert the syringe into the nephrostomy tube opening, and instill 2 to 3 ml of saline solution into the tube.
- Slowly aspirate the solution back into the syringe. To avoid damaging the renal pelvis tissue, never pull back forcefully on the plunger.
- If the solution doesn't return, remove the syringe from the tube and reattach it to the

Taping a nephrostomy tube

To tape a nephrostomy tube directly to the skin, cut a wide piece of hypoallergenic adhesive tape twice lengthwise to its midpoint.

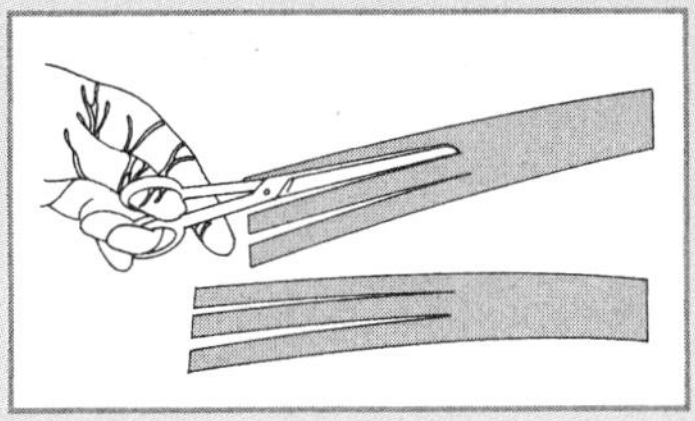

Apply the uncut end of the tape to the skin so that the midpoint meets the tube. Wrap the middle strip around the tube in spiral fashion. Tape the other two strips to the patient's skin on both sides of the tube.

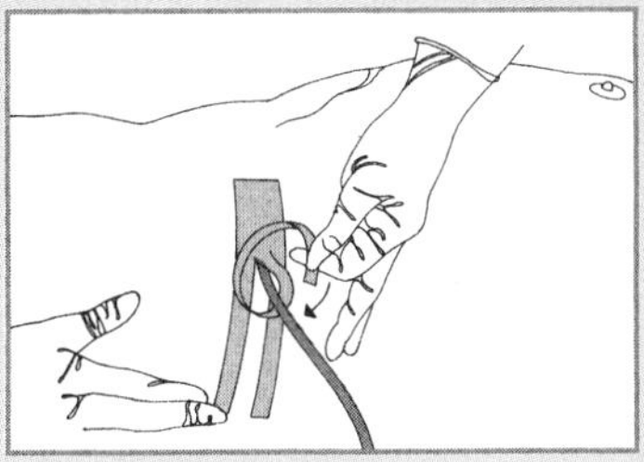

For greater security, repeat this step with a second piece of tape, applying it in the reverse direction. You may also apply two more strips of tape perpendicular to and over the first two pieces.

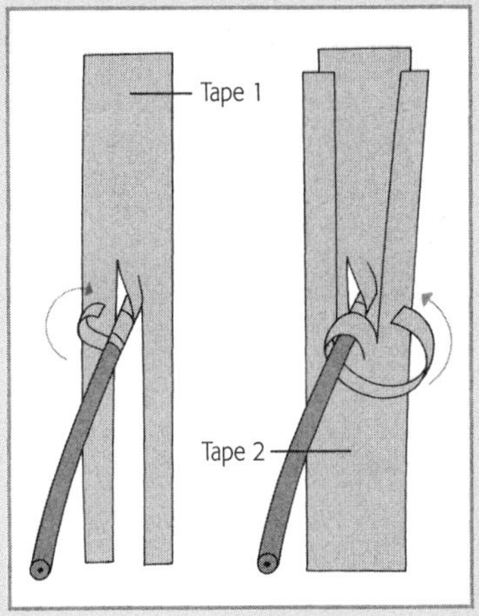

Always apply another strip of tape lower down on the tube in the direction of the drainage tube to further anchor the tube. Don't put tension on any sutures that prevent tube distention.

drainage tubing to allow the solution to drain by gravity.

- Dispose of all equipment appropriately.

Special considerations

- Change dressings once per day or more often if needed.

ALERT

Never irrigate a nephrostomy tube with more than 5 ml of solution because the capacity of the renal pelvis is usually between 4 and 8 ml. (*Remember*: The purpose of irrigation is to keep the tube patent, not to lavage the renal pelvis.)

- When necessary, irrigate a cystostomy tube as you would an indwelling urinary catheter. Be sure to perform the irrigation gently to avoid damaging any suture lines.
- Check a nephrostomy tube frequently for kinks or obstructions. Kinks are likely to occur if the patient lies on the insertion site. Suspect an obstruction when the amount of urine in the drainage bag decreases or the amount of urine around the insertion site increases. Pressure created by urine backing up in the tube can damage nephrons. Gently curve a cystostomy tube to prevent kinks.
- If a blood clot or mucus plug obstructs a nephrostomy or cystostomy tube, try milking the tube to restore its patency. With your nondominant hand, hold the tube se-

curely above the obstruction to avoid pulling the tube out of the incision. Then place the flat side of a closed hemostat under the tube, just above the obstruction, pinch the tube against the hemostat, and slide both your finger and the hemostat toward you, away from the patient.

- Typically, cystostomy tubes for postoperative urologic patients should be checked hourly for 24 hours to ensure adequate drainage and tube patency. To check tube patency, note the amount of urine in the drainage bag and check the patient's bladder for distention.

Complications

- Infection

Patient teaching

- Tell the home care patient to clean the insertion site with soap and water, check for skin breakdown, and change the dressing daily; then show him how to take these steps.
- Teach him how to change the leg bag or drainage bag. He can use a leg bag during the day and a larger drainage bag at night. Whether he uses a drainage bag or larger container, tell him to wash it daily with a 1:3 vinegar and water solution, rinse it with plain water, and dry it on a clothes hanger or over the towel rack. This prevents crystalline buildup.
- Encourage patients with unrestricted fluid intake to increase intake to at least 3 qt (3 L) per day to help flush the urinary system and reduce sediment formation.
- Stress the importance of reporting to the practitioner signs of infection (red skin or white, yellow, or green drainage at the insertion site) or tube displacement (drainage that smells like urine).

Documentation

Describe the color and amount of drainage from the nephrostomy or cystostomy tube, and record any color changes as they occur. Similarly, if the patient has more than one tube, describe the drainage (color, amount, and character) from each tube separately. If irrigation is necessary, record the amount and type of irrigant used and whether or not you obtained a complete return.

Neutropenic precautions

Unlike other types of precaution procedures, neutropenic precautions (also known as *protective precautions* and *reverse isolation*) guard the patient who's at increased risk for infection against contact with potential pathogens. These precautions are used primarily for patients with extensive noninfected burns, those who have leukopenia or a depressed immune system, and those receiving immunosuppressive treatments. (See *Conditions and treatments requiring neutropenic precautions*.)

Neutropenic precautions require a single room equipped with positive air pressure, if possible, to force suspended particles down and out of the room. The degree of precautions may range from using a single room, thorough hand-hygiene technique, and limitation of traffic into the room to more extensive precautions requiring the use of gowns, gloves, and masks by facility staff and visitors. The extent of neutropenic precautions may vary from facility to facility, depending on the reason for and the degree of the patient's immunosuppression.

To care for patients who have temporarily increased susceptibility, such as those who have undergone bone marrow transplantation, neutropenic precautions may also require a patient isolator unit and the use of sterile linens, gowns, gloves, and head and shoe coverings. In such cases, all other items taken into the room should be sterilized or disinfected. The patient's diet may also be modified to eliminate raw fruits and vegetables and to allow only cooked foods and possibly only sterile beverages.

Equipment

Gloves ♦ gowns ♦ masks ♦ neutropenic precautions door card

Gather any additional supplies, such as a thermometer, stethoscope, and blood

Conditions and treatments requiring neutropenic precautions

Condition or treatment	Precautionary period
Acquired immunodeficiency syndrome	Until white blood cell count reaches 1,000/ml or more, or according to your facility's guidelines
Agranulocytosis	Until remission
Burns, extensive noninfected	Until skin surface heals substantially
Dermatitis, noninfected vesicular, bullous, or eczematous disease (when severe and extensive)	Until skin surface heals substantially
Immunosuppressive therapy	Until patient's immunity is adequate
Lymphomas and leukemia, especially late stages of Hodgkin's disease or acute leukemia	Until clinical improvement is substantial

pressure cuff, so you don't have to leave the isolation room unnecessarily.

Preparation

- Keep supplies in a clean, enclosed cart or in an anteroom outside the room.

Key steps

- After placing the patient in a single room, explain isolation precautions to the patient and his family to ease patient anxiety and promote cooperation.
- Place a neutropenic precautions card on the door to caution those entering the room.
- Wash your hands with an antiseptic agent before putting on gloves, after removing gloves, and as indicated during patient care.
- Wear gloves and gown according to standard precautions, unless the patient's condition warrants a sterile gown, gloves, and a mask.
- Avoid transporting the patient out of the room; if he must be moved, make sure he wears a gown and mask. Notify the receiving department or area so that the precautions will be maintained and the patient will be returned to the room promptly.

Do's & don'ts

Don't allow visits by anyone known to be ill or infected.

Special considerations

Do's & don'ts

Don't perform invasive procedures, such as urethral catheterization, unless absolutely necessary because these procedures risk serious infection in the patient with impaired resistance.

- Instruct the housekeeping staff to put on gowns, gloves, and masks before entering the room; no ill or infected person should enter. They should follow the same requirements as the staff, depending on the patient's condition and facility policy.

- Make sure the room is cleaned with freshly prepared cleaning solutions. Because the patient doesn't have a contagious disease, materials leaving the room need no special precautions beyond standard precautions.

Complications

- None known

Documentation

Document the need for neutropenic precautions on the nursing care plan and as otherwise indicated by your facility.

O

Ommaya reservoir drug infusion

Also known as a *subcutaneous cerebrospinal fluid (CSF) reservoir,* an Ommaya reservoir allows delivery of long-term drug therapy to the CSF by way of the brain's ventricles. The reservoir spares the patient repeated lumbar punctures to administer chemotherapeutic drugs, analgesics, antibiotics, and antifungals. It's most commonly used for chemotherapy and pain management, specifically for treating central nervous system (CNS) leukemia, malignant CNS disease, and meningeal carcinomatosis.

The reservoir is a mushroom-shaped silicone apparatus with an attached catheter. It's surgically implanted beneath the patient's scalp in the nondominant lobe, and the catheter is threaded into the ventricle through a burr hole in the skull. (See *How the Ommaya reservoir works,* page 336.) Besides providing convenient, comparatively painless access to CSF, the Ommaya reservoir permits consistent and predictable drug distribution throughout the subarachnoid space and CNS. It also allows for measurement of intracranial pressure (ICP).

Before reservoir insertion, the patient may receive a local or general anesthetic, depending on his condition and the physician's preference. After an X-ray confirms placement of the reservoir, a pressure dressing is applied for 24 hours, followed by a gauze dressing for another day or two. The sutures may be removed in about 10 days. However, the reservoir can be used within 48 hours to deliver drugs, obtain CSF pressure measurements, drain CSF, and withdraw CSF specimens.

The physician usually injects drugs into the Ommaya reservoir, but a specially trained nurse may perform this procedure if allowed by your facility's policy and the state's nurse practice act. This sterile procedure usually takes 15 to 30 minutes.

Equipment

Preservative-free prescribed drug (at room temperature) ♦ sterile or chemotherapy gloves ♦ antiseptic solution ♦ sterile towel ♦ two 5- or 10-ml syringes ♦ 25G needle or 22G Huber needle ♦ sterile gauze pad ♦ collection tubes for CSF (if ordered) ♦ vial of bacteriostatic normal saline solution ♦ sterile labels ♦ sterile marker ♦ sterile tubes

Preparation

- Using the sterile towel, establish a sterile field near the patient.
- Label all medication and sterile tubes on and off the sterile field.
- Prepare a syringe with the preservative-free drug to be instilled and place it, the CSF collection tubes, and the normal saline solution on the sterile field.

Key steps

- If the patient is scheduled to receive an Ommaya reservoir, explain the procedure before reservoir insertion. Make sure the patient and his family understand the potential complications, and answer any questions they may have. Make sure that a consent form is signed. Reassure the pa-

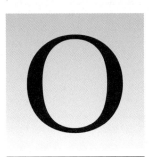

How the Ommaya reservoir works

To insert an Ommaya reservoir, the physician drills a burr hole and inserts the device's catheter through the patient's nondominant frontal lobe into the lateral ventricle. The reservoir, which has a self-sealing silicone injection dome, rests over the burr hole under a scalp flap. This creates a slight, soft bulge on the scalp about the size of a quarter. Usually, drugs are injected into the dome with a syringe.

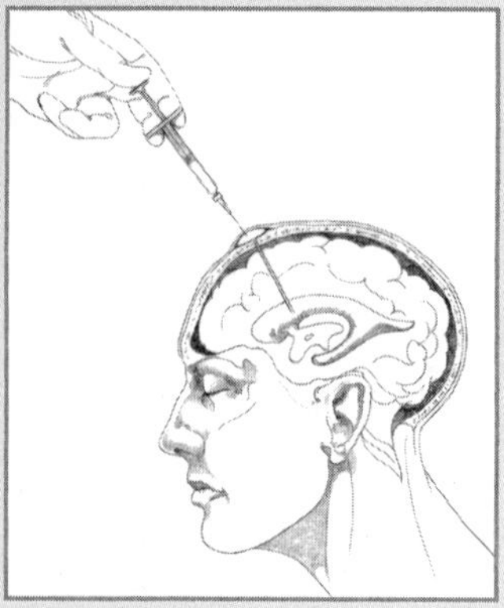

tient that any hair clipped for the implant will grow back and that only a coin-sized patch must remain clipped for injections. (Hair regrowth will be slower if the patient is receiving chemotherapy.)

Instilling medication

- Confirm the patient's identity using two patient identifiers according to facility policy.
- Obtain baseline vital signs.
- Position the patient so that he's either sitting or reclining. The head of the bed may be elevated or flat.
- Put on gloves and prepare the patient's scalp with the antiseptic solution. Use a gauze pad to move the patient's hair and expose the reservoir.
- Placing the 25G needle at a 45-degree angle, insert it into the reservoir and aspirate 3 ml of clear CSF into a syringe. (If the aspirate isn't clear, check with the physician before continuing.)
- Continue to aspirate as many milliliters of CSF as you will instill of the drug. Then detach the syringe from the needle hub, attach the drug syringe, and instill the medication slowly, monitoring for headache, nausea, and dizziness. (Some facilities use the CSF instead of a preservative-free diluent to deliver the drug.)
- Instruct the patient to lie quietly for 15 to 30 minutes after the procedure. This may prevent meningeal irritation leading to nausea and vomiting.
- Cover the site with a sterile dressing, and apply gentle pressure for a moment or two until superficial bleeding stops.
- Monitor the patient for adverse drug reactions and signs of increased ICP, such as nausea, vomiting, pain, and dizziness. Assess for adverse reactions every 30 minutes for 2 hours, then every hour for 2 hours and, finally, every 4 hours.

Special considerations

- The practitioner may prescribe an antiemetic to be administered 30 minutes before the procedure to control nausea and vomiting.
- After the reservoir is implanted, the patient may resume normal activities. Instruct him to protect the site from bumps and traumatic injury while the incision heals. Tell him that unless complications develop, the reservoir may function for years.

Complications

- Infection
- Catheter migration or blockage causing symptoms of increased ICP

Patient teaching

- Instruct the patient and his family to notify the practitioner if signs of infection develop at the insertion site (for example, redness, swelling, tenderness, and drainage) or if the patient develops headache, neck stiffness, or fever, which may indicate a systemic infection.

Documentation

Record the appearance of the reservoir insertion site before and after access, the patient's tolerance of the procedure, the amount of CSF withdrawn and its appearance, and the name and dose of the drug instilled.

Oral drug administration

Because oral administration is usually the safest, most convenient, and least expensive method, most drugs are administered by this route. Drugs for oral administration are available in many forms: tablets, enteric-coated tablets, capsules, syrups, elixirs, oils, liquids, suspensions, powders, and granules. Some require special preparation before administration, such as mixing with juice to make them more palatable; oils, powders, and granules most often require such preparation.

Sometimes oral drugs are prescribed in higher dosages than their parenteral equivalents because after absorption through the GI system, they're immediately broken down by the liver before they reach the systemic circulation.

Oral administration is contraindicated for unconscious patients; it may also be contraindicated in patients with nausea and vomiting and in those unable to swallow.

Equipment

Patient's medication record and chart ♦ prescribed medication ♦ medication cup ♦ appropriate vehicle, such as jelly or applesauce, for crushed pills commonly used with children or elderly patients, and juice, water, or milk for liquid medications plus drinking straw ♦ optional: mortar and pestle for crushing pills

Key steps

- Verify the order on the patient's medication record by checking it against the prescriber's order.
- Wash your hands.
- Check the label on the medication three times before administering it to make sure you'll be giving the prescribed medication. Check when you take the container from the shelf or drawer, again before you pour the medication into the medication cup, and again before returning the container to the shelf or drawer. If you're administering a unit-dose medication, check the label for the final time at the patient's bedside immediately after pouring the medication and before discarding the wrapper.
- Confirm the patient's identity using two patient identifiers according to facility policy.
- If your facility utilizes a bar code scanning system, be sure to scan your ID badge, the patient's ID bracelet, and the medication's bar code.
- Assess the patient's condition, including level of consciousness and vital signs, as needed. Changes in the patient's condition may warrant withholding medication. For example, you may need to withhold a medication that will slow the patient's heart rate if his apical pulse rate is less than 60 beats/minute.
- Give the patient his medication and an appropriate vehicle or liquid, as needed, to aid swallowing, minimize adverse effects, or promote absorption. For example, cyclophosphamide (Cytoxan) is given with fluids to minimize adverse effects; antitussive cough syrup is given without a fluid to avoid diluting its soothing effect on the throat. If appropriate, crush the medication to facilitate swallowing.
- Stay with the patient until he has swallowed the drug. If he seems confused or disoriented, check his mouth to make sure he has swallowed it. Return and reassess the patient's response within 1 hour after giving the medication.

Special considerations

- Make sure you have a written order for every medication given. Verbal orders should be signed by the prescriber within the specified time period. (Hospitals usually require a signature within 24 hours; long-term care facilities, within 48 hours.)
- Notify the prescriber about any medication withheld, unless instructions to withhold are already written.

Measuring liquid medications

To pour liquids, hold the medication cup at eye level. Use your thumb to mark off the correct level on the cup. Then set the cup down and read the bottom of the meniscus at eye level to ensure accuracy. If you've poured too much medication into the cup, discard the excess. Don't return it to the bottle.

Here are a few additional tips:

- Hold the container so that the medication flows from the side opposite the label so it won't run down the container and stain or obscure the label. Remove drips from the lip of the bottle first and then from the sides, using a clean, damp paper towel.
- For a liquid measured in drops, use only the dropper supplied with the medication.

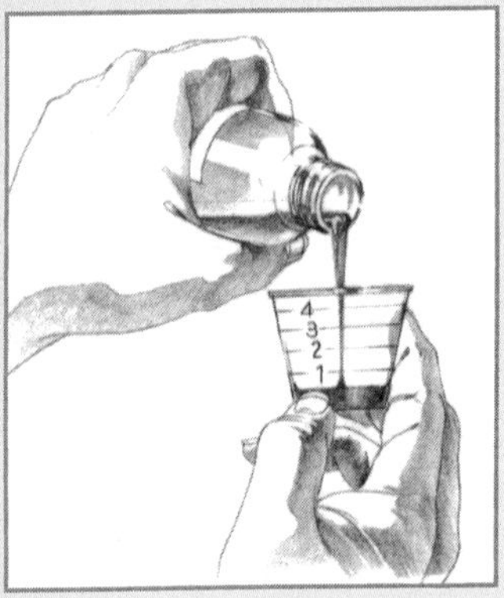

- Use care in measuring out the prescribed dose of liquid oral medication. (See *Measuring liquid medications*.)

DO'S & DON'TS

Don't give medication from a poorly labeled or unlabeled container. Don't attempt to label or reinforce drug labels yourself. This must be done by a pharmacist.

- Never give a medication poured by someone else. Never allow your medication cart or tray out of your sight. This prevents anyone from rearranging the medications or taking one without your knowledge. Never return unwrapped or prepared medications to stock containers. Instead, dispose of them and notify the pharmacy. Keep in mind that the disposal of any opioid drug must be cosigned by another nurse, as mandated by law.
- If the patient questions you about his medication or the dosage, check his medication record again. If the medication is correct, reassure him. Make sure you tell him about any changes in his medication or dosage. Instruct him, as appropriate, about possible adverse effects. Ask him to report anything he thinks may be an adverse effect.
- To avoid damaging or staining the patient's teeth, administer acid or iron preparations through a straw. An unpleasant-tasting liquid can usually be made more palatable if taken through a straw because the liquid contacts fewer taste buds.
- If the patient can't swallow a whole tablet or capsule, ask the pharmacist if the drug is available in liquid form or if it can be administered by another route. If not, ask him if you can crush the tablet or open the capsule and mix it with food. Keep in mind that many enteric-coated or time-release medications and gelatin capsules shouldn't be crushed. Remember to contact the prescriber for an order to change the administration route when necessary.
- Oral medications are relatively easy to give to infants because of their natural sucking instinct and, in infants under 4 months old, their undeveloped sense of taste.

Complications

- None known

Patient teaching

- Instruct the patient, as appropriate, about possible adverse effects.
- Advise the patient that his drugs must be taken as prescribed.
- For home administration, teach the patient any necessary preparation.

Documentation

Note the drug administered, dose, date and time, and patient's reaction, if any. If the patient refuses a drug, document the refusal and notify the charge nurse and the patient's practitioner, as needed. Also note if a drug was omitted or withheld for other reasons, such as radiology or laboratory tests, or if, in your judgment, the drug was contraindicated at the ordered time. Sign out all opioids given on the appropriate opioids central record.

Oronasopharyngeal suction

Oronasopharyngeal suction removes secretions from the pharynx by a suction catheter inserted through the mouth or nostril. Performed to maintain a patent airway, this procedure helps the patient who can't clear his airway effectively with coughing and expectoration such as the unconscious or severely debilitated patient. The procedure should be done as often as necessary, depending on the patient's condition.

Oronasopharyngeal suction is an aseptic procedure that requires sterile equipment. However, clean technique may be used for a tonsil-tip suction device. In fact, an alert patient can use a tonsil-tip suction device himself to remove secretions.

Nasopharyngeal suctioning should be used with caution in patients who have nasopharyngeal bleeding or spinal fluid leakage into the nasopharyngeal area, in trauma patients, in patients receiving anticoagulant therapy, and in those who have blood diseases because these conditions increase the risk of bleeding.

Equipment

Wall suction or portable suction apparatus ♦ collection bottle ♦ connecting tubing ♦ water-soluble lubricant ♦ sterile normal saline solution ♦ disposable sterile container ♦ sterile suction catheter (#12 or #14 French catheter for an adult, #8 or #10 French catheter for a child, or pediatric feeding tube for an infant) ♦ sterile gloves ♦ clean gloves ♦ nasopharyngeal or oropharyngeal airway (optional for frequent suctioning) ♦ overbed table or bedside stand ♦ waterproof trash bag ♦ mask and goggles or face shield ♦ optional: tongue blade, tonsil-tip suction device

A commercially prepared kit contains a sterile catheter, disposable container, and sterile gloves.

Preparation

- Before beginning, check your facility's policy to determine whether a practitioner's order is required for oronasopharyngeal suctioning.
- Review the patient's arterial blood gas or oxygen saturation values, and check his vital signs.
- Evaluate the patient's ability to cough and deep breathe to determine his ability to move secretions up the tracheobronchial tree.
- Check the patient's history for a deviated septum, nasal polyps, nasal obstruction, traumatic injury, epistaxis, or mucosal swelling.
- If no contraindications exist, gather and place the suction equipment on the patient's overbed table or bedside stand.
- Position the table or stand on your preferred side of the bed to facilitate suctioning.
- Attach the collection bottle to the suctioning unit, and attach the connecting tubing to it.
- Date and then open the bottle of sterile normal saline solution.
- Open the waterproof trash bag.

Key steps

- Confirm the patient's identity using two patient identifiers according to facility policy.
- Explain the procedure to the patient, even if he's unresponsive. Inform him that suctioning may stimulate transient coughing or gagging, but tell him that coughing helps to mobilize secretions. Reassure him throughout the procedure to minimize anxiety and fear, which can increase oxygen consumption. Assess nasal patency.
- Wash your hands.

Airway clearance tips

Deep breathing and coughing are vital for removing secretions from the airways. Other techniques used to help clear the airways include diaphragmatic breathing and forced expiration. Here's how to teach these techniques to your patients.

Diaphragmatic breathing

First, tell the patient to lie in a supine position, with his head elevated 15 to 20 degrees on a pillow. Tell him to place one hand on his abdomen and then inhale so that he can feel his abdomen rise.

Next, instruct the patient to exhale slowly through his nose—or, even better, through pursed lips—while letting his abdomen collapse. Explain that this action decreases his respiratory rate and increases his tidal volume.

Suggest that the patient perform this exercise for 30 minutes several times per day. After he becomes accustomed to the position and has learned to breathe using his diaphragm, he may apply abdominal weights of 9 to 11 lb (4 to 5 kg).

To enhance the effectiveness of exercise, the patient may also manually compress the lower costal margins, perform straight-leg lifts, and coordinate the breathing technique with a physical activity such as walking.

Forced expiration

Explain to the patient that forced expiration (also known as *huff coughing*) helps clear secretions while causing less traumatic injury than does a cough. To perform the technique, tell the patient to forcefully expire without closing his glottis, starting with a middle to low lung volume. Tell him to follow this expiration with a period of diaphragmatic breathing and relaxation.

- Assess the patient for other signs of respiratory compromise, such as labored breathing, tachypnea, or cyanosis.
- Place the patient in semi-Fowler's or high Fowler's position, if tolerated, to promote lung expansion and effective coughing.
- Put on goggles and a mask or a face shield.
- Turn on the suction from the wall or portable suction apparatus, and set the pressure according to your facility's policy. Occlude the end of the connecting tubing to check suction pressure.
- Using strict sterile technique, open the suction catheter kit or the packages containing the sterile catheter, container, and gloves. Put on the gloves; consider your dominant hand sterile and your nondominant hand nonsterile. Using your nondominant hand, pour the saline solution into the sterile container.
- With your nondominant hand, place a small amount of water-soluble lubricant on the sterile area. The lubricant is used to facilitate passage of the catheter during nasopharyngeal suctioning.
- Pick up the catheter with your dominant (sterile) hand and attach it to the connecting tubing. Use your nondominant hand to control the suction valve while your dominant hand manipulates the catheter.
- Instruct the patient to cough and breathe slowly and deeply several times before beginning suction. Coughing helps loosen secretions and may decrease the amount of suction necessary, while deep breathing helps minimize or prevent hypoxia. (See *Airway clearance tips*.)

Nasal insertion

- Raise the tip of the patient's nose with your nondominant hand to straighten the passageway and facilitate catheter insertion. Without applying suction, gently insert the sterile suction catheter into the patient's nostril. Roll the catheter between your fingers to help it advance through the turbinates. Continue to advance the catheter approximately 5″ to 6″ (12.5 to 15 cm) until you reach the pool of secretions or the patient begins to cough.

Oral insertion

- Without applying suction, gently insert the catheter into the patient's mouth. Advance it 3″ to 4″ (7.5 to 10 cm) along the side of the patient's mouth until you reach the pool of secretions or the patient begins to cough. Suction both sides of the patient's mouth and pharyngeal area.
- Using intermittent suction, withdraw the catheter from either the mouth or the nose with a continuous rotating motion to minimize invagination of the mucosa into the catheter's tip and side ports. Apply suction for no longer than 10 to 15 seconds at a time to minimize tissue trauma and hypoxia.
- Between passes, wrap the catheter around your dominant hand to prevent contamination.
- If secretions are thick, clear the catheter lumen by dipping it in sterile normal saline solution and applying suction.
- Repeat the procedure a second time, if necessary.
- After completing suctioning, pull your sterile glove off over the coiled catheter and discard it and the nonsterile glove along with the container of water.
- Flush the connecting tubing with sterile normal saline solution.
- Replace the reusable items so they're ready for the next suctioning, and wash your hands.
- Assist the patient with mouth care.

Special considerations

- If the patient has no history of nasal problems, alternate suctioning between nostrils to minimize traumatic injury. If repeated oronasopharyngeal suctioning is required, the use of a nasopharyngeal or oropharyngeal airway will help with catheter insertion, reduce traumatic injury, and promote a patent airway. To facilitate catheter insertion for oropharyngeal suctioning, depress the patient's tongue with a tongue blade, or ask another nurse to do so. This helps you to visualize the back of the throat and also prevents the patient from biting the catheter.
- If the patient has excessive oral secretions, consider using a tonsil-tip catheter because this allows the patient to remove oral secretions independently.
- Let the patient rest after suctioning while you continue to observe him. The frequency and duration of suctioning depend on the patient's tolerance of the procedure and on any complications.
- Remember that oronasopharyngeal suctioning is just one component of bronchial hygiene. The patient's lungs should be auscultated before suctioning to determine the presence of secretions in the airways.
- Perform suctioning only when necessary and when other methods of removing secretions haven't been effective.

Complications

- Increased dyspnea
- Bloody aspirate
- Hypoxia

Patient teaching

- Oronasopharyngeal suctioning may be performed in the home using a portable suction machine. Under these circumstances, suctioning is a clean rather than a sterile procedure. Properly cleaned catheters can be reused, putting less financial strain on patients.
- Catheters should be cleaned by first washing them in water with a detergent, followed by one of the following: a 60-minute soak in a solution of vinegar and water with an acetic acid content of 1.25% and greater, quaternary ammonium compound, glutaraldehyde, or boiling when equipment can withstand it. The catheters should then be rinsed with normal saline solution or tap water.
- Whether the patient requires disposable or reusable suction equipment, you should make sure that the patient and his caregivers have received proper teaching and support.
- Teach the patient proper coughing techniques and tell him to drink lots of fluids to help facilitate the removal of secretions.

Documentation

Record the date, time, reason for suctioning, and technique used; amount, color, consistency, and odor (if any) of the secretions; the patient's respiratory status before and after the procedure; any complications and interventions taken; and the patient's tolerance of the procedure.

Oropharyngeal airway insertion and care

An oropharyngeal airway, a curved rubber or plastic device, is inserted into the mouth to the posterior pharynx to establish or maintain a patent airway. In an unconscious patient, the tongue usually obstructs the posterior pharynx. The oropharyngeal airway conforms to the curvature of the palate, removing the obstruction and allowing air to pass around and through the tube. It also facilitates oropharyngeal suctioning and is intended for short-term use, as in the postanesthesia or postictal stage. It may be left in place longer as an airway adjunct to prevent the orally intubated patient from biting the endotracheal tube.

The oropharyngeal airway isn't the airway of choice for the patient with loose or avulsed teeth or recent oral surgery. Inserting this airway in the conscious or semiconscious patient may stimulate vomiting, laryngospasm, and retching as a result of gag reflex stimulation; therefore, you'll usually insert the airway only in an unconscious patient.

Equipment

Insertion

Oral airway of appropriate size ♦ tongue blade ♦ padded tongue blade ♦ gloves ♦ optional: suction equipment, handheld resuscitation bag or oxygen-powered breathing device

Cleaning

Hydrogen peroxide ♦ water ♦ basin ♦ optional: pipe cleaner

Reflex testing

Cotton-tipped applicator

Preparation

- Select an oral airway of appropriate size for your patient; an oversized airway can obstruct breathing by depressing the epiglottis into the laryngeal opening. Usually, you'll select a small size (size 1 or 2) for an infant or child, a medium size (size 4 or 5) for an average adult, and a large size (size 6) for a large adult.
- Be sure to confirm the correct size of the airway by placing the airway flange beside the patient's cheek, parallel to his front teeth. If the airway is the right size, the airway curve should reach to the angle of the jaw.

Key steps

- Explain the procedure to the patient even though he may not appear to be alert. Provide privacy and put on gloves to prevent contact with body fluids. If the patient is wearing dentures, remove them so they don't cause further airway obstruction.
- Suction the patient, if necessary.
- Place the patient in the supine position with his neck hyperextended if this isn't contraindicated.
- Insert the airway using the cross-finger or tongue blade technique. (See *Inserting an oral airway*.)
- Auscultate the lungs to ensure adequate ventilation.
- After the airway is inserted, position the patient on his side to decrease the risk of aspiration of vomitus.
- Perform mouth care every 2 to 4 hours, as needed. Begin by holding the patient's jaws open with a padded tongue blade and gently removing the airway. Place the airway in a basin, and rinse it with hydrogen peroxide and then water. If secretions remain, use a pipe cleaner to remove them. Complete standard mouth care, and reinsert the airway.
- While the airway is removed for mouth care, observe the mouth's mucous membranes because tissue irritation or ulceration can result from prolonged airway use.
- Frequently check the position of the airway to ensure correct placement.
- When the patient regains consciousness and can swallow, remove the airway by pulling it outward and downward, following the mouth's natural curvature. After the airway is removed, test the patient's cough and gag reflexes to ensure that re-

moval of the airway wasn't premature and that the patient can maintain his own airway.

- To test for the gag reflex, use a cotton-tipped applicator to touch both sides of the posterior pharynx. To test for the cough reflex, gently touch the posterior oropharynx with the cotton-tipped applicator.

Special considerations

- Bilateral breath sounds on auscultation indicate that the airway is the proper size and in the correct position.
- Avoid taping the airway in place because untaping it could delay airway removal, thus increasing the patient's risk of aspiration.
- Evaluate the patient's behavior to provide the cue for airway removal. The patient is likely to gag or cough as he becomes more alert, indicating that he no longer needs the airway.

Complications

- Tooth damage or loss, tissue damage, and bleeding
- Complete airway obstruction
- Aggravation of upper airway obstruction

ACTION STAT!

Immediately after inserting the airway, check for respirations. If respirations are absent or inadequate, initiate artificial positive-pressure ventilation by using a mouth-to-mask technique, a handheld resuscitation bag, or an oxygen-powered breathing device.

Documentation

Record the date and time of the airway's insertion, size of the airway, removal and cleaning of the airway, condition of mucous membranes, any suctioning, any adverse reactions and interventions taken, and the patient's tolerance of the procedure. Also document breath sounds and respiratory assessment findings.

Inserting an oral airway

Unless this position is contraindicated, hyperextend the patient's head (as shown below) before using either the cross-finger or tongue blade insertion method.

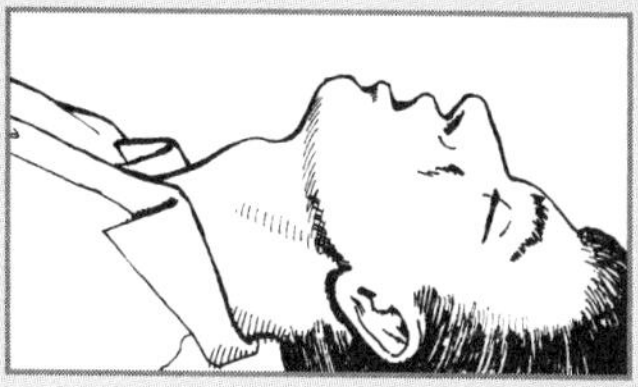

To insert an oral airway using the cross-finger method, place your thumb on the patient's lower teeth and your index finger on his upper teeth. Gently open his mouth by pushing his teeth apart (as shown below).

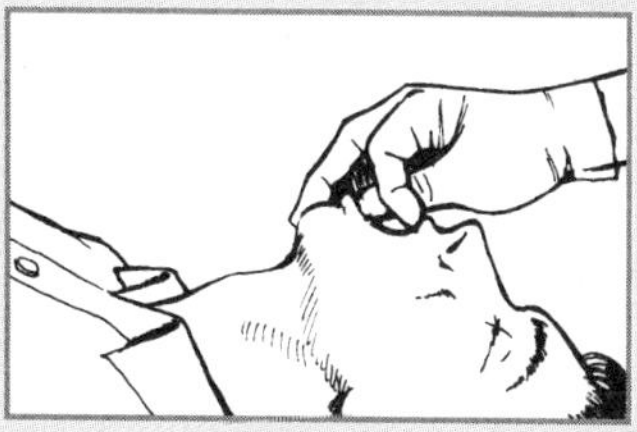

Insert the airway upside down to avoid pushing the tongue toward the pharynx, and slide it over the tongue toward the back of the mouth. Rotate the airway as it approaches the posterior wall of the pharynx so that it points downward (as shown below).

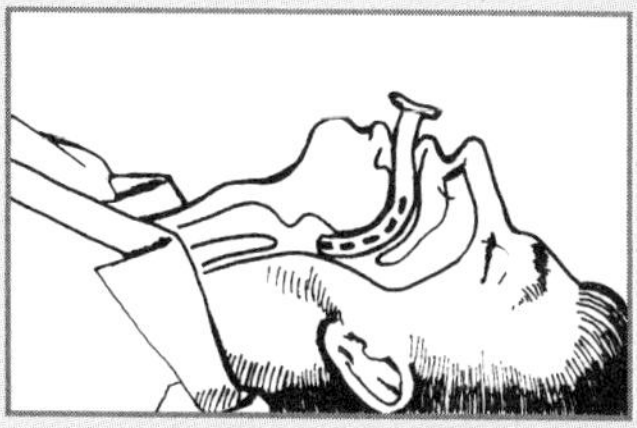

To use the tongue blade technique, open the patient's mouth and depress his tongue with the blade. Guide the airway over the back of the tongue as you did for the cross-finger technique.

Oxygen administration

A patient will need oxygen therapy when hypoxemia results from a respiratory or cardiac emergency or an increase in metabolic function.

In a respiratory emergency, oxygen administration enables the patient to reduce his ventilatory effort. When such conditions as atelectasis or acute respiratory distress syndrome impair diffusion or when lung volumes are decreased from alveolar hypoventilation, this procedure boosts alveolar oxygen levels.

In a cardiac emergency, oxygen therapy helps meet the increased myocardial workload as the heart tries to compensate for hypoxemia. Oxygen administration is particularly important for a patient whose myocardium is already compromised—perhaps from a myocardial infarction or cardiac arrhythmia.

When metabolic demand is high (for example, in cases of massive trauma, burns, or high fever), oxygen administration supplies the body with enough oxygen to meet its cellular needs. This procedure also increases oxygenation in the patient with a reduced blood oxygen-carrying capacity, perhaps from carbon monoxide poisoning or sickle cell crisis.

The adequacy of oxygen therapy is determined by arterial blood gas (ABG) analysis, oximetry monitoring, and clinical examination. The patient's disease, physical condition, and age will help determine the most appropriate method of administration.

Equipment

The equipment needed depends on the type of delivery system ordered. (See *Guide to oxygen delivery systems.*)

Oxygen source (wall unit, cylinder, liquid tank, or concentrator) ♦ flowmeter adapter, if using a wall unit, or a pressure-reduction gauge, if using a cylinder ♦ sterile humidity bottle and adapters ♦ sterile distilled water ♦ OXYGEN PRECAUTION sign ♦ appropriate oxygen delivery system (nasal cannula, simple mask, partial rebreather mask, or nonrebreather mask for low-flow and variable oxygen concentrations; a Venturi mask, aerosol mask, T tube, tracheostomy collar, tent, or oxygen hood for high-flow and specific oxygen concentrations) ♦ small- and large-diameter connection tubing ♦ flashlight (for nasal cannula) ♦ water-soluble lubricant ♦ gauze pads and tape (for oxygen masks) ♦ jet adapter for Venturi mask (if adding humidity) ♦ optional: oxygen analyzer

Preparation

- Although a respiratory therapist is typically responsible for setting up, maintaining, and managing the equipment, you'll need a working knowledge of the oxygen system being used.
- Check the oxygen outlet port to verify flow.
- Pinch the tubing near the prongs to ensure that an audible alarm will sound if the oxygen flow stops.

Key steps

- Confirm the patient's identity using two patient identifiers according to facility policy.
- Assess the patient's condition. In an emergency, verify that he has an open airway before administering oxygen.
- Explain the procedure to the patient, and let him know why he needs oxygen to ensure his cooperation.
- Check the patient's room to make sure it's safe for oxygen administration.

DEVICE SAFETY

Whenever possible, replace electrical devices with nonelectrical ones.

ALERT

If the patient is a child and is in an oxygen tent, remove all toys that may produce a spark. Oxygen supports combustion, and the smallest spark can cause a fire.

- Place an OXYGEN PRECAUTION sign over the patient's bed and on the door to his room.

Guide to oxygen delivery systems

Patients may receive oxygen through one of several administration systems. Each has its own benefits, drawbacks, and indications for use. The advantages and disadvantages of each system are compared below.

Nasal cannula

Oxygen is delivered through plastic cannulas placed in the patient's nostrils.

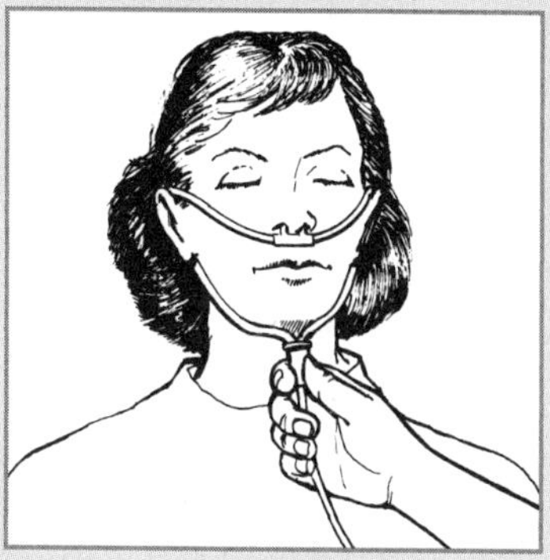

Advantages: Safe and simple, comfortable and easily tolerated, nasal prongs can be shaped to fit any face, effective for low oxygen concentrations, inexpensive and disposable, allows movement, eating, and talking

Disadvantages: Can't deliver concentrations higher than 40%, can't be used in patients with complete nasal obstruction, may cause headaches or dry mucous membranes if flow rate exceeds 6 L/minute, can dislodge easily

Administration guidelines: Ensure patency of the patient's nostrils with a flashlight. If patent, hook the cannula tubing behind the patient's ears and under the chin. Slide the adjuster upward under the chin to secure the tubing. If using an elastic strap to secure the cannula, position it over the ears and around the back of the head. Avoid applying it too tightly, which can result in excess pressure on facial structures and cannula occlusion as well. With a nasal cannula, oral breathers achieve the same oxygen delivery as nasal breathers.

Simple mask

Oxygen flows through an entry port at the bottom of the mask and exits through large holes on the sides of the mask.

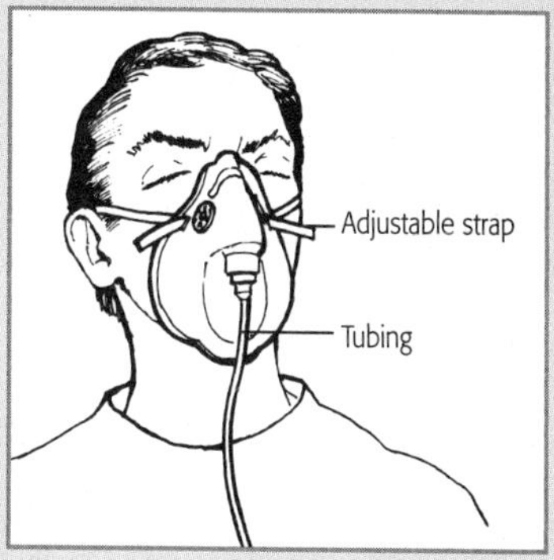

Advantages: Can deliver concentrations of 40% to 60%

Disadvantages: Hot and confining, may irritate patient's skin, interferes with talking and eating, impractical for long-term therapy because of imprecision, tight seal required for higher oxygen concentration may cause discomfort

Administration guidelines: Select the mask size that offers the best fit. Place the mask over the patient's nose, mouth, and chin, and mold the flexible metal edge to the bridge of the nose. Adjust the elastic band around the head to hold the mask firmly but comfortably over the cheeks, chin, and bridge of the nose. For elderly or cachectic patients with sunken cheeks, tape gauze pads to the mask over the cheek area to try to create an airtight seal. Without this seal, room air dilutes the oxygen, preventing delivery of the prescribed concentration. A minimum of 5 L/minute is required in all masks to flush expired carbon dioxide from the mask so that the patient doesn't rebreathe it.

(continued)

Guide to oxygen delivery systems *(continued)*

Nonrebreather mask

On inhalation, the one-way valve opens, directing oxygen from a reservoir bag into the mask. On exhalation, gas exits the mask through the one-way expiratory valve and enters the atmosphere. The patient only breathes air from the bag.

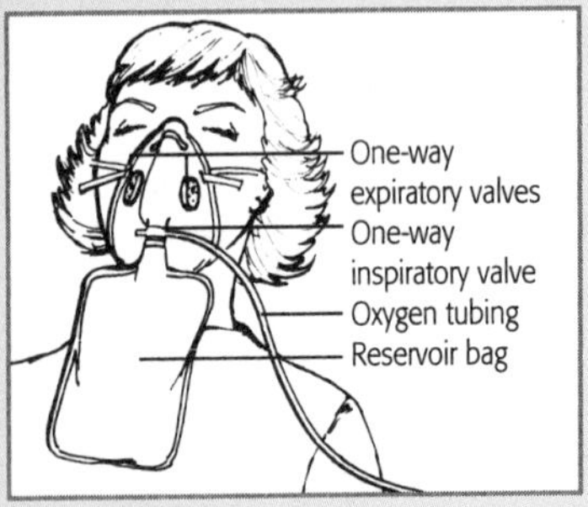

Advantages: Delivers the highest possible oxygen concentration (60% to 90%) short of intubation and mechanical ventilation, effective for short-term therapy, doesn't dry mucous membranes, can be converted to a partial rebreather mask, if necessary, by removing the one-way valve

Disadvantages: Requires a tight seal that may cause discomfort and be difficult to maintain, may irritate the patient's skin, interferes with talking and eating, impractical for long-term therapy

Administration guidelines: Follow procedures listed for the simple mask. Make sure the mask fits very snugly and the one-way valves are secure and functioning. Because the mask excludes room air, valve malfunction can cause carbon dioxide buildup and suffocate an unconscious patient. If the reservoir bag collapses more than slightly during inspiration, raise the flow rate until you see only a slight deflation. Marked or complete deflation indicates an insufficient flow rate. Keep the reservoir bag from twisting or kinking. Ensure free expansion by making sure the bag lies outside the patient's gown and bedcovers.

CPAP mask

This system allows the spontaneously breathing patient to receive continuous positive airway pressure (CPAP) with or without an artificial airway.

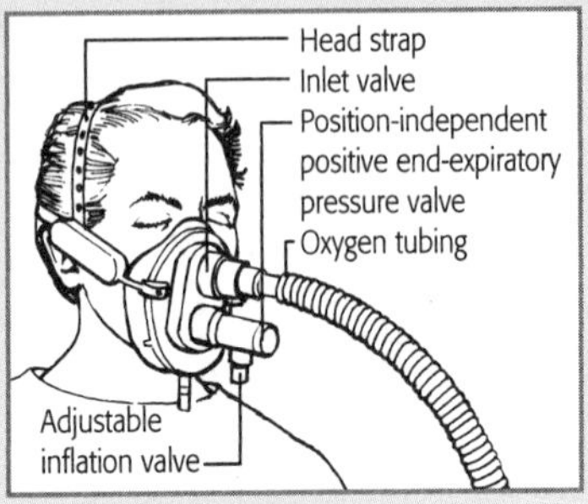

Advantages: Noninvasively improves arterial oxygenation by increasing functional residual capacity, alleviates the need for intubation, allows the patient to talk and cough without interrupting positive pressure

Disadvantages: Requires a tight fit that may cause discomfort, interferes with eating and talking, heightened risk of aspiration if the patient vomits, increased risk of pneumothorax, diminished cardiac output, and gastric distention; contraindicated in patients with chronic obstructive pulmonary disease, bullous lung disease, low cardiac output, or tension pneumothorax

Administration guidelines: Place one strap behind the patient's head and the other strap over his head to ensure a snug fit. Attach one latex strap to the connector prong on one side of the mask. Then, use one hand to position the mask on the patient's face while using the other hand to connect the strap to the other side of the mask. After the mask is applied, assess the patient's respiratory, circulatory, and GI function every hour. Watch for signs of pneumothorax, decreased cardiac output, a drop in blood pressure, and gastric distention.

Guide to oxygen delivery systems *(continued)*

Venturi mask

The mask is connected to a Venturi device, which mixes a specific volume of air and oxygen.

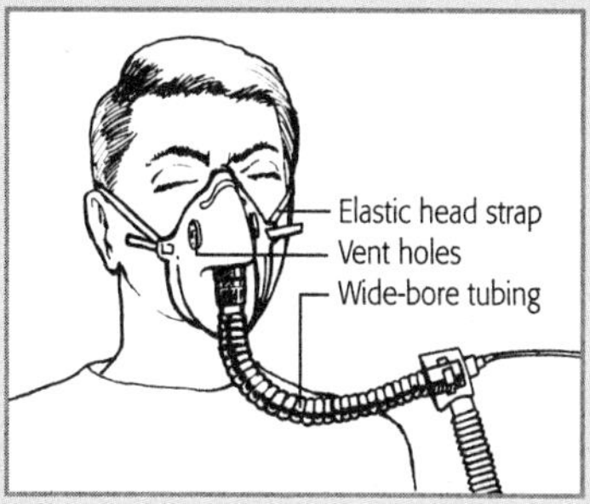

Advantages: Delivers highly accurate oxygen concentration despite patient's respiratory pattern because the same amount of air is always entrained, has dilute jets that can be changed or a dial that changes oxygen concentration, doesn't dry mucous membranes, allows addition of humidity or aerosol

Disadvantages: Confining and may irritate skin, interferes with eating and talking, condensate possibly collecting and dripping on the patient if humidification is used, possible oxygen concentration alteration if mask fits loosely, tubing kinks, oxygen intake ports become blocked, flow is insufficient, or patient is hyperpneic

Administration guidelines: Make sure the oxygen flow rate is set at the amount specified on each mask and the Venturi valve is set for the desired fraction of inspired oxygen.

Aerosols

A face mask, hood, tent, or tracheostomy tube or collar is connected to wide-bore tubing that receives aerosolized oxygen from a jet nebulizer. The jet nebulizer, which is attached near the oxygen source, adjusts air entrainment in a manner similar to the Venturi device.

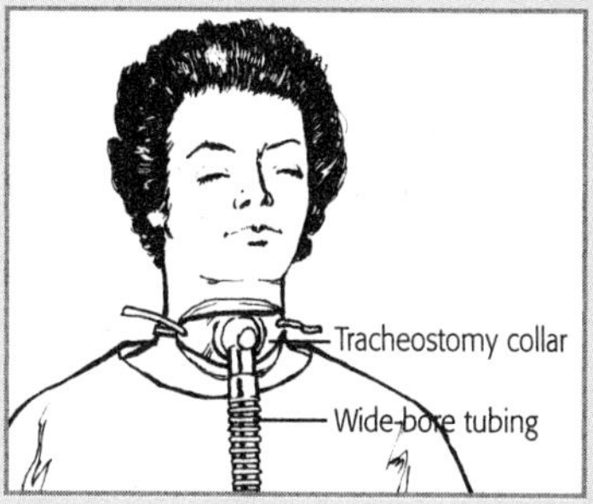

Advantages: Administers high humidity, allows gas to be heated (when delivered through artificial airway) or cooled (when delivered through a tent)

Disadvantages: Condensate collected in the tracheostomy collar or T tube possibly draining into the tracheostomy, weight of the T tube possibly putting stress on the tracheostomy tube

Administration guidelines: Guidelines vary with the type of nebulizer used: the ultrasonic, large-volume, small-volume, or in-line. When using a high-output nebulizer, watch for signs of overhydration, pulmonary edema, crackles, and electrolyte imbalance.

- Help place the oxygen delivery device on the patient. Make sure that it fits properly and that it's stable.
- Monitor the patient's response to oxygen therapy. Check his ABG values during initial adjustments of oxygen flow. When the patient is stabilized, you may use pulse oximetry instead. Check the patient frequently for signs of hypoxia, such as decreased level of consciousness, increased heart rate, arrhythmias, restlessness, perspiration, dyspnea, accessory muscle use, yawning or flared nostrils, cyanosis, and cool, clammy skin.
- Check the patient's skin to prevent skin breakdown on pressure points from the oxygen delivery device. Wipe moisture or

Types of home oxygen therapy

Oxygen therapy can be administered at home using an oxygen tank, an oxygen concentrator, or liquid oxygen.

Oxygen tank

Commonly used for patients who need oxygen on a standby basis or who need a ventilator at home, the oxygen tank has several disadvantages, including its cumbersome design and the need for frequent refills. Because oxygen is stored under high pressure, the oxygen tank also poses a potential hazard.

Oxygen concentrator

The oxygen concentrator extracts oxygen molecules from room air. It can be used for low oxygen flow (less than 4 L/minute) and doesn't need to be refilled with oxygen. However, because the oxygen concentrator runs on electricity, it won't function during a power failure.

Liquid oxygen

Liquid oxygen is commonly used by patients who are oxygen-dependent but still mobile. The system includes a large liquid reservoir for home use. When the patient wants to leave the house, he fills a portable unit worn over the shoulder; this supplies oxygen for up to several hours, depending on the liter flow.

---

perspiration from the patient's face and from the mask as needed.

- If the patient is receiving oxygen at a concentration above 60% for more than 24 hours, watch carefully for signs and symptoms of oxygen toxicity (fatigue, lethargy, weakness, restlessness, nausea, vomiting, anorexia, coughing, and dyspnea progressing to severe dyspnea, tachypnea, tachycardia, decreased breath sounds, crackles, and cyanosis). Remind the patient to cough and deep breathe frequently to prevent atelectasis. Also, to prevent the development of serious lung damage, measure ABG values repeatedly to determine whether high oxygen concentrations are still necessary.

Special considerations

ALERT

Never administer oxygen by nasal cannula at more than 2 L/minute to a patient with chronic lung disease unless you have a specific order to do so because he may have become dependent on a state of hypercapnia and hypoxia to stimulate his breathing, and supplemental oxygen could cause him to stop breathing. However, long-term oxygen therapy of 12 to 17 hours daily may help the patient with chronic lung disease sleep better, survive longer, and experience a reduced incidence of pulmonary hypertension.

- When monitoring a patient's response to a change in oxygen flow, check the pulse oximetry monitor or measure ABG values 20 to 30 minutes after adjusting the flow. In the interim, monitor the patient closely for an adverse response to the change in oxygen flow.

Complications

- Oxygen toxicity

Patient teaching

- Before discharging a patient who will receive oxygen therapy at home, make sure that you know the types of oxygen therapy, the kinds of services that are available, and the service schedules offered by local home suppliers. Together with the practitioner and the patient, choose the device best suited to the patient. (See *Types of home oxygen therapy*.)
- If the patient is receiving transtracheal oxygen therapy, teach him how to properly clean and care for the catheter. Advise him

to keep the skin surrounding the insertion site clean and dry to prevent infection.

- No matter which device the patient uses, you'll need to evaluate his and his family members' ability and motivation to administer oxygen therapy at home. Make sure that they understand the reason the patient is receiving oxygen and the safety issues involved in oxygen administration. Teach them how to properly use and clean the equipment and supplies.
- If the patient will be discharged with oxygen for the first time, make sure that his health insurance covers home oxygen. If it doesn't, find out what criteria he must meet to obtain coverage. Without a third-party payer, the patient may not be able to afford home oxygen therapy.

Documentation

Record the date and time of oxygen administration, the delivery device used, oxygen flow rate, patient's vital signs, skin color, respiratory effort, breath sounds, subjective patient response before and after initiation of therapy, and any patient or family teaching.

PQ

Pacemaker (permanent) insertion and care

Designed to operate for 3 to 20 years, a permanent pacemaker is a self-contained device. The cardiologist implants the pacemaker in a pocket beneath the patient's skin. This is usually done in the operating room or cardiac catheterization laboratory. Nursing responsibilities involve monitoring the electrocardiogram (ECG) and maintaining sterile technique.

Today, permanent pacemakers function in the demand mode, allowing the patient's heart to beat on its own but preventing it from falling below a preset rate. Pacing electrodes can be placed in the atria, in the ventricles, or in both chambers (atrioventricular sequential, dual chamber). (See *Understanding pacemaker codes.*) The most common pacing codes are VVI for single-chamber pacing and DDD for dual-chamber pacing. To keep the patient healthy and active, newer-generation pacemakers are specially designed to increase the heart rate with exercise and to pace both ventricles together.

Candidates for permanent pacemakers include patients with myocardial infarction and persistent bradyarrhythmia and patients with complete heart block or slow ventricular rates stemming from congenital or degenerative heart disease or cardiac surgery. Patients with Stokes-Adams syndrome as well as those with Wolff-Parkinson-White syndrome or sick sinus syndrome, may also benefit from permanent pacemaker implantation.

A biventricular pacemaker is also available for patients with heart failure. This device differs from a standard pacemaker in that it has three leads instead of one or two. One lead is placed in the right atrium, one in the right ventricle, and one in the left ventricle. The leads simultaneously stimulate the right and left ventricles, allowing the ventricles to coordinate their pumping action and making the heart more efficient.

Equipment

Sphygmomanometer ♦ stethoscope ♦ ECG monitor and strip-chart recorder ♦ sterile dressing tray ♦ antiseptic ointment ♦ clippers ♦ sterile gauze dressing ♦ hypoallergenic tape ♦ antibiotics ♦ analgesics ♦ sedatives ♦ alcohol pads ♦ emergency resuscitation equipment ♦ sterile gown and mask ♦ I.V. line for emergency medications

Key steps

- Confirm the patient's identity using two patient identifiers according to your facility's policy.
- Explain the procedure to the patient. Provide and review literature from the manufacturer or the American Heart Association so he can learn about the pacemaker and how it works. Emphasize that the pacemaker merely augments his natural heart rate.
- Make sure the patient or a responsible family member signs a consent form, and

Understanding pacemaker codes

A permanent pacemaker's three-letter (or sometimes five-letter) code simply refers to how it's programmed. The first letter represents the chamber that's paced; the second letter, the chamber that's sensed; and the third letter, how the pulse generator responds.

First letter	Second letter	Third letter
A = atrium	A = atrium	I = inhibited
V = ventricle	V = ventricle	T = triggered
D = dual (both chambers)	D = dual (both chambers)	D = dual (inhibited and triggered)
O = not applicable	O = not applicable	O = not applicable

Examples of two common programming codes are:

DDD
Pace: atrium and ventricle
Sense: atrium and ventricle
Response: inhibited and triggered
This is a fully automatic, or universal, pacemaker.

VVI
Pace: ventricle
Sense: ventricle
Response: inhibited
This is a demand pacemaker, inhibited.

ask the patient if he's allergic to anesthetics or iodine.

Preoperative care

- For pacemaker insertion, clip the hair on the patient's chest from the axilla to the midline and from the clavicle to the nipple line on the side selected by the physician.
- Establish an I.V. line at a keep-vein-open rate so that you can administer emergency drugs if the patient experiences ventricular arrhythmia.
- Obtain baseline vital signs and a baseline ECG.
- Provide sedation as ordered.

Perioperative care

- If you'll be present to monitor arrhythmias during the procedure, put on a gown and mask.
- Connect the ECG monitor to the patient, and run a baseline rhythm strip. Make sure the machine has enough paper to run additional rhythm strips during the procedure.
- In transvenous placement, the cardiologist, guided by a fluoroscope, passes the electrode catheter through the cephalic or external jugular vein and positions it in the right ventricle. He attaches the catheter to the pulse generator, inserts this into the chest wall, and sutures it closed.

Postoperative care

- Monitor the patient's ECG to check for arrhythmias and to ensure correct pacemaker functioning.
- Monitor the I.V. flow rate; the I.V. line is usually kept in place for 24 to 48 hours postoperatively to allow for possible emergency treatment of arrhythmias.
- Check the dressing for signs of bleeding and infection (swelling, redness, or exudate). The physician may order prophylactic antibiotics for up to 7 days after the implantation.
- Change the dressing and apply antiseptic ointment at least once every 24 to 48 hours, or according to physician's orders and facility policy. If the dressing becomes soiled or the site is exposed to air, change the dressing immediately, regardless of when you last changed it.
- Check vital signs and level of consciousness (LOC) every 15 minutes for the first hour, every hour for the next 4 hours, every 4 hours for the next 48 hours, and then once every shift.

Teaching about permanent pacemakers

If your patient is going home with a permanent pacemaker, be sure to teach him about daily care, safety and activity guidelines, and other precautions.

Daily care

- Clean your pacemaker site gently with soap and water when you take a shower or bath. Leave the incision exposed to the air.
- Inspect your skin around the incision. A slight bulge is normal but call your practitioner if you feel discomfort or notice swelling, redness, a discharge, or other problems.
- Check your pulse for 1 minute as your nurse or practitioner showed you—on the side of your neck, inside your elbow, or on the thumb side of your wrist. Your pulse rate should be the same as your pacemaker rate or faster. Contact your practitioner if you think your heart is beating too fast or too slow.
- Take your medications, including those for pain, as prescribed. Even with a pacemaker, you still need the medication your practitioner ordered.

Safety and activity

- Keep your pacemaker instruction booklet handy, and carry your pacemaker identification card at all times. This card has your pacemaker model number and other information needed by health care personnel who treat you.
- You can resume most of your usual activities when you feel comfortable doing so, but don't drive until the practitioner gives you permission. Also avoid heavy lifting and stretching exercises for at least 4 weeks or as directed by your practitioner.
- Try to use both arms equally to prevent stiffness. Check with your practitioner before you golf, swim, play tennis, or perform other strenuous activities.

Electromagnetic interference

- Pacemakers are designed and insulated to eliminate most electrical interference. You can safely operate common household electrical devices, including microwave ovens, razors, and sewing machines. You can ride in or operate a motor vehicle without it affecting your pacemaker.
- Take care to avoid direct contact with large running motors, high-powered CB radios and other similar equipment, welding machinery, and radar devices.
- If your pacemaker activates the metal detector in an airport, show your pacemaker identification card to the security official.
- Because the metal in your pacemaker makes you ineligible for certain diagnostic studies such as magnetic resonance imaging, be sure to inform your practitioners, dentist, and other health care personnel that you have a pacemaker.

Special precautions

- If you feel light-headed or dizzy when you're near electrical equipment, moving away from the device should restore normal pacemaker function. Ask your practitioner about particular electrical devices.
- Notify your practitioner if you experience signs of pacemaker failure, such as palpitations, a fast heart rate, a slow heart rate (5 to 10 beats less than the pacemaker's setting), dizziness, fainting, shortness of breath, swollen ankles or feet, anxiety, forgetfulness, or confusion.

Checkups

- Be sure to schedule and keep regular appointments with your practitioner.
- If your practitioner checks your pacemaker status by telephone, keep your transmission schedule and instructions in a handy place.

- Confused, elderly patients with second-degree heart block won't show immediate improvement in LOC.

ACTION STAT!

Watch for signs and symptoms of a perforated ventricle, with resultant cardiac tamponade: persistent hiccups, distant heart sounds, pulsus paradoxus, hypotension with narrow pulse pressure, increased venous pressure, cyanosis, distended jugular veins, decreased urine output, restlessness, or complaints of fullness in the chest. If the patient develops any of these, notify the physician immediately.

Special considerations

- Watch for signs of pacemaker malfunction.

Complications

- Infection, lead displacement, a perforated ventricle, cardiac tamponade, or lead fracture and disconnection

Patient teaching

- On discharge, provide the patient with an identification card that lists the pacemaker type and manufacturer, serial number, pacemaker rate setting, date implanted, and physician's name. (See *Teaching about permanent pacemakers*.) The markings, along with the shape of the generator, may assist in determining the manufacturer of the generator and pacemaker battery. This may be helpful if the patient has lost the permanent pacemaker identification card.

Documentation

Document the type of pacemaker used, the serial number and the manufacturer's name, the pacing rate, the date of implantation, and the physician's name. Note whether the pacemaker successfully treated the patient's arrhythmias and the condition of the incision site.

Pacemaker (temporary) insertion and care

Usually inserted in an emergency, a temporary pacemaker consists of an external, battery-powered pulse generator and a lead or electrode system. Four types of temporary pacemakers exist: transcutaneous, transvenous, transthoracic, and epicardial.

In a life-threatening situation, when time is critical, a transcutaneous pacemaker is the best choice. This device works by sending an electrical impulse from the pulse generator to the patient's heart by way of two electrodes, which are placed on the front and back of the patient's chest. Transcutaneous pacing is quick and effective, but it's used only until the physician can institute transvenous pacing.

In addition to being more comfortable for the patient, a transvenous pacemaker is more reliable than a transcutaneous pacemaker. Transvenous pacing involves threading an electrode catheter through a vein into the patient's right atrium or right ventricle. The electrode then attaches to an external pulse generator. As a result, the pulse generator can provide an electrical stimulus directly to the endocardium. This is the most common type of pacemaker.

During cardiac surgery, the surgeon may insert electrodes through the epicardium of the right ventricle and, if he wants to institute atrioventricular sequential pacing, the right atrium. From there, the electrodes pass through the chest wall, where they remain available if temporary pacing becomes necessary. This is called *epicardial pacing*.

In addition to helping to correct conduction disturbances, a temporary pacemaker may help diagnose conduction abnormalities. For example, during a cardiac catheterization or electrophysiology study, a physician may use a temporary pacemaker to localize conduction defects. In the process, he may also learn whether the patient risks developing an arrhythmia.

Among the contraindications to pacemaker therapy are pulseless electrical activity and ventricular fibrillation.

Equipment

Transcutaneous pacing

Transcutaneous pacing generator ♦ transcutaneous pacing electrodes ♦ cardiac monitor ♦ optional: electric clippers

Transvenous pacing

All equipment listed for temporary pacing ♦ bridging cable ♦ percutaneous introducer tray or venous cutdown tray ♦ sterile gowns ♦ linen-saver pad ♦ antimicrobial soap ♦ alcohol pads ♦ vial of 1% lidocaine (Xylocaine) ♦ 5-ml syringe ♦ fluoroscopy equipment, if necessary ♦ fenestrated drape ♦ prepackaged cutdown tray (for antecubital vein placement only) ♦ sutures ♦ receptacle for infectious wastes

Epicardial pacing

All equipment listed for temporary pacing ♦ atrial epicardial wires ♦ ventricular epicardial wires ♦ sterile rubber finger cot ♦ sterile dressing materials (if the wires won't be connected to a pulse generator)

All other types of temporary pacing

Temporary pacemaker generator with new battery ♦ guide wire or introducer ♦ electrode catheter ♦ sterile gloves ♦ sterile dressings ♦ adhesive tape ♦ antiseptic solution ♦ nonconducting tape or rubber surgical glove ♦ pouch for external pulse generator ♦ emergency cardiac drugs ♦ intubation equipment ♦ defibrillator ♦ cardiac monitor with strip-chart recorder ♦ equipment to start a peripheral I.V. line, if appropriate ♦ I.V. fluids ♦ sedative ♦ optional: elastic bandage or gauze strips, restraints

Key steps

- If applicable, explain the procedure to the patient.

Transcutaneous pacing

- If necessary, clip the hair over the areas of electrode placement.

DO'S & DON'TS

Don't shave the area. If you nick the skin, the current from the pulse generator could cause discomfort and the nicks could become irritated or infected after the electrodes are applied.

- Attach monitoring electrodes to the patient in lead I, II, or III position. Do this even if the patient is already on telemetry monitoring because you'll need to connect the electrodes to the pacemaker. If you select the lead II position, adjust the left leg (LL) electrode placement to accommodate the anterior pacing electrode and the patient's anatomy.
- Plug the patient cable into the electrocardiogram (ECG) input connection on the front of the pacing generator. Set the selector switch to the MONITOR ON position.
- You should see the ECG waveform on the monitor. Adjust the R-wave beeper volume to a suitable level and activate the alarm by pressing the ALARM ON button. Set the alarm for 10 to 20 beats lower and 20 to 30 beats higher than the intrinsic rate.
- Press the START/STOP button for a printout of the waveform.
- Now you're ready to apply the two pacing electrodes. First, make sure the patient's skin is clean and dry to ensure good skin contact.
- Pull off the protective strip from the posterior electrode (marked BACK) and apply the electrode on the left side of the back, just below the scapula and to the left of the spine.
- The anterior pacing electrode (marked FRONT) has two protective strips—one covering the jellied area and one covering the outer rim. Expose the jellied area and apply it to the skin in the anterior position—to the left side of the precordium in the usual V2 to V5 position. Move this electrode around to get the best waveform. Then expose the electrode's outer rim and firmly press it to the skin. (See *Proper electrode placement for a temporary pacemaker.*)
- Now you're ready to pace the heart. After making sure the energy output in milliamperes (mA) is on 0, connect the electrode cable to the monitor output cable.

- Check the waveform, looking for a tall QRS complex in lead II.
- Next, turn the selector switch to PACER ON. Tell the patient that he may feel a thumping or twitching sensation. Reassure him that you'll give him medication if he can't tolerate the discomfort.
- Now set the rate dial to 10 to 20 beats higher than the patient's intrinsic rhythm. Look for pacer artifact or spikes, which will appear as you increase the rate. If the patient doesn't have an intrinsic rhythm, set the rate at 60.
- Slowly increase the amount of energy delivered to the heart by adjusting the OUTPUT mA dial. Do this until capture is achieved—you'll see a pacer spike followed by a widened QRS complex that resembles a premature ventricular contraction. This is the pacing threshold. To ensure consistent capture, increase output by 10%. Don't go any higher because you could cause the patient needless discomfort.
- With full capture, the patient's heart rate should be approximately the same as the pacemaker rate set on the machine. The usual pacing threshold is between 40 and 80 mA.

Proper electrode placement for a temporary pacemaker

Place the pacing electrodes for a noninvasive temporary pacemaker at heart level on the patient's chest and back, with the heart lying between them. This placement ensures that the electrical stimulus will travel to the heart in the shortest distance.

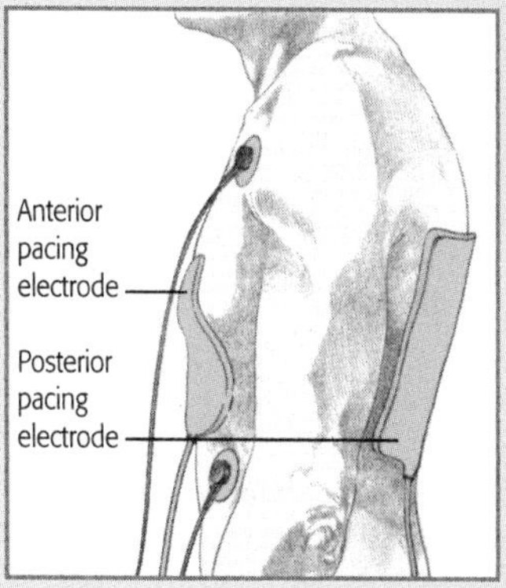

Transvenous pacing

- Check the patient's history for hypersensitivity to local anesthetics. Then attach the cardiac monitor to the patient and obtain a baseline assessment, including the patient's vital signs, skin color, level of consciousness (LOC), heart rate and rhythm, and emotional state. Next, insert a peripheral I.V. line if the patient doesn't already have one. Begin an I.V. infusion of dextrose 5% in water at a keep-vein-open rate.
- Insert a new battery into the external pacemaker generator, and test it to make sure it has a strong charge. Connect the bridging cable to the generator, and align the positive and negative poles. This cable allows slack between the electrode catheter and the generator, reducing the risk of accidental catheter displacement.
- Place the patient in the supine position. If necessary, clip the hair around the insertion site. Next, open the supply tray while maintaining a sterile field. Label all medications, medication containers, and other solutions on and off the sterile field. Using sterile technique, clean the insertion site with antimicrobial soap and then wipe the area with antiseptic solution. Cover the insertion site with a fenestrated drape. Because fluoroscopy may be used during the placement of leadwires, put on a protective apron.
- After anesthetizing the insertion site, the physician will puncture the brachial, femoral, subclavian, or jugular vein. Then he'll insert a guide wire or an introducer and advance the electrode catheter.
- As the catheter advances, watch the cardiac monitor. When the electrode catheter reaches the right atrium, you'll notice large P waves and small QRS complexes. Then, as the catheter reaches the right ventricle, the P waves will become smaller while the QRS complexes enlarge. When the catheter touches the right ventricular endocardium, expect to see elevated ST segments,

Handling pacemaker malfunction

Occasionally, a temporary pacemaker may fail to function appropriately. When this occurs, you'll need to take immediate action to correct the problem. Below you'll learn which steps to take when your patient's pacemaker falls to pace, capture, or sense intrinsic beats.

Failure to pace

Failure to pace occurs when the pacemaker either doesn't fire (as shown below) or fires too often. The pulse generator may not be working properly, or it may not be conducting the impulse to the patient.

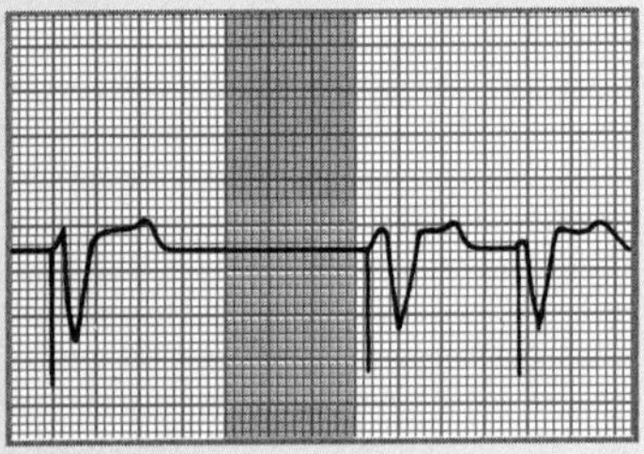

Nursing interventions

- If the pacing or sensing indicator flashes, check the connections to the cable and the position of the pacing electrode in the patient (by X-ray). The cable may have come loose, or the electrode may have been dislodged, pulled out, or broken.
- If the pulse generator is turned on but the indicators still aren't flashing, change the battery. If that doesn't help, use a different pulse generator.
- Check the settings if the pacemaker is firing too rapidly. If they're correct, or if altering them (according to facility policy or the practitioner's order) doesn't help, change the pulse generator.

Failure to capture

In failure to capture, you see pacemaker spikes but the heart isn't responding (as shown below). This may be caused by changes in the pacing threshold from ischemia, an electrolyte imbalance (high or low potassium or magnesium levels), acidosis, an adverse reaction to a medication, a perforated ventricle, fibrosis, or the position of the electrode.

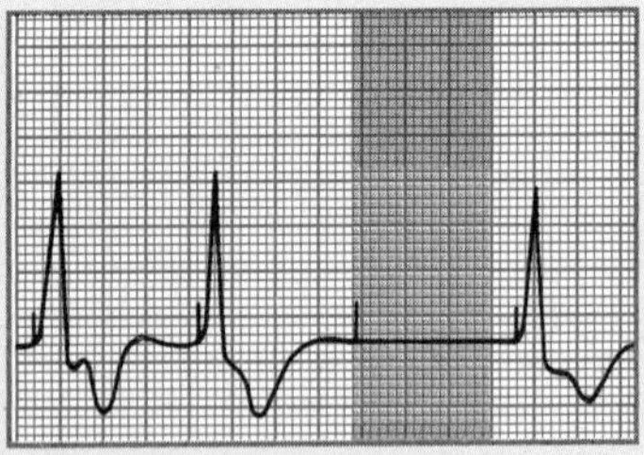

Nursing interventions

- If the patient's condition has changed, notify the practitioner and ask him for new settings.
- If pacemaker settings are altered by the patient or others, return them to their correct positions. Then make sure the face of the pacemaker is covered with a plastic shield. Also, tell the patient or others not to touch the dials.
- If the heart isn't responding, try any or all of these suggestions: Carefully check all connections; increase the milliamperes slowly (according to your facility's policy or the practitioner's order); turn the patient on his left side, then on his right (if turning him to the left didn't help); reverse the cable in the pulse generator so the positive electrode wire is in the negative terminal and the negative electrode wire is in the positive terminal; schedule an anteroposterior or lateral chest X-ray to determine the position of the electrode.

Failure to sense intrinsic beats

Failure to sense intrinsic beats could cause ventricular tachycardia or ventricular fibrillation if the pacemaker fires on the vulnerable T wave. This could be caused by the pacemaker sensing an external stimulus as a QRS complex, which could lead to asystole, or by the pacemaker not being sensitive enough, which means it could fire anywhere within the cardiac cycle (as shown below).

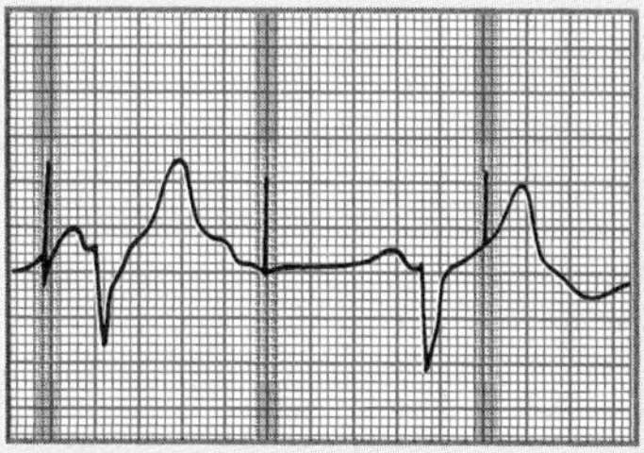

Nursing interventions

- If the pacing is undersensing, turn the sensitivity control completely to the right. If it's oversensing, turn it slightly to the left.
- If the pacemaker isn't functioning correctly, change the battery or the pulse generator.
- Remove items in the room causing electromechanical interference (razors, radios, cautery devices, and so on). Check the ground wires on the bed and other equipment for obvious damage. Unplug each piece and see if the interference stops. When you locate the cause, notify the staff engineer and ask him to check it.
- If the pacemaker is still firing on the T wave and all else has failed, turn off the pacemaker. Make sure atropine is available in case the patient's heart rate drops. Be prepared to call a code and institute cardiopulmonary resuscitation, if necessary.

premature ventricular contractions, or both.

- When the electrode catheter is in the right ventricle, it will send an impulse to the myocardium, causing depolarization. If the patient needs atrial pacing, either alone or with ventricular pacing, the physician may place an electrode in the right atrium.
- Meanwhile, continuously monitor the patient's cardiac status and treat any arrhythmias, as appropriate. Also assess the patient for jaw pain and earache; these symptoms indicate that the electrode catheter has missed the superior vena cava and has moved into the neck instead.
- When the electrode catheter is in place, attach the catheter leads to the bridging cable, lining up the positive and negative poles.
- Check the battery's charge by pressing the BATTERY TEST button.
- Set the pacemaker as ordered.
- The physician will then suture the catheter to the insertion site. Afterward, put on sterile gloves and apply a sterile dressing to the site. Label the dressing with the date and time of application.

Epicardial pacing

- During your preoperative teaching, inform the patient that epicardial pacemaker wires may be placed during cardiac surgery.
- During cardiac surgery, the physician will hook epicardial wires into the epicardium just before the end of the surgery. Depending on the patient's condition, the physician may insert either atrial or ventricular wires, or both.
- If indicated, connect the electrode catheter to the generator, lining up the positive and negative poles. Set the pacemaker as ordered.
- If the wires won't be connected to an external pulse generator, place them in a sterile rubber finger cot. Then cover both the wires and the insertion site with a sterile, occlusive dressing. This will help protect the patient from microshock as well as infection.

Special considerations

DEVICE SAFETY

Take care to prevent microshock. This includes warning the patient not to use any electrical equipment that isn't grounded, such as telephones, electric shavers, televisions, or lamps.

- Other safety measures you'll want to take include placing a plastic cover supplied by the manufacturer over the pacemaker controls to avoid an accidental setting change. Also, insulate the pacemaker by covering all exposed metal parts, such as electrode connections and pacemaker terminals, with nonconducting tape, or place the pacing unit in a dry, rubber surgical glove. If the patient is disoriented or uncooperative, use restraints to prevent accidental removal of pacemaker wires. If the patient needs emergency defibrillation, make sure the pacemaker can withstand the procedure. If you're unsure, disconnect the pulse generator to avoid damage.
- When using a transcutaneous pacemaker, don't place the electrodes over a bony area because bone conducts current poorly. With female patients, place the anterior electrode under the patient's breast but not over her diaphragm. If the physician inserts the electrode through the brachial or femoral vein, immobilize the patient's arm or leg to avoid putting stress on the pacing wires.
- After insertion of any temporary pacemaker, assess the patient's vital signs, skin color, LOC, and peripheral pulses to determine the effectiveness of the paced rhythm. Perform a 12-lead ECG to serve as a baseline, and then perform additional ECGs daily or with clinical changes. Also, if possible, obtain a rhythm strip before, during, and after pacemaker placement; any time that pacemaker settings are changed; and whenever the patient receives treatment because of a complication due to the pacemaker.
- Continuously monitor the ECG reading, noting capture, sensing, rate, intrinsic beats, and competition of paced and intrinsic rhythms. If the pacemaker is sensing correctly, the sense indicator on the pulse generator should flash with each beat. (See *Handling pacemaker malfunction*, pages 356 and 357.)
- Record the date and time of pacemaker insertion, the type of pacemaker, the reason for insertion, and the patient's response. Note the pacemaker settings. Document any complications and the interventions taken.
- If the patient has epicardial pacing wires in place, clean the insertion site with antiseptic solution and change the dressing daily. At the same time, monitor the site for signs of infection. Always keep the pulse generator nearby in case pacing becomes necessary.

Complications

- Microshock, equipment failure, and competitive or fatal arrhythmias
- Pneumothorax or hemothorax, cardiac perforation and tamponade, diaphragmatic stimulation, pulmonary embolism, thrombophlebitis, and infection
- Venous spasm, thrombophlebitis, or lead displacement resulting if the cardiologist threads the electrode through the antecubital or femoral vein
- Skin breakdown and muscle pain and twitching when the pacemaker fires with transcutaneous pacemakers
- Pneumothorax, cardiac tamponade, emboli, sepsis, lacerations of the myocardium or coronary artery, and perforations of a cardiac chamber with transthoracic pacemakers
- Infection, cardiac arrest, and diaphragmatic stimulation with epicardial pacemakers

Documentation

Record the reason for pacing, the time it started, and the locations of the electrodes. For a transvenous pacemaker, note the date, the time, and reason for the temporary pacemaker.

For any temporary pacemaker, record the pacemaker settings. Note the patient's response to the procedure, along with any complications and the interventions taken. If possible, obtain rhythm strips before, during, and after pacemaker placement, and whenever pacemaker settings are changed or when the patient receives treatment for a complication caused by the pacemaker. As you monitor the patient, record his response to temporary pacing and note any changes in his condition.

Pain management

Pain is defined as the sensory and emotional experience associated with actual or potential tissue damage. Thus, pain includes not only the perception of an uncomfortable stimulus, but also the response to that perception.

In health care, the physician's role is to identify and treat the cause of pain, and prescribe medications and other interventions to relieve pain, whereas nurses have traditionally been responsible for assessing and managing a patient's pain.

According to the Joint Commission standards, health care facilities are required to develop policies and procedures for pain control, which include developing policies and procedures supporting the appropriate use of analgesics and other pain control therapies. Health care providers are expected to be knowledgeable about pain assessment and management. The new standards also state that:

- Pain should be assessed on admission and regularly reassessed.
- Patients should be informed of relevant providers in pain assessment and management.
- Patients and their families should be educated regarding their roles in pain management as well as the potential limitations and adverse effects of pain treatments.
- Pain assessment should include personal, cultural, spiritual, and ethnic beliefs.
- Patients will be involved in making care decisions.
- Routine and as-needed analgesics are to be administered.

Several interventions can be used to manage pain. These include analgesics, emotional support, comfort measures, and cognitive techniques to distract the patient. Severe pain usually requires an opioid analgesic. Invasive measures, such as epidural analgesia or patient-controlled analgesia (PCA), may also be required. (See *Understanding patient-controlled analgesia,* page 360.)

Equipment

Pain assessment tool or scale ♦ oral hygiene supplies ♦ water ♦ nonopioid analgesic (such as aspirin or acetaminophen [Tylenol]) ♦ optional: PCA device; mild opioid (such as oxycodone [Oxycontin] or codeine); strong opioid (such as methadone [Dolophine], levorphanol [Levo-Dromoran], morphine [Duramorph], or hydromorphone [Dilaudid])

Key steps

- Confirm the patient's identity using two patient identifiers according to facility policy.
- Explain to the patient how pain medications work together with other pain-management therapies to provide relief. Explain that management aims to keep pain at a low level to permit optimal bodily function.
- Assess the patient's pain by using a pain assessment tool or scale or by asking him key questions and noting his response to the pain. For instance, ask him to describe its duration, severity, and source. Look for physiologic or behavioral clues to the pain's severity. (See *Assessing pain,* page 361.)
- Develop nursing diagnoses. Appropriate nursing diagnostic categories include acute or chronic pain, anxiety, activity intolerance, fear, risk for injury, deficient knowledge, and powerlessness.
- Work with the patient to develop a nursing care plan using interventions appropriate to his lifestyle. These may include prescribed medications, emotional support, comfort measures, cognitive techniques, and education about pain and its management. Emphasize the importance of maintaining good bowel habits, respiratory functions, and mobility because pain may exacerbate any problems in these areas.
- Implement your care plan. Because individuals respond to pain differently, you'll find that what works for one person may not work for another.

Understanding patient-controlled analgesia

In patient-controlled analgesia (PCA), the patient controls I.V. delivery of an analgesic (usually morphine [Duramorph]) by pressing the button on a delivery device. In this way, he receives analgesia at the level he needs and at the time he needs it. The device prevents the patient from accidentally overdosing by imposing a lockout time between doses—usually 6 to 10 minutes. During this interval, the patient won't receive any analgesic, even if he pushes the button.

The device is a reusable, battery-operated peristaltic action pump that delivers a drug dose when the patient presses a button at the end of a cord.

Indications and advantages

Indicated for a patient who needs parenteral analgesia, PCA therapy is typically given to a postoperative patient (trauma, orthopedic, cesarean birth) and to a terminal cancer patient and others with chronic diseases. To receive PCA therapy, a patient must be mentally alert and able to understand and comply with instructions and procedures and have no history of allergy to the analgesic. A patient ineligible for therapy is one with limited respiratory reserve, a history of drug abuse or chronic sedative or tranquilizer use, or a psychiatric disorder. PCA therapy's advantages include:

- no need for I.M. analgesics
- pain relief tailored to each patient's size and pain tolerance
- a sense of control over pain
- ability to sleep at night with minimal daytime drowsiness
- lower opioid use compared with patients not on PCA
- improved postoperative deep breathing, coughing, and ambulation.

PCA setup

To set up a PCA system, the practitioner's order should include:

- a loading dose, given by I.V. push at the start of PCA therapy (typically, morphine)
- the appropriate lockout interval
- the maintenance dose (basal dose)
- the amount the patient will receive when he activates the device (typically, 10 mg of meperidine [Demerol] or 1 mg of morphine)
- the maximum amount the patient can receive within a specified time (if an adjustable device is used).

Nursing considerations

Because the primary adverse effect of analgesics is respiratory depression, monitor the patient's respiratory rate routinely. Also, check for infiltration into the subcutaneous tissues and for catheter occlusion, which may cause the drug to back up in the primary I.V. tubing. If the analgesic nauseates the patient, you may need to administer an antiemetic drug.

Before the patient starts using the PCA device, teach him how it works. Then have the patient practice with a sample device. Explain that he should take enough analgesic to relieve acute pain but not enough to induce drowsiness.

During therapy, monitor and record the amount of analgesic infused, the patient's respiratory rate, and the patient's assessment of pain relief. If the patient reports insufficient pain relief, notify the practitioner.

Giving medications

- If the patient is allowed oral intake, begin with a nonopioid analgesic, such as acetaminophen or aspirin, every 4 to 6 hours as ordered.
- If the patient needs more relief than a nonopioid analgesic provides, you may give a mild opioid (such as oxycodone or codeine) as ordered.
- If the patient needs still more pain relief, you may administer a strong opioid (such as methadone, levorphanol, morphine, or hydromorphone) as prescribed. Administer oral medications if possible. Check the

Assessing pain

To assess pain properly, you'll need to consider the patient's description and your own observations of the patient's physical and behavioral responses. Start by asking the following series of key questions (bearing in mind that the patient's responses will be shaped by his prior experiences, self-image, and beliefs about his condition):

- Where's the pain located? How long does it last? How often does it occur?
- Can you describe the pain?
- What relieves the pain or makes it worse?

Ask the patient to rate his pain on a scale of 0 to 10, with 0 denoting lack of pain and 10 denoting the worst pain level. This helps the patient verbally evaluate pain therapies. Observe the patient's behavioral and physiologic responses to pain. Physiologic responses may be sympathetic or parasympathetic.

Behavioral responses

Behavioral responses include altered body position, moaning, sighing, grimacing, withdrawal, crying, restlessness, muscle twitching, and immobility.

Sympathetic responses

Sympathetic responses are commonly associated with mild to moderate pain and include pallor, elevated blood pressure, dilated pupils, skeletal muscle tension, dyspnea, tachycardia, and diaphoresis.

Parasympathetic responses

Parasympathetic responses are commonly associated with severe, deep pain and include pallor, decreased blood pressure, bradycardia, nausea and vomiting, weakness, dizziness, and loss of consciousness.

Assess pain at least every 2 hours and during rest, during activity, and through the night when pain commonly surges. Ability to sleep doesn't indicate absence of pain.

appropriate drug information for each medication given.

- If ordered, teach the patient how to use a PCA device. Such a device can help the patient manage his pain and decrease his anxiety.

Providing emotional support

- Show your concern by spending time talking with the patient. Because of his pain and his inability to manage it, he may be anxious and frustrated. Such feelings can worsen his pain.

Performing comfort measures

- Periodically reposition the patient to reduce muscle spasms and tension and to relieve pressure on bony prominences. Increasing the angle of the bed can reduce pull on an abdominal incision, diminishing pain. If appropriate, elevate a limb to reduce swelling, inflammation, and pain.
- Give the patient a back massage to help reduce tense muscles.
- Perform passive range-of-motion exercises to prevent stiffness and further loss of mobility, relax tense muscles, and provide comfort.
- Provide oral hygiene. Keep a fresh water glass or cup at the bedside because many pain medications tend to dry the mouth.
- Wash the patient's face and hands to soothe him, which may reduce his perception of pain.

Using cognitive therapy

- Help the patient enhance the effect of analgesics by using such techniques as distraction, guided imagery, deep breathing, and relaxation. You can easily use these "mind-over-pain" techniques at the bedside. Choose the method the patient prefers. If possible, start these techniques when the patient feels little or no pain. If he feels persistent pain, begin with short, simple exercises. Before beginning, dim the lights, remove the patient's restrictive

Visual pain rating scale

You can evaluate pain in a nonverbal manner for pediatric patients ages 3 and older and for adults with language difficulties. One instrument is the Wong-Baker FACES pain rating scale; another, two simple faces such as the ones shown below. Ask the patient to choose the face that describes how he's feeling—either happy because he has no pain, or sad because he has some or a lot of pain. Alternatively, to pinpoint varying levels of pain, you can ask the patient to draw a face.

clothing, and eliminate noise from the environment.

- For distraction, have the patient recall a pleasant experience or focus his attention on an enjoyable activity. For instance, have him use music as a distraction by turning on the radio when the pain begins. Tell him to close his eyes and concentrate on listening, raising or lowering the volume as his pain increases or subsides. Note, however, that distraction is usually effective only against brief episodes of pain lasting less than 5 minutes.
- For guided imagery, help the patient concentrate on a peaceful, pleasant image such as walking on the beach. Encourage him to concentrate on the details of the image he has selected by asking about its sight, sound, smell, taste, and touch. The positive emotions evoked by this exercise minimize pain.
- For deep breathing, have the patient stare at an object, then slowly inhale and exhale as he counts aloud to maintain a comfortable rate and rhythm. Tell him to concentrate on the rise and fall of his abdomen. Encourage him to feel more and more weightless with each breath while he concentrates on the rhythm of his breathing or on any restful image.
- For muscle relaxation, have the patient focus on a particular muscle group. Ask him to tense the muscles and note the sensation. After 5 to 7 seconds, tell him to relax the muscles and concentrate on the relaxed state. Tell him to note the difference between the tense and relaxed states. After he tenses and relaxes one muscle group, have him proceed to another and another until he has covered his entire body.

Special considerations

- Evaluate your patient's response to pain management. If he's still in pain, reassess him and alter your care plan as appropriate.
- Remind the patient that results of cognitive therapy techniques improve with practice. Help him through the initial sessions.
- Remember that patients receiving opioid analgesics are at risk for developing tolerance, dependence, or addiction. Patients with acute pain may have a smaller risk of dependence or addiction than patients with chronic pain.
- If a patient receiving an opioid analgesic experiences abstinence syndrome when the drug is withdrawn abruptly, suspect physical dependence. The signs and symptoms include anxiety, irritability, chills and hot flashes, excessive salivation and tearing, rhinorrhea, sweating, nausea, vomiting, and seizures. These signs and symptoms are likely to begin in 6 to 12 hours and to peak in 24 to 72 hours. To reduce the risk of dependence, discontinue an opioid by decreasing the dose gradually each day. You may switch to an oral opioid and decrease its dose gradually.
- If a patient becomes addicted, his behavior will be characterized by compulsive drug use and a craving for the drug to experience effects other than pain relief. A patient demonstrating such behavior usually has a preexisting problem that's exacerbated by the opioid use. Discuss the addicted patient's problem with supportive personnel, and make appropriate referrals to experts.

- During periods of intense pain, the patient's ability to concentrate diminishes. If your patient is in severe pain, help him to select a cognitive technique that's simple to use. After he selects a technique, encourage him to use it consistently.
- If your patient has dementia or some other cognitive impairment, don't assume that he can't understand a pain scale or communicate about his pain. Experiment with several pain scales, a scale featuring faces such as the Wong-Baker FACES scale is a good choice for many cognitively impaired patients and those with limited language skills. (See *Visual pain rating scale*.)

Complications

- Respiratory depression (the most serious), sedation, constipation, nausea, and vomiting with analgesics

Patient teaching

- Reinforce the alternative therapy methods the patient has learned.
- Teach the patient distraction, guided imagery, deep breathing, and relaxation techniques, as appropriate.

Documentation

Document each step of the nursing process. Describe the subjective information you elicited from the patient, using his own words. Note the location, quality, and duration of the pain as well as any precipitating factors.

Record your nursing diagnoses, and include the pain-relief method selected. Use a flow sheet to document pain assessment findings. Summarize your actions and the patient's response, including vital signs. If the patient's pain wasn't relieved, note alternative treatments to consider the next time pain occurs. Record any complications of drug therapy.

PAP and PAWP monitoring

Continuous pulmonary artery pressure (PAP) and intermittent pulmonary artery wedge pressure (PAWP) measurements provide important information about left ventricular function and preload. You can use this information not only for monitoring but also for aiding diagnosis, refining your assessment, guiding interventions, and projecting patient outcomes.

Nearly all acutely ill patients are candidates for PAP monitoring—especially those who are hemodynamically unstable, who need fluid management or continuous cardiopulmonary assessment, or who are receiving multiple or frequently administered cardioactive drugs. It's also crucial for patients with shock, trauma, pulmonary or cardiac disease, or multiorgan disease.

The original PAP monitoring catheter, the Swan-Ganz catheter, is commonly referred to as a pulmonary artery (PA) catheter. Current versions have up to six lumens, allowing more hemodynamic information to be gathered. In addition to distal and proximal lumens used to measure pressures, a PA catheter has a balloon inflation lumen that inflates the balloon for PAWP measurement and a thermistor connector lumen that allows cardiac output measurement. Some catheters also have a pacemaker wire lumen that provides a port for pacemaker electrodes and measures continuous mixed venous oxygen saturation. (See *PA catheters: Basic to complex,* page 364.)

Fluoroscopy usually isn't required during catheter insertion because the catheter is flow directed, following venous blood flow from the right heart chambers into the pulmonary artery. Also, the pulmonary artery, right atrium, and right ventricle produce characteristic pressures and waveforms that can be observed on the monitor to help track catheter-tip location. Marks on the catheter shaft, with 10-cm graduations, assist tracking by showing how far the catheter is inserted.

The PA catheter is inserted into the heart's right side with the distal tip lying in the pulmonary artery. Left-sided pressures can be assessed indirectly.

No specific contraindications for PAP monitoring exist. However, some patients undergoing it require special precautions. These include elderly patients with pulmonary hypertension, those with left

PA catheters: Basic to complex

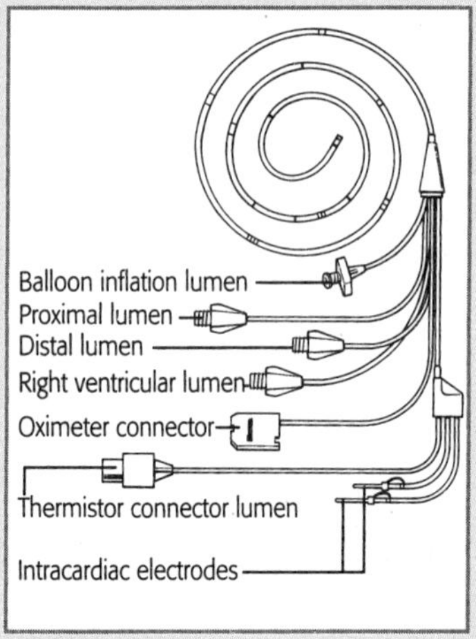

Depending on the intended use, a pulmonary artery (PA) catheter may be simple or complex. The basic PA catheter has a distal and proximal lumen, a thermistor, and a balloon inflation gate valve. The *distal lumen,* which exits into the pulmonary artery, monitors PA pressure. Its hub usually is marked "P distal" or is color-coded yellow. The *proximal lumen* exits in the right atrium or vena cava, depending on the size of the patient's heart. It monitors right atrial pressure and can be used as the injected solution lumen for cardiac output determination and for infusing solutions. The proximal lumen hub is usually marked "Proximal" or is color-coded blue.

The thermistor, located 1½" (3.8 cm) from the distal tip, measures temperature (aiding core temperature evaluation) and allows cardiac output measurement. The thermistor connector attaches to a cardiac output connector cable, then to a cardiac output monitor. Typically, it's red.

The balloon inflation gate valve is used for inflating the balloon tip with air. A stopcock connection, typically color-coded red, may be used.

Additional lumens

Some PA catheters have additional lumens used to obtain other hemodynamic data or permit certain interventions. For instance, *a proximal infusion port,* which exits in the right atrium or vena cava, allows additional fluid administration. *A right ventricular lumen,* exiting in the right ventricle, allows fluid administration, right ventricular pressure measurement, or use of a temporary ventricular pacing lead.

Some catheters have additional right atrial and right ventricular lumens for atrioventricular pacing. A right ventricular ejection fraction test-response thermistor, with pulmonary artery and right ventricular sensing electrodes, allows volumetric and ejection fraction measurements. Fiber-optic filaments, such as those used in pulse oximetry, exit into the pulmonary artery and permit measurement of continuous mixed venous oxygen saturation.

---

bundle-branch heart block, and those for whom a systemic infection would be life-threatening.

Equipment

Balloon-tipped, flow-directed PA catheter ♦ prepared pressure transducer system ♦ alcohol pads ♦ medication-added label ♦ monitor and monitor cable ♦ I.V. pole with transducer mount ♦ emergency resuscitation equipment ♦ electrocardiogram (ECG) monitor ♦ ECG electrodes ♦ arm board (for antecubital insertion) ♦ lead aprons (if fluoroscope is necessary) ♦ sutures ♦ sterile 4" × 4" gauze pads or other dry, occlusive dressing material ♦ prepackaged introducer kit ♦ optional: dextrose 5% in water, electric clippers (for femoral insertion site)

If a prepackaged introducer kit is unavailable, obtain the following: an introducer (one size larger than the catheter) ♦ sterile tray containing instruments for procedure ♦ masks ♦ sterile gowns ♦ sterile gloves ♦ antiseptic solution ♦ sutures ♦ two 10-ml syringes ♦ local anesthetic (1% to 2% lidocaine) ♦ one 5-ml syringe ♦ 25G ½" needle ♦ 1" and 3" tape

Preparation

- To obtain reliable pressure values and clear waveforms, the pressure monitoring system and bedside monitor must be properly calibrated and zeroed.
- Make sure the monitor has the correct pressure modules; then calibrate it according to the manufacturer's instructions. (For instructions, see "Transducer system setup," page 544.)
- Turn the monitor on before gathering the equipment to give it time to warm up.
- Prepare the pressure monitoring system according to your facility's policy. Your facility's guidelines may also specify whether to mount the transducer on the I.V. pole or tape it to the patient and whether to add heparin to the flush.
- To manage any complications from catheter insertion, make sure to have emergency resuscitation equipment on hand (defibrillator, oxygen, and supplies for intubation and emergency drug administration).
- Prepare a sterile field for insertion of the introducer and catheter.
- Label all medications, medication containers, and solutions on and off the sterile field.

Key steps

- Check the patient's chart for heparin sensitivity, which contraindicates adding heparin to the flush solution.
- Confirm the patient's identity using two patient identifiers according to facility policy. If the patient is alert, explain the procedure to him to reduce his anxiety. Reassure him that the catheter poses little danger and rarely causes pain. Tell him that if he feels pain at the introducer insertion site, the physician will order an analgesic or a sedative.
- Be sure to tell the patient and his family not to be alarmed if they see the pressure waveform on the monitor "move around." Explain that the cause is usually artifact.

Positioning the patient for catheter placement

- Position the patient at the proper height and angle. If the physician will use a superior approach for percutaneous insertion (most commonly using the internal jugular or subclavian vein), place the patient flat or in a slight Trendelenburg position. Remove the patient's pillow to help engorge the vessel and prevent air embolism. Turn his head to the side opposite the insertion site.
- If the physician will use an inferior approach to access a femoral vein, position the patient flat. Be aware that with this approach, certain catheters are harder to insert and may require more manipulation.

Preparing the catheter

- Maintain sterile technique and use standard precautions throughout catheter preparation and insertion.
- Wash your hands. Then clean the insertion site with an antiseptic solution and drape it.
- Put on a mask. Help the physician put on a sterile mask, gown, and gloves.
- Open the outer packaging of the catheter, revealing the inner sterile wrapping. Using sterile technique, the physician opens the inner wrapping and picks up the catheter. Take the catheter lumen hubs as he hands them to you.
- To remove air from the catheter and verify its patency, flush the catheter. In the more common flushing method, you connect the syringes aseptically to the appropriate pressure lines, and then flush them before insertion. This method makes pressure waveforms easier to identify on the monitor during insertion.
- Alternatively, you may flush the lumens after catheter insertion with sterile I.V. solution from sterile syringes attached to the lumens. Leave the filled syringes on during insertion.
- If the system has multiple pressure lines (such as a distal line to monitor PAP and a proximal line to monitor right atrial pressure), make sure the distal PA lumen hub is attached to the pressure line that will be observed on the monitor. Inadvertently attaching the distal PA line to the proximal lumen hub will prevent the proper waveform from appearing during insertion.
- Observe the diastolic values carefully during insertion. Make sure the scale is appropriate for lower pressures. A scale of 0

to 25 mm Hg or 0 to 50 mm Hg (more common) is preferred. (With a higher scale, such as 0 to 100 or 0 to 250 mm Hg, waveforms appear too small and the location of the catheter tip will be hard to identify.)

- To verify the integrity of the balloon, the physician inflates it with air (usually 1.5 cc) before handing you the lumens to attach to the pressure monitoring system. He then observes the balloon for symmetrical shape. He may also submerge it in a small, sterile basin filled with sterile water and observe it for bubbles, which indicate a leak.

Inserting the catheter

- Assist the physician as he inserts the introducer to access the vessel. He may perform a cutdown or (more commonly) insert the catheter percutaneously, as with a modified Seldinger technique.
- After the introducer is placed, and the catheter lumens are flushed, the physician inserts the catheter through the introducer. In the internal jugular or subclavian approach, he inserts the catheter into the end of the introducer sheath with the balloon deflated, directing the curl of the catheter toward the patient's midline.
- As insertion begins, observe the bedside monitor for waveform variations. (See *Normal PA waveforms*.)
- When the catheter exits the end of the introducer sheath and reaches the junction of the superior vena cava and right atrium (at the 15- to 20-cm mark on the catheter shaft), the monitor shows oscillations that correspond to the patient's respirations. The balloon is then inflated with the recommended volume of air to allow normal blood flow and aid catheter insertion.
- Using a gentle, smooth motion, the physician advances the catheter through the heart chambers, moving rapidly to the pulmonary artery because prolonged manipulation may reduce catheter stiffness.
- When the mark on the catheter shaft reaches 15 to 20 cm, the catheter enters the right atrium. The waveform shows two small, upright waves; pressure is low (between 2 and 4 mm Hg). Read pressure values in the mean mode because systolic and diastolic values are similar.
- The physician advances the catheter into the right ventricle, working quickly to minimize irritation. The waveform now shows sharp systolic upstrokes and lower diastolic dips. Depending on the size of the patient's heart, the catheter should reach the 30- to 35-cm mark. (The smaller the heart, the shorter the catheter length needed to reach the right ventricle.) Record both systolic and diastolic pressures. Systolic pressure normally ranges from 15 to 25 mm Hg; diastolic pressure, from 0 to 8 mm Hg.
- As the catheter floats into the pulmonary artery, note that the upstroke from right ventricular systole is smoother, and systolic pressure is nearly the same as right ventricular systolic pressure. Record systolic, diastolic, and mean pressures (typically ranging from 8 to 15 mm Hg). A dicrotic notch on the diastolic portion of the waveform indicates pulmonic valve closure.

Wedging the catheter

- To obtain a wedge tracing, the physician lets the inflated balloon float downstream with the blood flow to a smaller, more distal branch of the pulmonary artery. Here, the catheter lodges, or wedges, causing occlusion of right ventricular and PA diastolic pressures. The tracing resembles the right atrial tracing because the catheter tip is recording left atrial pressure. The waveform shows two small uprises. Record PAWP in the mean mode (usually between 6 and 12 mm Hg).
- A PAWP waveform, or wedge tracing, appears when the catheter has been inserted 45 to 50 cm. (In a large heart, a longer catheter length—up to 55 cm—typically is required. However, a catheter should never be inserted more than 60 cm.) Usually, 30 to 45 seconds elapse from the time the physician inserts the introducer until the wedge tracing appears.
- The physician deflates the balloon, and the catheter drifts out of the wedge position and into the pulmonary artery, its normal resting place.

Normal PA waveforms

During pulmonary artery (PA) catheter insertion, the monitor shows various waveforms as the catheter advances through the heart chambers.

Right atrium

When the catheter tip enters the right atrium, the first heart chamber on its route, a waveform like the one shown at right appears on the monitor. Note the two small upright waves. The *a* waves represent left atrial contraction; the *v* waves, increased pressure or volume in the left atrium during left ventricular systole.

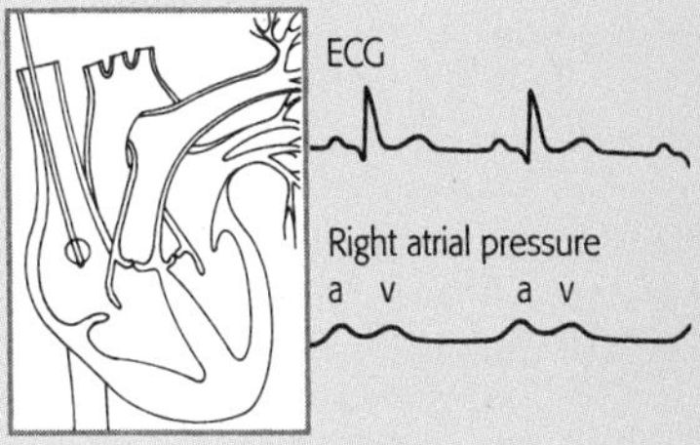

Right ventricle

As the catheter tip reaches the right ventricle, you'll see a waveform with sharp systolic upstrokes and lower diastolic dips.

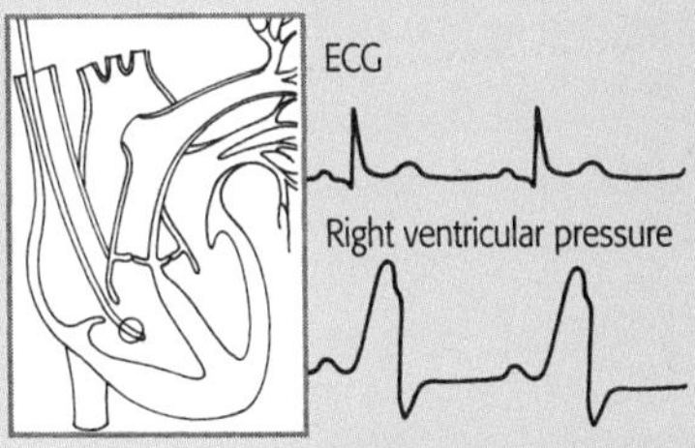

Pulmonary artery

The catheter then floats into the pulmonary artery, causing a waveform like the one shown at right. Note that the upstroke is smoother than on the right ventricular waveform. The dicrotic notch indicates pulmonic valve closure.

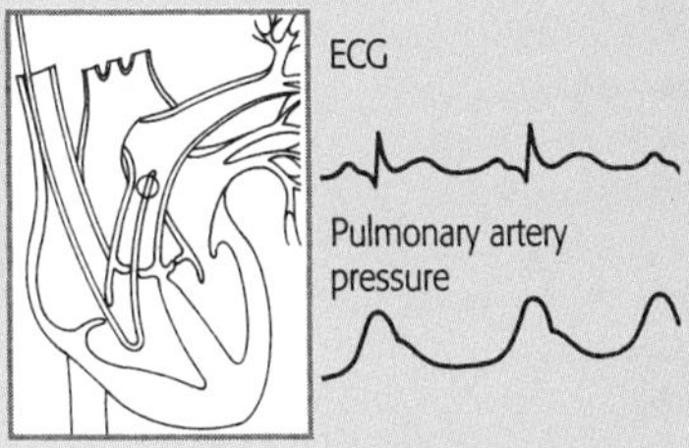

PAWP

Floating into a distal branch of the pulmonary artery, the balloon wedges where the vessel becomes too narrow for it to pass. The monitor now shows a pulmonary artery wedge pressure (PAWP) waveform, with two small uprises from left atrial systole and diastole. The balloon is then deflated and the catheter is left in the pulmonary artery. Observe for the return of the normal PA waveform.

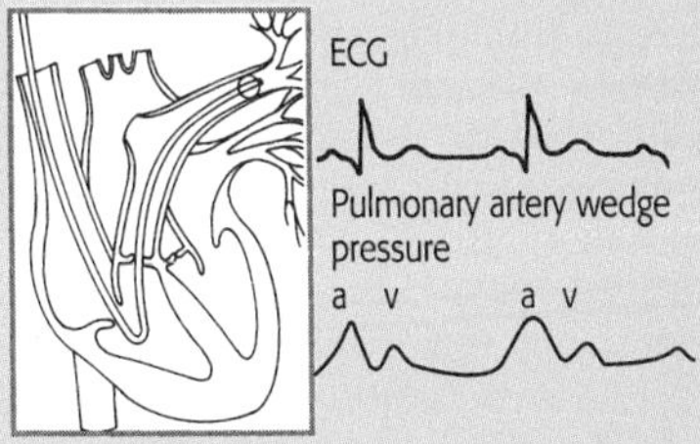

■ If the appropriate waveforms don't appear at the expected times during catheter insertion, the catheter may be coiled in the right atrium and ventricle. To correct this problem, deflate the balloon. To do this, unlock the gate valve or turn the stopcock to the ON position and then detach the syringe from the balloon inflation port. Back pressure in the pulmonary artery causes the balloon to deflate on its own. (Active air withdrawal may compromise balloon integrity.) To verify balloon deflation, observe the monitor for return of the PA tracing.
■ Typically, the physician orders a portable chest X-ray to confirm catheter position.
■ Apply a sterile occlusive dressing to the insertion site.

Obtaining intermittent PAP values

■ After inserting the catheter and recording initial pressure readings, record subsequent PAP values and monitor waveforms. These values will be used to calculate other important hemodynamic indices. To ensure accurate values, make sure the transducer is properly leveled and zeroed at the phlebostatic axis.
■ If possible, obtain PAP values at end expiration (when the patient completely exhales). At this time, intrathoracic pressure approaches atmospheric pressure and has the least effect on PAP. If you obtain a reading during other phases of the respiratory cycle, respiratory interference may occur. For instance, during inspiration, when intrathoracic pressure drops, PAP may be false-low because the negative pressure is transmitted to the catheter. During expiration, when intrathoracic pressure rises, PAP may be false-high.
■ For patients with a rapid respiratory rate and subsequent variations, you may have trouble identifying end expiration. The monitor displays an average of the digital readings obtained over time, as well as those readings obtained during a full respiratory cycle. If possible, obtain a printout. Use the averaged values obtained through the full respiratory cycle. To analyze trends accurately, be sure to record values at consistent times during the respiratory cycle.

Taking a PAWP reading

■ PAWP is recorded by inflating the balloon and letting it float in a distal artery. Some facilities allow only practitioners or specially trained nurses to take a PAWP reading because of the risk of PA rupture—a rare but life-threatening complication. If your facility permits you to perform this procedure, do so with extreme caution and make sure you're thoroughly familiar with intracardiac waveform interpretation.
■ To begin, verify that the transducer is properly leveled and zeroed. Detach the syringe from the balloon inflation hub. Draw 1.5 cc of air into the syringe, and then reattach the syringe to the hub. Watching the monitor, inject the air through the hub slowly and smoothly. When you see a wedge tracing on the monitor, immediately stop inflating the balloon. Never inflate the balloon beyond the volume needed to obtain a wedge tracing.
■ Take the pressure reading at end expiration. Note the amount of air needed to change the PA tracing to a wedge tracing (normally, 1.25 to 1.5 cc). If the wedge tracing appeared with the injection of less than 1.25 cc, suspect that the catheter has migrated into a more distal branch and requires repositioning. If the balloon is in a more distal branch, the tracings may move up the oscilloscope, indicating that the catheter tip is recording balloon pressure rather than PAWP. This may lead to PA rupture.
■ Detach the syringe from the balloon inflation port and allow the balloon to deflate on its own. Observe the waveform tracing and make sure the tracing returns from the wedge tracing to the normal PA tracing.

Removing the catheter

■ To assist the practitioner, inspect the chest X-ray for signs of catheter kinking or knotting. (In some states, you may be permitted to remove a PA catheter yourself under an advanced collaborative standard of practice.)
■ Obtain the patient's baseline vital signs, and note the ECG pattern.

- Explain the procedure to the patient. Place the head of the bed flat, unless ordered otherwise. If the catheter was inserted using a superior approach, turn the patient's head to the side opposite the insertion site. Gently remove the dressing.
- The physician will remove any sutures securing the catheter. However, if he wants to leave the introducer in place after catheter removal, he won't remove the sutures used to secure it.
- Turn all stopcocks off to the patient. (You may turn stopcocks on to the distal port if you wish to observe waveforms. However, use caution because this may cause an air embolism.)
- The physician puts on sterile gloves. After verifying that the balloon is deflated, he withdraws the catheter slowly and smoothly. If he feels any resistance, he'll stop immediately.
- Watch the ECG monitor for arrhythmias.
- If the introducer was removed, apply pressure to the site, and check it frequently for signs of bleeding. Dress the site again, as necessary. If the introducer is left in place, observe the diaphragm for any blood backflow, which verifies the integrity of the hemostasis valve.
- Return all equipment to the appropriate location. You may turn off the bedside pressure modules but leave the ECG module on.
- Reassure the patient and his family that he'll be observed closely. Make sure he understands that the catheter was removed because his condition has improved and he no longer needs it.

Special considerations

- Advise the patient to use caution when moving about in bed to avoid dislodging the catheter.
- Never leave the balloon inflated because this may cause pulmonary infarction. To determine if the balloon is inflated, check the monitor for a wedge tracing, which indicates inflation. (A PA tracing confirms balloon deflation.)
- Never inflate the balloon with more than the recommended air volume (specified on the catheter shaft) because this may cause loss of elasticity or balloon rupture. With appropriate inflation volume, the balloon floats easily through the heart chambers and rests in the main branch of the pulmonary artery, producing accurate waveforms. Never inflate the balloon with fluids because they may not be able to be retrieved from inside the balloon, preventing deflation.
- Be aware that the catheter may slip back into the right ventricle. Because the tip may irritate the ventricle, check the monitor for a right ventricular waveform to detect this problem promptly.
- To minimize valvular trauma, make sure the balloon is deflated whenever the catheter is withdrawn from the pulmonary artery to the right ventricle or from the right ventricle to the right atrium.
- Change the dressing whenever it's moist, every 24 to 48 hours, or according to your facility's policy. Change the catheter every 72 hours, the pressure tubing every 48 hours, and the flush solution every 24 hours.

Complications

- PA perforation, pulmonary infarction, catheter knotting, local or systemic infection, cardiac arrhythmias, and heparin-induced thrombocytopenia

Documentation

Document the date and time of catheter insertion, the physician who performed the procedure, the catheter insertion site, pressure waveforms and values for the various heart chambers, balloon inflation volume required to obtain a wedge tracing, any arrhythmias occurring during or after the procedure, type of flush solution used and its heparin concentration (if any), type of dressing applied, and the patient's tolerance of the procedure. Remember to initial and date the dressing.

After catheter removal, document the patient's tolerance for the removal procedure, and note any problems encountered during removal.

Passe-Muir valve use

Patients with a tracheostomy tube can't speak because the cuffed tracheostomy

Passe-Muir valve

These illustrations show how the one-way valve is open during inspiration and closed after expiration.

Front view

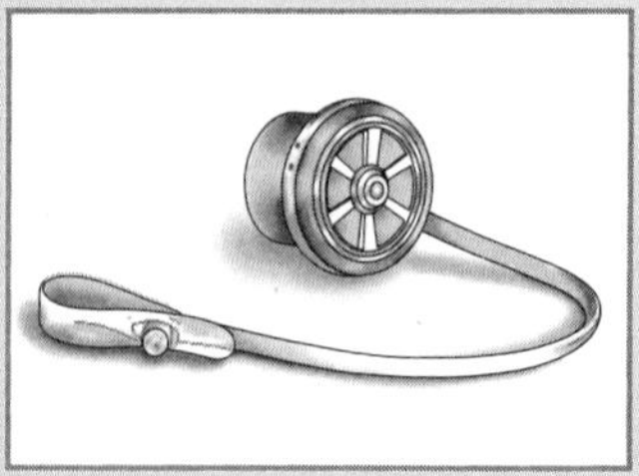

Side view

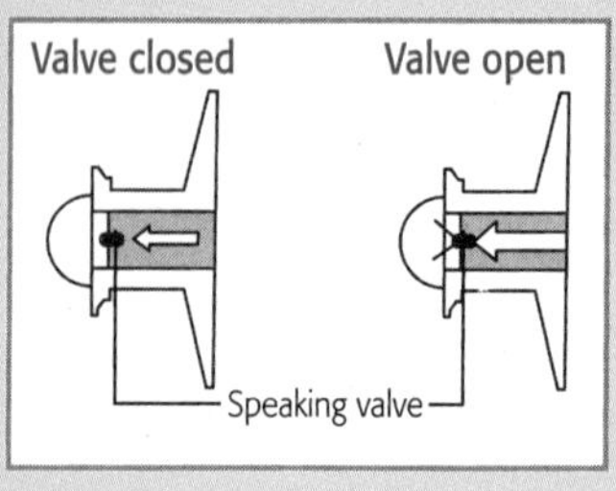

tube that directs air into the lungs expels air through the tracheostomy tube rather than the vocal cords, mouth, and nose. A Passe-Muir valve (PMV) is a positive-closure, one-way speaking valve that opens upon inspiration and closes after expiration, redirecting exhaled air around the tube, through the vocal cords, allowing the patient to speak. (See *Passe-Muir valve*.)

To function safely when using a PMV, the tracheostomy cuff must be completely deflated to enable the patient to exhale, or the tracheostomy tube must be cuffless.

Short- and long-term adult, pediatric, and infant tracheostomy and ventilator-dependent patients may benefit from the use of a speaking valve. A PMV should always be used with the assistance of a speech-language pathologist who should assess cognitive, language, and oral motor function and may evaluate swallowing status and risk of aspiration.

A practitioner's order is required for placement of the PMV and sometimes for cuff deflation.

Equipment

Appropriate-sized ventilator speaking valve ♦ gloves ♦ suction equipment ♦ 10-ml luer-lock syringe ♦ instruction booklet ♦ cuff-deflation warning signs

Key steps

- Explain the procedure to the patient. Provide written instructions, as needed.
- If this is the patient's first wearing experience, an initial trial should be coordinated with the respiratory therapist and speech-language pathologist.
- Elevate the head of the patient's bed about 45 degrees.
- The tracheostomy cuff must be completely deflated before valve is placed.
- Put on gloves and deflate the cuff slowly so he can get used to using his upper airways again. Attach a 10-ml syringe to the tracheostomy tube's pilot balloon and remove the air until air can no longer be extracted and a vacuum is created.
- Suction the trachea and oral cavity as needed.
- Hold the valve between your fingers. For a patient who isn't ventilator-dependent, attach the valve to the hub of the existing tracheostomy hub with a quarter-turn twist.
- After the valve is in place, encourage him to relax and concentrate on exhaling through his mouth and nose.
- Have him count aloud to 10, or speak, as he becomes comfortable breathing with the valve in place. The speech-language pathologist can facilitate voice production and speech.
- The aqua-colored PMV 007 is more convenient for ventilator-dependent patients because it's tapered to fit into disposable ventilator tubing. Insert the PMV into the end of the wide-mouth, short flex tubing.
- Connect the other end of the short flex tubing to the ventilator tubing.
- Then attach the PMV (connected to the short flex tubing) and the ventilator tubing to the closed-suction system.

- The PMV can also be attached between the swivel adapter and the short flex tubing and ventilator tubing.
- Post cuff-deflation warning signs in the room and label the tracheostomy pilot balloon to remind health care providers to reinflate the pilot balloon after removing the PMV.
- Gently twist the PMV to remove it; restore the original setup, then return ventilator settings to original levels and reinflate the pilot balloon cuff. Always remember to reinflate the tracheostomy cuff after removing the PMV.

Special considerations

- For maximum airflow around the tube, the tube shouldn't be larger than two-thirds the size of the tracheal lumen.

DO'S & DON'TS

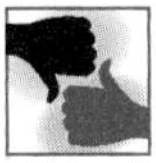

Don't place the PMV on the tracheostomy tube before deflating the cuff; the patient won't be able to breathe.

- The nurse and respiratory therapist are responsible for monitoring the patient's response to the PMV by evaluating blood pressure, heart rate, and respiratory status.
- Make sure that the patient is involved in the decision to use the ventilator speaking valve; make sure he understands how it functions and what to expect.
- If he's anxious, especially during cuff deflation, he may be unwilling to use the valve; provide emotional support.
- If he can't tolerate the valve initially; troubleshoot to determine the cause.
- To correct, try repositioning the patient, using a smaller tracheostomy tube, changing to a cuffless tube, or correcting airway obstruction. Some patients have to build tolerance, wearing the valve a few minutes at a time at first.
- If repeated trials fail, the speech-language pathologist should assess the patient for other communication options.

ALERT

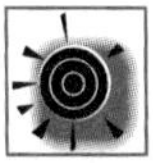

Remove the PMV if the patient shows signs of distress: significant change in blood pressure or heart rate, increased respiratory rate, dyspnea, diaphoresis, anxiety, uncontrollable coughing, or arterial oxygen saturation less than 90%. Reassess the patient before trying the valve again.

Complications

- None known

Patient teaching

- Explain the procedure to the patient. Provide written instructions, as needed.
- Instruct the patient and his family on the proper use of the PMV valve.
- Teach the patient and his family signs of distress, such as difficulty breathing, anxiety, sweating, and uncontrolled coughing. Tell them to call the patient's practitioner if any of these signs occur.

Documentation

Note the patient's response to the procedure. Record how long the PMV has been in place. Document respiratory and hemodynamic status. Document secretion management and note the patient's ability to vocalize.

Perineal care

Care of external genitalia and the anal area should be performed during the daily bath and, if necessary, at bedtime and after urination and bowel movements. Perineal care promotes cleanliness and prevents infection. It removes irritating and odorous secretions, such as smegma, that collect under the foreskin of the penis and on the inner surface of the labia. For the patient with perineal skin breakdown, frequent bathing followed by application of ointment or cream aids healing. Standard precautions must be followed when providing perineal care.

Equipment

Gloves ♦ washcloths ♦ clean basin ♦ mild soap ♦ bath towel or bath blanket ♦ toilet tissue ♦ linen-saver pad ♦ trash bag ♦ peri bottle ♦ antiseptic soap ♦ petroleum jelly ♦ zinc oxide cream ♦ vitamin A and D ointment ♦ ABD pad ♦ optional: bedpan

Preparation

- Following genital or rectal surgery, you may need to use sterile supplies, including sterile gloves, gauze, and cotton balls.
- Obtain ointment or cream, as needed.
- Fill the basin two-thirds full with warm water.
- Fill the peri bottle with warm water, if needed.

Key steps

- Assemble equipment at the patient's bedside and provide privacy.
- Wash your hands and put on gloves.
- Explain the procedure to the patient.
- Adjust the bed to a comfortable working height to prevent back strain; lower the head of the bed, if allowed.
- Help the patient to a supine position.
- Place a linen-saver pad under the patient's buttocks to protect the bed from stains and moisture.

Perineal care for the female patient

- To minimize the patient's exposure, place the bath blanket over her with the corners head to foot and side to side.
- Wrap each leg with a side corner, tucking it under the hip.
- Fold back the corner between the legs to expose the perineum.
- Ask the patient to bend her knees slightly and spread her legs.
- Separate her labia with one hand and wash with the other, using downward strokes from the front to the back of the perineum to prevent intestinal organisms from contaminating the urethra or vagina.
- Avoid the area around the anus, and use a clean section of washcloth for each stroke by folding each used section inward. This prevents the spread of contaminated secretions or discharge.
- Using a clean washcloth, rinse thoroughly from front to back; soap residue can cause skin irritation.
- Pat the area dry with a bath towel because moisture can also cause skin irritation and discomfort.
- Apply ordered ointments or creams.
- Turn the patient on her side to Sims' position, if possible, to expose the anal area.
- Clean, rinse, and dry the anal area, starting at the posterior vaginal opening and wiping from front to back.

Perineal care for the male patient

- Drape the patient's legs to minimize exposure of the genital area.
- Hold the shaft of the penis with one hand and wash with the other, beginning at the tip and working in a circular motion from the center to the periphery to avoid introducing microorganisms into the urethra.
- Use a clean section of washcloth for each stroke to prevent spread of contaminated secretions or discharge.
- Rinse thoroughly, using the same circular motion.
- For the uncircumcised patient, gently retract the foreskin and clean beneath it. Rinse well but don't dry because moisture provides lubrication and prevents friction when replacing the foreskin. Replace the foreskin to avoid constriction of the penis, which causes edema and tissue damage.
- Wash the rest of the penis, using downward strokes toward the scrotum.
- Rinse well and pat dry with a bath towel.
- Handle the scrotum gently to avoid causing discomfort.
- Turn the patient on his side. Clean the bottom of the scrotum and the anal area.
- Rinse well and pat dry.

After providing perineal care

- Reposition and make the patient comfortable.
- Remove the bath blanket and linen-saver pad.
- Replace the bed linens.
- Clean and return the basin and dispose of soiled articles, including gloves.

Special considerations

- Give perineal care in a matter-of-fact way to minimize embarrassment.
- If the patient is incontinent, first remove excess feces with toilet tissue.

- Position him on a bedpan, and add a small amount of antiseptic soap to a peri bottle to eliminate odor.
- Irrigate the perineal area to remove any remaining fecal matter.
- After cleaning the perineum, apply ointment or cream (petroleum jelly, zinc oxide cream, or vitamin A and D ointment) to prevent skin breakdown.
- To reduce the number of linen changes, tuck an ABD pad between the patient's buttocks to absorb oozing feces.

Complications

- None known

Patient teaching

- Teach family members the proper techniques for providing perineal care. Have them provide a return demonstration if time permits.

Documentation

Record perineal care and special treatments. Note need for continued treatment, if necessary, in your care plan. Describe perineal skin condition and odor or discharge.

Peripheral I.V. line insertion

Peripheral I.V. catheter insertion involves selection of a venipuncture device and an insertion site, application of a tourniquet, preparation of the site, and venipuncture. Selection of a venipuncture device and site depends on the type of solution to be used; frequency and duration of infusion; patency and location of accessible veins; the patient's age, size, and condition; and, when possible, the patient's preference.

If possible, choose a vein in the nondominant arm or hand. Preferred venipuncture sites are the cephalic and basilic veins in the lower arm and the veins in the dorsum of the hand; least favorable are the leg and foot veins because of the increased risk of thrombophlebitis. Antecubital veins can be used if no other venous access is available.

A peripheral catheter allows administration of fluids, medication, blood, and blood components and maintains I.V. access to the patient. Insertion is contraindicated in a sclerotic vein, an edematous or impaired arm or hand, or a postmastectomy arm and in patients with a mastectomy, burns, or an arteriovenous fistula. Subsequent venipunctures should be performed proximal to a previously used or injured vein.

Equipment

Alcohol pads or other approved antimicrobial solution such as chlorhexidine swabs ♦ gloves ♦ tourniquet (rubber tubing or a blood pressure cuff) ♦ I.V. access devices ♦ I.V. solution with attached and primed administration set ♦ I.V. pole ♦ sharps container ♦ gauze pads or a transparent semipermeable dressing ♦ 1″ hypoallergenic tape ♦ optional: arm board, roller gauze, tube gauze, warm packs, scissors, catheter securement device

Commercial venipuncture kits come with or without an I.V. access device. (See *Comparing basic venous access devices,* page 374.) In many facilities, venipuncture equipment is kept on a tray or cart, allowing choice of correct access devices and easy replacement of contaminated items.

Preparation

- Check the information on the label of the I.V. solution container, including the patient's name and room number, type of solution, time and date of its preparation, preparer's name, and ordered infusion rate.
- Compare the prescriber's orders with the solution label to verify that the solution is the correct one.
- Then select the smallest-gauge device that's appropriate for the infusion (unless subsequent therapy will require a larger one). Smaller gauges cause less trauma to veins, allow greater blood flow around their tips, and reduce the risk of phlebitis.
- If you're using a winged infusion set, connect the adapter to the administration set, and unclamp the line until fluid flows from the open end of the needle cover.

Comparing basic venous access devices

Use the chart below to compare the two major types of venous access devices.

Over-the-needle catheter

Purpose

- Long-term therapy for the active or agitated patient

Advantages

- Inadvertent puncture of vein less likely than with a winged infusion set
- More comfortable for the patient
- Radiopaque thread for easy location
- Syringe attached to some units that permits easy check of blood return and prevents air from entering the vessel on insertion
- Safety needles that prevent accidental needle sticks
- Activity-restricting device, such as arm board, rarely required

Disadvantages

- Difficult to insert
- Extra care required to ensure that needle and catheter are inserted into vein

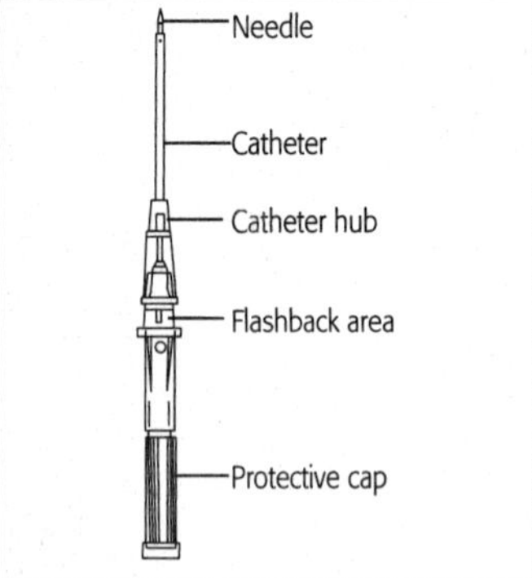

Winged infusion set

Purpose

- Short-term therapy (such as single-dose infusion) for cooperative adult patient
- Therapy of any duration for an infant or a child or for an elderly patient with fragile or sclerotic veins

Advantages

- Easiest intravascular device to insert because needle is thin-walled and extremely sharp
- Ideal for nonirritating I.V. push drugs

Disadvantage

- Risk of infiltration increases as duration of use increases

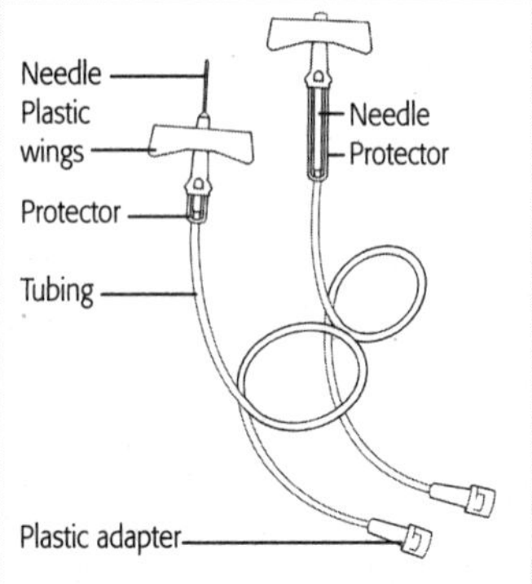

- Then close the clamp and place the needle on a sterile surface, such as the inside of its packaging.
- If you're using a catheter device, open its package to allow easy access.

Key steps

- Place the I.V. pole in the proper slot in the patient's bed frame. If you're using a portable I.V. pole, position it close to the frame.
- Hang the I.V. solution with attached primed administration set on the I.V. pole.

■ Confirm the patient's identity using two patient identifiers according to facility policy.
■ Wash your hands thoroughly. Then explain the procedure to the patient to ensure his cooperation and reduce anxiety. Anxiety can cause a vasomotor response resulting in venous constriction.

Selecting the site

■ Select the puncture site. If long-term therapy is anticipated, start with a vein at the most distal site so that you can move proximally as needed for subsequent I.V. insertion sites. For infusion of an irritating medication, choose a large vein distal to any nearby joint. Make sure the intended vein can accommodate the cannula.
■ Place the patient in a comfortable, reclining position, leaving the arm in a dependent position to increase venous fill of the lower arms and hands. If the patient's skin is cold, warm it by rubbing and stroking the arm, or cover the entire arm with warm packs or submerge in warm water for 5 to 10 minutes.

Applying the tourniquet

■ Apply a tourniquet about 6″ (15 cm) above the intended puncture site to dilate the vein (as shown below). Check for a radial pulse. If it isn't present, release the tourniquet and reapply it with less tension to prevent arterial occlusion.

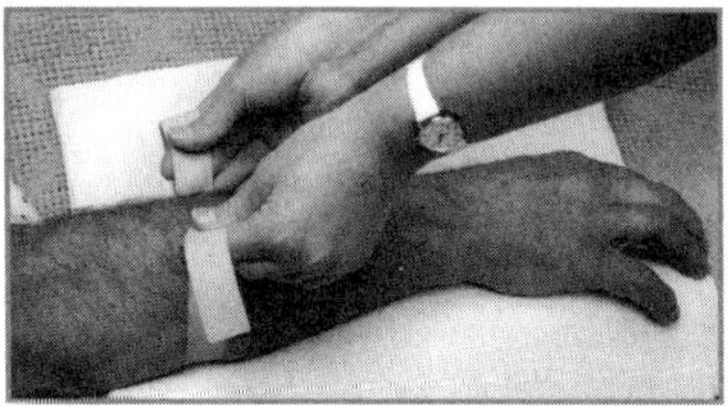

■ Lightly palpate the vein with the index and middle fingers of your nondominant hand. Stretch the skin to anchor the vein. If the vein feels hard or ropelike, select another.
■ If the vein is easily palpable but not sufficiently dilated, one or more of the following techniques may help raise the vein. Place the extremity in a dependent position for several seconds, and gently tap your finger over the vein or rub or stroke the skin upward toward the tourniquet. If you have selected a vein in the arm or hand, tell the patient to open and close his fist several times.
■ Leave the tourniquet in place for no longer than 3 minutes. If you can't find a suitable vein and prepare the site in that time, release the tourniquet for a few minutes. Then reapply it and continue the procedure.

Preparing the site

■ Put on gloves. Clip the hair around the insertion site if needed. Clean the site with alcohol pads or another approved antimicrobial solution, according to facility policy.

Use a vigorous side-to-side motion (as shown below) to remove flora that would otherwise be introduced into the vascular system with the venipuncture. Allow the antimicrobial solution to dry.

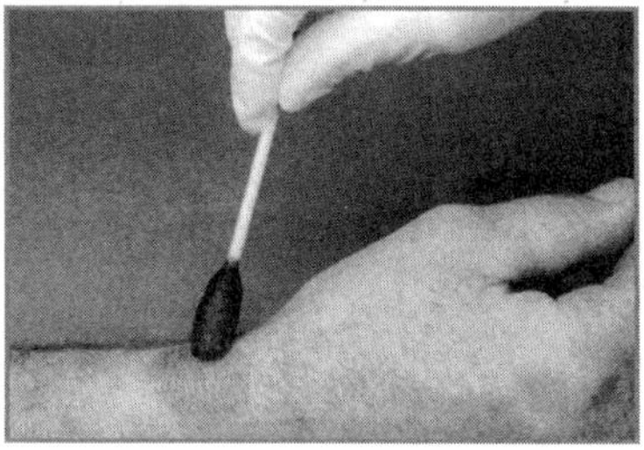

■ If ordered, administer a local anesthetic. Make sure the patient isn't sensitive to lidocaine.
■ Lightly press the vein with the thumb of your nondominant hand about 1½″ (3.8 cm) from the intended insertion site. The vein should feel round, firm, fully engorged, and resilient.
■ Grasp the access cannula. If you're using a winged infusion set, hold the short edges of the wings (with the needle's bevel facing upward) between the thumb and forefinger of your dominant hand. Then squeeze the wings together. If you're using an over-the-needle cannula, grasp the plastic hub with your dominant hand, remove the cover, and examine the cannula tip. If the edge isn't smooth, discard and replace the device.

■ Using the thumb of your nondominant hand, stretch the skin taut below the puncture site to stabilize the vein (as shown below).

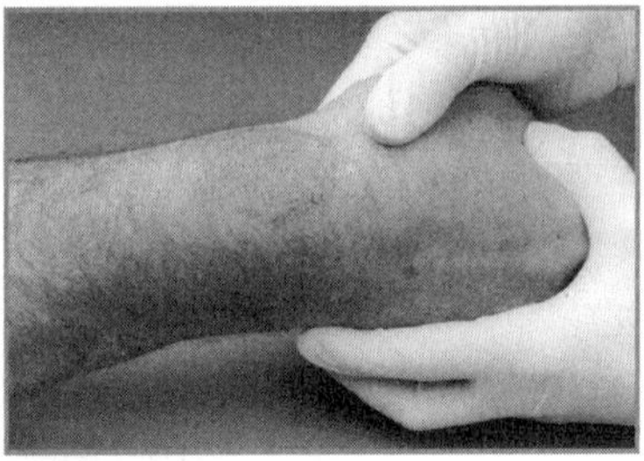

■ Tell the patient that you are about to insert the device.

■ Hold the needle bevel up and enter the skin directly over the vein at a 0- to 15-degree angle (as shown below).

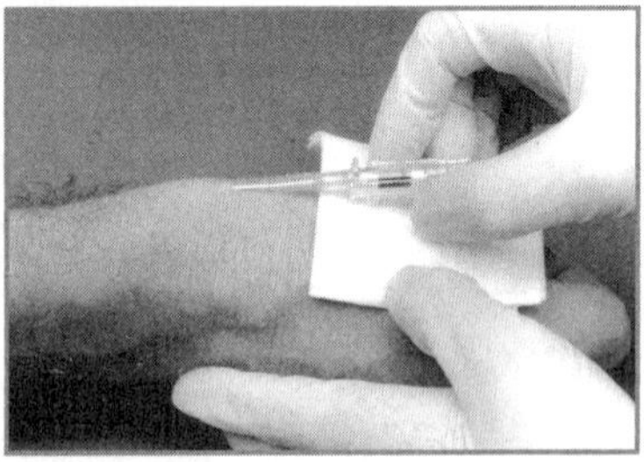

■ Aggressively push the needle directly through the skin and into the vein in one motion. Check the flashback chamber behind the hub for blood return, signifying that the vein has been properly accessed. (You may not see a blood return in a small vein.)

■ Then level the insertion device slightly by lifting the tip of the device up to prevent puncturing the back wall of the vein with the access device.

■ If you're using a winged infusion set, advance the needle fully, if possible, and hold it in place. Release the tourniquet, open the administration set clamp slightly, and check for free flow or infiltration.

■ If you're using an over-the-needle cannula, advance the device to at least one-half of its length to ensure that the cannula itself—not just the introducer needle—has entered the vein. Then remove the tourniquet.

■ Grasp the cannula hub to hold it in the vein, and withdraw the needle. As you withdraw it, press lightly on the catheter tip to prevent bleeding (as shown below).

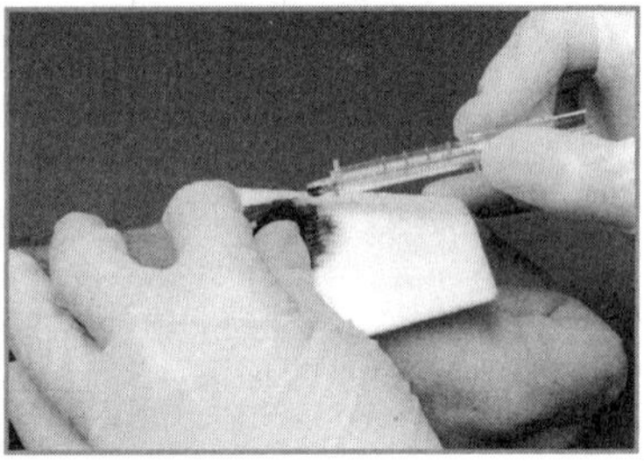

■ Advance the cannula up to the hub or until you meet resistance.

■ To advance the cannula while infusing I.V. solution, release the tourniquet and remove the inner needle. Using sterile technique, attach the I.V. tubing and begin the infusion. While stabilizing the vein with one hand, use the other to advance the catheter into the vein. When the catheter is advanced, decrease the I.V. flow rate. This method reduces the risk of puncturing the vein's opposite wall because the catheter is advanced without the steel needle and because the rapid flow dilates the vein.

■ To advance the cannula before starting the infusion, first release the tourniquet. While stabilizing the vein and needle with one hand, use the other to advance the catheter off the needle and further into the vein up to the hub (as shown below). Next, remove the inner needle and, using sterile technique, quickly attach the I.V. tubing. This method usually results in less blood being spilled.

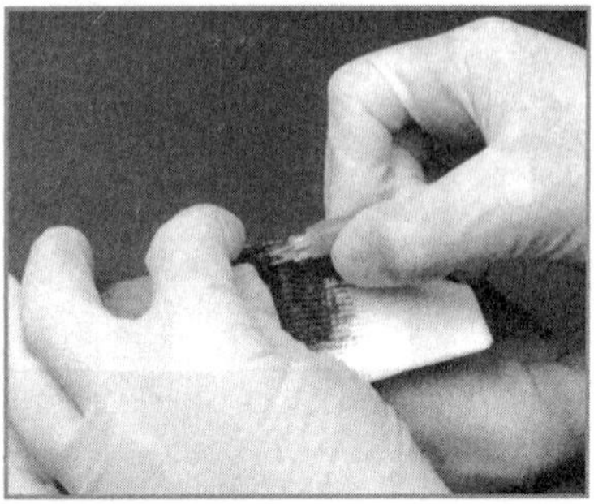

Dressing the site

- After the venous access device has been inserted, clean the skin completely. Dispose of the needle in a sharps container. Then regulate the flow rate.
- You may use a transparent semipermeable dressing to secure the device. (See *How to apply a transparent semipermeable dressing*.)
- If you don't use a transparent dressing, cover the site with a sterile gauze pad or small adhesive bandage.
- Loop the I.V. tubing on the patient's limb, and secure the tubing with tape. The loop allows some slack to prevent dislodgment of the cannula from tension on the line. (See *Methods of taping a venous access site*, page 378.)
- You may also use a catheter securement device to secure the device. Follow the manufacturer's directions for applying the device.
- Label the last piece of tape with the type, gauge of needle, and length of cannula; date and time of insertion; and your initials. Adjust the flow rate as ordered.
- If the puncture site is near a movable joint, place an arm board under the joint and secure it with roller gauze or tape to provide stability because excessive movement can dislodge the venous access device and increase the risk of thrombophlebitis and infection.
- When an arm board is used, check frequently for impaired circulation distal to the infusion site.

How to apply a transparent semipermeable dressing

To secure the I.V. insertion site, you can apply a transparent semipermeable dressing as follows:

- Make sure the insertion site is clean and dry.
- Remove the dressing from the package and, using sterile technique, remove the protective seal. Avoid touching the sterile surface.
- Place the dressing directly over the insertion site and the hub, as shown below. Don't cover the tubing. Also, don't stretch the dressing because doing so may cause itching.

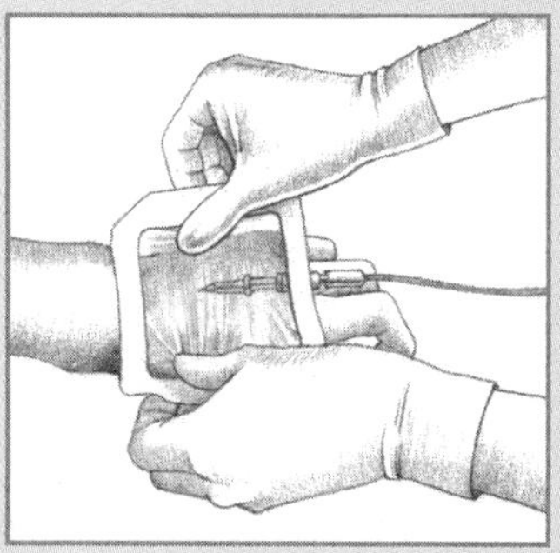

- Tuck the dressing around and under the cannula hub to make the site impervious to microorganisms.
- To remove the dressing, grasp one corner, and then lift and stretch it. If removal is difficult, try loosening the edges with alcohol or water.

Removing a peripheral I.V. line

- A peripheral I.V. line is removed on completion of therapy, for cannula site changes, and for suspected infection or infiltration; the procedure usually requires gloves, a sterile gauze pad, and an adhesive bandage.
- To remove the I.V. line, first clamp the I.V. tubing to stop the flow of solution. Then gently remove the transparent dressing and all tape from the skin.
- Using sterile technique, open the gauze pad and adhesive bandage and place them within reach. Put on gloves. Hold the sterile gauze pad over the puncture site with one hand, and use your other hand to withdraw the cannula slowly and smoothly, keeping it parallel to the skin. (Inspect the cannula tip; if it isn't smooth, assess the patient immediately, and notify the practitioner.)
- Using the gauze pad, apply firm pressure over the puncture site for 1 to 2 minutes after removal or until bleeding has stopped.

Methods of taping a venous access site

If you'll be using tape to secure the access device to the insertion site, use one of the basic methods described below. Use sterile tape if you'll be placing a transparent dressing over the tape.

Chevron method

- Cut a long strip of ½" tape and place it sticky side up under the cannula and parallel to the short strip of tape.
- Cross the ends of the tape over the cannula so that the tape sticks to the patient's skin (as shown below).
- Apply a piece of 1" tape across the two wings of the chevron.
- Loop the tubing and secure it with another piece of 1" tape. When the dressing is secured, apply a label. On the label, write the date and time of insertion, type and gauge of the needle, and your initials.

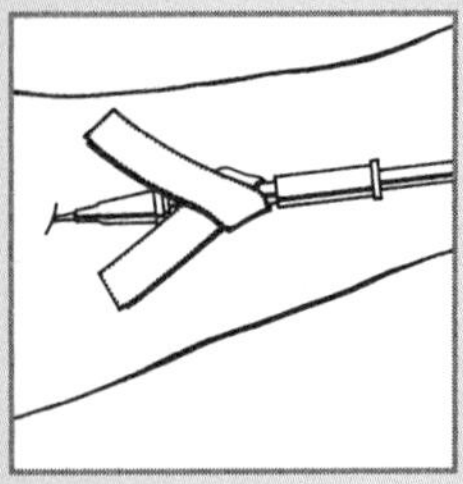

U method

- Cut a 2" (5 cm) strip of ½" tape. With the sticky side up, place it under the hub of the cannula.
- Bring each side of the tape up, folding it over the wings of the cannula in a U shape (as shown). Press it down parallel to the hub.
- Apply tape to stabilize the catheter.
- When a dressing is secured, apply a label. On the label, write the date and time of insertion, type and gauge of the needle or cannula, and your initials.

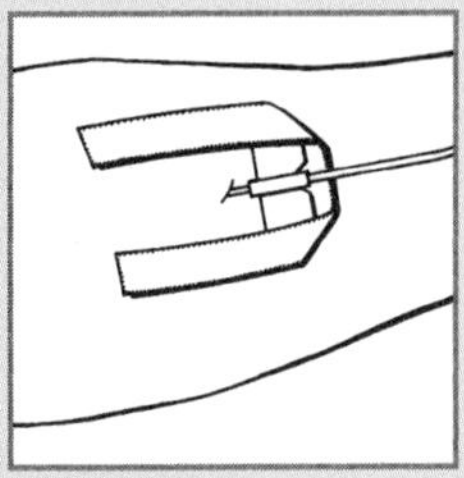

H method

- Cut three strips of 1" tape.
- Place one strip of tape over each wing, keeping the tape parallel to the cannula (as shown).
- Now place the other strip of tape perpendicular to the first two. Put it either directly on top of the wings or just below the wings, directly on top of the tubing.
- Make sure the cannula is secure; then apply a dressing and a label. On the label, write the date and time of insertion, type and gauge of needle or cannula, and your initials.

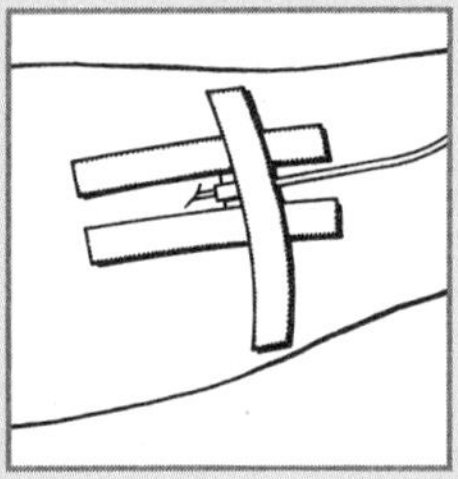

- Clean the site and apply the adhesive bandage or, if blood oozes, apply a pressure bandage.
- If drainage appears at the puncture site, swab the tip of the device across an agar plate or cut the tip into a sterile container using sterile scissors and send it to the laboratory to be cultured according to your facility's policy. (A draining site may be infected.) Then clean the area, apply a sterile dressing, and notify the practitioner.
- Instruct the patient to restrict activity for about 10 minutes and to leave the dressing in place for at least 1 hour. If the patient experiences lingering tenderness at the site, apply warm packs and notify the practitioner.

Special considerations

- Apply the tourniquet carefully to avoid pinching the skin. If necessary, apply it over the patient's gown. Make sure skin preparation materials are at room temperature to avoid vasoconstriction resulting from lower temperatures.

- If the patient is allergic to iodine-containing compounds, clean the skin with alcohol.
- If you fail to see blood flashback after the needle enters the vein, pull back slightly and rotate the device. If you still fail to see flashback, remove the cannula and try again or proceed according to your facility's policy.
- Change a gauze or transparent dressing whenever you change the administration set (every 48 to 72 hours or according to your facility's policy).
- Be sure to rotate the I.V. site every 72 hours or according to facility policy.

Complications

- Infection, phlebitis, and embolism from the catheter; circulatory overload, infiltration, sepsis, and allergic reaction from the solution (see *Risks of peripheral I.V. therapy,* pages 380 to 387)

Patient teaching

- Most patients who receive I.V. therapy at home have a central venous line. But if you're caring for a patient going home with a peripheral line, you should teach him how to care for the I.V. site and identify certain complications.
- If the patient must observe movement restrictions, make sure he understands them.
- Teach the patient how to examine the site, and instruct him to notify the practitioner or home care nurse if redness, swelling, or discomfort develops or if the dressing becomes moist.
- Also tell the patient to report any problems with the I.V. line, for instance, if the solution stops infusing or if an alarm goes off on an infusion pump. Explain that the I.V. site will be changed at established intervals by a home care nurse.
- If the patient is using an intermittent infusion device at home, teach him how and when to flush it. Finally, teach the patient to document daily whether the I.V. site is free from pain, swelling, and redness.

Documentation

In your notes or on the appropriate I.V. sheets, record the date and time of the venipuncture; type, gauge, and length of the cannula; anatomic location of the insertion site; and reason the site was changed.

Also document the number of attempts at venipuncture (if you made more than one), type and flow rate of the I.V. solution, name and amount of medication in the solution (if any), any adverse reactions and actions taken to correct them, patient teaching and evidence of patient understanding, and your initials.

Peripheral I.V line maintenance

Routine maintenance of I.V. sites and systems includes regular assessment and rotation of the site and periodic changes of the dressing, tubing, and solution. These measures help prevent complications, such as thrombophlebitis and infection. They should be performed according to facility policy.

Typically, I.V. dressings are changed when the device is changed or whenever the dressing becomes wet, soiled, or nonocclusive. I.V. tubing is changed every 48 to 72 hours or according to your facility's policy, and I.V. solution is changed every 24 hours or as needed. The site should be assessed every 4 hours if a transparent semipermeable dressing is used or with every dressing change otherwise and should be rotated every 72 hours. Sometimes limited venous access prevents frequent site changes; if so, be sure to assess the site frequently.

Equipment

Dressing changes

Sterile gloves ♦ antimicrobial or alcohol pads ♦ antimicrobial ointment ♦ adhesive bandage ♦ sterile 2″ × 2″ gauze pad, or transparent semipermeable dressing ♦ 1″ adhesive tape

(Text continues on page 386.)

Risks of peripheral I.V. therapy

Complication	Signs and symptoms	Possible causes
Local complications Phlebitis	▪ Tenderness at tip of and proximal to venous access device ▪ Redness at tip of cannula and along vein ▪ Puffy area over vein ▪ Vein hard on palpation ▪ Elevated temperature	▪ Poor blood flow around venous access device ▪ Friction from cannula movement in vein ▪ Venous access device left in vein too long ▪ Drug or solution with high or low pH or high osmolarity
Extravasation	▪ Swelling at and above I.V. site (may extend along entire limb) ▪ Discomfort, burning, or pain at site (may be painless) ▪ Tight feeling at site ▪ Decreased skin temperature around site ▪ Blanching at site ▪ Continuing fluid infusion even when vein is occluded (although rate may decrease)	▪ Venous access device dislodged from vein, or perforated vein
Cannula dislodgment	▪ Loose tape ▪ Cannula partly backed out of vein ▪ Solution infiltrating	▪ Loosened tape, or tubing snagged in bed linens, resulting in partial retraction of cannula; pulled out by confused patient
Occlusion	▪ Infusion doesn't flow ▪ Infusion pump alarms, indicating occlusion	▪ I.V. flow interrupted ▪ Heparin lock not flushed ▪ Blood backflow in line when patient walks ▪ Line clamped too long
Pain at I.V. site	▪ Pain during infusion ▪ Possible blanching if vasospasm occurs ▪ Red skin over vein during infusion	▪ Solution with high or low pH or high osmolarity, such as phenytoin, and some antibiotics (vancomycin, erythromycin, and nafcillin)

Nursing interventions

- Remove venous access device.
- Apply warm soaks.
- Notify practitioner if patient has a fever.
- Document patient's condition and your interventions.

Prevention

- Restart infusion using larger vein for irrigating solution, or restart with smaller-gauge device.
- Tape device securely.

- Stop infusion. Infiltrate site with an antidote, if appropriate.
- Apply ice (early) or warm soaks (later). Elevate limb.
- Check for pulse and capillary refill periodically.
- Restart infusion above infiltration site or in another limb.
- Document patient's condition and your interventions.

Prevention

- Check I.V. site frequently.
- Don't obscure area above site with tape.
- Teach patient to observe I.V. site and report pain or swelling.

- If no infiltration occurs, retape without pushing cannula back into vein. If pulled out, apply pressure to I.V. site with sterile dressing.

Prevention

- Tape venipuncture device securely on insertion.

- Use mild flush injection. Don't force it. If unsuccessful, reinsert I.V. line.

Prevention

- Maintain I.V. flow rate.
- Flush promptly after intermittent piggyback administration.
- Have patient walk with his arm bent at the elbow.

- Decrease the flow rate.
- Try using an electronic flow device.

Prevention

- Dilute solutions before administration. For example, give antibiotics in 250-ml solution rather than 100-ml solution. If drug has low pH, ask pharmacist if drug can be buffered with sodium bicarbonate. (Refer to your facility's policy.)
- If long-term therapy of irritating drug is planned, ask practitioner to use central I.V. line.

(continued)

Risks of peripheral I.V. therapy *(continued)*

Complication	Signs and symptoms	Possible causes
Hematoma	▪ Tenderness at venipuncture site ▪ Bruised area around site ▪ Inability to advance or flush I.V. line	▪ Vein punctured through opposite wall at time of insertion ▪ Leakage of blood from needle displacement ▪ Inadequate pressure applied when cannula is discontinued
Severed cannula	▪ Leakage from cannula shaft	▪ Cannula inadvertently cut by scissors ▪ Reinsertion of needle into cannula
Venous spasm	▪ Pain along vein ▪ Flow rate sluggish when clamp completely open ▪ Blanched skin over vein	▪ Severe vein irritation from irritating drugs or fluids ▪ Administration of cold fluids or blood ▪ Very rapid flow rate (with fluids at room temperature)
Vasovagal reaction	▪ Sudden collapse of vein during venipuncture ▪ Sudden pallor, sweating, faintness, dizziness, and nausea ▪ Decreased blood pressure	▪ Vasospasm from anxiety or pain
Thrombosis	▪ Painful, reddened, and swollen vein ▪ Sluggish or stopped I.V. flow	▪ Injury to endothelial cells of vein wall, allowing platelets to adhere and thrombi to form
Thrombophlebitis	▪ Severe discomfort ▪ Reddened, swollen, and hardened vein	▪ Thrombosis and inflammation

Nursing interventions

- Remove venous access device.
- Apply pressure and warm soaks to affected area.
- Recheck for bleeding.
- Document patient's condition and your interventions.

Prevention

- Choose a vein that can accommodate the size of venous access device.
- Release tourniquet as soon as insertion is successful.

- If broken part is visible, attempt to retrieve it. If unsuccessful, notify the practitioner.
- If portion of cannula enters bloodstream, place tourniquet above I.V. site.
- Notify practitioner and radiology department.
- Document patient's condition and your interventions.

Prevention

- Don't use scissors around I.V. site.
- Never reinsert needle into cannula.
- Remove unsuccessfully inserted cannula and needle together.

- Apply warm soaks over vein and surrounding area.
- Decrease flow rate.

Prevention

- Use a blood warmer for blood or packed red blood cells.

- Lower head of bed.
- Have patient take deep breaths.
- Check vital signs.

Prevention

- Prepare patient for therapy.
- Use local anesthetic.

- Remove venous access device; restart infusion in opposite limb if possible.
- Apply warm soaks.
- Watch for I.V. therapy–related infection; thrombi provide an excellent environment for bacterial growth.

Prevention

- Use proper venipuncture techniques to reduce injury to vein.

- Same as for thrombosis.

Prevention

- Check site frequently. Remove venous access device at first sign of redness and tenderness.

(continued)

Risks of peripheral I.V. therapy *(continued)*

Complication	Signs and symptoms	Possible causes
Nerve, tendon, or ligament damage	▪ Extreme pain (similar to electric shock when nerve is punctured) ▪ Numbness and muscle contraction ▪ Delayed effects, including paralysis, numbness, and deformity	▪ Improper venipuncture technique, resulting in injury to surrounding nerves, tendons, or ligaments ▪ Tight taping or improper splinting with arm board
Systemic complications Systemic infection (septicemia or bacteremia)	▪ Fever, chills, and malaise for no apparent reason ▪ Contaminated I.V. site, usually with no visible signs of infection at site	▪ Failure to maintain sterile technique during insertion or site care ▪ Severe phlebitis, which can set up ideal conditions for organism growth ▪ Poor taping that permits venous access device to move, which can introduce organisms into bloodstream ▪ Prolonged indwelling time of device ▪ Weak immune system
Allergic reaction	▪ Itching ▪ Watery eyes and nose ▪ Bronchospasm ▪ Wheezing ▪ Urticarial rash ▪ Edema at I.V. site ▪ Anaphylactic reaction (flushing, chills, anxiety, itching, palpitations, paresthesia, wheezing, seizures, cardiac arrest) after exposure	▪ Allergens such as medications
Circulatory overload	▪ Discomfort ▪ Jugular vein engorgement ▪ Respiratory distress ▪ Increased blood pressure ▪ Crackles ▪ Increased difference between fluid intake and output	▪ Roller clamp loosened to allow runon infusion ▪ Flow rate too rapid ▪ Miscalculation of fluid requirements

Nursing interventions

- Stop procedure.

Prevention

- Don't repeatedly penetrate tissues with venous access device.
- Don't apply excessive pressure when taping; don't encircle limb with tape.
- Pad arm boards and tape securing arm boards, if possible.

- Notify the practitioner.
- Administer medications as prescribed.
- Culture the site and device.
- Monitor vital signs.

Prevention

- Use scrupulous sterile technique when handling solutions and tubing, inserting venous access device, and discontinuing infusion.
- Secure all connections.
- Change I.V. solutions, tubing, and venous access device at recommended times.
- Use I.V. filters.

- If reaction occurs, stop infusion immediately.
- Maintain a patent airway.
- Notify the practitioner.
- Administer antihistaminic steroid, anti-inflammatory, and antipyretic drugs, as prescribed.
- Give epinephrine as prescribed. Repeat as needed and prescribed.
- Administer cortisone if prescribed.

Prevention

- Obtain patient's allergy history. Be aware of crossallergies.
- Assist with test dosing.
- Monitor patient carefully during first 15 minutes of administration of a new drug.

- Raise the head of the bed.
- Administer oxygen as needed.
- Notify the practitioner.
- Administer medications (probably furosemide) as prescribed.

Prevention

- Use pump, controller, or rate minder for elderly or compromised patients.
- Recheck calculations of fluid requirements.
- Monitor infusion frequently.

(continued)

Risks of peripheral I.V. therapy *(continued)*

Complication	Signs and symptoms	Possible causes
Air embolism	▪ Respiratory distress ▪ Unequal breath sounds ▪ Weak pulse ▪ Increased central venous pressure ▪ Decreased blood pressure ▪ Loss of consciousness	▪ Solution container empty ▪ Solution container empties, and added container pushes air down the line (if line wasn't purged first) ▪ Tubing disconnected

Solution changes

Solution container ♦ alcohol pad

Tubing changes

I.V. administration set ♦ gloves ♦ sterile 2″ × 2″ gauze pad ♦ adhesive tape for labeling ♦ optional: hemostats

Commercial kits containing the equipment for dressing changes are available.

Preparation

▪ If your facility keeps I.V. equipment and dressings in a tray or cart, have it nearby, if possible, because you may have to select a new venipuncture site, depending on the current site's condition.

▪ If you're changing both the solution and the tubing, attach and prime the I.V. administration set before entering the patient's room.

Key steps

▪ Wash your hands thoroughly to prevent the spread of microorganisms. Remember to wear sterile gloves whenever working near the venipuncture site.

▪ Explain the procedure to the patient to allay his fears and ensure cooperation.

Changing the dressing

▪ Remove the old dressing, open all supply packages, and put on gloves.

▪ Hold the cannula in place with your nondominant hand to prevent accidental movement or dislodgment, which could puncture the vein and cause infiltration.

▪ Assess the venipuncture site for signs of infection (redness and pain at the puncture site), infiltration (coolness, blanching, and edema at the site), and thrombophlebitis (redness, firmness, pain along the path of the vein, and edema). If any such signs are present, cover the area with a sterile 2″ × 2″ gauze pad and remove the catheter or needle. Apply pressure to the area until the bleeding stops, and apply an adhesive bandage. Then, using fresh equipment and solution, start the I.V. in another appropriate site, preferably on the opposite extremity.

▪ If the venipuncture site is intact, stabilize the cannula and carefully clean around the puncture site with an antimicrobial pad. Work in a circular motion outward from the site to avoid introducing bacteria into the clean area. Allow the area to dry completely.

▪ Apply antimicrobial ointment and cover the site with a transparent semipermeable dressing. The transparent dressing allows visualization of the insertion site and maintains sterility. It's placed over the insertion site to halfway up the cannula.

Changing the solution

▪ Wash your hands.

▪ Inspect the new solution container for cracks, leaks, and other damage. Check

Nursing interventions

- Discontinue infusion.
- Place patient on his left side in Trendelenburg's position.
- Administer oxygen.
- Notify the practitioner.
- Document patient's condition and your interventions.

Prevention

- Purge tubing of air completely before starting infusion.
- Use air-detection device on pump or air-eliminating filter proximal to I.V. site.
- Secure connections.

the solution for discoloration, turbidity, and particulates. Note the date and time the solution was mixed and its expiration date.

- Clamp the tubing when inverting it to prevent air from entering the tubing. Keep the drip chamber half full.
- If you're replacing a bag, remove the seal or tab from the new bag and remove the old bag from the pole. Remove the spike, insert it into the new bag, and adjust the flow rate.
- If you're replacing a bottle, remove the cap and seal from the new bottle and wipe the rubber port with an alcohol pad. Clamp the line, remove the spike from the old bottle, and insert the spike into the new bottle. Then hang the new bottle and adjust the flow rate.

Changing the tubing

- Reduce the I.V. flow rate, remove the old spike from the container, and hang it on the I.V. pole. Place the cover of the new spike loosely over the old one.
- Keeping the old spike in an upright position above the patient's heart level, insert the new spike into the I.V. container (as shown top of next column).

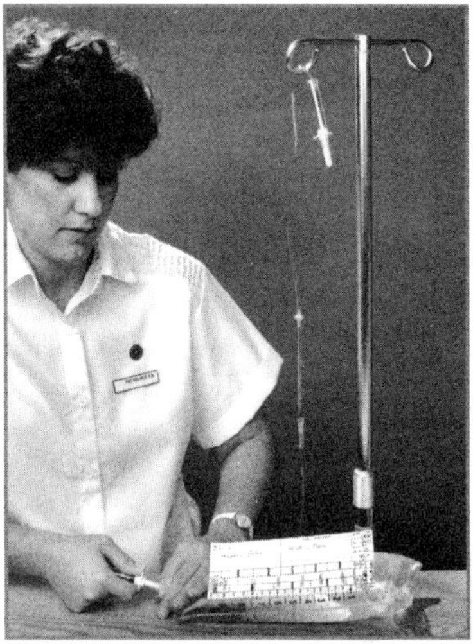

- Prime the system. Hang the new I.V. container and primed set on the pole, and grasp the new adapter in one hand. Then stop the flow rate in the old tubing.
- Put on sterile gloves.
- Place a sterile gauze pad under the needle or cannula hub to create a sterile field. Press one of your fingers over the cannula to prevent bleeding.
- Gently disconnect the old tubing (as shown top of next page), being careful not to dislodge or move the I.V. device. (If you have trouble disconnecting the old tubing, use a hemostat to hold the hub securely while twisting the tubing to remove

it. Or use one hemostat on the venipuncture device and another on the hard plastic end of the tubing. Then pull the hemostats in opposite directions. Don't clamp the hemostats shut; this could crack the tubing adapter or the venipuncture device.)

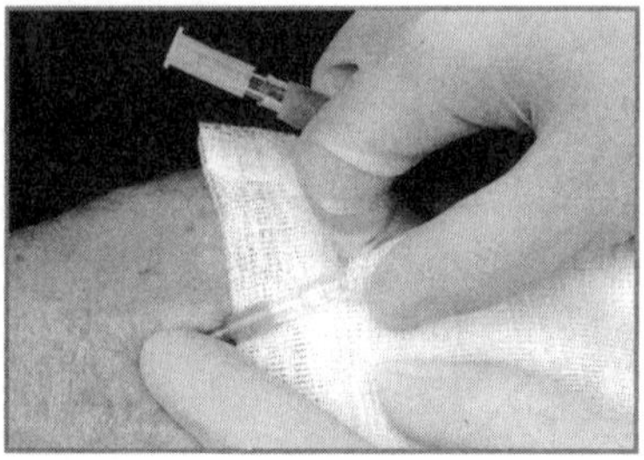

- Remove the protective cap from the new tubing, and connect the new adapter to the cannula. Hold the hub securely to prevent dislodging the needle or cannula tip.
- Observe for blood backflow into the new tubing to verify that the needle or cannula is still in place. (You may not be able to do this with small-gauge cannulas.)
- Adjust the clamp to maintain the appropriate flow rate.
- Retape the cannula hub and I.V. tubing, and recheck the I.V. flow rate because taping may alter it.
- Label the new tubing and container with the date and time. Label the solution container with a time strip (as shown below).

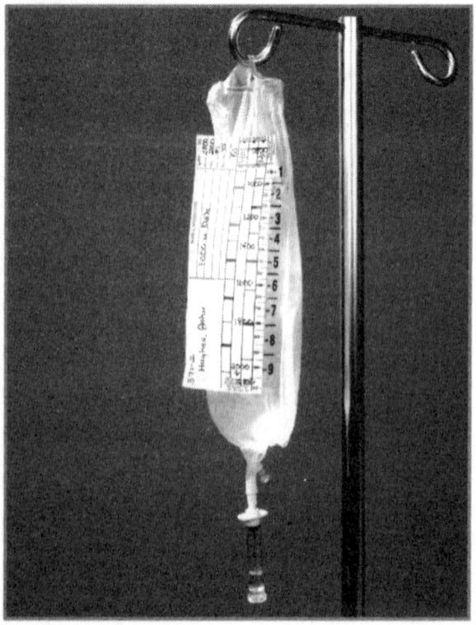

Special considerations

- Check the prescribed I.V. flow rate before each solution change to prevent errors.
- If you crack the adapter or hub (or if you accidentally dislodge the cannula from the vein), remove the cannula. Apply pressure and an adhesive bandage to stop any bleeding. Perform a venipuncture at another site and restart the I.V.

Complications

- Air embolism
- Infection

Documentation

Record the time, date, and rate and type of solution (and any additives) on the I.V. flowchart. Also record this information, dressing or tubing changes, and appearance of the site in your notes.

Peripherally inserted central catheters

Peripheral central venous (CV) therapy involves the insertion of a catheter into a peripheral vein instead of a central vein, but the catheter tip still lies in the CV circulation. A peripherally inserted central catheter (PICC) usually enters at the basilic vein and terminates in the subclavian vein or superior vena cava. A specially trained nurse may insert PICCs. New catheters have longer needles and smaller lumens, facilitating this procedure. For a patient who needs CV therapy for 1 to 6 months or who requires repeated venous access, a PICC may be the best option.

PICCs are commonly used in home I.V. therapy but may also be used with chest injury; chest, neck, or shoulder burns; compromised respiratory function; proximity of a surgical site to the CV line placement site; and if a physician isn't available to insert a CV line. With any of these conditions, a PICC helps avoid complications that may occur with a CV line.

Infusions commonly given by a PICC include total parenteral nutrition, chemotherapy, antibiotics, opioids, and analgesics. PICC therapy works best when introduced early in treatment; it shouldn't be considered as a last resort for patients with sclerotic or repeatedly punctured veins.

Before PICC insertion, anatomical measurements should be taken to determine the length of the catheter required to ensure full advancement of the catheter with tip placement in the superior vena cava. PICCs may range from 16G to 23G in diameter and from 16″ to 24″ (40.5 to 61 cm) in length.

The patient receiving PICC therapy must have a peripheral vein large enough to accept a 14G or 16G introducer needle and a 3.8G to 4.8G catheter.

Site selection should be routinely initiated in the region of the antecubital fossa; veins that should be considered for PICC insertion are the cephalic, basilic, and median cubital veins.

If your state nurse practice act permits, you may insert a PICC if you show sufficient knowledge of vascular access devices. To prove your competence in PICC insertion, it's recommended that you complete an 8-hour workshop and demonstrate three successful catheter insertions. You may have to demonstrate competence every year.

Equipment

Catheter insertion kit ♦ antiseptic solution ♦ 3-ml vial of heparin (100 units/ml) ♦ injection port with short extension tubing ♦ sterile and clean measuring tape ♦ vial of normal saline solution ♦ sterile gauze pads ♦ tape ♦ linen-saver pad ♦ sterile drapes ♦ tourniquet ♦ sterile transparent semipermeable dressing ♦ sterile marker ♦ sterile labels ♦ two pairs of sterile gloves ♦ sterile gown ♦ mask ♦ goggles

Preparation

- Gather the necessary supplies.
- If you're administering PICC therapy in the patient's home, bring the equipment listed above with you.

Key steps

- Confirm the patient's identity using two patient identifiers according to facility policy.
- Describe the procedure to the patient and answer her questions.
- Wash your hands.
- Prepare the sterile field and label all medications, medication containers, and other solutions on and off the sterile field.

Inserting a PICC

- Place the tourniquet on the patient's arm, and assess the antecubital fossa. Select the insertion site.
- Remove the tourniquet.
- Determine catheter tip placement or the spot at which the catheter tip will rest after insertion.
- For placement in the superior vena cava, measure the distance from the insertion site to the shoulder and from the shoulder to the sternal notch. Then add 3″ (7.6 cm) to the measurement (as shown below).

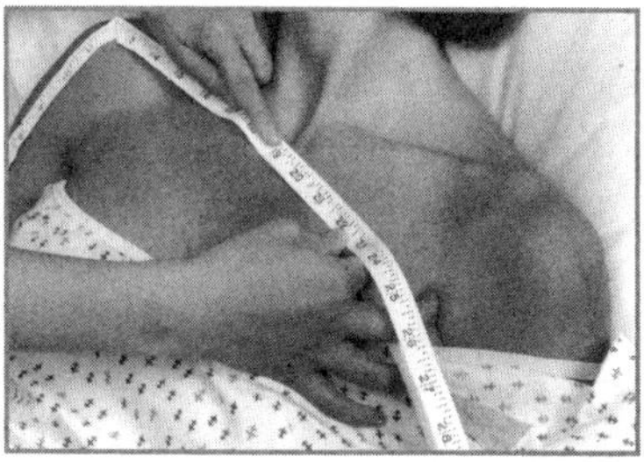

- Have the patient lie in a supine position with her arm at a 90-degree angle to her body. Place a linen-saver pad under her arm.
- Open the PICC tray and drop the rest of the sterile items onto the sterile field. Put on the sterile gown, mask, goggles, and gloves.
- Using the sterile measuring tape, cut the distal end of the catheter according to the manufacturer's recommendations and guidelines, using the equipment provided by the manufacturer (as shown below).

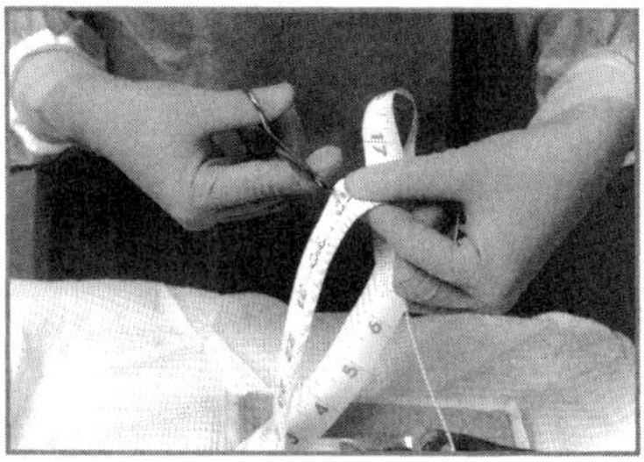

- Using sterile technique, withdraw 5 ml of the normal saline solution and flush the extension tubing and the cap (as shown below).

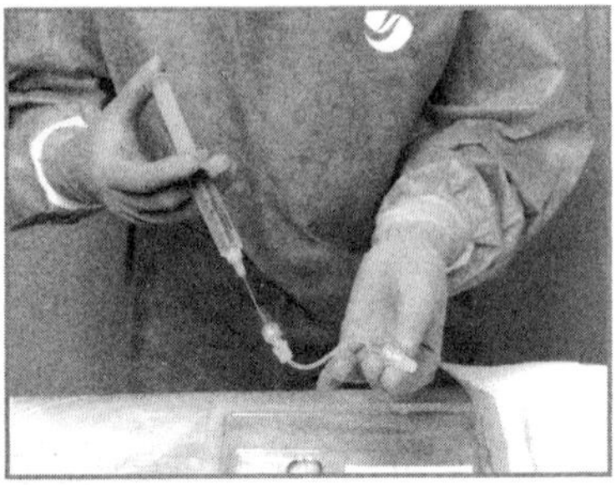

- Remove the needle from the syringe. Attach the syringe to the hub of the catheter and flush (as shown below).

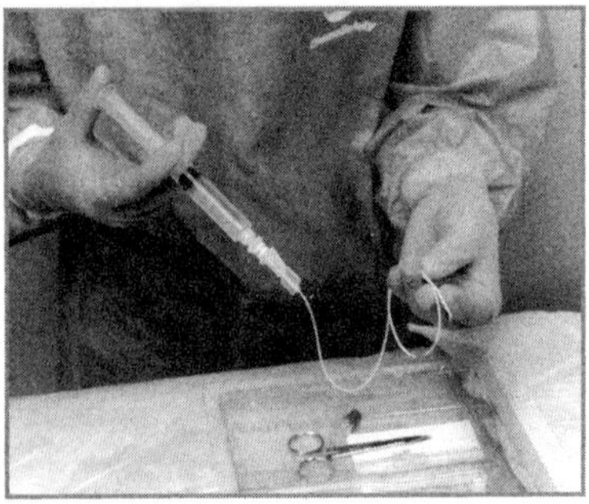

- Prepare the insertion site using an antiseptic solution. Follow the manufacturer's recommendations for proper cleaning techniques depending on solution used. Allow the area to dry. Be sure not to touch the intended insertion site. Take your gloves off. Then apply the tourniquet about 4″ (10 cm) above the antecubital fossa.
- Put on a new pair of sterile gloves. Then place a sterile drape under the patient's arm and another on top of her arm. Drop a sterile 4″ × 4″ gauze pad over the tourniquet.
- Stabilize the patient's vein. Insert the catheter introducer at a 10-degree angle directly into the vein (as shown top of next column).

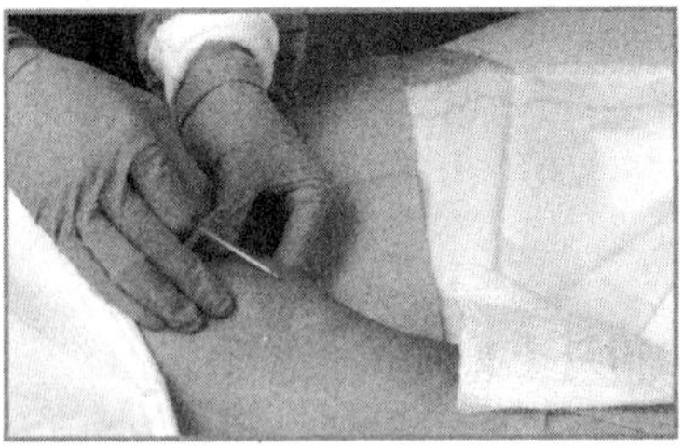

- After successful vein entry, you should see a blood return in the flashback chamber. Without changing the needle's position, gently advance the plastic introducer sheath until you're sure the tip is well within the vein.
- Carefully withdraw the needle while holding the introducer still. To minimize blood loss, try applying finger pressure on the vein just beyond the distal end of the introducer sheath (as shown below).

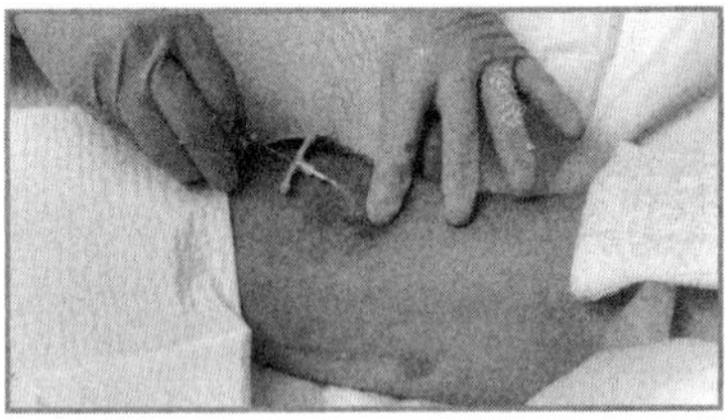

- Using sterile forceps, insert the catheter into the introducer sheath, and advance it into the vein 2″ to 4″ (5 to 10 cm) (as shown below).

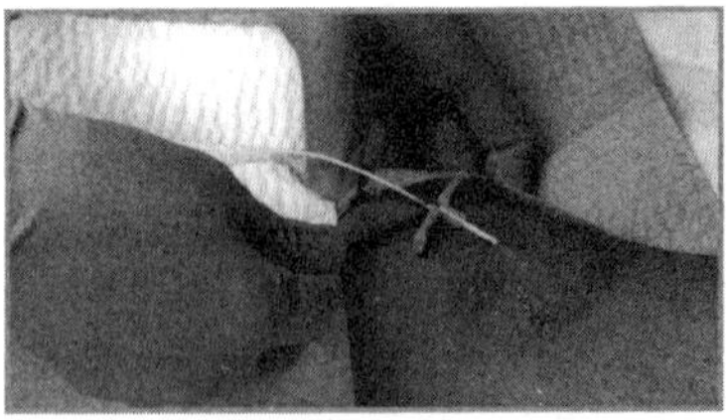

- Remove the tourniquet using a sterile 4″ × 4″ gauze pad.
- When you've advanced the catheter to the shoulder, ask the patient to turn her head toward the affected arm and place her chin on her chest. This will occlude the jugular vein and ease the catheter's advancement into the subclavian vein.
- Advance the catheter until about 4″ remain. Then pull the introducer sheath out

of the vein and away from the venipuncture site (as shown below).

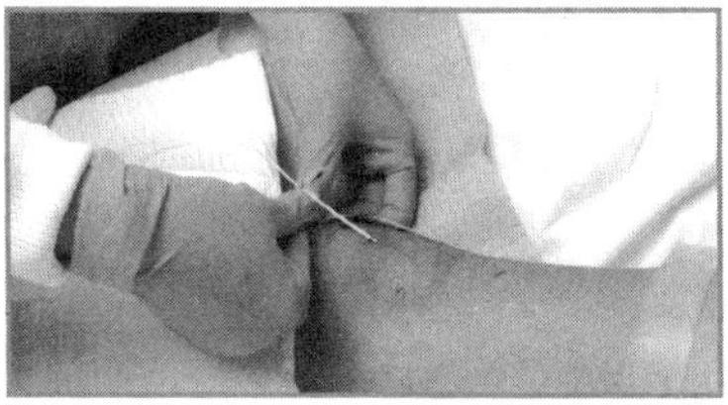

- Grasp the tabs of the introducer sheath, and flex them toward its distal end to split the sheath.
- Pull the tabs apart and away from the catheter until the sheath is completely split (as shown below). Discard the sheath.

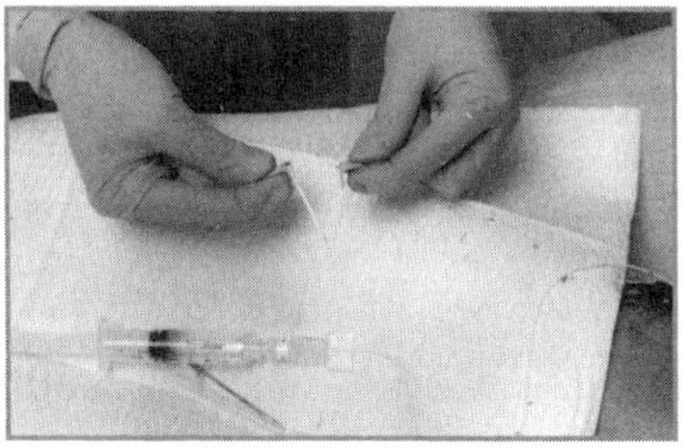

- Continue to advance the catheter until it's completely inserted. Flush with normal saline solution followed by heparin, according to your facility's policy.
- With the patient's arm below heart level, remove the syringe. Connect the capped extension set to the catheter hub.
- Apply a sterile 2″ × 2″ gauze pad directly over the site and a sterile transparent semipermeable dressing over that. Leave this dressing in place for 24 hours.
- After the initial 24 hours, apply a new sterile transparent semipermeable dressing. The gauze pad is no longer necessary. You can place adhesive strips over the catheter wings.
- Flush with heparin, according to facility policy.

Administering drugs

- As with any CV line, be sure to check for blood return and flush with normal saline solution before administering a drug through a PICC line.
- Clamp the 7″ (17.8-cm) extension tubing, and connect the empty syringe to the tubing. Release the clamp and aspirate slowly to verify blood return. Flush with 3 ml of normal saline solution in a 10-ml syringe, then administer the drug.
- After giving the drug, flush again with 3 ml of normal saline solution in a 10-ml syringe. (Remember to flush with normal saline solution between infusions of incompatible drugs or fluids.)

Changing the dressing

- Change the dressing every 2 to 7 days and more frequently if the integrity of the dressing becomes compromised. If possible, choose a transparent semipermeable dressing, which has a high moisture-vapor transmission rate. Use sterile technique.
- Wash your hands and assemble the necessary supplies. Position the patient with her arm extended away from her body at a 45- to 90-degree angle so that the insertion site is below heart level to reduce the risk of air embolism. Put on a sterile mask.
- Open a package of sterile gloves and use the inside of the package as a sterile field. Then open the transparent semipermeable dressing and drop it onto the field. Put on clean gloves, and remove the old dressing by holding your left thumb on the catheter and stretching the dressing parallel to the skin. Repeat the last step with your right thumb holding the catheter. Free the remaining section of the dressing from the catheter by peeling toward the insertion site from the distal end to the proximal end to prevent catheter dislodgment. Remove the clean gloves.
- Put on sterile gloves. Clean the area thoroughly with three alcohol swabs or other approved antimicrobial solution, starting at the insertion site and working outward from the site. Repeat the step three times with 2% chlorhexidine swabs and allow to dry.
- Apply the dressing carefully. Secure the tubing to the edge of the dressing over the tape with ¼″ adhesive tape.

Removing a PICC

- You'll remove a PICC when therapy is complete, if the catheter becomes damaged or broken and can't be repaired or, possibly, if the line becomes occluded. Measure the catheter after you remove it to ensure that the line has been removed intact.

- Assemble the necessary equipment at the patient's bedside.
- Explain the procedure to the patient. Wash your hands. Place a linen-saver pad under the patient's arm.
- Remove the tape holding the extension tubing. Open two sterile gauze pads on a clean, flat surface. Put on clean gloves. Stabilize the catheter at the hub with one hand. Without dislodging the catheter, use your other hand to gently remove the dressing by pulling it toward the insertion site.
- Next, withdraw the catheter with smooth, gentle pressure in small increments. It should come out easily. If you feel resistance, stop. Apply slight tension to the line by taping it down. Then try to remove it again in a few minutes. If you still feel resistance, notify the practitioner for further instructions.
- After you successfully remove the catheter, apply manual pressure to the site with a sterile gauze pad for 1 minute.
- Measure and inspect the catheter. If a part has broken off during removal, notify the practitioner immediately and monitor the patient for signs of distress.
- Cover the site with antiseptic ointment, and tape a new folded gauze pad in place. Dispose of used items properly, and wash your hands.

Special considerations

- For a patient receiving intermittent PICC therapy, flush the catheter with 6 ml of normal saline solution and 3 ml of heparin (100 units/ml) after each use. For catheters that aren't being used routinely, flushing every 12 hours with 3 ml (100 units/ml) of heparin will maintain patency.
- You can use a declotting agent to clear a clotted PICC, but make sure that you read the manufacturer's recommendations first and follow your facility's policy.
- Remember to add an extension set to all PICCs so you can start and stop an infusion away from the insertion site. An extension set will also make using a PICC easier for the patient who will be administering infusions herself.
- If a patient will be receiving blood or blood products through the PICC, use at least an 18G cannula.
- Assess the catheter insertion site through the transparent semipermeable dressing every 24 hours. Look at the catheter and cannula pathway, and check for bleeding, redness, drainage, and swelling. Ask the patient if she's having pain associated with therapy. Although oozing is common for the first 24 hours after insertion, excessive bleeding after that should be evaluated.

ALERT

If a portion of the catheter breaks during removal, immediately apply a tourniquet to the upper arm, close to the axilla, to prevent advancement of the catheter piece into the right atrium. Then check the patient's radial pulse. If you don't detect the radial pulse, the tourniquet is too tight. Keep the tourniquet in place until an X-ray can be obtained, the practitioner is notified, and surgical retrieval is attempted.

Complications

- Catheter breakage on removal
- Air embolism
- Catheter tip migration
- Catheter occlusion

Documentation

Document the entire procedure, including problems with catheter placement. Also document the size, length, and type of catheter as well as the insertion location.

Peritoneal dialysis

Peritoneal dialysis is indicated for patients with chronic renal failure who have cardiovascular instability, vascular access problems that prevent hemodialysis, fluid overload, or electrolyte imbalances. In this procedure, dialysate—the solution instilled into the peritoneal cavity by a catheter—draws waste products, excess fluid, and electrolytes from the blood across the semipermeable peritoneal membrane. After a prescribed period, the dialysate is drained from the peritoneal cavity, removing impurities with it. The dialysis procedure is then repeated, using a new dialysate each time, until waste removal is complete and fluid, electrolyte, and acid-base balance has been restored.

The catheter is inserted in the operating room or at the patient's bedside with a nurse assisting. With special preparation, the nurse may perform dialysis, either manually or using an automatic or semiautomatic cycle machine.

Equipment

Catheter placement and dialysis

Prescribed dialysate (in 1- or 2-L bottles or bags as ordered) ♦ warmer, heating pad, or water bath ♦ at least three face masks ♦ medication, such as heparin, if ordered ♦ dialysis administration set with drainage bag ♦ two pairs of sterile gloves ♦ I.V. pole ♦ fenestrated sterile drape ♦ vial of 1% or 2% lidocaine ♦ antimicrobial pads ♦ 3-ml syringe with 25G 1″ needle scalpel (with #11 blade) ♦ ordered type of multi-eyed, nylon, peritoneal catheter (see *Comparing peritoneal dialysis catheters,* page 394) ♦ peritoneal stylet ♦ sutures or hypoallergenic tape ♦ povidone-iodine solution (to prepare abdomen) ♦ precut drain dressings ♦ protective cap for catheter ♦ small, sterile plastic clamp ♦ 4″ × 4″ gauze pads ♦ sterile labels ♦ sterile marker ♦ optional: 10-ml syringe with 22G ½″ needle, protein or potassium supplement, specimen container, label, laboratory request form

Dressing changes

One pair of sterile gloves ♦ 10 sterile cotton-tipped applicators or sterile 2″ × 2″ gauze pads ♦ antimicrobial ointment ♦ two precut drain dressings ♦ adhesive tape ♦ antimicrobial solution or normal saline solution ♦ two sterile 4″ × 4″ gauze pads

All equipment must be sterile. Commercially packaged dialysis kits or trays are available.

Preparation

- Bring all equipment to the patient's bedside.
- Make sure that the dialysate is at body temperature. This decreases patient discomfort during the procedure and reduces vasoconstriction of the peritoneal capillaries. Dilated capillaries enhance blood flow to the peritoneal membrane surface, increasing waste clearance into the peritoneal cavity. Place the container in a warmer or water bath, or wrap it in a heating pad set at 98.6° F (37° C) for 30 to 60 minutes to warm the solution.

Key steps

- Confirm the patient's identity using two patient identifiers according to your facility's policy.
- Explain the procedure to the patient. Assess and record his vital signs and weight to establish baseline levels.
- Review recent laboratory values (blood urea nitrogen, serum creatinine, sodium, potassium, and complete blood count).

Catheter placement and dialysis

- Have the patient try to urinate. This reduces the risk of bladder perforation during the insertion of the peritoneal catheter. If he can't urinate and you suspect that his bladder isn't empty, obtain an order for straight catheterization to empty his bladder.
- Place the patient in the supine position, and have him put on one of the sterile face masks.
- Wash your hands.
- Inspect the warmed dialysate, which should appear clear and colorless.
- Put on a sterile face mask. Prepare to add any prescribed medication to the dialysate, using strict sterile technique to avoid contaminating the solution. Label all medications, medication containers, and other solutions on and off the sterile field. Medications should be added immediately before the solution will be hung and used. Disinfect multiple-dose vials by soaking them in antimicrobial solution for 5 minutes. Heparin is typically added to the dialysate to prevent fibrin accumulation in the catheter.

Comparing peritoneal dialysis catheters

The first step in any type of peritoneal dialysis is insertion of a catheter to allow instillation of dialyzing solution. The surgeon may insert one of three different catheters described below.

Tenckhoff catheter

To implant a Tenckhoff catheter, the surgeon inserts the first 6¾" (17 cm) of the catheter into the patient's abdomen. The next 2¾" (7 cm) segment, which may have a Dacron cuff at one or both ends, is imbedded subcutaneously. Within a few days after insertion, the patient's tissues grow around the cuffs, forming a tight barrier against bacterial infiltration. The remaining 3⅞" (10 cm) of the catheter extends outside of the abdomen and is equipped with a metal adapter at the tip that connects to dialyzer tubing.

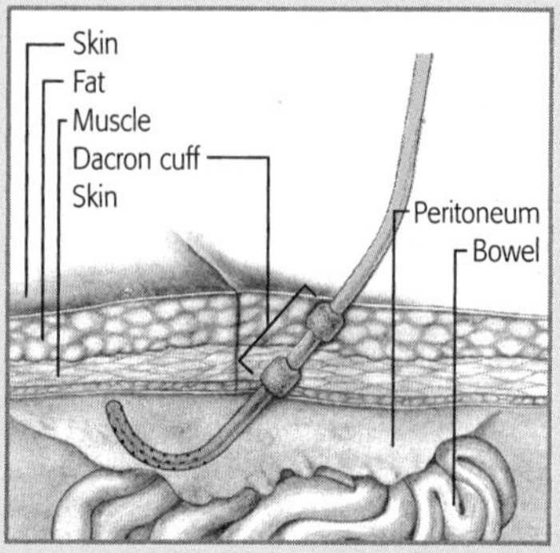

Flanged-collar catheter

To insert this type of catheter, the surgeon positions its flanged collar just below the dermis so that the device extends through the abdominal wall. He keeps the cuff's distal end from extending into the peritoneum, where it could cause adhesions.

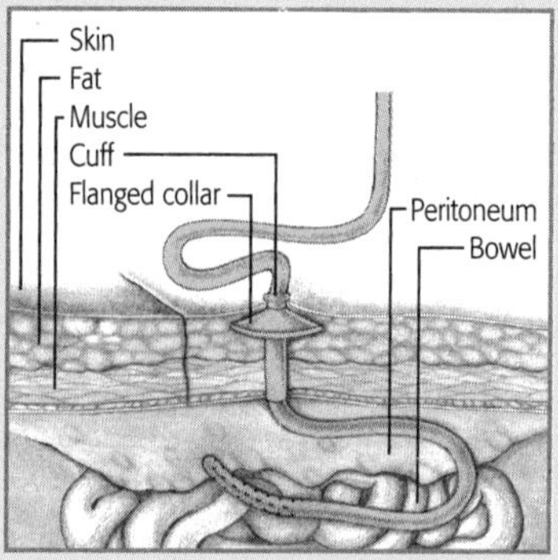

Column-disk peritoneal catheter

To insert a column-disk peritoneal catheter (CDPC), the surgeon rolls up the flexible disk section of the implant, inserts it into the peritoneal cavity, and retracts it against the abdominal wall. The implant's first cuff rests just outside the peritoneal membrane, while its second cuff rests just underneath the skin. Because the CDPC doesn't float freely in the peritoneal cavity, it keeps inflowing dialyzing solution from being directed at the sensitive organs, which increases patient comfort during dialysis.

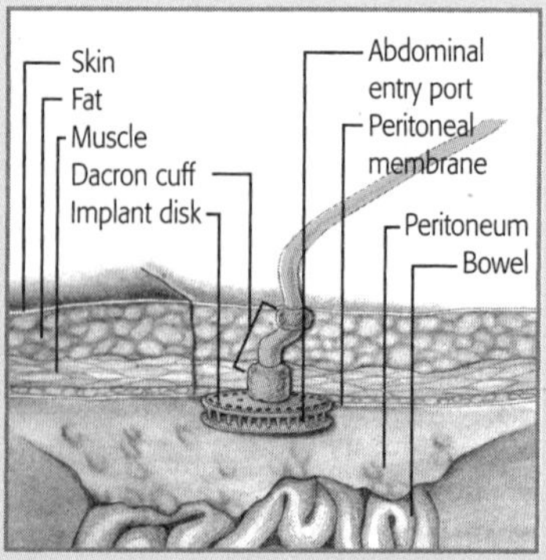

- Prepare the dialysis administration set as shown. (See *Setup for peritoneal dialysis.*)
- Close the clamps on all lines. Place the drainage bag below the patient to facilitate gravity drainage, and connect the drainage line to it. Connect the dialysate infusion lines to the bottles or bags of dialysate. Hang the bottles or bags on the I.V. pole at the patient's bedside. To prime the tubing, open the infusion lines and allow the solution to flow until all lines are primed. Close all clamps.
- At this point, the practitioner puts on a mask and a pair of sterile gloves. He cleans the patient's abdomen with povidone-iodine solution and drapes it with a sterile drape.
- Wipe the stopper of the lidocaine vial with povidone-iodine and allow it to dry. Invert the vial and hand it to the practitioner so he can withdraw the lidocaine, using the 3-ml syringe with the 25G 1″ needle.
- The practitioner anesthetizes a small area of the patient's abdomen below the umbilicus. He then makes a small incision with the scalpel, inserts the catheter into the peritoneal cavity—using the stylet to guide the catheter—and sutures or tapes the catheter in place.
- If the catheter is already in place, clean the site with antimicrobial solution in a circular outward motion, according to your facility's policy, before each dialysis treatment.
- Connect the catheter to the administration set, using strict sterile technique to prevent contamination of the catheter and the solution, which could cause peritonitis.
- Open the drain dressing and the 4″ × 4″ gauze pad packages. Put on the other pair of sterile gloves. Apply the precut drain dressings around the catheter. Cover them with the gauze pads and tape them securely.
- Unclamp the lines to the patient. Rapidly instill 500 ml of dialysate into the peritoneal cavity to test the catheter's patency.
- Clamp the lines to the patient. Immediately unclamp the lines to the drainage bag to allow fluid to drain into the bag. Outflow should be brisk.

Setup for peritoneal dialysis

This illustration shows the proper setup for peritoneal dialysis.

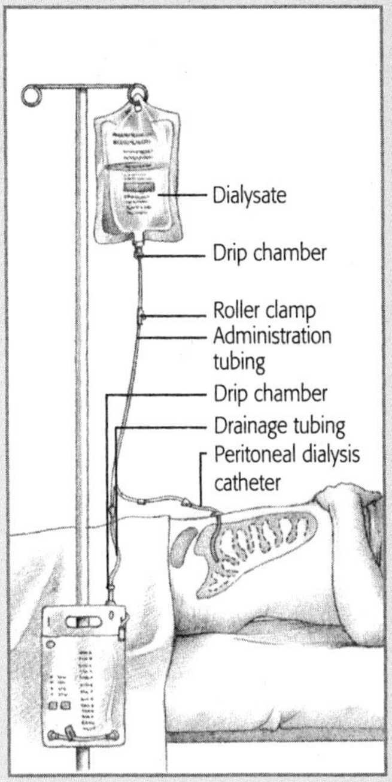

- Having established the catheter's patency, clamp the lines to the drainage bag and unclamp the lines to the patient to infuse the prescribed volume of solution over a period of 5 to 10 minutes. As soon as the dialysate container empties, clamp the lines to the patient to prevent air from entering the tubing.
- Allow the solution to dwell in the peritoneal cavity for the prescribed time (4 to 6 hours). This lets excess fluid, electrolytes, and accumulated wastes move from the blood through the peritoneal membrane and into the dialysate.
- Warm the solution for the next infusion.
- At the end of the prescribed dwell time, unclamp the line to the drainage bag and allow the solution to drain from the peri-

toneal cavity into the drainage bag (normally 30 to 40 minutes).

- Repeat the infusion-dwell-drain cycle immediately after outflow until the prescribed number of fluid exchanges has been completed.
- If the practitioner or your facility's policy requires a dialysate specimen, you'll usually collect one after every 10 infusion-dwell-drain cycles (always during the drain phase), after every 24-hour period, or as ordered. To do this, attach the 10-ml syringe to the 22G ½″ needle and insert it into the injection port on the drainage line, using strict sterile technique, and aspirate the drainage specimen. Transfer the specimen to the specimen container, label it appropriately, and send it to the laboratory with a laboratory request form.
- After completing the prescribed number of exchanges, clamp the catheter, and put on sterile gloves. Disconnect the administration set from the peritoneal catheter. Place the sterile protective cap over the catheter's distal end.
- Dispose of used equipment appropriately.

Dressing changes

- Explain the procedure to the patient and wash your hands.
- If necessary, carefully remove the old dressings to avoid putting tension on the catheter and accidentally dislodging it and to avoid introducing bacteria into the tract through the catheter's movement.
- Put on the sterile gloves.
- Saturate the sterile applicators or the 4″ × 4″ gauze pads with antimicrobial ointment, and clean the skin around the catheter, moving in concentric circles from the catheter site outward. Remove any crusted material carefully.
- Inspect the catheter site for drainage and the tissue around the site for redness and swelling.
- Apply antimicrobial ointment to the catheter site with a sterile gauze pad.
- Place two precut drain dressings around the catheter site. Tape the 4″ × 4″ gauze pads over them to secure the dressing.

Special considerations

- During and after dialysis, monitor the patient and his response to treatment. Peritoneal dialysis is usually contraindicated in the patient who has had extensive abdominal or bowel surgery or extensive abdominal trauma or who has severe vascular disease, obesity, or respiratory distress.
- Monitor the patient's vital signs every 10 to 15 minutes for the first 1 to 2 hours of exchanges, then every 2 to 4 hours, or more frequently if necessary. Notify the practitioner of abrupt changes in the patient's condition.
- To reduce the risk of peritonitis, use strict sterile technique during catheter insertion, dialysis, and dressing changes. All personnel in the room should wear masks whenever the dialysis system is opened or entered. Change the dressing at least every 24 hours or whenever it becomes wet or soiled. Frequent dressing changes will also help prevent skin excoriation from any leakage.
- To prevent respiratory distress, position the patient for maximal lung expansion. Promote lung expansion through turning and deep-breathing exercises.

ALERT

If the patient suffers severe respiratory distress during the dwell phase of dialysis, drain the peritoneal cavity and notify the practitioner. Monitor the patient on peritoneal dialysis who's being weaned from a ventilator.

- To prevent protein depletion, the practitioner may order a high-protein diet or protein supplement. He'll also monitor serum albumin levels.
- Dialysate is available in three concentrations: 4.25% dextrose, 2.5% dextrose, and 1.5% dextrose. The 4.25% solution usually removes the largest amount of fluid from the blood because its glucose concentration is highest. If the patient receives this concentrated solution, monitor him carefully to prevent excess fluid loss. Some of the glucose in the 4.25% solution may enter the patient's bloodstream, causing hyperglycemia severe enough to require an

insulin injection or an insulin addition to the dialysate.

- Patients with low serum potassium levels may require the addition of potassium to the dialysate solution to prevent further losses.
- Monitor fluid volume balance, blood pressure, and pulse to help prevent fluid imbalance. Assess fluid balance at the end of each infusion-dwell-drain cycle. Fluid balance is positive if less than the amount infused was recovered; it's negative if more than the amount infused was recovered. Notify the practitioner if the patient retains 500 ml or more of fluid for three consecutive cycles or if he loses at least 1 L of fluid for three consecutive cycles.
- Weigh the patient daily to help determine how much fluid is being removed during dialysis treatment. Note the time and any variations in the weighing technique next to his weight on his chart.
- If inflow and outflow are slow or absent, check the tubing for kinks. You can also try raising the I.V. pole or repositioning the patient to increase the inflow rate. Repositioning the patient or applying manual pressure to the lateral aspects of the patient's abdomen may also help increase drainage. If these maneuvers fail, notify the practitioner. Improper positioning of the catheter or an accumulation of fibrin may obstruct the catheter.
- Always examine outflow fluid (effluent) for color and clarity. Normally it's clear or pale yellow, but pink-tinged effluent may appear during the first three or four cycles. If the effluent remains pink-tinged or if it's grossly bloody, suspect bleeding into the peritoneal cavity and notify the practitioner. Notify the practitioner if the outflow contains feces, which suggests bowel perforation, or if it's cloudy, which suggests peritonitis. Obtain a specimen for culture and Gram stain. Send the specimen in a labeled specimen container to the laboratory with a laboratory request form.
- Patient discomfort at the start of the procedure is normal. If the patient experiences pain during the procedure, determine when it occurs, its quality and duration, and whether it radiates to other body parts. Notify the practitioner. Pain during infusion usually results from a dialysate that's too cool or acidic. Pain may also result from rapid inflow; slowing the inflow rate may reduce the pain. Severe, diffuse pain with rebound tenderness and cloudy effluent may indicate peritoneal infection. Pain that radiates to the shoulder commonly results from air accumulation under the diaphragm. Severe, persistent perineal or rectal pain can result from improper catheter placement.
- The patient undergoing peritoneal dialysis will require a great deal of assistance in his daily care. To minimize his discomfort, perform daily care during a drain phase in the cycle, when the patient's abdomen is less distended.

Complications

- Peritonitis
- Protein depletion
- Respiratory distress
- Constipation
- Excessive fluid loss from the use of 4.25% solution causing hypovolemia, hypotension, and shock; excessive fluid retention leading to blood volume expansion, hypertension, peripheral edema, and even pulmonary edema and heart failure
- Electrolyte imbalance and hyperglycemia

Patient teaching

- Teach the patient and his family how to use sterile technique throughout the procedure, especially for cleaning and dressing changes, to prevent complications such as peritonitis.
- Also teach them the signs and symptoms of peritonitis (cloudy fluid, fever, and abdominal pain and tenderness) and infection (redness and drainage). Stress the importance of notifying the practitioner immediately if such signs or symptoms arise.
- Inform the patient about the advantages of an automated continuous cycler for home use.
- Instruct the patient to record his weight and blood pressure daily and to check regularly for swelling of the extremities. Teach him to keep an accurate record of intake and output.

Documentation

Record the amount of dialysate infused and drained, any medications added to the solution, and the color and character of effluent. Record the patient's daily weight and fluid balance.

Use a peritoneal dialysis flowchart to compute total fluid balance after each exchange. Note the patient's vital signs and tolerance of the treatment and other pertinent observations.

Peritoneal dialysis, continuous ambulatory

Continuous ambulatory peritoneal dialysis (CAPD) requires insertion of a permanent peritoneal catheter, such as a Tenckhoff catheter, to circulate dialysate in the peritoneal cavity constantly. Inserted under local anesthetic, the catheter is sutured in place and its distal portion tunneled subcutaneously to the skin surface. There it serves as a port for the dialysate, which flows in and out of the peritoneal cavity by gravity. (See *Continuous ambulatory peritoneal dialysis: Three major steps*.)

CAPD is used most commonly for patients with end-stage renal disease. CAPD can be a welcome alternative to hemodialysis because it gives the patient more independence and requires less travel for treatments. It also provides more stable fluid and electrolyte levels than conventional hemodialysis.

Patients or family members can usually learn to perform CAPD after only 2 weeks of training. Also, because the patient can resume normal daily activities between solution changes, CAPD helps promote independence and a return to a near-normal lifestyle. It also costs less than hemodialysis.

Conditions that may prohibit CAPD include recent abdominal surgery, abdominal adhesions, an infected abdominal wall, diaphragmatic tears, ileus, and respiratory insufficiency.

Equipment

Infusing dialysate

Prescribed amount of dialysate (usually in 2-L bags) ♦ heating pad or commercial warmer ♦ three face masks ♦ 42″ (106.7-cm) connective tubing with drain clamp ♦ six to eight packages of sterile 4″ × 4″ gauze pads ♦ medication, if ordered ♦ antimicrobial pads ♦ hypoallergenic tape ♦ plastic snap-top container ♦ antimicrobial solution ♦ sterile basin ♦ container of alcohol ♦ sterile gloves ♦ belt or fabric pouch ♦ two sterile waterproof paper drapes (one fenestrated) ♦ optional: syringes, labeled specimen container

Discontinuing dialysis temporarily

Three sterile waterproof paper barriers (two fenestrated) ♦ 4″ × 4″ gauze pads (for cleaning and dressing the catheter) ♦ two face masks ♦ sterile basin ♦ hypoallergenic tape ♦ antimicrobial solution ♦ sterile gloves ♦ sterile rubber catheter cap

All equipment for infusing the dialysate and discontinuing the procedure must be sterile.

Commercially prepared sterile CAPD kits are available.

Preparation

- Check the concentration of the dialysate and compare it to the practitioner's order.
- Check the expiration date and appearance of the solution—it should be clear, not cloudy.
- Warm the solution to body temperature with a heating pad or a commercial warmer if one is available.

DO'S & DON'TS

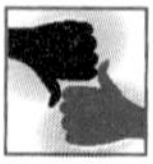

Don't warm the solution in a microwave oven because the temperature is unpredictable.

- To minimize the risk of contaminating the bag's port, leave the dialysate container's wrapper in place. This also keeps the bag dry, which makes examining it for leakage easier after you remove the wrapper.
- Wash your hands and put on a surgical mask.

Continuous ambulatory peritoneal dialysis: Three major steps

1. A bag of dialysate is attached to the tube entering the patient's abdominal area so the fluid flows into the peritoneal cavity.

2. While the dialysate remains in the peritoneal cavity, the patient can roll up the bag, place it under his shirt, and go about his normal activities.

3. Unrolling the bag and suspending it below the pelvis allows the dialysate to drain from the peritoneal cavity back into the bag.

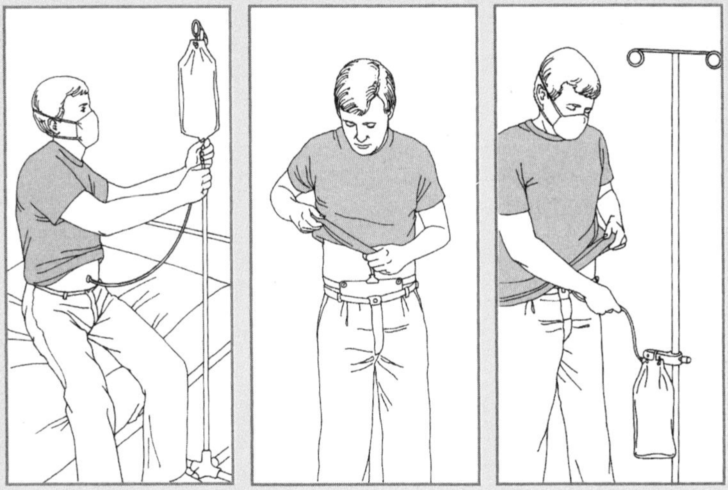

- Remove the dialysate container from the warming setup, and remove its protective wrapper. Squeeze the bag firmly to check for leaks.
- If ordered, use a syringe to add prescribed medication to the dialysate, using sterile technique to avoid contamination. (The ideal approach is to add medication under a laminar flow hood.)
- Disinfect multiple-dose vials in a 5-minute antimicrobial soak.
- Insert the connective tubing into the dialysate container.
- Open the drain clamp to prime the tube. Close the clamp.
- Place an antimicrobial pad on the dialysate container's port.
- Cover the port with a dry gauze pad, and secure the pad with tape.
- Remove and discard the surgical mask.
- Tear the tape so it will be ready to secure the new dressing.
- Commercial devices with povidone-iodine pads are available for covering the dialysate container and tubing connection.

Key steps

- Confirm the patient's identity using two patient identifiers according to your facility's policy.
- Weigh the patient to establish a baseline level. Weigh him at the same time every day to help monitor fluid balance.

Infusing dialysate

- Assemble all equipment at the patient's bedside, and explain the procedure to him. Prepare the sterile field by placing a waterproof, sterile paper drape on a dry surface near the patient. Take care to maintain the drape's sterility.

▪ Fill the snap-top container with antimicrobial solution, and place it on the sterile field. Place the basin on the sterile field. Place four pairs of sterile gauze pads in the sterile basin, and saturate them with the antimicrobial solution. Place the remaining gauze pads on the sterile field. Loosen the cap on the alcohol container, and place the cap next to the sterile field.
▪ Put on a clean surgical mask and provide one for the patient.
▪ Carefully remove the dressing covering the peritoneal catheter and discard it. Be careful not to touch the catheter or skin. Check skin integrity at the catheter site, and look for signs of infection such as purulent drainage. If drainage is present, obtain a swab specimen, put it in a labeled specimen container, and notify the practitioner.
▪ Put on the sterile gloves and palpate the insertion site and subcutaneous tunnel route for tenderness or pain. If these symptoms occur, notify the practitioner.
▪ Wrap one gauze pad saturated with antimicrobial solution around the distal end of the catheter, and leave it in place for 5 minutes. Clean the catheter and insertion site with the rest of the gauze pads, moving in concentric circles away from the insertion site. Use straight strokes to clean the catheter, beginning at the insertion site and moving outward. Use a clean area of the pad for each stroke. Loosen the catheter cap one notch and clean the exposed area. Place each used pad at the base of the catheter to help support it. After using the third pair of pads, place the fenestrated paper drape around the base of the catheter. Continue cleaning the catheter for another minute with one of the remaining pads soaked with antimicrobial.
▪ Remove the antimicrobial pad on the catheter cap, remove the cap, and use the remaining antimicrobial pad to clean the end of the catheter hub. Attach the connective tubing from the dialysate container to the catheter. Be sure to secure the luer-lock connector tightly.
▪ Open the drain clamp on the dialysate container to allow solution to enter the peritoneal cavity by gravity over a period of 5 to 10 minutes. Leave a small amount of fluid in the bag to make folding it easier. Close the drain clamp.
▪ Fold the bag and secure it with a belt, or tuck it in the patient's clothing or a small fabric pouch.
▪ After the prescribed dwell time (usually 4 to 6 hours), unfold the bag, open the clamp, and allow peritoneal fluid to drain back into the bag by gravity.
▪ When drainage is complete, attach a new bag of dialysate and repeat the infusion.
▪ Discard used supplies appropriately.

Discontinuing dialysis temporarily

▪ Wash your hands, put on a surgical mask, and provide one for the patient. Explain the procedure to him.
▪ Using sterile gloves, remove and discard the dressing over the peritoneal catheter.
▪ Set up a sterile field next to the patient by covering a clean, dry surface with a waterproof drape. Be sure to maintain the drape's sterility. Place all equipment on the sterile field, and place the 4″ × 4″ gauze pads in the basin. Saturate them with the antimicrobial solution. Open the 4″ × 4″ gauze pads to be used as the dressing, and place them onto the sterile field. Tear pieces of tape as needed.
▪ Tape the dialysate tubing to the side rail of the bed to keep the catheter and tubing off the patient's abdomen.
▪ Change to another pair of sterile gloves. Place one of the fenestrated drapes around the base of the catheter.
▪ Use a pair of antimicrobial pads to clean about 6″ (15 cm) of the dialysis tubing. Clean for 1 minute, moving in one direction only, away from the catheter. Clean the catheter, moving from the insertion site to the junction of the catheter and dialysis tubing. Place used pads at the base of the catheter to prop it up. Use two more pairs of pads to clean the junction for a total of 3 minutes.
▪ Place the second fenestrated paper drape over the first at the base of the catheter. With the fourth pair of sponges, clean the junction of the catheter and 6″ of the dialysate tubing for another minute.
▪ Disconnect the dialysate tubing from the catheter. Pick up the catheter cap and fas-

ten it to the catheter, making sure that it fits securely over both notches of the hard plastic catheter tip.

- Clean the insertion site and a 2″ (5-cm) radius around it with antimicrobial pads, working from the insertion site outward. Let the skin air-dry before applying the dressing.
- Remove tape and discard used supplies appropriately.

Special considerations

- Absolute contraindications for CAPD include:
  - documented loss of peritoneal function or extensive abdominal adhesions that limit dialysate flow
  - physical or mental incapacity to perform peritoneal dialysis and no assistance available at home
  - mechanical defects that prevent effective dialysis, which can't be corrected, or increase the risk of infection (such as surgically irreparable hernia, omphalocele, gastroschisis, diaphragmatic hernia, and bladder extrophy).
- Relative contraindications for CAPD include:
  - fresh intra-abdominal foreign bodies (for example, 4-month wait after abdominal vascular prostheses, recent ventricular-peritoneal shunt)
  - peritoneal leaks or infection, or infection of the abdominal wall or skin
  - body size limitations—either a patient who's too small to tolerate adequate dialysate, or a patient who's too large to be effectively dialyzed
  - inability to tolerate the necessary volumes of dialysate for peritoneal dialysis to be successful
  - inflammatory or ischemic bowel disease, or recurrent episodes of diverticulitis
  - morbid obesity in short individuals, or patients suffering from severe malnutrition.
- If inflow and outflow are slow or absent, check the tubing for kinks. You can also try raising the solution or repositioning (turning from side to side) the patient to increase the inflow rate. Repositioning the patient or applying manual pressure to the lateral aspects of the patient's abdomen may also help increase drainage.

Complications

- Peritonitis
- Excessive fluid loss
- Excessive fluid retention

Patient teaching

- Upon discharge, discuss the importance of compliance with therapy. Inform the patient that skipping treatments has been shown to increase the risk of hospitalization and death. Assist the patient with setting up and adjusting his CAPD schedule.
- Teach the patient and his family how to use sterile technique throughout the procedure, especially for cleaning and dressing changes, to prevent complications such as peritonitis.
- Inform the patient about the advantages of an automated continuous cycler system for home use. (See *Continuous-cycle peritoneal dialysis,* page 402.)
- Teach the patient and his family the signs and symptoms of peritonitis—cloudy fluid, fever, and abdominal pain and tenderness—and stress the importance of notifying the practitioner immediately if such signs or symptoms arise. Tell them to call the practitioner if redness and drainage occur; these are also signs of infection.
- Instruct the patient to record his weight and blood pressure daily and to check regularly for swelling of the extremities. Teach him to keep an accurate record of intake and output.

Documentation

Record the type and amount of fluid instilled and returned for each exchange, the time and duration of the exchange, and medications added to the dialysate. Note the color and clarity of the returned exchange fluid and check it for mucus, pus, and blood. Note any discrepancy in the balance of fluid intake and output as well as signs of fluid imbalance, such as weight changes, decreased breath sounds, peripheral edema, ascites, and changes in skin turgor. Record the patient's weight, blood pressure, and pulse rate after his last fluid exchange for the day.

Continuous-cycle peritoneal dialysis

Continuous ambulatory peritoneal dialysis is easier for the patient who uses an automated continuous cycler system. When set up, the system runs the dialysis treatment automatically until all the dialysate is infused. The system remains closed throughout the treatment, which reduces the risk of contamination. Continuous-cycle peritoneal dialysis (CCPD) can be performed while the patient is awake or asleep. The system's alarms warn about general system, dialysate, and patient problems.

The cycler can be set to an intermittent or continuous dialysate schedule at home or in a health care facility. The patient typically initiates CCPD at bedtime and undergoes three to seven exchanges, according to his prescription. On awakening, the patient infuses the prescribed dialysis volume, disconnects himself from the unit, and carries the dialysate in his peritoneal cavity during the day.

The continuous cycler follows the same sterile care and maintenance procedures as the manual method.

Postmortem care

Postmortem care usually begins after a practitioner certifies the patient's death. After the patient dies, care includes preparing him for family viewing, arranging transportation to the morgue or funeral home, and determining the disposition of his belongings.

Nurses should check for the presence of family, identify the next of kin, and determine if the family has been informed of the patient's death. Postmortem care entails supporting the patient's family and friends. The nurse should observe the family's response, realize that there's no "right" way to grieve, and decide whether the family needs time alone with the patient or would feel more comfortable with a staff member in the room. Respect of ethnic and cultural differences toward death aids in the grieving process. Discussing and inquiring about cultural or spiritual practices in regard to preparation of the body helps increase the family's sense of control.

If the patient died under mysterious or violent circumstances, it's important for the nurse to explain that an autopsy must be performed. If it has already been done, she should prepare the family for the appearance of the body before viewing.

Families that wish to be involved in postmortem care should be encouraged to participate. Allowing the family to assist can facilitate the grieving process and acknowledgment of death.

Equipment

Gauze or soft string ties ♦ gloves ♦ chin straps ♦ ABD pads ♦ cotton balls ♦ plastic shroud or body wrap ♦ three identification tags ♦ adhesive bandages to cover wounds or punctures ♦ plastic bag for patient's belongings ♦ water-filled basin ♦ soap ♦ towels ♦ washcloths ♦ morgue stretcher ♦ protective equipment

A commercial morgue pack usually contains gauze or string ties, chin straps, a shroud, and identification tags.

Key steps

- Document auxiliary equipment, such as a mechanical ventilator, still present. Put on gloves.
- Put on protective equipment according to standard precautions.
- Place the body in the supine position, arms at sides and head on a pillow. Then elevate the head of the bed slightly to prevent discoloration caused by blood settling in the face.
- If the patient wore dentures and your facility's policy permits, gently insert them; then close the mouth. Close the eyes by gently pressing on the lids with your fingertips. If they don't stay closed, place moist cotton balls on the eyelids for a few minutes, and then try again to close them. Place a folded towel under the chin to keep the jaw closed.

- Remove all indwelling urinary catheters, tubes, and tape, and apply adhesive bandages to puncture sites. Replace soiled dressings.
- Collect all the patient's valuables to prevent loss. If you can't remove a ring, cover it with gauze, tape it in place, and tie the gauze to the wrist to prevent slippage and subsequent loss.
- Clean the body thoroughly, using soap, a basin, and washcloths. Place one or more ABD pads between the buttocks to absorb rectal discharge or drainage.
- Cover the body up to the chin with a clean sheet.
- Offer comfort and emotional support to the family and intimate friends. Ask if they wish to see the body. If they do, allow them to do so in privacy. Ask if they would prefer to leave the patient's jewelry on the body.
- After the family leaves, remove the towel under the chin, pad the chin, wrap straps under it, and tie the straps loosely on top of the head. Then pad the wrists and ankles to prevent bruises, and tie them together with gauze or soft string ties.
- Fill out the three identification tags. Each tag should include the deceased patient's name, room and bed numbers, date and time of death, and practitioner's name. Tie one tag to the deceased patient's hand or foot, but don't remove his identification bracelet to ensure correct identification.
- Place the shroud or body wrap on the morgue stretcher and, with assistance, transfer the body to the stretcher. Wrap the body, and tie the shroud or wrap with the string provided. Then attach another identification tag, and cover the shroud or wrap with a clean sheet. If a shroud or wrap isn't available, dress the deceased patient in a clean gown and cover the body with a sheet.
- Place the deceased patient's personal belongings, including valuables, in a bag and attach the third identification tag to it.
- If the patient died of an infectious disease, label the body according to your facility's policy.
- Close the doors of adjoining rooms if possible. Then take the body to the morgue. Use corridors that aren't crowded and, if possible, use a service elevator.

Special considerations

- Give the deceased patient's personal belongings to his family or take them to the morgue. If you give the family jewelry or money, make sure that a coworker is present as a witness. Obtain the signature of an adult family member to verify receipt of valuables or to state their preference that jewelry remain on the patient.
- Offer emotional support to the deceased patient's family and friends and to the patient's roommate, if appropriate.

Complications

- None known

Documentation

Although the extent of documentation varies among facilities, always record the disposition of the patient's possessions, especially jewelry and money. Also note the date and time the deceased patient was transported to the morgue.

Postoperative care

Postoperative care begins when the patient arrives in the postanesthesia care unit (PACU) and continues as he moves on to the short procedure unit, medical-surgical unit, or critical care area. Postoperative care aims to minimize complications by early detection and prompt treatment of the condition, such as postoperative pain, inadequate oxygenation, or other adverse physiologic effects.

Recovery from general anesthesia takes longer than induction because the anesthetic is retained in fat and muscle. Fat has a meager blood supply; thus, it releases the anesthetic slowly, providing enough anesthesia to maintain adequate blood and brain levels during surgery. The patient's recovery time varies with his amount of body fat, his overall condition, his premedication regimen, and the type, dosage, and duration of anesthesia. The effects of anesthesia and surgery can place the patient at risk for various physiologic disorders.

During the postoperative phase, the nurse is initially responsible for assessing the patient's physical status and monitoring changes that occur during the recovery process. When the patient's condition stabilizes, nursing care focuses on returning the patient to a functional level of wellness as soon as possible within the limitations created by surgery. The speed of a patient's recovery depends on how effectively the nurse can anticipate potential complications, begin the necessary preventive and supportive measures, and involve the patient's family in the recovery process. Facilitating communication among the patient, family, and members of the health care team is also the nurse's responsibility.

If the patient is discharged home after surgery, it's the nurse's responsibility to help the patient and his family translate instructions on the discharge sheet into useful ways to deal with practical matters at home. Areas to be discussed include food, bowel movements, resumption of sexual activity, wound care, driving, return to work, and medications. Each patient's care plan should be individualized to improve wellness and to maximize independence.

Equipment

Thermometer ♦ watch with second hand ♦ stethoscope ♦ sphygmomanometer ♦ postoperative flowchart or other documentation tool

Preparation

- Assemble the necessary equipment needed at the patient's bedside.

Key steps

- Obtain the patient's record from the PACU nurse. This should include a summary of operative procedures and pertinent findings, type of anesthesia, vital signs (preoperative, intraoperative, and postoperative), medical history, medication history (including preoperative, intraoperative, and postoperative medications), fluid therapy (including estimated blood loss, type and number of drains, catheters, and characteristics of drainage), and notes on the condition of the surgical wound. If the patient had vascular surgery, for example, knowing the location and duration of blood vessel clamping can prevent postoperative complications.
- Confirm the patient's identity using two patient identifiers according to your facility's policy.
- Transfer the patient from the PACU stretcher to the bed and position him properly. Get coworkers to help. Never try to move a patient alone; it's best to have three or four people assisting, with one supporting the patient's head. If the patient has had orthopedic surgery, one person should move only the affected extremity. If the patient is in skeletal traction, you may receive special orders for moving him. If this occurs, have one coworker move the weights as you and another coworker move the patient.
- When moving the patient, keep transfer movements smooth to minimize pain and postoperative complications and avoid back strain among team members.
- Make the patient comfortable and raise the bed's side rails to ensure his safety.
- Assess the patient's level of consciousness, skin color, and mucous membranes.
- Monitor the patient's respiratory status by assessing his airway. Note breathing rate and depth, and auscultate for breath sounds. Administer oxygen, and initiate oximetry to monitor oxygen saturation, if ordered.
- Monitor the patient's pulse rate. It should be strong and easily palpable. The heart rate should be within 20% of the preoperative rate.
- Compare postoperative blood pressure to preoperative blood pressure. It should be within 20% of the preoperative level unless the patient suffered a hypotensive episode during surgery.
- Assess the patient's temperature because anesthesia lowers body temperature. Body temperature should be at least 95° F (35° C). If it's lower, apply blankets to warm the patient.
- Assess the patient's infusion sites for redness, pain, swelling, or drainage.
- Assess surgical wound dressings; they should be clean and dry. If they're soiled, assess the characteristics of the drainage and outline the soiled area. Note the date

and time of assessment on the dressing. Assess the soiled area frequently; if it enlarges, reinforce the dressing and alert the practitioner.

- Note the presence and condition of any drains and tubes. Note the color, type, odor, and amount of drainage. Make sure that all drains are properly connected and free from kinks and obstructions.
- If the patient has had vascular or orthopedic surgery, assess the appropriate extremity or all extremities, depending on the surgical procedure. Assess color, temperature, sensation, movement, and presence and quality of pulses, and notify the practitioner of any abnormalities.
- As the patient recovers from anesthesia, monitor his respiratory and cardiovascular status closely. Stay alert for signs of airway obstruction and hypoventilation caused by laryngospasm or for sedation, which can lead to hypoxemia. Cardiovascular complications—such as arrhythmias or hypotension—may result from the anesthetic agent or the operative procedure.
- Encourage coughing and deep-breathing exercises. However, don't encourage them if the patient has just had nasal, ophthalmic, or neurologic surgery to avoid increasing intracranial pressure.
- Administer postoperative medications, such as antibiotics, analgesics, antiemetics, or reversal agents, as ordered and as appropriate.
- Remove all fluids from the patient's bedside until he's alert enough to eat and drink. Before giving him liquids, assess his gag reflex to prevent aspiration. To do this, lightly touch the back of his throat with a cotton swab—the patient will gag if the reflex has returned. Do this test quickly to prevent a vagal reaction.

Special considerations

- Fear, pain, anxiety, hypothermia, confusion, and immobility can upset the patient and jeopardize his safety and postoperative status. Offer emotional support to the patient and his family. Keep in mind that the patient who has lost a body part or who has been diagnosed with an incurable disease will need ongoing emotional support. Refer him and his family for counseling as needed.
- As the patient recovers from general anesthesia, reflexes appear in reverse order to that in which they disappeared. Hearing recovers first, so avoid holding inappropriate conversations.
- The patient under general anesthesia can't protect his own airway because the muscles are relaxed. As he recovers, cough and gag reflexes return. If he can lift his head without assistance, he can usually breathe on his own.
- If the patient received spinal anesthesia, he'll need to remain in a supine position with the bed adjusted to between 0 and 20 degrees for at least 6 hours to reduce the risk of headache from leakage of cerebrospinal fluid. The patient won't be able to move his legs, so be sure to reassure him that sensation and mobility will return.
- If the patient has had epidural anesthesia for postoperative pain control, monitor his respiratory status closely. Respiratory arrest may result from paralysis of the diaphragm by the anesthetic. He may also suffer nausea, vomiting, or itching.
- If the patient will be using a patient-controlled analgesia (PCA) unit, make sure he understands how to use it. Caution him to activate it only when he has pain, not when he feels sleepy or is pain-free. Review your facility's criteria for PCA use.

Complications

- Arrhythmias, hypotension, hypovolemia, septicemia, septic shock, atelectasis, pneumonia, thrombophlebitis, pulmonary embolism, urine retention, wound infection, wound dehiscence, evisceration, abdominal distention, paralytic ileus, constipation, altered body image, or postoperative psychosis

Documentation

Document the patient's vital signs on the appropriate flowchart. Record the condition of dressings, drains, and characteristics of drainage. Document all interventions taken to alleviate pain and anxiety and the patient's responses to them. Document complications and interventions taken.

Preoperative care

Preoperative care begins when surgery is planned and ends with the administration of anesthesia. This phase of care includes a preoperative interview and assessment to collect baseline subjective and objective data from the patient and his family; diagnostic tests, such as urinalysis, electrocardiogram, and chest radiography; preoperative teaching; securing informed consent from the patient; and physical preparation.

During the preoperative phase, the nurse performs a thorough assessment of the patient's emotional and physical status, to determine teaching needs and to identify patients at risk for surgery, and documents baseline data for future comparisons. The nursing goals in preparing the patient for surgery are reducing his anxiety, ensuring his safety, and identifying and decreasing the potential risks of complications of surgery.

Anxiety can interfere with the effectiveness of anesthesia and the patient's ability to actively participate in his care. Providing information about what will occur during surgery and sensations the patient can expect to feel helps to decrease anxiety. Demonstrating a caring attitude toward the patient and his family increases trust, reduces fear, and establishes a therapeutic relationship.

Informed consent is required by law to help protect the patient's rights, autonomy, and privacy. Failure to obtain informed consent can result in assault and battery or negligence charges against the health care providers. The surgeon should provide the patient with information regarding the extent and type of surgery, alternative therapies, and usual risks and benefits. A consent form that includes all of this information must be signed by the patient and a witness, verifying that the patient has received the required information.

The nurse is usually responsible for making sure the consent form is signed. The nurse also promotes patient safety by restricting activity after administration of sedatives and by completing a preoperative checklist to make sure that all procedures are carried out.

Equipment

Thermometer ♦ sphygmomanometer ♦ stethoscope ♦ watch with second hand ♦ weight scale ♦ tape measure

Preparation

- Assemble all equipment needed at the patient's bedside or in the admission area.

Key steps

- Confirm the patient's identity using two patient identifiers according to your facility's policy.
- If the patient is having same-day surgery, make sure that he knows ahead of time not to eat or drink anything before surgery. Follow your facility's policy for the time frame that the patient may not eat or drink before the procedure, which can range from 4 to 8 hours. Confirm with him what time he's scheduled to arrive at the health care facility, and tell him to leave all jewelry and valuables at home. Also make sure that the patient has arranged for someone to accompany him home after surgery.
- Obtain a health history and assess the patient's knowledge, perceptions, and expectations about the surgery. Ask about previous medical and surgical interventions. Also determine the patient's psychosocial needs; ask about occupational well-being, financial matters, support systems, mental status, and cultural beliefs. Use your facility's preoperative surgical assessment database, if available, to gather this information. Obtain a drug history. Ask about current prescription and over-the-counter medications and about known allergies to foods, drugs, and latex.
- Obtain the patient's height, weight, and vital signs.
- Identify risk factors that may interfere with a positive expected outcome. Be sure to consider age, general health, medications, mobility, nutritional status, fluid and electrolyte disturbances, and lifestyle. Also consider the primary disorder's duration, location, and nature and the extent of the surgical procedure.

- Explain preoperative procedures to the patient. Include typical events that he can expect and the sensations he can expect to experience. Discuss equipment that may be used postoperatively, such as nasogastric tubes and I.V. equipment. Explain the typical incision, dressings, and staples or sutures that will be used. Preoperative teaching can help reduce postoperative anxiety and pain, increase patient compliance, hasten recovery, and decrease length of stay.
- Talk the patient through the sequence of events from operating room to recovery room (postanesthesia care unit [PACU]) and back to the patient's room. He may be transferred from the PACU to an intensive care unit or surgical care unit. The patient may also benefit from a tour of the areas he'll see during the perioperative events.
- Tell the patient that when he goes to the operating room, he may have to wait a short time in the holding area. Explain that the surgeons and nurses will wear surgical dress, and even though they'll be observing him closely, they won't talk to him very much. Explain that minimal conversation will help the preoperative medication take effect.
- When discussing transfer procedures and techniques, describe sensations the patient will experience. Tell him that he'll be taken to the operating room on a stretcher and transferred from the stretcher to the operating room table. For his own safety, he'll be held securely to the table with soft restraints. The operating room nurses will check his vital signs frequently.
- Warn the patient that the operating room may feel cool. Electrodes may be put on his chest to monitor his heart rate during surgery. Describe the drowsy floating sensation he'll feel as the anesthetic takes effect. Tell him it's important that he relax at this time.
- Tell the patient about exercises that he may be expected to perform after surgery, such as deep breathing, coughing (while splinting the incision if necessary), limb exercises, and movement and ambulation to minimize respiratory and circulatory complications. If the patient will undergo ophthalmic or neurologic surgery, he won't be asked to cough because coughing increases intracranial pressure.
- On the day of surgery, important interventions include giving morning care, verifying that the patient has signed an informed consent form, administering ordered preoperative medications, completing the preoperative checklist and chart, and providing support to the patient and his family.
- Make sure that the surgical site has been verified by the surgeon and witnessed by the patient. The surgeon should identify the site by placing his initials with a permanent marker on the appropriate site with the assistance of the patient.
- Other immediate preoperative interventions may include preparing the GI tract (restricting food and fluids before surgery) to reduce vomiting and the risk of aspiration, cleaning the lower GI tract of fecal material by enemas before abdominal or GI surgery, or giving antibiotics for 2 or 3 days preoperatively to prevent contamination of the peritoneal cavity by GI bacteria.
- Just before the patient is moved to the surgical area, make sure he's wearing a hospital gown, his identification band is in place, and his vital signs have been recorded. Check to see that hairpins, nail polish, and jewelry have been removed. Note whether dentures, contact lenses, or prosthetic devices have been removed or left in place.

Special considerations

- Preoperative medications must be given on time to enhance the effect of ordered anesthesia. The patient should take nothing by mouth preoperatively. Don't give oral medications unless ordered. Be sure to raise the bed's side rails immediately after giving preoperative medications.
- If family or others are present, direct them to the appropriate waiting area and offer support as needed.

Complications

- None known

Documentation

Complete the preoperative checklist used by your facility. Record all nursing care measures and preoperative medications, results of diagnostic tests, and the time the patient is transferred to the surgical area. The chart and the surgical checklist must accompany the patient to surgery.

Pressure dressing application

For effective control of capillary or small-vein bleeding, temporary application of pressure directly over a wound may be achieved with a bulk dressing held by a glove-protected hand, bound into place with a pressure bandage, or held under pressure by an inflated air splint. A pressure dressing requires frequent checks for wound drainage to determine its effectiveness in controlling bleeding.

Pressure dressing may be prescribed for patients with fluid volume deficit, impaired skin integrity, impaired tissue integrity, or altered tissue perfusion.

Equipment

Two or more sterile gauze pads ♦ roller gauze ♦ adhesive tape ♦ clean disposable gloves ♦ metric ruler

Preparation

- Obtain the pressure dressing quickly to avoid excessive blood loss.
- Use clean cloth for the dressing if sterile gauze pads are unavailable.

Key steps

- Quickly explain the procedure to the patient to help decrease his anxiety, and put on gloves.
- Elevate the injured body part to help reduce bleeding.
- Place enough gauze pads over the wound to cover it. Don't clean the wound until the bleeding stops.
- For an extremity or a trunk wound, hold the dressing firmly over the wound and wrap the roller gauze tightly across it and around the body part to provide pressure on the wound. Secure the bandage with adhesive tape.
- To apply a dressing to the neck, the shoulder, or another location that can't be tightly wrapped, don't use roller gauze. Instead, apply tape directly over the dressings to provide the necessary pressure at the wound site.
- Check the patient's pulse, temperature, and skin condition distal to the wound site because excessive pressure can obstruct normal circulation.
- Check the dressing frequently to monitor wound drainage. Use the metric standard of measurement to determine the amount of drainage, and document these serial measurements for later reference.

DO'S & DON'TS

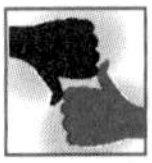

Don't circle a potentially wet dressing with ink because this provides no permanent documentation in the medical record and also runs the risk of contaminating the dressing.

- If the dressing becomes saturated, don't remove it because this will interfere with the pressure. Instead, apply an additional dressing over the saturated one and continue to monitor and record drainage.
- Obtain additional medical care as soon as possible.

Special considerations

- Apply pressure directly to the wound with your gloved hand if sterile gauze pads and clean cloth are unavailable.
- Avoid using an elastic bandage to bind the dressing because it can't be wrapped tightly enough to create pressure on the wound site.

Complications

- Impaired circulation

Documentation

When the bleeding is controlled, record the date and time of dressing application, presence or absence of distal pulses, integrity of distal skin, amount of wound drainage, and complications.

Pressure ulcer care

A pressure ulcer is a lesion caused by unrelieved pressure that results in damage to underlying tissues. Most pressure ulcers develop over bony prominences, where friction and shearing force combine with pressure to break down skin and underlying tissues. Approximately 95% of pressure ulcers occur in the lower part of the body, with the sacrum or the heel being the two most frequent sites that experience skin breakdown.

Successful pressure ulcer treatment involves relieving pressure, restoring circulation and, if possible, resolving or managing related disorders. Typically, the effectiveness and duration of treatment depend on the pressure ulcer's characteristics. (See *Assessing pressure ulcers,* page 410.) Preventive strategies include recognizing the risk, decreasing the effects of pressure, assessing nutritional status, avoiding excessive bedrest, and preserving skin integrity.

Treatment includes methods to decrease pressure, such as frequent repositioning to shorten pressure duration, and the use of special equipment to reduce pressure intensity. Treatment may involve special pressure-reducing devices, such as beds, mattresses, mattress overlays, and chair cushions. Other therapeutic measures include decreasing risk factors and use of topical treatments, wound cleaning, debridement, and the use of dressings to support moist wound healing. (See *Topical agents for pressure ulcers,* page 411.)

Nurses usually perform or coordinate treatments, according to facility policy. The procedures detailed below address cleaning and dressing the pressure ulcer. Always follow the standard precautions guidelines of the Centers for Disease Control and Prevention.

Equipment

Hypoallergenic tape or elastic netting ♦ overbed table ♦ piston-type irrigating system ♦ two pairs of gloves ♦ normal saline solution, as ordered ♦ sterile 4″ × 4″ gauze pads ♦ sterile cotton swabs ♦ selected topical dressing ♦ linen-saver pads ♦ impervious plastic trash bag ♦ disposable wound-measuring device (a square, transparent card with concentric circles arranged in bull's-eye fashion and bordered with a straight-edge ruler)

Preparation

- Assemble equipment at the patient's bedside.
- Cut the tape into strips for securing dressings.
- Loosen the lids on cleaning solutions and medications for easy removal.
- Loosen existing dressing edges and tapes before putting on gloves.
- Attach an impervious plastic trash bag to the bedside table to hold used dressings and refuse.

Key steps

- Confirm the patient's identity using two patient identifiers according to your facility's policy.
- Premedicate the patient if necessary.
- Before a dressing change, wash your hands, and review the principles of standard precautions.

Cleaning the pressure ulcer

- Provide privacy, and explain the procedure to the patient to allay his fears and promote cooperation.
- Position the patient to increase his comfort, but make sure his position allows easy access to the pressure ulcer site.
- Cover the bed linens with a linen-saver pad to prevent soiling.
- Open the normal saline solution container and the piston syringe. Carefully pour normal saline solution into an irrigation container to avoid splashing. (This container may be clean or sterile, depending on your facility's policy.) Put the piston syringe into the opening provided in the irrigation container.
- Open the packages of supplies.
- Put on gloves to remove the old dressing and expose the pressure ulcer. Discard the soiled dressing in the impervious plastic trash bag to avoid contaminating the sterile field and spreading infection.
- Inspect the wound. Note the color, amount, and odor of drainage and necrotic debris. Measure the wound perimeter with the disposable wound-measuring device (a square, transparent card with concentric circles arranged in bull's-eye fashion and bordered with a straight-edge ruler).

Assessing pressure ulcers

To select the most effective treatment for a pressure ulcer, you first need to assess its characteristics. The pressure ulcer stages described here reflect the anatomic depth of exposed tissue. Keep in mind that if the wound contains necrotic tissue, you won't be able to determine the stage until you can see the wound base.

Stage I

An ulcer at stage I is a nonblanchable erythema of intact skin. The heralding lesion of a pressure ulcer is persistent redness in lightly pigmented skin and persistent red, blue, or purple hues on darker skin. Other indicators include changes in temperature, consistency, or sensation.

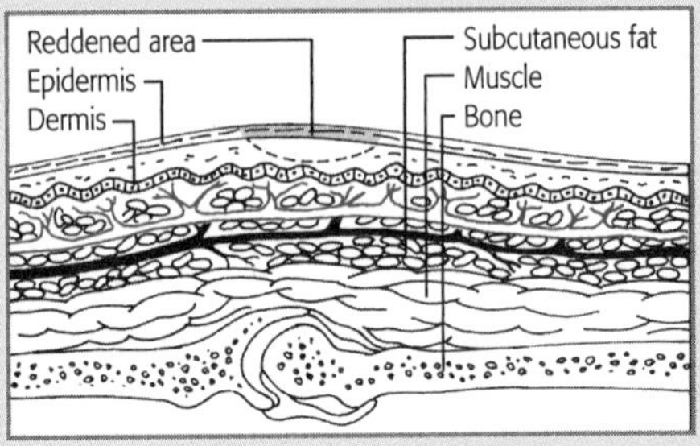

Stage II

Stage II is marked by partial-thickness skin loss involving the epidermis, dermis, or both. The ulcer is superficial and appears as an abrasion, blister, or shallow crater.

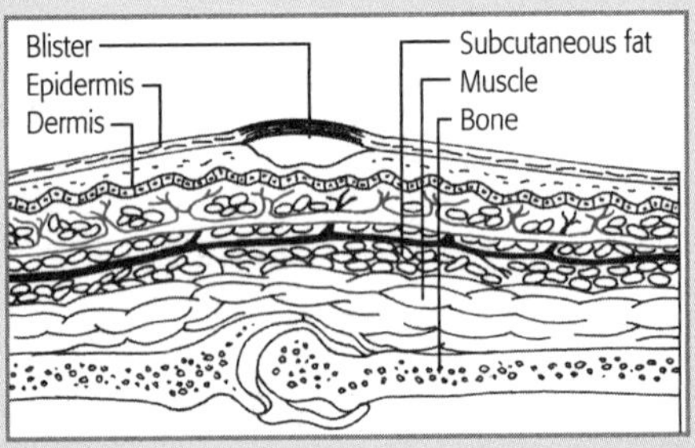

Stage III

At stage III, the ulcer constitutes a full-thickness wound penetrating the subcutaneous tissue, which may extend to—but not through—underlying fascia. The ulcer resembles a deep crater and may undermine adjacent tissue.

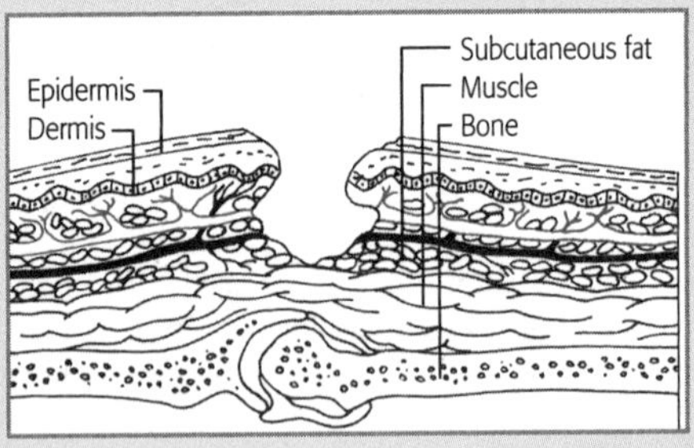

Stage IV

At stage IV, the ulcer extends through the skin, accompanied by extensive destruction, tissue necrosis, or damage to muscle, bone, or supporting structures (such as tendons and joint capsules).

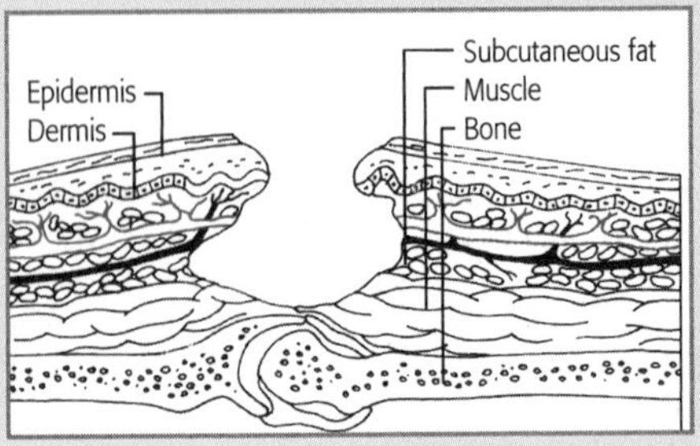

Topical agents for pressure ulcers

Topical agents	Nursing considerations
Antibiotics Silver sulfadiazine, triple antibiotics	▪ Consider a 2-week trial of topical antibiotics for clean or exudated pressure ulcers that aren't responding to moist-wound healing therapy.
Circulatory stimulants (Granulex, Proderm)	▪ Use these agents to promote blood flow. Both contain balsam of Peru and castor oil, but Granulex also contains trypsin, an enzyme that facilitates debridement.
Enzymes Collagenase (Santyl)	▪ Apply collagenase in thin layers after cleaning the wound with normal saline solution. ▪ Avoid concurrent use of collagenase with agents that decrease enzymatic activity, including detergents, hexachlorophene, antiseptics with heavy-metal ions, iodine, or such acid solutions as Burow's solution. ▪ Use collagenase cautiously near the patient's eyes. If contact occurs, flush the eyes repeatedly with normal saline solution or sterile water.
Exudate absorbers Dextranomer beads (Debrisan)	▪ Use dextranomer beads on secreting ulcers. Discontinue use when secretions stop. ▪ Clean—but don't dry—the ulcer before applying dextranomer beads. Don't use in tunneling ulcers. ▪ Remove gray-yellow beads (which indicate saturation) by irrigating with sterile water or normal saline solution. ▪ Use cautiously near the eyes. If contact occurs, flush the eyes repeatedly with normal saline solution or sterile water.
Isotonic solutions Normal saline solution	▪ This agent moisturizes tissue without injuring cells.

- Using the piston syringe, apply full force to irrigate the pressure ulcer to remove necrotic debris.
- Remove and discard your soiled gloves, and put on a fresh pair.
- Insert a gloved finger or sterile cotton swab into the wound to assess wound tunneling or undermining. Tunneling usually signals wound extension along fascial planes.
- Next, reassess the condition of the skin and the ulcer. Note the character of the clean wound bed and the surrounding skin.
- If you observe adherent necrotic material, notify a wound care specialist or a practitioner to ensure appropriate debridement. (See *Understanding pressure ulcer debridement*, page 412.)
- Prepare to apply the appropriate topical dressing. Directions for typical moist saline gauze, hydrocolloid, transparent, alginate, foam, and hydrogel dressings follow. For other dressings or topical agents, follow your facility's protocol or the supplier's instructions. (See *Choosing a pressure ulcer dressing*, page 413.)

Understanding pressure ulcer debridement

Because moist, necrotic tissue promotes the growth of pathologic organisms, removing such tissue aids pressure ulcer healing. A pressure ulcer can be debrided using various methods; the patient's condition and the goals of care determine which method to use. Sharp debridement is indicated for patients with an urgent need for debridement, such as those with sepsis or cellulitis; otherwise, another method—such as mechanical, enzymatic, or autolytic debridement—may be used. Sometimes several methods are used in combination.

Sharp debridement

The most rapid method, sharp debridement removes thick, adherent eschar and devitalized tissue through the use of a scalpel, scissors, or another sharp instrument. Small amounts of necrotic tissue can be debrided at the bedside; extensive amounts must be debrided in the operating room.

Mechanical debridement

Typically, mechanical debridement involves the use of wet-to-damp dressings. Gauze moistened with normal saline solution is applied to the wound and allowed to become damp. It's removed before it becomes completely dry. The goal is to debride the wound as the dressing is removed. Mechanical debridement has certain disadvantages; for example, it's typically painful and may take a long time to completely debride the ulcer.

Enzymatic debridement

Enzymatic debridement removes necrotic tissue by breaking down tissue elements. Topical enzymatic debriding agents are placed on the necrotic tissue. If eschar is present, it must be crosshatched to allow the enzyme to penetrate the tissue.

Autolytic debridement

Autolytic debridement involves the use of moisture-retentive dressings to cover the wound bed. Necrotic tissue is then removed through self-digestion of enzymes in the wound fluid. Although this method takes longer than other debridement methods, it's appropriate for patients who can't tolerate other methods. If the ulcer is infected, autolytic debridement isn't the treatment of choice.

Applying a moist saline gauze dressing

- Irrigate the pressure ulcer with normal saline solution. Blot the surrounding skin dry.
- Moisten the gauze dressing with saline solution.
- Gently place the dressing over the surface of the ulcer. To separate surfaces within the wound, gently place a dressing between opposing wound surfaces. To avoid damage to tissues, don't pack the gauze tightly.
- Change the dressing often enough to keep the wound moist.

Applying a hydrocolloid dressing

- Irrigate the pressure ulcer with normal saline solution. Blot the surrounding skin dry.
- Choose a clean, dry, presized dressing, or cut one to overlap the pressure ulcer by about 1" (2.5 cm). Remove the dressing from its package, pull the release paper from the adherent side of the dressing, and apply the dressing to the wound. To minimize irritation, carefully smooth out wrinkles as you apply the dressing.
- If the dressing's edges need to be secured with tape, apply a skin sealant to the intact skin around the ulcer. After the area dries, tape the dressing to the skin. The sealant protects the skin and promotes tape adher-

Choosing a pressure ulcer dressing

Choosing the proper dressing for a wound can be guided by four basic questions:

- What does the wound need (for example, does it need to be drained, protected, or kept moist)?
- What does the dressing do?
- How well does the product do it? (For example, if the wound is draining a large amount, how absorptive is the dressing?)
- What's available and practical?

Gauze dressings

Made of absorptive cotton or synthetic fabric, gauze dressings are permeable to water, water vapor, and oxygen and may be impregnated with petroleum jelly or another agent. When uncertain about which dressing to use, you may apply a gauze dressing moistened in normal saline solution until a wound specialist recommends definitive treatment.

Hydrocolloid dressings

Hydrocolloid dressings are adhesive, moldable wafers made of a carbohydrate-based material and usually have waterproof backings. They're impermeable to oxygen, water, and water vapor, and most have some absorptive properties.

Transparent film dressings

Clear, adherent, and nonabsorptive, transparent film dressings are polymer-based dressings permeable to oxygen and water vapor but not to water. Their transparency allows visual inspection. Because they can't absorb drainage, transparent film dressings are used on partial-thickness wounds with minimal exudate.

Alginate dressings

Made from seaweed, alginate dressings are nonwoven, absorptive dressings available as soft, white sterile pads or ropes. They absorb excessive exudate and may be used on infected wounds. As these dressings absorb exudate, they turn into a gel that keeps the wound bed moist and promotes healing. When exudate is no longer excessive, switch to another type of dressing.

Foam dressings

Foam dressings are spongelike polymer dressings that may be impregnated or coated with other materials. Somewhat absorptive, they may be adherent. These dressings promote moist wound healing and are useful when a nonadherent surface is desired.

Hydrogel dressings

Water-based and nonadherent, hydrogel dressings are polymer-based and have some absorptive properties. They're available as a gel in a tube, as flexible sheets, and as saturated gauze packing strips. They may have a cooling effect, which eases pain.

ence. Avoid using tension or pressure when applying the tape.

- Remove your gloves, and discard them in the impervious plastic trash bag. Dispose of refuse according to your facility's policy, and wash your hands.
- Change a hydrocolloid dressing every 2 to 7 days, as needed—for example, if the patient complains of pain, the dressing no longer adheres, or leakage occurs.

Applying a transparent dressing

- Irrigate the pressure ulcer with normal saline solution. Blot the surrounding skin dry.
- Clean and dry the wound as described above.
- Select a dressing to overlap the ulcer by 2″ (5 cm).
- Gently lay the dressing over the ulcer. To prevent shearing force, don't stretch the dressing. Press firmly on the edges of the

dressing to promote adherence. Although this type of dressing is self-adhesive, you may have to tape the edges to prevent them from curling.

- If necessary, aspirate accumulated fluid with a 21G needle and syringe. After aspirating the pocket of fluid, clean the aspiration site with an alcohol pad, and cover it with another strip of transparent dressing.
- Change the dressing every 3 to 7 days, depending on the amount of drainage.

Applying an alginate dressing

- Irrigate the pressure ulcer with normal saline solution. Blot the surrounding skin dry.
- Apply the alginate dressing to the ulcer surface. Cover the area with a second dressing (such as gauze pads), as ordered. Secure the dressing with tape or elastic netting.
- If the wound is draining heavily, change the dressing once or twice daily for the first 3 to 5 days. As drainage decreases, change the dressing less frequently—every 2 to 4 days or as ordered. When the drainage stops or the wound bed looks dry, stop using alginate dressing.

Applying a foam dressing

- Irrigate the pressure ulcer with normal saline solution. Blot the surrounding skin dry.
- Gently lay the foam dressing over the ulcer.
- Use tape, elastic netting, or gauze to hold the dressing in place.
- Change the dressing when the foam no longer absorbs the exudate.

Applying a hydrogel dressing

- Irrigate the pressure ulcer with normal saline solution. Blot the surrounding skin dry.
- Apply gel to the wound bed.
- Cover the area with a second dressing.
- Change the dressing daily, or as needed, to keep the wound bed moist.
- If the dressing you select comes in sheet form, cut the dressing to match the wound base; otherwise, the intact surrounding skin can become macerated.
- Hydrogel dressings also come in prepackaged, saturated gauze for wounds that require "dead space" to be filled. Follow the manufacturer's directions for usage.

Preventing pressure ulcers

- Turn and reposition the patient every 1 to 2 hours, unless contraindicated. For a patient who can't turn himself or who's turned on a schedule, use a pressure-reducing device, such as air, gel, or a 4" (10.2 cm) foam mattress overlay. Low- or high-air-loss therapy may be indicated to reduce excessive pressure and promote evaporation of excess moisture. As appropriate, implement active or passive range-of-motion exercises to relieve pressure and promote circulation. To save time, combine these exercises with bathing, if applicable.
- When turning the patient, lift him, rather than slide him, because sliding increases friction and shear. Use a turning sheet, and get help from coworkers if necessary.
- Use pillows to position your patient and increase his comfort. Be sure to eliminate sheet wrinkles that could increase pressure and cause discomfort.
- Post a turning schedule at the patient's bedside. Adapt position changes to his situation. Emphasize the importance of regular position changes to the patient and his family, and encourage their participation in treatment and prevention of pressure ulcers by having them perform a position change correctly after you have demonstrated how.
- Avoid placing the patient directly on the trochanter. Instead, position him on his side, at an angle of about 30 degrees.
- Except for brief periods, avoid raising the head of the bed more than 30 degrees to prevent shearing pressure.
- Direct the patient confined to a chair or wheelchair to shift his weight every 15 minutes to promote blood flow to compressed tissues. Show a paraplegic patient how to shift his weight by doing push-ups in the wheelchair. If the patient needs your help, sit next to him, and help him shift his weight to one buttock for 60 seconds, then repeat the procedure on the other

side. Provide him with pressure-relieving cushions, as appropriate. However, avoid seating the patient on a rubber or plastic doughnut, which can increase localized pressure at vulnerable points.
- Adjust or pad appliances, casts, or splints, as needed, to ensure proper fit and avoid increased pressure and impaired circulation.
- Tell the patient to avoid heat lamps and harsh soaps because they dry the skin. Applying lotion after bathing will help keep his skin moist. Tell him to avoid vigorous massage because it can damage capillaries.
- If the patient's condition permits, recommend a diet that includes adequate calories, protein, and vitamins. Dietary therapy may involve nutritional consultation, food supplements, enteral feeding, or total parenteral nutrition.
- If diarrhea develops or if the patient is incontinent, clean and dry soiled skin. Apply a protective moisture barrier to prevent skin maceration.
- Make sure the patient, family members, and caregivers learn pressure ulcer prevention and treatment strategies so that they understand the importance of care, the choices that are available, the rationales for treatments, and their role in selecting goals and shaping the care plan.

Special considerations

DO'S & DON'TS

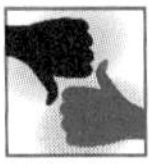

Don't use elbow and heel protectors that fasten with a single narrow strap. The strap may impair neurovascular function in the involved hand or foot.

- Avoid using artificial sheepskin. It doesn't reduce pressure and may create a false sense of security.
- Repair of stage III and IV ulcers may require surgical intervention—such as direct closure, skin grafting, or flaps—depending on the patient's needs. They also may be treated with growth factors, electrical stimulation, heat therapy, or vacuum-assisted wound closure.

Complications

- Infection causing foul-smelling drainage, persistent pain, severe erythema, induration, and elevated skin and body temperatures; advancing infection or cellulitis leading to septicemia; severe erythema signaling worsening cellulitis indicating that the offending organisms have invaded the tissue and are no longer localized

Patient teaching

- If the patient is at risk for pressure ulcers or has a pressure ulcer, teach him and his family the importance of prevention, position changes, and treatment at home.

Documentation

Record the date and time of initial and subsequent treatments. Note the specific treatment given. Detail preventive strategies performed. Document the pressure ulcer's location and size (length, width, and depth); color and appearance of the wound bed; amount, odor, color, and consistency of drainage; and the condition of the surrounding skin. Reassess pressure ulcers at least weekly.

Update the care plan as required. Note changes in the condition or size of the pressure ulcer and any elevation of skin temperature on the clinical record. Document when the practitioner was notified of pertinent abnormal observations. Record the patient's temperature daily on the graphic sheet to allow easy assessment of body temperature patterns.

Prone positioning

Prone positioning is a therapeutic maneuver to improve oxygenation and pulmonary mechanics in patients with acute lung injury or acute respiratory distress syndrome (ARDS). Also known as *proning*, the procedure involves physically turning a patient from a supine position (on the back) to a facedown position (prone position). This positioning may improve oxygenation in patients by shifting blood flow to regions of the lung that are better ventilated. With the appropriate equipment, prone positioning may also facilitate better movement of the diaphragm by allowing the abdomen to expand more fully.

The criteria for prone positioning frequently include:

- acute onset of respiratory failure
- hypoxemia, specifically a PaO_2/FIO_2 ratio of 300 or less for acute lung injury or a PaO_2/FIO_2 ratio of 200 or less for ARDS
- radiological evidence of diffuse bilateral pulmonary infiltrates.

Proning equipment, such as a lightweight, cushioned frame that straps to the front of the patient before turning, has helped to minimize the risks associated with moving patients and maintaining them in the prone position for several hours at a time.

Prone positioning is usually performed for 6 or more hours per day, for as long as 10 days, until the requirement for a high concentration of inspired oxygen resolves. Aside from early intervention, factors predictive of patients' responses aren't consistent among studies, and patients' initial responses aren't always predictive of their subsequent responses. Patients with extrapulmonary ARDS (such as ARDS due to multiple trauma) appear to respond consistently to prone positioning. Although research has demonstrated improved oxygenation with proning, it's unclear whether the survival rate is increased.

The procedure is indicated to support mechanically ventilated patients with ARDS, who require high concentrations of inspired oxygen. Prone positioning may correct severe hypoxemia and help maintain adequate oxygenation (PO_2 greater than 60%) while avoiding ventilator-induced lung injury.

Prone positioning is contraindicated in patients whose heads can't be supported in a facedown position, or those who can't tolerate a head down position. Relative contraindications include:

- increased intracranial pressure
- spinal instability
- unstable bone fractures
- multiple trauma
- left ventricular failure (nonpulmonary respiratory failure)
- shock
- abdominal compartment syndrome or abdominal surgery
- patients who are extremely obese (more than 300 lb [136 kg])
- pregnancy.

Hemodynamically unstable patients (systolic blood pressure less than 90 mm Hg) despite aggressive fluid resuscitation and vasopressors should be thoroughly evaluated before being placed in the prone position.

Equipment

Vollman Prone Positioner (Hill-Rom), or other prone-positioning device ♦ gloves ♦ personal protective equipment, as appropriate

Preparation

- Clean the positioner according to your facility's policy between positioning turns and when discontinuing prone positioning.

Key steps

- Assess the patient's hemodynamic status to determine whether the patient will be able to tolerate the prone position.
- Assess the patient's neurologic status prior to prone positioning. Generally, the patient will be heavily sedated. Although agitation isn't a contraindication for proning, it must be managed effectively.
- Determine whether the patient's size and weight will allow turning him on a generally narrow intensive care bed. Consider obtaining a wider specialty bed if needed.

Preparing the patient

- Explain the purpose and procedure of prone positioning to the patient and his family.

Before turning the patient

- Wash your hands and put on gloves or other protective wear, as appropriate.
- Provide eye care, including lubrication and horizontal taping of the patient's eyelids, if indicated.
- Make sure the patient's tongue is inside his mouth; if edematous or protruding, insert a bite block.

- Secure the patient's endotracheal (ET) tube or tracheotomy tube to prevent dislodgment.
- Perform anterior body wound care and dressing changes.
- Empty ileostomy or colostomy drainage bags.
- Remove anterior chest wall electrocardiogram monitoring leads, while ensuring ability to monitor the patient's cardiac rate and rhythm. These leads will be repositioned onto the patient's back once he's prone.
- Make sure that the brake of the bed is engaged. Attach the surface of the prone positioner to the bed frame, as recommended by the manufacturer.
- Position staff appropriately; a minimum of three people is required: one on either side of the bed and one at the head of the bed.

ALERT

The staff member at the head of the bed is responsible for monitoring the ET tube and mechanical ventilator tubing.

- Adjust all patient tubing and invasive monitoring lines to prevent dislodgment, kinking, disconnection, or contact with the patient's body during the turning procedure and while the patient remains in the prone position.

ALERT

Place all lines inserted in the upper torso over the right or left shoulder, with the exception of chest tubes, which are placed at the foot of the bed. All lines inserted in the lower torso are positioned at the foot of the bed.

- Turn the patient's face away from the ventilator, placing the ET tubing on the side of the patient's face that's turned away from the ventilator. Loop the remaining tubing above the patient's head. These maneuvers prevent disconnection of the ventilator tubing or kinking of the ET tube during proning.
- Place the straps of the prone positioner under the patient's head, chest, and pelvic area.
- Attach the prone-positioning device to the patient by placing the frame on top of the patient.
- Position the nonmovable chest piece, which acts as a marker for the proper device placement, so that it's resting between the patient's clavicles and sixth ribs.

ALERT

If the patient has a short neck or limited neck range of motion (ROM), align the chest piece lower, at the third intercostal space; move both headpieces up to the top of the frame so that only the forehead is supported by the head cushion and the chin is suspended to reduce the risk of skin breakdown.

- Adjust the pelvic piece of the device so that it rests ½″ (1.3 cm) above the iliac crest.
- Evaluate the distance between the chest and pelvic pieces to ensure suspension of the abdomen, while preventing bowing of the patient's back.
- Adjust the chin and forehead pieces of the device so that facial support is provided in either a facedown or side-lying position without interfering with the ET tube.
- Secure the positioning device to the patient, by fastening all the soft adjustable straps on one side before tightening them on the opposite side. Once secured, lift the positioner to ensure a secure fit.
- To help ensure a secure fit, look for cushion compression. If the frame isn't tightly secured, shear and friction injuries to the chest and pelvic area may occur.

Turning the patient

- Lower the side rails of the bed, and move the patient to the edge of the bed farthest away from the ventilator by using a draw sheet. The person closest to the patient maintains body contact with the bed at all times, serving as a side rail.
- Tuck the straps attached to the steel bar closest to the center of the bed underneath the patient. Then tuck the patient's arm

and hand that are resting in the center of the bed under the buttocks. Cross the leg closest to the edge of the bed over the opposite leg at the ankle, which will help with forward motion when the turning process begins.
- If the patient's arm can't be straightened to tuck under his buttocks, tuck his arm into the open space between the chest and pelvic pads.
- Turn the patient toward the ventilator at a 45-degree angle.

Do's & don'ts

Always turn the patient in the direction of the mechanical ventilator.

- The person on the side of the bed with the ventilator grasps the upper steel bar. The person on the other side of the bed grasps the lower steel bar or turning straps of the device.
- Lift the patient by the frame into the prone position on the count of three.
- Gently move the patient's tucked arm and hand so they're parallel to his body and comfortable.

Do's & don'ts

To prevent placing stress on the shoulder capsule, don't extend the patient's arm to a 90-degree angle.

- Loosen the straps if the patient is clinically stable.
- Keeping the straps securely fastened in an unstable patient allows for rapid supine repositioning in an emergency.
- Support the patient's feet with a pillow or towel roll to provide correct flexion while in the prone position.
- Pad the patient's elbows to prevent ulnar nerve compression.
- Monitor the patient's response to proning using vital signs, pulse oximetry, and mixed venous oxygen saturation. During the initial proning, arterial blood gases should be obtained within 30 minutes of proning and within 30 minutes prior to returning the patient to the supine position.
- Reposition the patient's head hourly while in the prone position to prevent facial breakdown. As one person lifts the patient's head, the second person moves the headpieces to provide head support in a different position.
- Provide ROM to shoulders, arms, and legs every 2 hours.

Returning the patient to the supine position

- Securely fasten positioning device straps.
- Position the patient on the edge of the bed closest to the ventilator.
- Adjust all patient tubing and monitoring lines to prevent dislodgment.
- Straighten the patient's arms and rest them on either side. Cross the leg closest to the edge of the bed over the opposite leg.
- Using the steel bars of the device, turn the patient to a 45-degree angle away from the ventilator, and then roll him to the supine position.
- Position the patient's arms parallel to his body.
- Unfasten the positioning device, and remove it from the patient.

Special considerations

- A practitioner's order is usually required before prone positioning of a critically ill patient.
- The procedure requires special training and established guidelines to ensure patient safety.
- Not all patients with ARDS respond favorably to prone positioning, and the benefit sometimes decreases over time.
- Patients may require increased sedation during proning.
- The prone-positioning schedule is generally determined by the patient's ability to maintain improvements in $Pa{O_2}$ while in the prone position.
- Use capnography, if possible, to verify correct ET tube placement during proning.
- Reposition the patient every 4 to 6 hours to prevent pressure-related injury.
- Discontinue the procedure when the patient no longer demonstrates improved oxygenation with the position change.

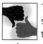

- Lateral rotation therapy is strongly recommended with prone positioning.

Complications

- Inadvertent ET extubation
- Airway obstruction
- Decreased oxygen saturation
- Apical atelectasis
- Obstructed chest tube
- Pressure injuries on the weight-bearing parts of the body, including the knees and chest
- Hemodynamic instability
- Dislodgment of central venous access
- Transient arrhythmias
- Reversible dependent edema of the face (forehead, eyelids, conjunctiva, lips, and tongue) and anterior chest wall
- Contractures
- Enteral feeding intolerance
- Aspiration of enteral feeding when repositioned supine
- Corneal ulceration

ALERT

Critically ill patients with active intra-abdominal processes, regardless of position, are at risk for sepsis and septic shock.

Documentation

Document the patient's response to therapy, ability to tolerate the turning procedure, length of time in the position, positioning schedule. Also document monitoring, complications, and interventions.

Pulse assessment

The pulse is a recurring wave of blood created by contraction of the left ventricle. It can be palpated where an artery crosses over bone on firm tissue. In a healthy person, pulse reflects the heartbeat, meaning that the pulse rate and the rate of ventricular contractions are the same.

In adults and children older than age 3, the radial artery in the wrist is the most common palpation site. (See *Pulse points,* page 420.) In infants and children younger than age 3, the best practice is to listen to the heart itself rather than palpate a pulse. Because auscultation is done at the heart's apex, this is called the *apical pulse.*

Assessment of the pulse should include the rate (number of beats per minute), rhythm (pattern or regularity of the beats), and volume (amount of blood pumped with each beat). If the pulse is faint or weak, use a Doppler ultrasound blood flow detector, if available. (See "Doppler use," page 135.) If the pulse is regular, count the rate for 30 seconds and multiply by two; however, if the pulse is irregular, the best practice is to count the rate for a full minute.

Equipment

Watch with second hand ♦ stethoscope (for auscultating apical pulse) ♦ Doppler ultrasound blood flow detector, if necessary ♦ alcohol pad

Preparation

- If you aren't using your own stethoscope, disinfect the earpieces with an alcohol pad before and after use to prevent cross-contamination.

Key steps

- Confirm the patient's identity using two patient identifiers according to your facility's policy.
- Wash your hands, and tell the patient you intend to take his pulse.
- Make sure that the patient is comfortable and relaxed because an awkward, uncomfortable position may affect the heart rate.

Taking a radial pulse

- Place the patient in a sitting or supine position, with his arm at his side or across his chest.
- Gently press your index, middle, and ring fingers on the radial artery, inside the patient's wrist. You should feel a pulse with only moderate pressure; excessive pressure may obstruct blood flow distal to the pulse site.

DO'S & DON'TS

Don't use your thumb to take the patient's pulse because you

Pulse points

Shown here are anatomic locations where an artery crosses bone or firm tissue that can be palpated for a pulse.

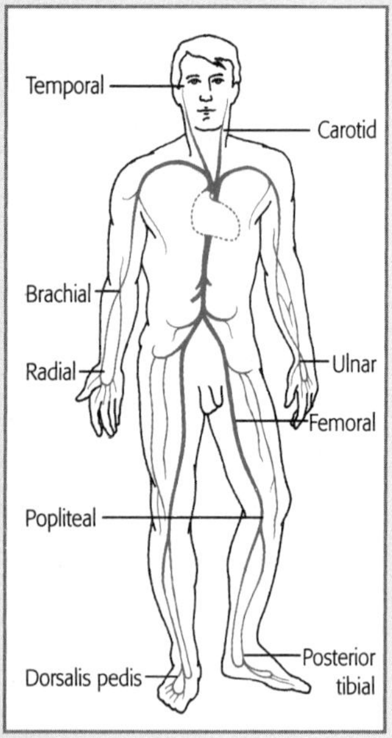

may mistake your thumb's own strong pulse for the patient's pulse.

- After locating the pulse, count the beats for 60 seconds, or count for 30 seconds and multiply by 2. Counting for a full minute provides a more accurate picture of irregularities.
- While counting the rate, assess pulse rhythm and volume by noting the pattern and strength of the beats. If you detect an irregularity, repeat the count, and note whether it occurs in a pattern or randomly. If you're still in doubt, take an apical pulse. (See *Identifying pulse patterns*.)

Taking an apical pulse

- Help the patient to a supine position and drape him if necessary.
- Warm the diaphragm or bell of the stethoscope in your hand. Placing a cold stethoscope against the skin may startle the patient and momentarily increase his heart rate. Keep in mind that the bell transmits low-pitched sounds more effectively than the diaphragm.
- Place the diaphragm or bell of the stethoscope over the apex of the heart (normally located at the fifth intercostal space left of the midclavicular line). Count the beats for 60 seconds, and note their rhythm, volume, and intensity (loudness).
- Remove the stethoscope and make the patient comfortable.

Taking an apical-radial pulse

- Two nurses work together to obtain the apical-radial pulse; one palpates the radial pulse while the other nurse auscultates the apical pulse with a stethoscope. Both must use the same watch when counting beats.
- Help the patient to a supine position and drape him if necessary.
- Locate the apical and radial pulses.
- Determine a time to begin counting. Then each nurse counts beats for 60 seconds.

Special considerations

- When the peripheral pulse is irregular, take an apical pulse to measure the heartbeat more directly. If the pulse is faint or weak, use a Doppler ultrasound blood flow detector if available.
- If another nurse isn't available for an apical-radial pulse assessment, hold the stethoscope in place with the hand that holds the watch while palpating the radial pulse with the other hand. You can then feel any discrepancies between the apical and radial pulses.

Complications

- None known

Patient teaching

- Teach the patient and family members the correct way to take a pulse and when to call the practitioner.

Documentation

Record the site, pulse rate, rhythm, and volume as well as the time of measurement. "Full" or "bounding" describes a pulse of increased volume; "weak" or

Identifying pulse patterns

Type	Rate	Rhythm (per 3 seconds)	Causes and incidence
Normal	60 to 80 beats/minute; in neonates, 120 to 140 beats/minute	● ● ● ●	■ Varies with such factors as age, physical activity, and gender (men usually have lower pulse rates than women)
Tachycardia	More than 100 beats/minute	●●●●●●●●	■ Accompanies stimulation of the sympathetic nervous system by emotional stress (such as anger, fear, or anxiety) or the use of certain drugs such as caffeine ■ May result from exercise and from certain health conditions, such as heart failure, anemia, and fever (which increases oxygen requirements and therefore pulse rate)
Bradycardia	Fewer than 60 beats/minute	● ● ●	■ Accompanies stimulation of the parasympathetic nervous system by use of certain drugs, especially digoxin, and such conditions as cerebral hemorrhage and heart block ■ May also be present in fit athletes
Irregular	Uneven time intervals between beats (for example, periods of regular rhythm interrupted by pauses or premature beats)	●●●● ●●●	■ May indicate cardiac irritability, hypoxia, digoxin toxicity, potassium imbalance, or sometimes more serious arrhythmias if premature beats occur frequently ■ Occasionally premature beats occurring, which are normal

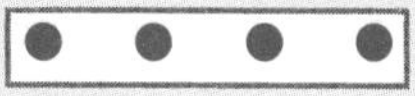

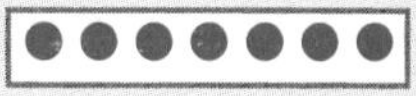

"thready," decreased volume. When recording the apical pulse, include intensity of heart sounds. When recording the apical-radial pulse, chart the rate according to the pulse site—for example, apical-radial pulse of 80/76.

Pulse and ear oximetry

Performed intermittently or continuously, oximetry is a relatively simple procedure used to monitor arterial oxygen saturation noninvasively. Arterial oxygen saturation values obtained by pulse oximeters are denoted with the symbol Spo_2, whereas invasively measured arterial oxygen saturation values are denoted by the symbol Sao_2.

In this procedure, two diodes send red and infrared light through a pulsating arterial vascular bed such as the one in the fingertip. A photodetector slipped over the finger measures the transmitted light as it passes through the vascular bed, detects the relative amount of color absorbed by arterial blood, and calculates the exact mixed venous oxygen saturation without interference from surrounding venous blood, skin, connective tissue, or bone. Ear oximetry works by monitoring the transmission of light waves through the vascular bed of a patient's earlobe. Results will be inaccurate if the patient's earlobe is poorly perfused, as in the case of a patient with a low cardiac output. (See *How oximetry works*.)

Equipment

Oximeter ♦ finger or ear transducer probe ♦ alcohol pads ♦ nail polish remover, if necessary

Preparation

- Review the manufacturer's instructions for assembling the oximeter.
- Choose the appropriate probe for the site you're using.

Key steps

- Confirm the patient's identity using two patient identifiers according to your facility's policy.
- Explain the procedure to the patient.
- Validate pulse oximetry readings by comparing Spo_2 readings with Sao_2 values obtained by arterial blood gas (ABG) analysis. Obtain these two measurements simultaneously at the beginning of pulse oximetry monitoring, and then reevaluate periodically according to the patient's condition.
- If pulse oximetry readings are being monitored continuously, set the high and low alarms according to the patient's clinical condition.

Pulse oximetry

- Select a finger for the test. Although the index finger is commonly used, a smaller finger may be selected if the patient's fingers are too large for the equipment. Make sure that the patient isn't wearing false fingernails, and remove any nail polish from the test finger. Place the transducer (photodetector) probe over the patient's finger so that light beams and sensors oppose each other. If the patient has long fingernails, position the probe perpendicular to the finger, if possible, or clip the fingernail. Always position the patient's hand at heart level to eliminate venous pulsations and to promote accurate readings.

ALERT

If you're testing a neonate or small infant, use probes specifically designed for them. For a large infant, use a probe that fits on the great toe and secure it to the foot.

- Turn on the power switch. If the device is working properly, a beep will sound, a display will light momentarily, and the pulse searchlight will flash. Initially, the Spo_2 and pulse rate displays will show stationary zeros. After four to six heartbeats, the displays will supply information with each beat and the pulse amplitude indicator will begin tracking the pulse.

How oximetry works

The pulse oximeter allows noninvasive monitoring of the percentage of hemoglobin saturated by oxygen, or Spo_2, levels by measuring the absorption (amplitude) of light waves as they pass through areas of the body that are highly perfused by arterial blood. Oximetry also monitors pulse rate and amplitude.

Light-emitting diodes in a transducer (photodetector) attached to the patient's body (shown here on the index finger) send red and infrared light beams through tissue. The photodetector records the relative amount of each color absorbed by arterial blood and transmits the data to a monitor, which displays the information with each heartbeat. If the Spo_2 level or pulse rate varies from preset limits, the monitor triggers visual and audible alarms.

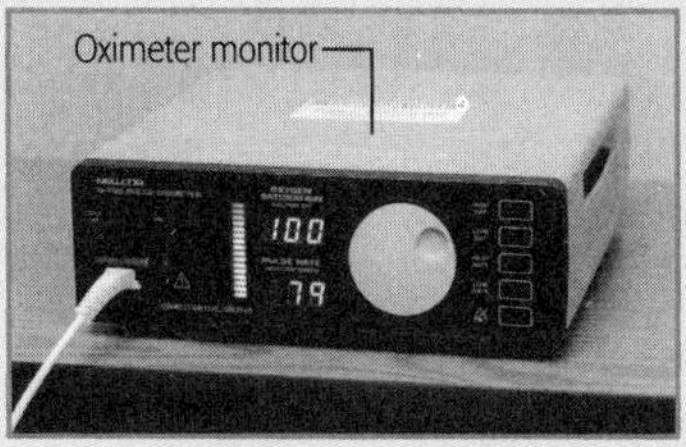

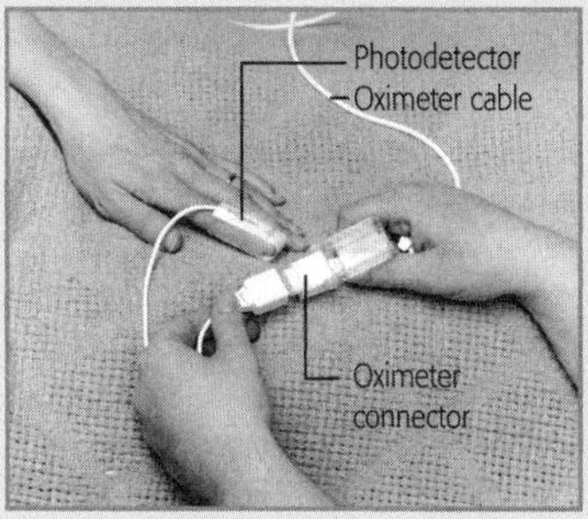

Ear oximetry

- Using an alcohol pad, massage the patient's earlobe for 10 to 20 seconds. Mild erythema indicates adequate vascularization. Following the manufacturer's instructions, attach the ear probe to the patient's earlobe or pinna. Use the ear probe stabilizer for prolonged or exercise testing. Be sure to establish good contact on the ear because an unstable probe may set off the low-perfusion alarm. After the probe has been attached for a few seconds, a saturation reading and pulse waveform will appear on the oximeter's screen.
- Leave the ear probe in place for 3 or more minutes, until readings stabilize at the highest point, or take three separate readings and average them. Make sure that you revascularize the patient's earlobe each time.
- After the procedure, remove the probe, turn off and unplug the unit, and clean the probe by gently rubbing it with an alcohol pad.

Special considerations

- Use clinical judgment in evaluating pulse oximetry readings. Validate the readings with a clinical assessment of the patient.
- If oximetry has been performed properly, readings are typically accurate. However, certain factors may interfere with accuracy. For example, an elevated bilirubin level may falsely lower Spo_2 readings, while elevated carboxyhemoglobin or methemoglobin levels (such as occur in heavy smokers and urban dwellers) can cause a falsely elevated Spo_2 reading.
- Certain intravascular substances, such as lipid emulsions and dyes, can also prevent accurate readings. Other factors that may interfere with accurate results include excessive light (for example, from phototherapy, surgical lamps, direct sunlight, and excessive ambient lighting), excessive patient movement, excessive ear pigment, hypothermia, hypotension, and vasoconstriction.
- Pulse oximetry may be used to monitor Spo_2 during respiratory arrest. Because pulse oximetry relies on perfusion, it shouldn't be used during cardiac arrest.

DEVICE SAFETY

Diagnosing pulse oximeter problems

To maintain a continuous display of arterial oxygen saturation (Spo_2) levels, you'll need to keep the monitoring site clean and dry. Make sure that the skin doesn't become irritated from adhesives used to keep disposable probes in place. You may need to change the site if this happens. Disposable probes that irritate the skin can also be replaced by nondisposable models that don't need tape.

Another common problem with pulse oximeters is the failure of the devices to obtain a signal. Your first reaction if this happens should be to check the patient's vital signs. If they're sufficient to produce a signal, check for the following problems.

Venous pulsations

Erroneous readings may be obtained if the pulse oximeter detects venous pulsations. This may occur in patients with tricuspid insufficiency, pulmonary hypertension, or if a finger probe is taped too tightly to the finger.

Poor concentration

See if the sensors are properly aligned. Make sure that the wires are intact and securely fastened and that the pulse oximeter is plugged into a power source.

Inadequate or intermittent blood flow to the site

Check the patient's pulse rate and capillary refill time and take corrective action if blood flow to the site is decreased. This may mean loosening restraints, removing tight-fitting clothes, taking off a blood pressure cuff, or checking arterial and I.V. lines. If none of these interventions work, you may need to find an alternate site. Finding a site with proper circulation may also prove challenging when a patient is receiving vasoconstrictive drugs.

Equipment malfunction

If you think the equipment might be malfunctioning, remove the pulse oximeter from the patient, set the alarm limits at 85% and 100%, and try the instrument on yourself or another healthy person. This will tell you if it's working correctly.

Penumbra effect

The penumbra effect may occur when an adult oximetry probe is placed on an infant's or a small child's finger. Because of a different path length of tissue for each of the wavelengths, the oximeter can underread or overread the Spo_2 level. To avoid the penumbra effect, use probes specifically designed for infants and children.

- Know whether your facility's policy allows nurses to initiate pulse oximetry without a practitioner's order.
- If the patient has compromised circulation in his extremities, you can place a photodetector across the bridge of his nose.
- If Spo_2 is used to guide weaning the patient from forced inspiratory oxygen, obtain an ABG analysis occasionally to correlate Spo_2 readings with Sao_2 levels.
- If an automatic blood pressure cuff is used on the same extremity that's used for measuring Spo_2, the cuff will interfere with Spo_2 readings during inflation.
- If light is a problem, cover the probes; if patient movement is a problem, move the probe or select a different probe; and if ear pigment is a problem, reposition the probe, revascularize the site, or use a finger probe. (See *Diagnosing pulse oximeter problems*.)
- Normal Spo_2 readings for ear and pulse oximetry are 95% to 100% for adults and 93% to 100% by 1 hour after birth for healthy, full-term neonates. Lower levels may indicate hypoxemia, which warrants intervention. For such patients, follow

your facility's policy or the practitioner's order, which may include increasing oxygen therapy. If Spo_2 readings decrease suddenly, perform a clinical assessment of the patient. Notify the practitioner of any significant change in the patient's condition.

- When the Sao_2 level is greater than 80%, pulse oximetry is highly accurate in healthy people. In patients on mechanical ventilation, however, accuracy is reduced when the Sao_2 level is 90% or lower.

Complications

- None known

Patient teaching

- If the patient will be using pulse oximetry at home, teach him and any family members how to use the equipment and when to call the practitioner.

Documentation

Document the procedure, including the date, time, procedure type, oximetry measurement, and any action taken. Chart other relevant patient assessments performed to validate the oximetry reading. Record the inspired oxygen concentrated and the type of oxygen delivery device used. Record ABG values obtained. Record readings in appropriate flowcharts, if indicated.

R

Radiation implant therapy

In radiation implant therapy, also called *brachytherapy,* the practitioner uses implants of radioactive isotopes (encapsulated in seeds, needles, or sutures) to deliver ionizing radiation within a body cavity or interstitially to a tumor site. Implants can deliver a continuous radiation dose over several hours or days to a specific site while minimizing exposure to adjacent tissues. The implants may be permanent or temporary. Isotopes used to treat cancers include cesium 137, gold 198, iodine 125, iridium 192, palladium 103, and phosphorus 32. (See *Radioisotopes and their uses.*)

Common implant sites include the brain, breast, cervix, endometrium, lung, neck, oral cavity, prostate, and vagina. Radiation implant therapy is commonly combined with external radiation therapy (or *teletherapy*) for increased effectiveness.

For treatment, the patient is usually placed in a private room (with its own bathroom) located as far away from high-traffic areas as practical. If monitoring shows an increased radiation hazard, adjacent rooms and hallways may also need to be restricted. Consult your facility's radiation safety policy for specific guidelines.

Equipment

Film badge or pocket dosimeter ♦ radiation precaution sign for door ♦ radiation precaution warning labels ♦ masking tape ♦ lead-lined container ♦ long-handled forceps ♦ male T-binder and two sanitary napkins with safety pin (if Burnett applicator is being used) ♦ optional: lead shield and lead strip

Preparation

- Place the lead-lined container and long-handled forceps in a corner of the patient's room.
- Mark a "safe line" on the floor with masking tape 6′ (1.8 m) from the patient's bed to warn visitors to keep clear of the patient to minimize their radiation exposure.
- If desired, place a portable lead shield in the back of the room to use when providing care.
- Place an emergency tracheotomy tray in the room if an implant will be inserted in the oral cavity or neck.

Key steps

- Explain the treatment and its goals to the patient. Before treatment begins, review radiation safety procedures, visitation policies, potential adverse effects, and interventions for those effects. Also review long-term concerns and home care issues.
- Place the radiation precaution sign on the door.
- Check to see that informed consent has been obtained.
- Ensure that all laboratory tests are performed before beginning treatment. If laboratory work is required during treatment, the badged technician obtains the specimen, labels the collection tube with a radioactive precaution label, and alerts the laboratory personnel before bringing it.

Radioisotopes and their uses

Radioisotopes are unstable elements that emit three kinds of energy particles as they "decay" to a stable state. These particles are ranked by their penetrating power.

Alpha particles possess the lowest energy level and are easily stopped by a sheet of paper. More powerful beta particles can be stopped by the skin's surface. Gamma rays, the most powerful, can be stopped only by dense shielding such as lead. Some isotopes commonly used in cancer treatments are described below.

Isotope and indications	Description	Nursing considerations
Cesium 137 (^{137}Cs) Gynecologic cancers	▪ 30-year half-life ▪ Emits gamma particles ▪ Encased in steel capsules that are placed in the patient temporarily in the operating room	▪ Elevate the head of the bed no more than 45 degrees. ▪ Encourage fluids and implement a low-residue diet. ▪ Encourage quiet activities; enforce strict bed rest as ordered.
Gold 198 (^{198}Au) Localized male genitourinary tumors	▪ 3-day half-life ▪ Emits gamma particles ▪ Permanently implanted as tiny seeds directly into the tumor or tumor bed	▪ If a seed is dislodged and found, call the radiation oncology department for disposal.
Iodine 125 (^{125}I) Localized or unresectable tumors; slow-growing tumors; recurrent disease	▪ 60-day half-life ▪ Emits gamma particles ▪ Permanently implanted as tiny seeds or sutures directly into the tumor or tumor bed	▪ Because seeds may become dislodged, no linens, body fluids, instruments, or utensils may leave the patient's room until they're monitored. ▪ If a seed is dislodged and found, call the radiation oncology department; use long-handled forceps to put it in a lead-lined container in the room. ▪ Monitor body fluids to detect displaced seeds. Give the patient a 24-hour urine container that can be closed.
Iridium 192 (^{192}Ir) Localized or unresectable tumors	▪ 74-day half-life ▪ Emits gamma particles ▪ Temporarily implanted as seeds strung inside special catheters that are implanted around the tumor	▪ If a catheter is dislodged, call the radiation oncology department; use long-handled forceps to put the implant in a lead-lined container in the room.

(continued)

Radioisotopes and their uses *(continued)*

Isotope and indications	Description	Nursing considerations
Palladium 103 (^{103}Pd) Superficial, localized, or unresectable intrathoracic or intra-abdominal tumors	■ 17-day half-life ■ Emits gamma particles ■ Permanently implanted as seeds in the tumor or tumor bed	■ See Special considerations for ^{125}I therapy.
Phosphorus 32 (^{32}P) Polycythemia, leukemia, bone metastasis, and malignant ascites	■ 14-day half-life ■ Emits beta particles ■ Used as an I.V. solution rather than an implant because of its low energy level	■ Patients receiving ^{32}P are placed in a private room with a separate bathroom.

If urine tests are needed for phosphorus 32 therapy, ask the radiation oncology department or laboratory technician how to transport the specimens safely.

■ Affix a radiation precaution warning label to the patient's identification wristband.

■ Affix warning labels to the patient's chart and Kardex to ensure staff awareness of the patient's radioactive status.

■ Wear a film badge or dosimeter at waist level during the entire shift. Turn in the radiation badge monthly or according to facility protocol. Pocket dosimeters measure immediate exposures. In many centers, these measurements aren't part of the permanent exposure record but are used to ensure that nurses receive the lowest possible exposure.

■ Each nurse must have a personal, nontransferable film badge or ring badge. Badges document each person's cumulative lifetime radiation exposure. Only primary caregivers are badged and allowed into the patient's room.

■ To minimize exposure to radiation, use the three principles of time, distance, and shielding: Time—plan to give care in the shortest time possible. Less time equals less exposure. Distance—work as far away from the radiation source as possible. Give care from the side opposite the implant or from a position allowing the greatest working distance possible. The intensity of radiation exposure varies inversely as the square of the distance from the source. Shielding—use a portable shield if needed and desired.

■ Provide essential nursing care only; omit bed baths. If ordered, provide perineal care, making sure that wipes, sanitary pads, and similar items are bagged correctly and monitored. (Refer to facility radiation policy.)

■ Dressing changes over an implanted area must be supervised by the radiation technician or another designated caregiver.

■ Before discharge, a patient's temporary implant must be removed and properly stored by the radiation oncology department. A patient with a permanent implant may not be released until his radioactivity level is less than 5 millirems/hour at 1 m.

Special considerations

■ Nurses and visitors who are pregnant or trying to conceive or father a child must not attend patients receiving radiation implant therapy because the gonads and developing embryo and fetus are highly susceptible to the damaging effects of ionizing radiation.

■ All visitors should limit the time they spend with the patient and stay at least 6′ (1.8 m) away.

- If the patient must be moved out of his room, notify the appropriate department of the patient's status to give receiving personnel time to make appropriate preparations to receive the patient. When moving the patient, ensure that the route is clear of equipment and other people and that the elevator, if there is one, is keyed and ready to receive the patient. Move the patient in a bed or wheelchair, accompanied by two badged caregivers. If the patient is delayed along the way, stand as far away from the bed as possible until you can continue.
- If the patient is scheduled for multiple procedures, communicate with all departments to group the patient's activities and limit his time out of his room.
- The patient's room must be monitored daily by the radiation oncology department, and disposables must be monitored and removed according to facility guidelines.
- If an implant becomes dislodged, notify the radiation oncology department staff, and follow their instructions. Typically, the dislodged implant is collected with long-handled forceps and placed in a lead-shielded canister.
- If a code is called on a patient with an implant, follow your facility's code procedures as well as these steps: Notify the code team of the patient's radioactive status to exclude any team member who's pregnant or trying to conceive or father a child. Also notify the radiation oncology department. Cover the implant site with a strip of lead shielding if possible. Don't allow anything to leave the patient's room until it's monitored for radiation. The primary care nurse must remain in the room (as far from the patient as possible) to act as a resource person for the patient and to provide film badges or dosimeters to code team members.
- If a patient with an implant dies on the unit, notify the radiation oncology department so they can remove a temporary implant and store it properly. If the implant was permanent, radiation oncology staff members will determine which precautions to follow before postmortem care can be provided and before the body can be moved to the morgue.
- Encourage the patient and family members to keep in contact with the radiation oncology department and to call them if concerns or physical changes occur.

Complications

- Dislodgment of the radiation source or applicator, tissue fibrosis, xerostomia, radiation pneumonitis, muscle atrophy, sterility, vaginal dryness or stenosis, fistulas, hypothyroidism, altered bowel habits, infection, airway obstruction, diarrhea, cystitis, myelosuppression, neurotoxicity, and secondary cancers

Patient teaching

- Provide the patient and his family with radiation oncology department contact information.
- Tell the patient who has had a cervical implant to expect slight to moderate vaginal bleeding after being discharged. This flow normally changes color from pink to brown to white. Instruct her to notify the practitioner if bleeding increases, persists for more than 48 hours, or has a foul odor.
- Explain to the patient that she may resume most normal activities but should avoid sexual intercourse and the use of tampons until after her follow-up visit to the practitioner (about 6 weeks after discharge).
- Instruct her to take showers rather than baths for 2 weeks, to avoid douching unless allowed by the practitioner, and to avoid activities that cause abdominal strain for 6 weeks.
- Refer the patient for sexual or psychological counseling if needed.

Documentation

Record radiation precautions taken during treatment, adverse effects of therapy, teaching given to the patient and his family and their responses to it, the patient's tolerance of isolation procedures and the family's compliance with procedures, and referrals to local cancer services.

Radiation therapy, external

About 60% of all cancer patients are treated with some form of external radiation therapy. Also called *radiotherapy,* this treatment delivers X-rays or gamma rays directly to the cancer site. Its effects are local because only the area being treated experiences direct effects.

Radiation doses are based on the type, stage, and location of the tumor as well as on the patient's size, condition, and overall treatment goals. Doses are given in increments, usually three to five times per week, until the total dose is reached.

The goals of radiation therapy include cure, in which the cancer is completely destroyed and not expected to recur; control, in which the cancer doesn't progress or regress but is expected to progress at some later time; or palliation, in which radiation is given to relieve symptoms caused by the cancer (such as bone pain, bleeding, and headache).

External beam radiation therapy is delivered by machines that aim a concentrated beam of high-energy particles (photons and gamma rays) at the target site. Two types of machines are commonly used: units containing cobalt or cesium as radioactive sources for gamma rays, and linear accelerators that use electricity to produce X-rays. Linear accelerators produce high energy with great penetrating ability. Some (known as orthovoltage machines) produce less powerful electron beams that may be used for superficial tumors.

Radiation therapy may be augmented by chemotherapy, brachytherapy (radiation implant therapy), or surgery as needed.

Equipment

Radiation therapy machine ♦ film badge or pocket dosimeter

Key steps

- Explain the treatment to the patient and his family. Review the treatment goals, and discuss the range of potential adverse effects as well as interventions to minimize them. Also discuss possible long-term complications and treatment issues. Educate the patient and his family about local cancer services.
- Make sure the radiation oncology department has obtained informed consent.
- Review the patient's clinical record for recent laboratory and imaging results, and alert the radiation oncology staff to any abnormalities or other pertinent results (such as myelosuppression, paraneoplastic syndromes, oncologic emergencies, and tumor progression).
- Transport the patient to the radiation oncology department.
- The patient begins by undergoing simulation (treatment planning), in which the target area is mapped out on his body using a machine similar to the radiation therapy machine. Then the target area is marked in ink on his body to ensure accurate treatments.
- The physician and radiation oncologist determine the duration and frequency of treatments, depending on the patient's body size, size of portal, extent and location of cancer, and treatment goals.
- The patient is positioned on the treatment table beneath the machine. Treatments last from a few seconds to a few minutes. Reassure the patient that he won't feel anything and won't be radioactive. After treatment is complete, the patient may return home or to his room.

Special considerations

- Explain to the patient that the full benefit of radiation treatments may not occur until several weeks or months after treatments begin. Instruct him to report long-term adverse effects.
- Adverse effects arise gradually and diminish gradually after treatments. They may be acute, subacute (accumulating as treatment progresses), chronic (following treatment), or long-term (arising months to years after treatment).

Complications

- Adverse effects localized to the area of treatment and their severity depending on the total radiation dose, underlying organ sensitivity, and the patient's overall condition

- Common acute and subacute adverse effects including altered skin integrity, altered GI and genitourinary function, altered fertility and sexual function, altered bone marrow production, fatigue, and alopecia
- Chronic and long-term complications or adverse effects including radiation pneumonitis, neuropathy, skin and muscle atrophy, telangiectasia, fistulas, altered endocrine function, and secondary cancers
- Other complications including headache, alopecia, xerostomia, dysphagia, stomatitis, altered skin integrity (wet or dry desquamation), nausea, vomiting, heartburn, diarrhea, cystitis, and fatigue

Patient teaching

- Instruct the patient and his family about proper skin care and management of possible adverse effects.
- Emphasize the importance of keeping follow-up appointments with the practitioner.
- Refer the patient to a support group, such as a local chapter of the American Cancer Society.
- Instruct the patient to leave target area markings intact.

Documentation

Record radiation precautions taken during treatment; interventions used and their effectiveness; grading of adverse effects; teaching given to the patient and his family and their responses to it; the patient's tolerance of isolation procedures and the family's compliance with procedures; discharge plans and teaching; and referrals to local cancer services, if any.

Radioactive iodine therapy

Because the thyroid gland concentrates iodine, radioactive iodine 131 (^{131}I) can be used to treat thyroid cancer. Usually administered orally, this isotope is used to treat postoperative residual cancer, recurrent disease, inoperable primary thyroid tumors, invasion of the thyroid capsule, and thyroid ablation as well as cancers that have metastasized to cervical or mediastinal lymph nodes or other distant sites.

Because ^{131}I is absorbed systemically, all body secretions, especially urine, must be considered radioactive. For ^{131}I treatments, the patient usually is placed in a private room (with its own bathroom) located as far away from high-traffic areas as practical. Adjacent rooms and hallways may also need to be restricted. Consult your facility's radiation safety policy for specific guidelines.

In lower doses, ^{131}I also may be used to treat hyperthyroidism. Most patients receive this treatment on an outpatient basis and are sent home with appropriate home care instructions.

Equipment

Film badges, pocket dosimeters, or ring badges ♦ radiation precaution sign for door ♦ radiation precaution warning labels ♦ waterproof gowns ♦ clear and red plastic bags for contaminated articles ♦ plastic wrap ♦ absorbent plastic-lined pads ♦ masking tape ♦ rubber gloves ♦ trash cans ♦ optional: portable lead shield

Preparation

- Assemble all necessary equipment in the patient's room.
- Keep an emergency tracheotomy tray just outside the room or in a handy place at the nurses' station.
- Place the radiation precaution sign on the door.
- Affix warning labels to the patient's chart and Kardex to ensure staff awareness of the patient's radioactive status.
- Place an absorbent plastic-lined pad on the bathroom floor and under the sink; if the patient's room is carpeted, cover it with such a pad as well. Place an additional pad over the bedside table. Secure plastic wrap over the telephone, television controls, bed controls, mattress, call bell, and toilet. These measures prevent radioactive contamination of working surfaces.
- Keep large trash cans in the room lined with plastic bags (two clear bags inserted inside an outer red bag). Monitor all objects before they leave the room.

■ Notify the dietitian to supply foods and beverages only in disposable containers and with disposable utensils.

Key steps

■ Explain the procedure and review treatment goals with the patient and his family. Before treatment begins, review the facility's radiation safety procedures and visitation policies, potential adverse effects, interventions, and home care procedures.

■ Verify that the physician has obtained informed consent.

■ Check for allergies to iodine-containing substances, such as contrast media and shellfish. Review the medication history for thyroid-containing or thyroid-altering drugs and for lithium carbonate, which may increase ^{131}I uptake.

■ Review the patient's health history for vomiting, diarrhea, productive cough, and sinus drainage, which could increase the risk of radioactive secretions.

■ If necessary, remove the patient's dentures to avoid contaminating them and to reduce radioactive secretions. Tell him that they'll be replaced 48 hours after treatment.

■ Affix a radiation precaution warning label to the patient's identification wristband.

■ Encourage the patient to use the toilet rather than a bedpan or urinal and to flush it three times after each use to reduce radiation levels.

■ Tell the patient to remain in his room except for tests or procedures. Allow him to ambulate in the room.

■ Unless contraindicated, instruct the patient to increase his fluid intake to 3 qt (3 L) daily.

■ Encourage the patient to chew or suck on hard candy to keep salivary glands stimulated and prevent them from becoming inflamed (which may develop in the first 24 hours).

■ Make sure that all laboratory tests are performed before beginning treatment. If laboratory work is required, the badged laboratory technician obtains the specimen, labels the collection tube with a radiation precaution warning label, and alerts the laboratory personnel before transporting it. If urine tests are needed, ask the radiation oncology department or laboratory technician how to transport the specimens safely.

■ Wear a film badge or dosimeter at waist level during the entire shift. Turn in the radiation badge monthly or according to your facility's protocol, and be sure to record your exposures accurately. Pocket dosimeters measure immediate exposures. These measurements may not be part of the permanent exposure record but help to ensure that nurses receive the lowest possible exposure.

■ Each nurse must have a personal, nontransferable film badge or ring badge. Badges document each person's cumulative lifetime radiation exposure. Only primary caregivers are badged and allowed into the patient's room.

■ Wear gloves to touch the patient or objects in his room.

■ Allow visitors to stay no longer than 30 minutes every 24 hours with the patient. Stress that no visitors will be allowed who are pregnant or trying to conceive or father a child.

ALERT

Visitors younger than age 18 aren't allowed.

■ Restrict direct contact to no longer than 30 minutes or 20 millirems per day. If the patient is receiving 200 millicuries of ^{131}I, remain with him only 2 to 4 minutes, and stand no closer than 1′ (30 cm) away. If standing 3′ (1 m) away, the time limit is 20 minutes; if standing 5′ (1.5 m) away, the limit is 30 minutes.

■ Give essential nursing care only; omit bed baths. If ordered, provide perineal care, making sure that wipes, sanitary pads, and similar items are bagged correctly.

■ If the patient vomits or urinates on the floor, notify the nuclear medicine department, and use nondisposable rubber gloves when cleaning the floor. After cleanup, wash your gloved hands, remove the gloves and leave them in the room, and then rewash your hands.

- If the patient must be moved from his room, notify the appropriate department of his status so that receiving personnel can make appropriate arrangements to receive him. When moving the patient, ensure that the route is clear of equipment and other people and that the elevator, if there is one, is keyed and ready to receive the patient. Move the patient in a bed or wheelchair, accompanied by two badged caregivers. If delayed, stand as far away from him as possible until you can continue.
- The patient's room must be cleaned by the radiation oncology department, not by housekeeping. The room must be monitored daily, and disposables must be monitored and removed according to facility guidelines.
- At discharge, schedule the patient for a follow-up examination. Also arrange for a whole-body scan about 7 to 10 days after ^{131}I treatment.
- Inform the patient and his family of community support services for patients with cancer.

Special considerations

- Nurses and visitors who are pregnant or trying to conceive or father a child must not attend or visit patients receiving ^{131}I therapy because the gonads and developing embryo and fetus are highly susceptible to the damaging effects of ionizing radiation.
- If a code is called on a patient undergoing ^{131}I therapy, follow your facility's code procedures as well as these steps: Notify the code team of the patient's radioactive status to exclude any team member who's pregnant or trying to conceive or father a child. Also notify the radiation oncology department. Don't allow anything out of the patient's room until it's monitored. The primary care nurse must remain in the room (as far as possible from the patient) to act as a resource person and to provide film badges or dosimeters to code team members.
- If the patient dies on the unit, notify the radiology safety officer, who will determine which precautions to follow before postmortem care is provided and before the body can be removed to the morgue.

Complications

- Myelosuppression in those undergoing repeated ^{131}I treatments
- Radiation pulmonary fibrosis developing if extensive lung metastasis was present when ^{131}I was administered
- Other complications including nausea, vomiting, headache, radiation thyroiditis, fever, salivary gland inflammation, and pain and swelling at metastatic sites

Patient teaching

- Instruct the patient to report long-term adverse reactions. In particular, review signs and symptoms of hypothyroidism and hyperthyroidism. Also ask him to report signs and symptoms of thyroid cancer, such as enlarged lymph nodes, dyspnea, bone pain, nausea, vomiting, and abdominal discomfort.
- Although the patient's radiation level at discharge will be safe, suggest that he take extra precautions during the first week at home, such as using separate eating utensils, sleeping in a separate bedroom, and avoiding body contact.
- Sexual intercourse may be resumed 1 week after ^{131}I treatment, However, urge a female patient to avoid pregnancy for 6 months after treatment, and tell a male patient to avoid impregnating his partner for 3 months after treatment.

Documentation

Record radiation precautions taken during treatment, teaching given to the patient and his family, the patient's tolerance of (and the family's compliance with) isolation procedures, and referrals to local cancer counseling services.

Reality orientation

Reality orientation is used to help a confused person retain or regain an awareness of his own identity, surroundings, and correct time reference. It also encourages socialization, reinforces socially acceptable behavior, encourages independence in activities of daily living, and helps to build confidence, dignity, and self-esteem.

Two categories of people may benefit from reality orientation. One category includes patients who are confused or disoriented from any cause, regardless of their age or diagnosis. The patient's confusion can result from such factors as arteriosclerosis, sensory deprivation, overmedication, metabolic imbalance, nutritional deficiency, or emotional stress. The other category includes patients who are oriented but face a stressful situation, which could cause confusion. Examples are changes in living arrangements, surgery, loss of a spouse, or even vision or hearing problems. Both groups are encountered in all areas of nursing, including extended care, medical-surgical, and psychiatric units as well as urgent care and clinic settings.

Equipment

Reality orientation props such as clocks ♦ directional signs ♦ pictures ♦ cards ♦ mementos ♦ bulletin boards ♦ newspapers ♦ magazines ♦ televisions ♦ radios ♦ night lights ♦ calendars ♦ mirrors ♦ paintings

The above equipment should be used throughout the patient's environment, such as in hallways, rooms, and dining rooms, to aid in orientation as the patient moves about.

DO'S & DON'TS

Label orientation tools using large lettering for patients with vision deficits.

Key steps

- Assess the patient's current orientation status by observing for specific behaviors, such as wandering, getting lost, using rambling speech, or withdrawing from social situations. Ask questions about time, place, and person as well as recent and remote memories.
- If the patient is confused, use reality orientation props, and orient him through verbal interaction. For example, say, "Mr. George, look at the calendar; today is Monday. Your wife will come to visit you on Wednesday." Or, "This is your bed, Mrs. Peters. See your name on the end of the bed?" Orient the patient frequently, in every interaction, 24 hours per day.
- Teach family members and visitors how to reorient the patient.
- Ensure consistency in all interventions by establishing and maintaining a regular routine for daily activities and by avoiding changes of room, unit, or furniture.
- Address the patient by his correct title and full name to promote self-esteem, dignity, and orientation.
- Always identify yourself and your role, and state what you expect the patient to do. Explain one step at a time, employing good eye contact, touch, and a positive attitude.
- Provide a calm environment, but recognize that it's also important to plan for and provide some stimulation to prevent monotony.
- Socialize and talk with the patient, and relate time, place, and person to current activities.
- Give praise and recognition, such as a smile, warm handshake, pat on the back, or sincere verbal praise, for each positive response. Positive reinforcement helps to improve self-esteem and increases the likelihood that the positive response will be repeated.
- Encourage the patient to take an interest in his personal appearance by using a mirror to maintain awareness of his body image. Encourage self-care within the patient's known limitations.
- Correct rambling speech or actions. Offer reminders in a nonthreatening and noncritical way.

Special considerations

- Patients who need reality orientation are found in all age-groups, but primarily are elderly patients.

Complications

- None known

Patient teaching

- Explain reality orientation to the patient's family and how to continue reality orientation at home, if necessary.

Documentation

Document all interventions as well as the patient's response in your progress notes. An interdisciplinary treatment care plan should also be written with attainable goals and interventions. Update this as needed according to facility policy.

Rectal suppository or ointment administration

A rectal suppository is a small, solid, medicated mass, usually cone-shaped, with a cocoa butter or glycerin base. It may be inserted to stimulate peristalsis and defecation or to relieve pain, vomiting, and local irritation. Rectal suppositories commonly contain drugs that reduce fever, induce relaxation, interact poorly with digestive enzymes, or have a taste too offensive for oral use. They melt at body temperature and are absorbed slowly.

Because insertion of a rectal suppository may stimulate the vagus nerve, this procedure is contraindicated in patients with potential cardiac arrhythmias. It may have to be avoided in patients with recent rectal or prostate surgery because of the risk of local trauma or discomfort during insertion.

A rectal ointment is a semisolid medication used to produce local effects. It may be applied externally to the anus or internally to the rectum. Rectal ointments commonly contain drugs that reduce inflammation or relieve pain and itching.

Equipment

Rectal suppository or tube of ointment and applicator ♦ patient's medication ♦ record and chart ♦ gloves ♦ water-soluble lubricant ♦ 4″ × 4″ gauze pads ♦ optional: bedpan

Preparation

- Store rectal suppositories in the refrigerator until needed to prevent softening and, possibly, decreased effectiveness of the medication. A softened suppository is also difficult to handle and insert. To harden it again, hold the suppository (in its wrapper) under cold running water.

Key steps

- Verify the order on the patient's medication record by checking it against the prescriber's order.
- Make sure the label on the medication package agrees with the medication order. Read the label again before you open the wrapper and again as you remove the medication. Check the expiration date.
- Wash your hands with warm water and soap.
- Confirm the patient's identity using two patient identifiers according to facility policy.
- If your facility utilizes a bar code scanning system, be sure to scan your ID badge, the patient's ID bracelet, and the medication's bar code.
- Explain the procedure and the purpose of the medication to the patient.
- Provide privacy.

Inserting a rectal suppository

- Place the patient on his left side in Sims' position. Drape him with the bedcovers to expose only the buttocks.
- Put on gloves. Remove the suppository from its wrapper, and lubricate it with water-soluble lubricant.

DO'S & DON'TS

Don't use an oil-based lubricant, such as petroleum jelly, because it won't absorb through the rectal membranes.

- Lift the patient's upper buttock with your nondominant hand to expose the anus.
- Instruct the patient to take several deep breaths through his mouth to help relax the anal sphincters and reduce anxiety or discomfort during insertion.
- Using the index finger of your dominant hand, insert the suppository—tapered end first—about 3″ (7.6 cm), until you feel it pass the internal anal sphincter. Try to direct the tapered end toward the side of the rectum so that it contacts the membranes. (See *How to administer a rectal suppository or ointment,* page 436.)

How to administer a rectal suppository or ointment

When inserting a suppository, direct its tapered end toward the side of the rectum so that it contacts the membranes to encourage absorption of the medication.

When applying a rectal ointment internally, be sure to lubricate the applicator to minimize pain on insertion. Then direct the applicator tip toward the patient's umbilicus.

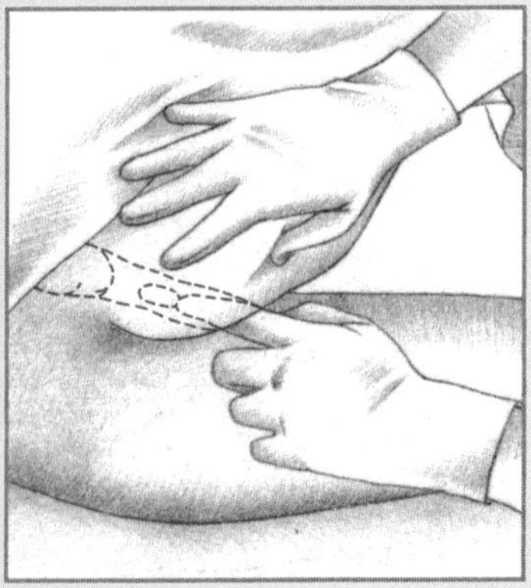

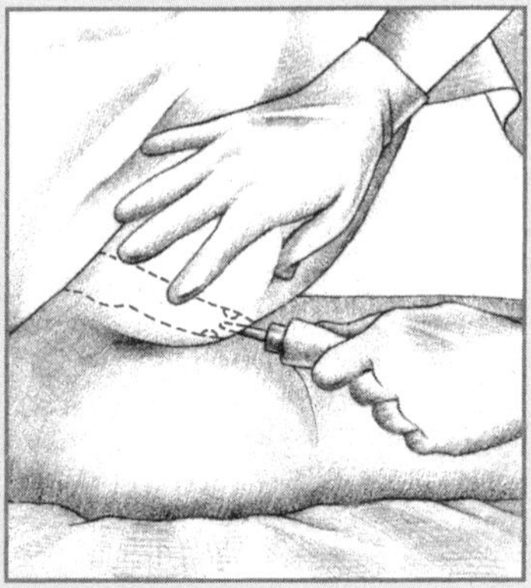

▪ After administration, ensure the patient's comfort. Encourage him to lie quietly and, if applicable, to retain the suppository for the appropriate length of time. A suppository administered to relieve constipation should be retained as long as possible (at least 20 minutes) to be effective. Press on the anus with a gauze pad if necessary until the urge to defecate passes.
▪ Remove and discard your gloves.

Applying rectal ointment

▪ Put on gloves.
▪ To apply externally, use gloves or a gauze pad to spread medication over the anal area.
▪ To apply internally, attach the applicator to the tube of ointment, and coat the applicator with water-soluble lubricant.
▪ Expect to use about 1″ (2.5 cm) of ointment. To gauge how much pressure to use during application, squeeze a small amount from the tube before you attach the applicator.
▪ Lift the patient's upper buttock with your nondominant hand to expose the anus.
▪ Instruct the patient to take several deep breaths through his mouth to relax the anal sphincters and reduce anxiety or discomfort during insertion.
▪ Gently insert the applicator, directing it toward the umbilicus.
▪ Slowly squeeze the tube to eject the medication.
▪ Remove the applicator, and place a folded 4″ × 4″ gauze pad between the patient's buttocks to absorb excess ointment.
▪ Detach the applicator from the tube, and recap the tube. Then clean the applicator thoroughly with soap and warm water.

Special considerations

▪ Because the intake of food and fluid stimulates peristalsis, a suppository for relieving constipation should be inserted about 30 minutes before mealtime to help soften the feces in the rectum and facilitate defecation. A medicated retention suppository should be inserted between meals.
▪ Instruct the patient to avoid expelling the suppository. If he has difficulty retaining it, place him on a bedpan.
▪ Make sure the patient's call bell is handy, and watch for his signal because he may be unable to suppress the urge to defecate. For example, a patient with proctitis has a

highly sensitive rectum and may not be able to retain a suppository for long.

- Be sure to inform the patient that the suppository may discolor his next bowel movement. Anusol suppositories, for example, can give feces a silver-gray pasty appearance.

Complications

- None known

Documentation

Record the administration time, dose, and patient's response.

Rectal tube insertion and removal

Whether GI hypomotility simply slows the normal release of gas and feces or results in paralytic ileus, inserting a rectal tube may relieve the discomfort of distention and flatus. Decreased motility may result from various medical or surgical conditions, certain medications (such as atropine sulfate), or even swallowed air. Conditions that contraindicate using a rectal tube include recent rectal or prostatic surgery, recent myocardial infarction, and diseases of the rectal mucosa.

Equipment

Stethoscope ♦ linen-saver pads ♦ drape ♦ water-soluble lubricant ♦ commercial kit or #22 to #32 French rectal tube of soft rubber or plastic ♦ container (emesis basin, plastic bag, or water bottle with vent) ♦ tape ♦ gloves

Key steps

- Bring all equipment to the patient's bedside, provide privacy, and wash your hands.
- Explain the procedure, and encourage the patient to relax.
- Check for abdominal distention. Using the stethoscope, auscultate for bowel sounds.
- Place the linen-saver pads under the patient's buttocks to absorb any drainage that may leak from the tube.
- Position the patient in the left-lateral Sims' position to facilitate rectal tube insertion.
- Put on gloves.
- Drape the patient's exposed buttocks.
- Lubricate the rectal tube tip with water-soluble lubricant to ease insertion and prevent rectal irritation.

DO'S & DON'TS

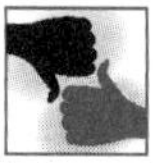

Don't use an oil-based lubricant, such as petroleum jelly, because it won't absorb through the rectal membranes.

- Lift the patient's right buttock to expose the anus.
- Insert the rectal tube tip into the anus, advancing the tube 2″ to 4″ (5 to 10 cm) into the rectum. Direct the tube toward the umbilicus along the anatomic course of the large intestine.
- As you insert the tube, tell the patient to breathe slowly and deeply, or suggest that he bear down as he would for a bowel movement to relax the anal sphincter and ease insertion.
- Using tape, secure the rectal tube to the buttocks. Then attach the tube to the container to collect possible leakage.
- Remove the tube after 15 to 20 minutes. If the patient reports continued discomfort or if gas wasn't expelled, you can repeat the procedure in 2 or 3 hours if ordered.
- Clean the patient, and replace soiled linens and the linen-saver pad. Make sure the patient feels as comfortable as possible. Again, check for abdominal distention and listen for bowel sounds.
- If you will reuse the equipment, clean it and store it in the bedside cabinet; otherwise discard the tube.

Special considerations

- Inform the patient about each step, and reassure him throughout the procedure to encourage cooperation and promote relaxation.
- Fastening a plastic bag (like a balloon) to the external end of the tube lets you observe gas expulsion. Leaving a rectal tube in place indefinitely does little to promote peristalsis, can reduce sphincter respon-

siveness, and may lead to permanent sphincter damage or pressure necrosis of the mucosa.

- Repeat insertion periodically to stimulate GI activity. If the tube fails to relieve distention, notify the practitioner.

Complications

- None known

Documentation

Record the date and time that you insert the tube. Write down the amount, color, and consistency of any evacuated matter. Describe the patient's abdomen—hard, distended, soft, or drumlike on percussion. Note bowel sounds before and after insertion.

Respiration assessment

Respiration is the interchange of gases between an organism and the medium in which it lives. External respiration, or breathing, is the exchange of oxygen and carbon dioxide between the atmosphere and the body. Internal respiration takes place throughout the body at the cellular level.

Four measures of respiration—rate, rhythm, depth, and sound—reflect the body's metabolic state, diaphragm and chest-muscle condition, and airway patency. Respiratory rate is recorded as the number of cycles (one inspiration and one expiration) per minute; rhythm, as the regularity of these cycles; depth, as the volume of air inhaled and exhaled with each respiration; and sound, as the audible digression from normal, effortless breathing. Breathing that's normal in rate and depth is called eupnea; abnormally slow respiration, bradypnea; and abnormally fast respiration, tachypnea. Apnea is the absence of respiration.

Equipment

Watch with a second hand

Key steps

- The best time to assess your patient's respirations is immediately after taking the pulse rate. Keep your fingertips over the radial artery, and don't tell the patient you're counting respirations. If you tell him, he'll become conscious of his respirations, and the rate may change.
- Count respirations by observing the rise and fall of the patient's chest as he breathes. Alternatively, position the patient's opposite arm across his chest and count respirations by feeling its rise and fall. Consider one rise and one fall as one respiration.
- Count respirations for 30 seconds, and multiply by 2, or count for 60 seconds if respirations are irregular to account for variations in respiratory rate and pattern.
- As you count respirations, stay alert for and record such breath sounds as stertor, stridor, wheezing, or an expiratory grunt. Stertor is a snoring sound resulting from secretions in the trachea and large bronchi; listen for it in patients who are comatose or have a neurologic disorder. Stridor is an inspiratory crowing sound associated with upper airway obstruction in laryngitis, croup, or the presence of a foreign body.

ALERT

When listening for stridor in infants and children with croup, also observe for sternal, substernal, or intercostal retractions.

- Wheezing is caused by partial obstruction in the smaller bronchi and bronchioles. This high-pitched, musical sound is common in patients with emphysema or asthma.

ALERT

In infants, an expiratory grunt indicates imminent respiratory distress. In older patients, an expiratory grunt may result from partial airway obstruction or neuromuscular reflex.

- Watch the patient's chest movements and listen to his breathing to determine the rhythm and sound of his respirations. (See *Identifying respiratory patterns*.)

Identifying respiratory patterns

Type	Characteristics	Pattern	Possible causes
Apnea	Periodic absence of breathing	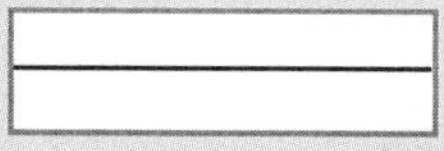	▪ Mechanical airway obstruction ▪ Conditions affecting the brain's respiratory center in the lateral medulla oblongata
Apneustic respirations	Prolonged, gasping inspiration followed by extremely short, inefficient expiration	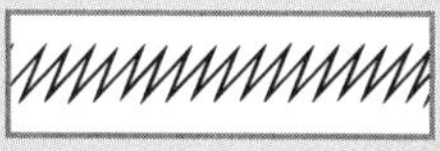	▪ Lesions of the respiratory center
Bradypnea	Slow, regular respirations of equal depth	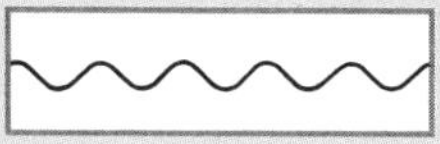	▪ Conditions affecting the respiratory center: tumors, metabolic disorders, respiratory decompensation; use of opiates and alcohol
Cheyne-Stokes respirations	Fast, deep respirations punctuated by periods of apnea lasting 20 to 60 seconds	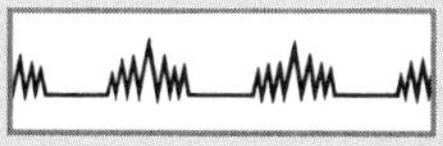	▪ Increased intracranial pressure, severe heart failure, renal failure, meningitis, drug overdose, cerebral anoxia
Eupnea	Normal rate and rhythm	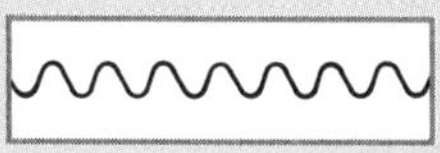	▪ Normal respiration
Kussmaul's respirations	Fast (over 20 breaths/minute), deep (resembling sighs), labored respirations without pause	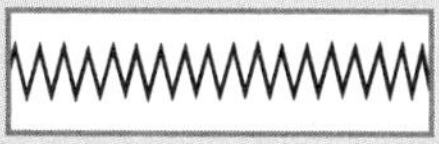	▪ Renal failure or metabolic acidosis, particularly diabetic ketoacidosis
Tachypnea	Rapid respirations (Rate rises with body temperature: about 4 breaths/minute for every degree Fahrenheit above normal.)	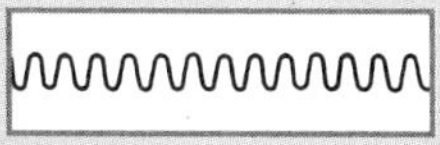	▪ Pneumonia, compensatory respiratory alkalosis, respiratory insufficiency, lesions of the respiratory center, salicylate poisoning

- Use a stethoscope to detect other breath sounds—such as crackles or rhonchi—or the lack of sound in the lungs.
- Observe chest movements for depth of respirations. If the patient inhales a small volume of air, record this as shallow; if he inhales a large volume, record this as deep.
- Observe the patient for accessory muscle use, such as the scalene, sternocleidomastoid, trapezius, and latissimus dorsi. Using these muscles reflects a weakness of the diaphragm and the external intercostal muscles—the major muscles of respiration.

Special considerations

ACTION STAT!

Respiratory rates of less than 8 breaths/minute or more than 40 breaths/minute are usually considered abnormal; report the sudden onset of such rates promptly to the practitioner.

- Observe the patient for signs of dyspnea, such as an anxious facial expression, flaring nostrils, a heaving chest wall, or cyanosis. To detect cyanosis, look for characteristic bluish discoloration in the nail beds or the lips, under the tongue, in the buccal mucosa, or in the conjunctiva.
- In assessing the patient's respiratory status, consider his personal and family history. Ask if he smokes and, if so, for how many years and how many packs per day.
- A child's respiratory rate may double in response to exercise, illness, or emotion. Normally, the rate for neonates is 30 to 80 breaths/minute; for toddlers, 20 to 40; and for children of school age and older, 15 to 25. Children usually reach the adult rate (12 to 20) at about age 15.

Complications

- None known

Documentation

Record the rate, depth, rhythm, and sound of the patient's respirations.

Restraints

Restraint is a method of physically restricting a person's freedom of movement, physical activity, or normal access to his body. This includes not only traditional restraints, such as limb or vest restraints, but also tightly tucked sheets or the use of side rails to prevent a patient from getting out of bed.

The Joint Commission has issued standards regarding the use of restraints. According to these standards, restraints are to be limited to emergencies in which the patient is at risk for harming himself or others and when other less restrictive measures have proved ineffective. One purpose of the revisions is to reduce the use of restraints. Restraints can cause numerous problems, including limited mobility, skin breakdown, impaired circulation, incontinence, psychological distress, and strangulation.

Equipment

Soft restraints

Restraint (vest, limb, mitt, belt, or body as needed) ♦ padding if needed ♦ restraint flow sheet

Leather restraints

Two wrist and two ankle leather restraints ♦ four straps ♦ key ♦ large gauze pads to cushion each extremity ♦ restraint flow sheet

Preparation

- Before entering the patient's room, make sure that the restraints are the correct size for the patient's build and weight.

DEVICE SAFETY

If you use leather restraints, make sure that the straps are unlocked and that the key fits the locks.

Key steps

- Follow Joint Commission and Centers for Medicare & Medicaid Services (CMS, formerly the Health Care Financing Administration [HCFA]) standards for applying restraints. Make sure that less restrictive measures have been tried before applying restraints.

■ When all other methods have failed to keep the patient from harming himself or others, apply restraints only as a last resort and for as short a time as possible. Choose a restraint that's the least restrictive to the patient.
■ Explain the need for restraints to the patient, and inform him of the conditions necessary for his release from restraints. Assure him that they're being used to protect him from injury rather than to punish him.
■ If necessary, obtain adequate assistance to manually restrain the patient before entering his room to apply restraints. Enlist the aid of several coworkers and organize their effort, giving each person a specific task—for example, one person explains the procedure to the patient and applies the restraints while the others immobilize the patient's arms and legs.
■ Within 1 hour of placing a patient in restraints, the patient should be evaluated by a licensed independent practitioner, and an order must be written for restraints. The order must be time limited; 4 hours for adults, 2 hours for patients ages 9 to 17, and 1 hour for patients younger than age 9. The original order expires in 24 hours.
■ To ensure safety, assess the patient every 2 hours or according to facility policy.
■ If the patient consented to have his family informed of his care, notify them of the use of restraints.

Applying a vest restraint

■ Assist the patient to a sitting position if his condition permits. Then slip the vest over his gown. Crisscross the cloth flaps at the front, placing the V-shaped opening at the patient's throat. Never crisscross the flaps in the back because this may cause the patient to choke if he tries to squirm out of the vest.
■ Pass the tab on one flap through the slot on the opposite flap. Then adjust the vest for the patient's comfort. You should be able to slip your fist between the vest and the patient. Avoid wrapping the vest too tightly because it may restrict respiration.
■ Tie all restraints securely to the frame of the bed, chair, or wheelchair and out of the patient's reach. Use a bow or a knot that can be released quickly and easily in an emergency. (See *Knots for securing soft restraints,* page 442.) Never tie a regular knot to secure the straps. Leave 1″ to 2″ (2.5 to 5 cm) of slack in the straps to allow room for movement.
■ After applying the vest, check the patient's respiratory rate and breath sounds regularly. Stay alert for signs of respiratory distress. Also, make sure that the vest hasn't tightened with the patient's movement. Loosen the vest frequently, if possible, so the patient can stretch, turn, and breathe deeply.

Applying a limb restraint

■ Wrap the patient's wrist or ankle with a padded restraint.
■ Pass the strap on the narrow end of the restraint through the slot in the broad end, and adjust for a snug fit, or fasten the buckle or hook-and-loop cuffs to fit the restraint. You should be able to slip one or two fingers between the restraint and the patient's skin. Avoid applying the restraint too tightly because it may impair circulation distal to the restraint.
■ Tie the restraint as described under "Applying a vest restraint."
■ After applying limb restraints, stay alert for signs of impaired circulation, movement, or sensation in the restrained extremity. If the skin appears blue or feels cold, or if the patient complains of a tingling sensation or numbness, loosen the restraint. Perform range-of-motion (ROM) exercises regularly to stimulate circulation and prevent contractures and resultant loss of mobility.
■ Release the restraint every 2 hours.

Applying a mitt restraint

■ Roll up a washcloth or gauze pad, and place it in the patient's palm. Have him form a loose fist, if possible; then pull the mitt over it, and secure the closure.
■ To restrict the patient's arm movement, attach the strap to the mitt, and tie it securely, using a bow or a knot that can be released quickly and easily in an emergency.

Knots for securing soft restraints

When securing soft restraints, use knots that can be released quickly and easily such as those shown below. Remember, never secure restraints to the bed's side rails.

Magnus hitch

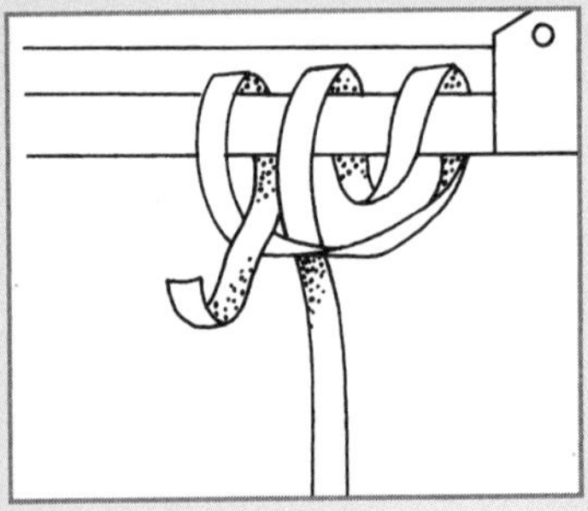

Clove hitch

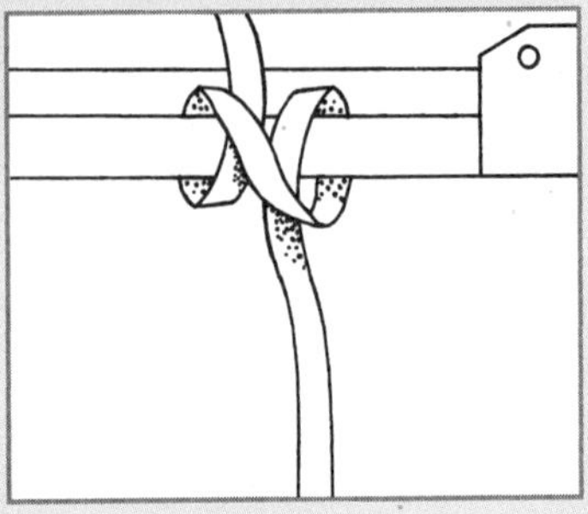

Loop

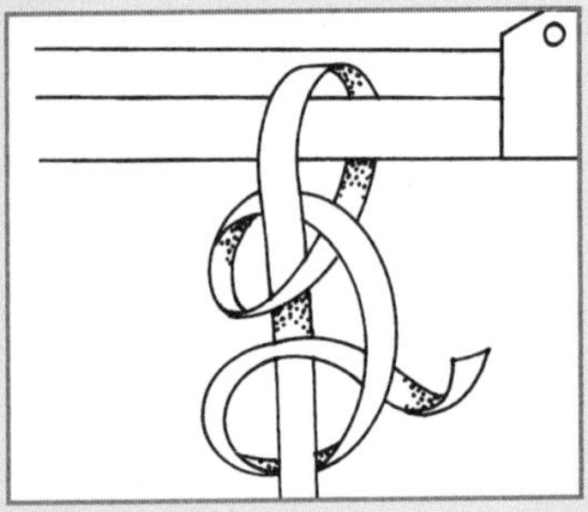

Reverse clove hitch

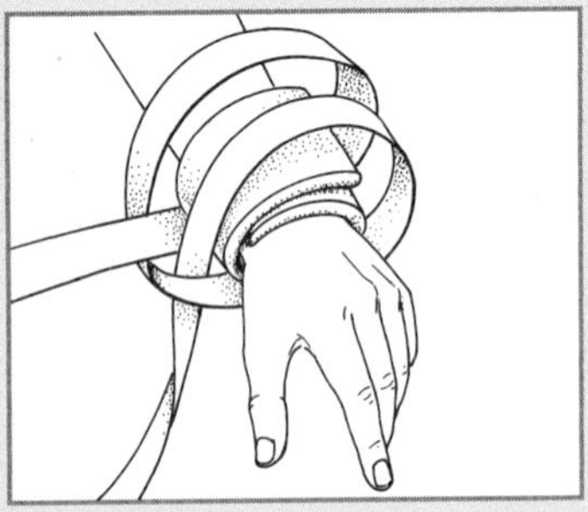

- When using mitts made of transparent mesh, check hand movement and skin color frequently to assess circulation. Remove the mitts every 2 hours to stimulate circulation, and perform passive ROM exercises to prevent contractures.

Applying a belt restraint

- Center the flannel pad of the belt on the bed. Then wrap the short strap of the belt around the bed frame, and fasten it under the bed.
- Position the patient on the pad. Then have him roll slightly to one side while you guide the long strap around his waist and through the slot in the pad.
- Wrap the long strap around the bed frame, and fasten it under the bed.
- After applying the belt, slip your hand between the patient and the belt to ensure a secure but comfortable fit. The belt is too loose if it can be raised to chest level; a belt that's too tight can cause abdominal discomfort.

Applying a body (Posey net) restraint

- Place the restraint flat on the bed, with arm and wrist cuffs facing down and the V at the head of the bed.
- Place the patient in the prone position on top of the restraint. Lift the V over the patient's head. Thread the chest belt through one of the loops in the V to ensure a snug fit.
- Secure straps around the patient's chest, thighs, and legs. Turn the patient on his

back and secure the straps to the bed frame. Then secure the straps around the patient's arms and wrists.

Applying leather restraints

- Place the patient in a supine position, holding each arm and leg securely. Immobilize the patient's arms and legs at the joints.
- Apply gauze pads to the patient's wrists and ankles to reduce friction. Wrap the restraint around the gauze pad.
- Insert the metal loop through the hole that gives the best fit. Apply the restraint securely, but not too tight.
- Thread the strap through the metal loop on the restraint, close the metal loop, and secure the strap to the bed frame, out of the patient's reach. Flex the patient's arm and leg slightly before locking the restraint. Place the key in an accessible location at the nurse's station.
- Provide emotional support and reassess the need for continued restraint use.
- Check the patient's vital signs at least every 2 hours. Remove or loosen the restraints, one at a time every hour to perform passive ROM exercises. Watch for signs of impaired circulation.

Special considerations

- Know the latest Joint Commission and CMS standards for restraint applications. Implement alternative strategies to reduce the need for restraints. Choose the least restrictive restraint, if necessary, for your patient.
- Provide for continuous patient monitoring in which a designated person can directly observe the patient at all times.
- Assess and assist the restrained patient every 15 minutes, including injuries caused by the restraint, nutrition, hydration, circulation, ROM, vital signs, hygiene, elimination, comfort, and physical and psychosocial status. Also assess whether the patient is ready to have restraints discontinued.
- When the patient is at risk for aspiration, restrain him on his side. Never secure all four restraints to one side of the bed because the patient may fall out of bed.
- When working to loosen the restraints, have a coworker on hand to assist in manually restraining the patient, if necessary.
- Don't apply a limb restraint above an I.V. site because the constriction may occlude the infusion or cause infiltration into surrounding tissue.
- Never secure restraints to the side rails because someone might inadvertently lower the rail before noticing the attached restraint. This could jerk the patient's limb or body, causing him discomfort and trauma. Never secure restraints to the fixed frame of the bed if the patient's position is to be changed.
- Don't restrain a patient in the prone position. This position limits his field of vision, intensifies feelings of helplessness and vulnerability, and impairs respiration, especially if the patient has been sedated.
- Because the restrained patient has limited mobility, his nutrition, elimination, and positioning become your responsibility. To prevent pressure ulcers, reposition him regularly, and pad bony prominences and other vulnerable areas.
- The condition of the restrained patient must be continually monitored, assessed, and evaluated. Release the restraints every hour; assess his pulse and skin condition, and perform ROM exercises. A restraint flow sheet must be used with hourly notations.

Complications

- Impaired respiration from reduced peripheral circulation caused by excessively tight limb restraints
- Skin breakdown from limb restraints
- Pneumonia, urine retention, constipation, and sensory deprivation due to long periods of immobility

Documentation

Document each episode of the use of restraints, including the date and time they were initiated. Record the circumstances resulting in the use of restraints and nonphysical interventions used first. Describe the rationale for the specific type of restraint used. Chart the name of the licensed independent practitioner who ordered the restraint. Include the conditions or behaviors necessary for discontinuing the restraint and whether these conditions were communicated to the patient. Document each in-person evaluation by the licensed independent practitioner. Record all assessments of the patient, including signs of injury, nutrition, hydration, circulation, ROM, vital signs, hygiene, elimination, comfort, physical and psychological status, and readiness for removing restraints. Record your interventions to help the patient meet the conditions for removing restraints. Note that the patient was continuously monitored. Document any injuries or complications, the name of the practitioner and the time notified of your interventions, and your actions.

Rotation beds

Because of their constant motion, rotation beds—such as the Roto Rest—promote postural drainage and peristalsis and help prevent the complications of immobility. These beds rotate from side to side in a cradlelike motion, achieving a maximum elevation of 62 degrees and full side-to-side turning approximately every 4½ minutes.

Because the bed holds the patient motionless, it's especially helpful for patients with spinal cord injury, multiple trauma, stroke, multiple sclerosis, coma, severe burns, hypostatic pneumonia, atelectasis, or other unilateral lung involvement causing poor ventilation and perfusion.

Rotation beds such as the Roto Rest bed can accommodate cervical traction devices and tongs. One type of Roto Rest bed has an access hatch underneath for the perineal area; another type has access hatches for the perineal, cervical, and thoracic areas. Both have arm and leg hatches that fold down to allow range-of-motion (ROM) exercises. Other features include variable angles of rotation, a fan, access for X-rays, and supports and clips for chest tubes, catheters, and drains. Racks beneath the bed hold X-ray plates in place for chest and spinal X-ray films. (See *Roto Rest bed*.)

Rotation beds are contraindicated for the patient who has severe claustrophobia or who has an unstable cervical fracture without neurologic deficit and the complications of immobility. Patient transfer and positioning on the bed should be performed by at least two persons to ensure the patient's safety.

The instructions given below apply to the Roto Rest bed.

Equipment

Rotation bed with appropriate accessories ♦ pillowcases or linen-saver pads ♦ flat sheet or padding

Preparation

- When using the Roto Rest bed, carefully inspect the bed, and run it through a complete cycle in both automatic and manual modes to ensure that it's working properly. If you're using the Mark I model, check the tightness of the set screws at the head of the bed.
- To prepare the bed for the patient, remove the counterbalance weights from the keel, and place them in the base frame's storage area.
- Release the connecting arm by pulling down on the cam handle and depressing the lower side of the footboard.
- Next, lock the table in the horizontal position, and place all side supports in the extreme lateral position by loosening the cam handles on the underside of the table. Slide the supports off the bed. Note that all supports and packs are labeled RIGHT or LEFT on the bottom to facilitate reassembly.
- Remove the knee packs by depressing the snap button and rotating and pulling the packs from the tube. Then remove the abductor packs (the Mark III model has only one) by depressing and sliding them toward the head of the bed.
- Next, loosen the foot and knee assemblies by lifting the cam handle at its base, and slide them to the foot of the bed.
- Finally, loosen the shoulder clamp assembly and knobs; swing the shoulder clamps to the vertical position, and retighten them.
- If you're using the Mark I model, remove the cervical, thoracic, and perineal packs. Cover them with pillowcases or linen-saver pads, smooth all wrinkles, and replace the packs.

Roto Rest bed

Driven by a silent motor, the Roto Rest bed turns the immobilized patient slowly and continuously, more than 300 times daily. The motion provides constant passive exercise and peristaltic stimulation without depriving the patient of sleep or risking further injury. The bed is radiolucent, permitting X-rays to be taken through it without moving the patient. It also has a built-in cooling fan, and allows access for surgery on the multiple-trauma patient without disrupting spinal alignment or traction.

The bed's hatches provide access to various parts of the patient's body. Arm hatches permit full range of motion and have holes for chest tubes. Leg hatches allow full hip extension. The perineal hatch provides access for bowel and bladder care, the thoracic hatch for chest auscultation and lumbar puncture, and the cervical hatch for wound care, bathing, and shampooing.

Top view

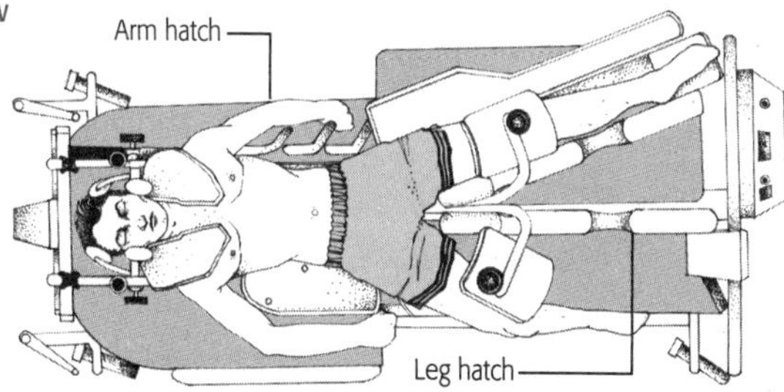

Back view

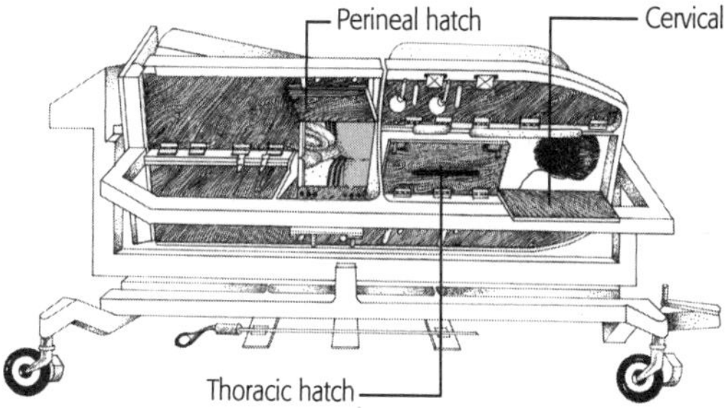

■ If you're using the Mark III model, remove the perineal pack, cover, and replace. Cover the upper half of the bed, which is a solid unit, with padding or a sheet. Install new disposable foam cushions for the patient's head, shoulders, and feet.

Key steps

■ If possible, show the patient the bed before use. Explain and demonstrate its operation, and reassure the patient that the bed will hold him securely.

■ Before positioning the patient on the bed, make sure it's turned off. Then place and lock the bed in the horizontal position, out of gear. Latch all hatches and lock the wheels.

■ Obtain assistance and transfer the patient. Move him gently to the center of the bed to prevent contact with the pillar posts and to ensure proper balance during bed operation. Smooth the pillowcase or linen-saver pad beneath his hips. Then place any tubes through the appropriate notches in the hatches, and ensure that any traction weights hang freely.

- Insert the thoracic side supports in their posts. Adjust the patient's longitudinal position to allow a 1" (2.5 cm) space between the axillae and the supports, thereby avoiding pressure on the axillary blood vessels and the brachial plexus. Push the supports against his chest, and lock the cam arms securely to provide support and ensure patient safety.
- Place the disposable supports under his legs to remove pressure from his heels and prevent pressure ulcers.
- Install and adjust the foot supports so that the patient's feet lie in the normal anatomic position, thereby helping to prevent footdrop. The foot supports should be in position for only 2 hours of every shift to prevent excessive pressure on the soles and toes.
- Place the abductor packs in the appropriate supports, allowing a 6" (15.2 cm) space between the packs and the patient's groin. Tighten the knobs on the bed's underside at the base of the support tubes.
- Install the leg side supports snugly against the patient's hips, and tighten the cam arms. Position the knee assemblies slightly above his knees, and tighten the cam arms. Then place your hand on the patient's knee and move the knee pack until it rests lightly on the top of your hand. Repeat for the other knee.
- Loosen the retaining rings on the crossbar, and slide the head and shoulder assembly laterally. The retaining rings maintain correct lateral position of the shoulder clamp assembly and head support pack.
- Carefully lower the head and shoulder assembly into place, and slide it to touch the patient's head.
- Place your hand on the patient's shoulder, and move the shoulder pack until it touches your hand. Tighten it in place. Repeat for the other shoulder. The 1" clearance between the shoulders and the packs prevents excess pressure, which can lead to pressure ulcers.
- Place the head pack close to, but not touching, the patient's ears (or tongs).
- Tighten the head and shoulder assembly securely so it won't lift off the bed. Position the restraining rings next to the shoulder assembly bracket and tighten them.
- Place the patient's arms on the disposable supports. Install the side arm supports, and secure the safety straps, placing one across the shoulder assembly and the other over the thoracic supports. If necessary, cover the patient with a flat sheet.
- Make sure all tubing is intact and secured so it won't be pulled out upon turning.

Balancing the bed

- Place one hand on the footboard to prevent the bed from turning rapidly if it's unbalanced. Then remove the locking pin. If the bed rotates to one side, reposition the patient in its center; if it tilts to the right, gently turn it slightly to the left, and slide the packs on the right side toward the patient; if it tilts to the left, reverse the process. If a large imbalance exists, you may have to adjust the packs on both sides.
- After the patient is centered, gently turn the bed to the 62-degree position.
- Measure the space between the patient's chest, hip, and thighs and the inside of the packs. If this space exceeds ½" (1.3 cm) for the Mark III model or 1" for the Mark I, return the bed to horizontal position, lock it in place, and slide the packs inward on both sides. If the space appears too tight, proceed as above, but slide both packs outward. Excessively loose packs cause the patient to slide from side to side during turning, possibly resulting in unnecessary movement at fracture sites, skin irritation from shearing force, and bed imbalance. Overly tight packs can place pressure on the patient during turning.
- After adjusting the packs, check the bed; balance it and make any necessary adjustments.
- If you're using the Mark III model bed, and the patient weighs more than 160 lb (72.6 kg), the bed may become top-heavy. To correct this, place counterbalance weights in the appropriate slots in the keel

of the bed. Add one weight for every 20 lb (9 kg) over 160, but remember that placement of weights doesn't replace correct patient positioning.

- If you're using the Mark I model, it may be necessary to add weights for the patient weighing less than 160 lb. Place one weight for each 20 lb less than 160 in the proper bracket at the foot of the bed.

Initiating automatic bed rotation

- Ensure that all packs are securely in place. Then hold the footboard firmly, and remove the locking pin to start the bed's motor. The bed will continue to rotate until the pin is reinserted.
- Raise the connecting arm cam handle until the connecting assembly snaps into place, locking the bed into automatic rotation.
- Remain with the patient for at least three complete turns from side to side to evaluate his comfort and safety. Observe his response and offer him emotional support.

Special considerations

- If the patient develops cardiac arrest while on the bed, perform cardiopulmonary resuscitation after taking the bed out of gear, locking it in horizontal position, removing the side arm support and the thoracic pack, lifting the shoulder assembly, and dropping the arm pack. Doing all these steps takes only 5 to 10 seconds. You won't need a cardiac board because of the bed's firm surface.
- If the electricity fails, lock the bed in horizontal or lateral position, and rotate it manually every 30 minutes to prevent pressure ulcers. If cervical traction causes the patient to slide upward, place the bed in reverse Trendelenburg's position; if extremity traction causes the patient to migrate toward the foot of the bed, use Trendelenburg's position.
- Lock the bed in the extreme lateral position for access to the back of the head, thorax, and buttocks through the appropriate hatches. Clean the mattress and nondisposable packs during patient care, and rinse them thoroughly to remove all soap residue. When replacing the packs and hatches, take care not to pinch the patient's skin between the packs. This can cause pain and tissue necrosis.
- Expect increased drainage from any pressure ulcers for the first few days the patient is on the bed because the motion helps debride necrotic tissue and improves local circulation.
- Perform or schedule daily ROM exercises, as ordered, because the bed allows full access to all extremities without disturbing spinal alignment. Drop the arm hatch for shoulder rotation, remove the thoracic packs for shoulder abduction, and drop the leg hatch and remove leg and knee packs for hip rotation and full leg motion.
- For female patients, tape an indwelling urinary catheter to the thigh before bringing it through the perineal hatch. For the male patient with spinal cord lesions, tape the catheter to the abdomen and then to the thigh to facilitate gravity drainage. Hang the drainage bag on the clips provided, and make sure it doesn't become caught between the bed frames during rotation.
- If the patient has a tracheal or endotracheal tube and is on mechanical ventilation, attach the tube support bracket between the cervical pack and the arm packs. Tape the connecting T tubing to the support, and run it beside the patient's head and off the center of the table to help prevent reflux of condensation.
- For the patient with pulmonary congestion or pneumonia, suction secretions more often during the first 12 to 24 hours on the bed because the motion will increase drainage. A vibrator is available for use under the thoracic hatch of the Mark I to help mobilize pulmonary secretions more quickly.

Complications

- Claustrophobia
- Pressure ulcers

Documentation

Record changes in the patient's condition and his response to therapy in your progress notes. Note turning times and ongoing care on the flowchart.

S

Seizure management

Seizures are paroxysmal events associated with abnormal electrical discharges of neurons in the brain. Partial seizures are usually confined to one cerebral hemisphere, involving a localized or focal area of the brain. Generalized seizures involve the entire brain. When a patient has a generalized seizure, nursing care aims to protect him from injury and prevent serious complications. Appropriate care also includes observation of seizure characteristics to help determine the area of the brain involved.

Patients considered at risk for seizures are those with a history of seizures and those with conditions that predispose them to seizures. Such conditions include metabolic abnormalities, such as hypocalcemia, hypoglycemia, and pyridoxine deficiency; brain tumors or other space-occupying lesions; infections, such as meningitis, encephalitis, and brain abscess; traumatic injury, especially if the dura mater was penetrated; ingestion of toxins, such as mercury, lead, or carbon monoxide; genetic abnormalities, such as tuberous sclerosis and phenylketonuria; perinatal injuries; and stroke. Patients at risk for seizures need precautionary measures to help prevent injury if a seizure occurs. (See *Precautions for generalized seizures.*)

Most major seizures (generalized or tonic-clonic) last only 1 to 2 minutes and demand little of the person observing the seizure. All that's needed is to let the seizure run its course, to ensure that the patient is in no physical danger, and to maintain a patent airway. However, a patient with status epilepticus, in which he experiences repeated seizures without regaining consciousness, requires immediate medical intervention.

Equipment

Oral airway ♦ suction equipment ♦ side rail pads ♦ seizure activity record ♦ additional equipment: I.V. line, normal saline solution, oxygen, endotracheal (ET) intubation equipment

Key steps

- If you're with the patient when he experiences an aura, help him into bed, raise the side rails, and adjust the bed flat. If he's away from his room, lower him to the floor, and place a pillow, blanket, or other soft material under his head to keep it from hitting the floor.
- Provide privacy if possible.
- When you have a patient in the hospital who has a known seizure history, maintain I.V. access or a saline lock so that if he does have a seizure, there's I.V. access to administer medications (for example, diazepam [Valium]).
- Stay with the patient during the seizure, and be ready to intervene if complications such as airway obstruction develop. If necessary, have another staff member obtain the appropriate equipment and notify the practitioner of the obstruction.
- Depending on facility policy, if the patient is in the beginning of the tonic phase of the seizure, you may insert an oral airway into his mouth so his tongue doesn't block his airway. If an oral airway isn't

Precautions for generalized seizures

Taking appropriate precautions will help you protect a patient from injury, aspiration, and airway obstruction should he have a seizure. Plan your precautions using information obtained from the patient's history. What kind of seizure has the patient had before? Is he aware of exacerbating factors? Sleep deprivation, missed doses of anticonvulsants, and even upper respiratory tract infections can increase seizure frequency in some people who have had seizures. Was his previous seizure an acute episode, or did it result from a chronic condition?

Equipment preparation

Based on answers provided in the patient's history, you can tailor your precautions to his needs. Start by gathering the appropriate equipment, including a hospital bed with full-length side rails, commercial side rail pads or six bath blankets (four for a crib), adhesive tape, an oral airway, and oral or nasal suction equipment.

Bedside preparation

Carry out the precautions you think appropriate for the patient. Remember that a patient with preexisting seizures who's being admitted for a change in medication, treatment of an infection, or detoxification may have an increased risk of seizures.

- Explain the reasons for the precautions to the patient.
- To protect the patient's limbs, head, and feet from injury if he has a seizure while in bed, cover the side rails, headboard, and footboard with side rail pads or bath blankets. If you use blankets, keep them in place with adhesive tape. Be sure to keep the side rails raised while the patient is in bed to prevent falls. Keep the bed in a low position to minimize any injuries that may occur if the patient climbs over the rails.
- Place an airway at the patient's bedside, or tape it to the wall above the bed, according to your facility's protocol. Keep suction equipment nearby in case you need to establish a patent airway. Explain to the patient how the airway will be used.
- If the patient has frequent or prolonged seizures, prepare an I.V. saline lock to facilitate administration of emergency medications.

available, don't try to hold his mouth open or place your hands inside because you may be bitten. After the patient's jaw becomes rigid, don't force the airway into place because you may break his teeth or cause another injury. Turn the patient to his side to allow secretions to drain and the tongue to fall forward.

DO'S & DON'TS

Don't force any objects into the patient's mouth unless his airway is compromised.

- Move hard or sharp objects out of the patient's way, and loosen his clothing.
- Don't forcibly restrain the patient or restrict his movements during the seizure because the force of the patient's movements against restraints could cause muscle strain or even joint dislocation.
- Continually assess the patient during the seizure. Observe the earliest symptom, such as head or eye deviation, as well as how the seizure progresses, what form it takes, and how long it lasts. Your description may help determine the seizure's type and cause.
- If this is the patient's first seizure, notify the practitioner immediately. If the patient has had seizures before, notify the practitioner only if the seizure activity is prolonged or if the patient fails to regain consciousness. (See *Understanding status epilepticus,* page 450.)

Understanding status epilepticus

Status epilepticus—a seizure state that continues unless interrupted by emergency interventions—can occur in all seizure types. The most life-threatening example is generalized tonic-clonic status epilepticus, a continuous generalized tonic-clonic seizure without intervening return of consciousness.

Status epilepticus, always an emergency, is accompanied by respiratory distress. It can result from abrupt withdrawal of anticonvulsant medications, hypoxic or metabolic encephalopathy, acute head trauma, or septicemia secondary to encephalitis or meningitis.

Emergency treatment of status epilepticus usually consists of diazepam (Valium), phenytoin (Dilantin), or phenobarbital (Solfoton), dextrose 50% in water I.V. (when seizures are secondary to hypoglycemia), and thiamine I.V. (in the presence of chronic alcoholism or withdrawal).

- If ordered, establish an I.V. line, and infuse normal saline solution at a keep-vein-open rate.
- If the seizure is prolonged and the patient becomes hypoxemic, administer oxygen as ordered. Some patients may require ET intubation.
- For the patient with diabetes, administer 50 ml of dextrose 50% in water by I.V. push as ordered. For the alcoholic patient, a 100-mg bolus of thiamine may be ordered to stop the seizure.
- After the seizure, turn the patient on his side, and apply suction if necessary to facilitate drainage of secretions and maintain a patent airway. Insert an oral airway if needed.
- Check for injuries.
- Reorient and reassure the patient as necessary.
- When the patient is comfortable and safe, document what happened during the seizure.
- Place side rail pads on the bed in case the patient experiences another seizure.
- After the seizure, monitor vital signs and mental status every 15 to 20 minutes for 2 hours.
- Ask the patient about his aura and activities preceding the seizure. The type of aura (auditory, visual, olfactory, gustatory, or somatic) helps pinpoint the site in the brain where the seizure originated.

Special considerations

- Because a seizure commonly indicates an underlying disorder such as meningitis or a metabolic or electrolyte imbalance, a complete diagnostic workup will be ordered if the cause of the seizure isn't evident.
- If you suspect a serious injury after the seizure, such as a fracture or deep laceration, notify the practitioner, and arrange for appropriate evaluation and treatment.
- After the seizure, complete a respiratory assessment, and notify the practitioner if you suspect a problem.
- Expect most patients to experience a postictal period of decreased mental status lasting 30 minutes to 24 hours. Reassure the patient that this doesn't indicate incipient brain damage.

Complications

- Injury including scrapes and bruises suffered from hitting objects during the seizure and traumatic injury to the tongue caused by biting
- Respiratory difficulty including aspiration, airway obstruction, and hypoxemia
- Decreased mental capability

Documentation

Document that the patient requires seizure precautions, and record all precautions taken. Record the date and the time the seizure began as well as its duration and any precipitating factors. Identify any sensation that may be considered an aura. If the seizure was preceded by an aura, have the patient describe what he experienced.

Record any involuntary behavior that occurred at the onset, such as lip smacking, chewing movements, or hand and eye movements. Describe where the movement began and the parts of the body involved. Note any progression or pattern to the activity. Document whether the patient's eyes deviated to one side and if the pupils changed in size, shape, equality, or reaction to light. Note if the patient's teeth were clenched or open. Record any incontinence, vomiting, or salivation that occurred during the seizure.

Note the patient's response to the seizure. Was he aware of what happened? Did he fall into a deep sleep following the seizure? Was he upset or ashamed? Note any medications given, any complications experienced during the seizure, and any interventions performed. Finally, note the patient's postseizure mental status.

Self-catheterization

Self-catheterization is performed by many patients who have some form of impaired or absent bladder function.

The two major advantages of self-catheterization are that patient independence is maintained and bladder control is regained. In addition, self-catheterization allows normal sexual intimacy without the fear of incontinence, decreases the chance of urinary reflux, reduces the use of aids and appliances and, in many cases, allows the patient to return to work.

Self-catheterization requires thorough and careful patient teaching. At home the patient will use clean technique for self-catheterization, but if the patient is hospitalized he must use sterile technique because of the increased risk of acquiring a nosocomial urinary tract infection (UTI).

Equipment

Rubber catheter ♦ washcloth, soap, and water ♦ small packet of water-soluble lubricant ♦ plastic storage bag ♦ optional: drainage container, paper towels, cornstarch, rubber or plastic sheets, gooseneck lamp, catheterization record, mirror

Preparation

- Instruct the patient to keep a supply of catheters at home and to use each catheter only once before cleaning it.
- Advise him to wash the used catheter in warm, soapy water, rinse it inside and out, then dry it with a clean towel and store it in a plastic bag until the next time it's needed. Because catheters become brittle with repeated use, tell the patient to check them often and to order a new supply well in advance.

Key steps

- Tell the patient to begin by trying to urinate into the toilet or, if a toilet isn't available or if he needs to measure urine quantity, into a drainage container. He should wash his hands thoroughly with soap and water and dry them.
- Demonstrate how the patient should perform the catheterization, explaining each step clearly and carefully. Position a gooseneck lamp nearby if room lighting is inadequate to make the urinary meatus clearly visible. Arrange the patient's clothing so that it's out of the way.

Teaching the female patient

- Demonstrate and explain to the female patient that she should separate the vaginal folds as widely as possible with the fingers of her nondominant hand to obtain a full view of the urinary meatus. She may need to use a mirror to visualize the meatus. Ask if she's right- or left-handed, and then tell her which is her nondominant hand. While holding her labia open with the nondominant hand, she should use the dominant hand to wash the perineal area thoroughly with a soapy washcloth, using downward strokes. Tell her to rinse the area with the washcloth, using downward strokes as well.
- Show her how to squeeze the lubricant onto the first 3″ (7.5 cm) of the catheter and then how to insert the catheter. (See *Teaching self-catheterization,* page 452.)
- When the urine stops draining, tell her to remove the catheter slowly, get dressed,

Teaching self-catheterization

Female patient

Instruct the female patient to hold the catheter in her dominant hand as if it were a pencil or a dart, about ½″ (1 cm) from its tip. Keeping the vaginal folds separated, she should slowly insert the lubricated catheter about 3″ (7.6 cm) into the urethra. Tell her to press down with her abdominal muscles to empty the bladder, allowing all urine to drain through the catheter and into the toilet or drainage container.

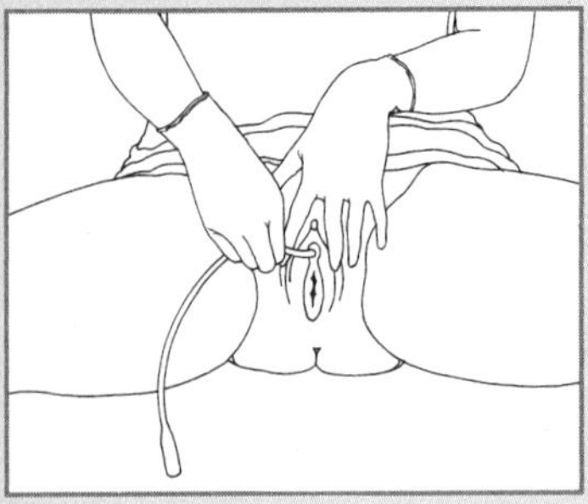

Male patient

Teach the male patient to hold his penis in his nondominant hand, at a right angle to his body. He should hold the catheter in his dominant hand as if it were a pencil or a dart and slowly insert it 7″ to 10″ (17.5 to 25 cm) into the urethra—until urine begins flowing. Then he should gently advance the catheter about 1″ (2.5 cm) farther, allowing all urine to drain into the toilet or drainage container.

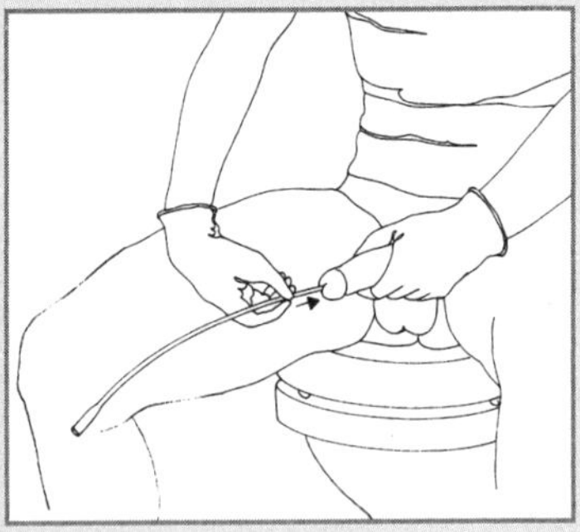

and wash the catheter with warm, soapy water. She should rinse it inside and out and dry it with a paper towel.

Teaching the male patient

- Instruct the male patient to wash and rinse the end of his penis thoroughly with soap and water, pulling back the foreskin if appropriate. He should keep the foreskin pulled back during the procedure.
- Show him how to squeeze lubricant onto a paper towel, and have him roll the first 7″ to 10″ (17.5 to 25 cm) of the catheter in the lubricant. Tell him that copious lubricant will make the procedure more comfortable for him. Show him how to insert the catheter.
- When the urine stops draining, tell him to remove the catheter slowly and, if necessary, pull the foreskin forward again. Have him get dressed and wash and dry the catheter as described above.

Special considerations

- Self-catheterization usually occurs every 4 to 6 hours around the clock (or more often at first).
- Keep in mind the difference between boiling and sterilization. Boiling kills bacteria, viruses, and fungi, but doesn't kill spores, whereas sterilization does. However, because catheter cleaning will be done in the patient's home, boiling provides sufficient safeguard against spreading infections.

Complications

- UTI or urine leakage due to overdistention of the bladder
- UTI from improper hand washing or equipment cleaning
- Urethral or bladder mucosa injury from incorrect catheter insertion

Patient teaching

- Impress upon the patient that the timing of catheterization is critical to prevent overdistention of the bladder, which can lead to infection.

- Teach female patients the body parts involved in self-catheterization: labia majora, labia minora, vagina, and urinary meatus.
- Advise the patient to hold off storing the cleaned catheters in a plastic bag until after they're completely dry to prevent growth of gram-negative organisms.
- Stress the importance of regulating fluid intake, as ordered, to prevent incontinence while maintaining adequate hydration. However, explain that incontinent episodes may occur occasionally. For managing incontinence, the practitioner or a home health care nurse can help develop a plan such as more frequent catheterizations. After an incontinent episode, tell the patient to wash with soap and water, pat himself dry with a towel, and expose the skin to the air for as long as possible. Bedding and furniture can be protected by covering them with rubber or plastic sheets and then covering the rubber or plastic with fabric.
- Stress the importance of taking medications as ordered to increase urine retention and help prevent incontinence. Advise the patient to avoid calcium-rich and phosphorus-rich foods, as ordered, to reduce the chance of renal calculus formation.

Documentation

Record the date and times of catheterization, character of urine (color, odor, clarity, presence of particles or blood), the amount of urine (increase, decrease, no change), and any problems encountered during the procedure. Note whether the patient has difficulty performing a return demonstration.

Sequential compression therapy

Sequential compression therapy is a safe, effective, noninvasive means of preventing deep vein thrombosis (DVT) in surgical patients at high risk for DVT. It massages the legs in a wavelike, milking motion that promotes blood flow and deters thrombosis. Sequential compression therapy counteracts blood stasis and coagulation changes—two of the three major factors that promote DVT. It reduces stasis by increasing peak blood flow velocity, helping to empty the femoral vein's valve cusps of pooled or static blood. The compressions cause an anticlotting effect by increasing fibrinolytic activity, which stimulates the release of a plasminogen activator.

Sequential compression therapy typically complements other preventive measures, such as antiembolism stockings and anticoagulant medications. Sequential compression sleeves and antiembolism stockings are commonly used preoperatively and postoperatively to prevent blood clots that tend to form during surgery. Preventive measures are continued for as long as the patient remains at risk. (See *Foot compression device,* page 454.)

Equipment

Measuring tape ♦ sizing chart for the brand of sleeves you're using ♦ pair of compression sleeves in correct size ♦ connecting tubing ♦ compression controller

Preparation

- To determine the proper size of sleeve, measure the circumference of the upper thigh (as shown below).

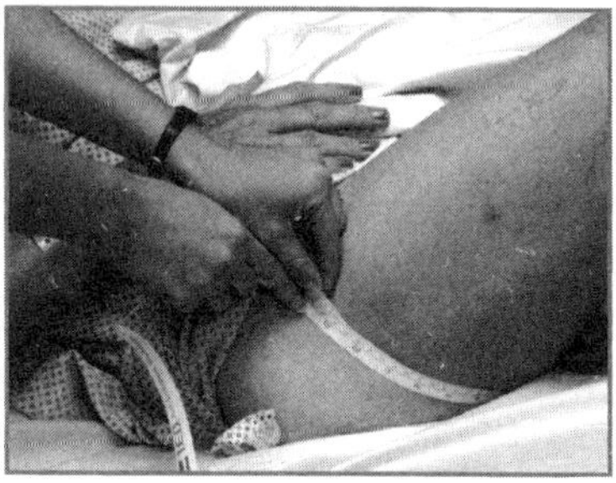

- Hold the tape snugly, but not tightly, under the patient's thigh at the gluteal furrow. Find the patient's thigh measurement on the sizing chart, and locate the corresponding size of the compression sleeve.
- Remove the compression sleeves from the package, and unfold them. Lay the unfolded sleeves on a flat surface with cotton lining facing up (as shown middle left of next page).

Foot compression device

There are times when the patient won't be able to use a sequential compression device due to a lower extremity fracture or a soft tissue injury. The patient may benefit from using a foot compression device, which is similar to the sequential compression device.

A foot compression device functions just as the sequential compression device but also helps to increase circulation and prevent blood clots. Recent studies are investigating the use of foot compression devices with venous stasis ulcers and peripheral arterial occlusive disease.

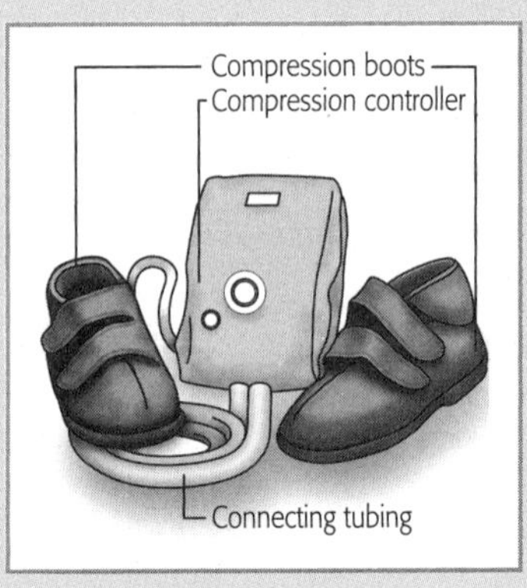

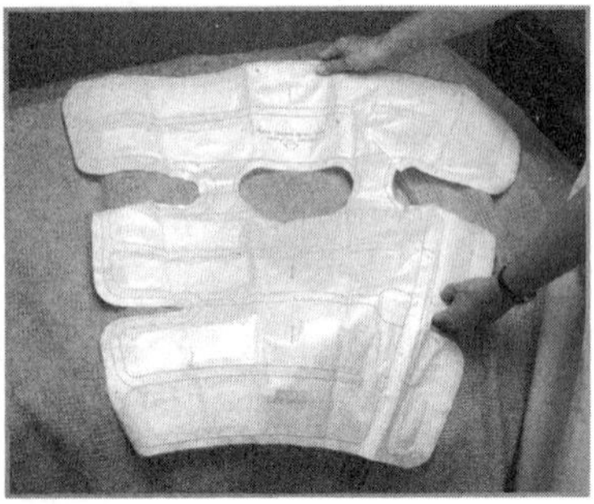

- Position the sleeve at the appropriate ankle or knee landmark.

Key steps

Applying the sleeves

- Place the patient's leg on the sleeve lining; position the back of the knee over the popliteal opening.
- Make sure that the back of the ankle is over the ankle marking.
- Starting at the side opposite the clear plastic tubing, wrap the sleeve snugly around his leg.
- Fasten the sleeve securely with the Velcro fasteners starting at the ankle, then moving to calf and thigh.
- Check the fit by inserting two fingers between the sleeve and the patient's leg at the knee opening.
- Using the same procedure, apply the second sleeve (as shown below).

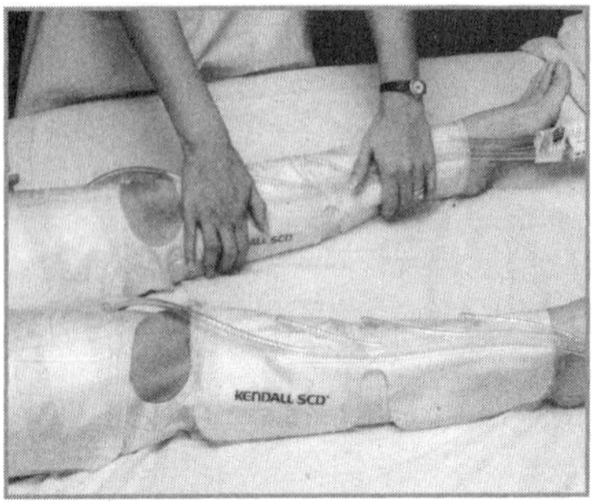

Operating the system

- Connect both sleeves to the tubing leading to the controller.
- Line up the blue arrows on the sleeve connector with the arrows on the tubing connectors, and push the ends together firmly.
- Listen for a click, signaling a firm connection. Make sure that the tubing isn't kinked.
- Plug the compression controller into the proper wall outlet. Turn the controller on.
- The controller automatically sets the compression sleeve pressure at 45 mm Hg, which is the midpoint of the normal range (35 to 55 mm Hg).
- Observe the patient to see how well he tolerates therapy.

- The green light on the AUDIBLE ALARM key should be lit.
- The compression sleeves should function continuously (24 hours daily) until the patient is fully ambulatory.
- Check sleeves once each shift to ensure proper fit and inflation.

Removing the sleeves

- You may remove the sleeves if the patient should walk, bathe, or leave the room for tests or other procedures. Reapply them immediately after these activities.
- To disconnect the sleeves from the tubing, depress the latches on each side of the connectors, and pull the connectors apart.
- Store the tubing and compression controller according to facility protocol.

Special considerations

- The compression controller has a mechanism to cool the patient.
- If a malfunction triggers the instrument's alarm, you'll hear beeping. The system shuts off whenever the alarm is activated.

Complications

- Pronounced leg deformity (decreased benefit)

Documentation

Record the date and time the device was applied. Note the type of sleeve used (knee- or thigh-length). Document the patient's response to and understanding of the procedure. Record the maximum sequential compression device inflation pressure and the patient's blood pressure. Note the reason for removal of sequential compression device along with length of time it was removed. Document the status of the alarm and cooling settings. Record the sleeve cooling mode status. Document proper application of the sleeves. Document assessments of skin and circulation of the lower extremities, including distal pulses. Provide rationale if only one leg sleeve is applied.

Skin biopsy

Skin biopsy is a diagnostic test in which a small piece of tissue is removed, under local anesthesia, from a lesion that's suspected of being malignant or from another dermatosis.

One of three techniques may be used: shave biopsy, punch biopsy, or excisional biopsy. Shave biopsy cuts the lesion above the skin line, which allows further biopsy of the site. Punch biopsy removes an oval core from the center of the lesion. Excisional biopsy removes the entire lesion and is indicated for rapidly expanding lesions; for sclerotic, bullous, or atrophic lesions; and for examination of the border of a lesion surrounding normal skin.

Lesions suspected of being malignant usually have changed color, size, or appearance or have failed to heal properly after injury. Fully developed lesions should be selected for biopsy whenever possible because they provide more diagnostic information than lesions that are resolving or in early stages of development. For example, if the skin shows blisters, the biopsy should include the most mature ones.

Normal skin consists of squamous epithelium (epidermis) and fibrous connective tissue (dermis). Histologic examination of the tissue specimen obtained during biopsy may reveal a benign or malignant lesion. Benign growths include cysts, seborrheic keratoses, warts, pigmented nevi (moles), keloids, dermatofibromas, and neurofibromas. Malignant tumors include basal cell carcinoma, squamous cell carcinoma, and malignant melanoma.

Equipment

Gloves ♦ #15 scalpel for shave or excisional biopsy ♦ local anesthetic ♦ specimen bottle containing 10% formaldehyde solution ♦ 4-0 sutures for punch or excisional biopsy ♦ adhesive bandage ♦ forceps ♦ laboratory specimen labels and laboratory biohazard transport bags

Key steps

- Confirm the patient's identity using two patient identifiers according to facility policy. Describe the procedure, and tell him who will perform it. Answer any questions he may have to ease anxiety and ensure cooperation.

- Inform the patient that he need not restrict food or fluids.
- Tell him that he'll receive a local anesthetic for pain.
- Inform him that the biopsy will take about 15 minutes and that the test results are usually available in 1 day.
- Have the patient or an appropriate family member sign a consent form.
- Check the patient's history for hypersensitivity to the local anesthetic.
- Position the patient comfortably, and clean the biopsy site before the local anesthetic is administered.
- Label all tubes on and off the sterile field.
- For a shave biopsy, the protruding growth is cut off at the skin line with a #15 scalpel. The tissue is placed immediately in a properly labeled specimen bottle containing 10% formaldehyde solution. Apply pressure to the area to stop the bleeding. Apply an adhesive bandage.
- For a punch biopsy, the skin surrounding the lesion is pulled taut, and the punch is firmly introduced into the lesion and rotated to obtain a tissue specimen. The plug is lifted with forceps or a needle and is severed as deeply into the fat layer as possible. The specimen is placed in a properly labeled specimen bottle containing 10% formaldehyde solution or in a sterile container if indicated. Closing the wound depends on the size of the punch: A 3-mm punch requires only an adhesive bandage, a 4-mm punch requires one suture, and a 6-mm punch requires two sutures.
- For an excisional biopsy, a #15 scalpel is used to excise the lesion; the incision is made as wide and as deep as necessary. The tissue specimen is removed and placed immediately in a properly labeled specimen bottle containing 10% formaldehyde solution. Apply pressure to the site to stop the bleeding. The wound is closed using a 4-0 suture. If the incision is large, a skin graft may be required.
- Check the biopsy site for bleeding.
- Label the specimen, and send the specimen to the laboratory immediately in a laboratory biohazard transport bag.
- If the patient experiences pain, administer analgesics.

Special considerations

- Characteristics of malignant lesions include change in color, size, or appearance or failure to heal properly after injury.

Complications

- Bleeding and infection of the surrounding tissue

Patient teaching

- Advise the patient going home with sutures to keep the area clean and as dry as possible.
- Tell him that facial sutures will be removed in 3 to 5 days and trunk sutures, in 7 to 14 days.
- Instruct the patient with adhesive strips to leave them in place for 14 to 21 days.

Documentation

Document the time and location where the specimen was obtained, the appearance of the specimen and site, and whether bleeding occurred at the biopsy site.

Skin graft care

A skin graft consists of healthy skin taken either from the patient (autograft) or a donor (allograft) and applied to an area of the patient's body damaged by burns, traumatic injury, or surgery. Care procedures for an autograft or an allograft are essentially the same. However, an autograft requires care for two sites on the patient: the graft site and the donor site.

Skin grafts are indicated where skin loss has occurred due to burns or for reconstructive purposes following trauma, infection (such as necrotizing fasciitis), malformation, deformity, congenitally deformed tissue, removal of malignant lesions, and plastic surgery in which direct closure by suturing isn't possible.

The graft itself may be one of several types: split-thickness, full-thickness, or pedicle-flap. (See *Understanding types of grafts*.) Successful grafting depends on various factors, including clean wound granulation with adequate vascularization, complete contact of the graft with the wound bed, sterile technique to prevent infection,

Understanding types of grafts

A burn patient may receive one or more of the graft types described here.

Split-thickness

The type used most commonly for covering open burns, a split-thickness graft includes the epidermis and part of the dermis. It may be applied as a sheet (usually on the face or neck to preserve the cosmetic result) or as a mesh. A mesh graft has tiny slits cut in it, which allow the graft to expand up to nine times its original size. Mesh grafts prevent fluids from collecting under the graft and typically are used over extensive full-thickness burns.

Full-thickness

A full-thickness graft includes the epidermis and the entire dermis. Consequently, the graft contains hair follicles, sweat glands, and sebaceous glands, which typically aren't included in split-thickness grafts. Full-thickness grafts usually are used for small burns that cause deep wounds.

Pedicle-flap

This full-thickness graft includes not only skin and subcutaneous tissue but also subcutaneous blood vessels, to ensure a continued blood supply to the graft. Pedicle-flap grafts may be used during reconstructive surgery to cover previous defects.

adequate graft immobilization, and skilled care.

The size and depth of the patient's burns determine whether the burns require grafting. Grafting usually occurs at the completion of wound debridement. The goal is to cover all wounds with an autograft or allograft within 2 weeks. With enzymatic debridement, grafting may be performed 5 to 7 days after debridement is complete; with surgical debridement, grafting can occur the same day as the surgery.

Depending on your facility's policy, a physician or specially trained nurse may change graft dressings. The dressings usually stay in place for 5 to 7 days after surgery to avoid disturbing the graft site. Meanwhile, the donor graft site needs diligent care. (See *Caring for a donor graft site* and *Postoperative graft care*, page 458.)

Equipment

Ordered analgesic ♦ clean and sterile gloves ♦ sterile gown ♦ cap ♦ mask ♦ sterile forceps ♦ sterile scissors ♦ sterile scalpel ♦ sterile 4″ × 4″ gauze pads ♦ Xeroflo gauze ♦ elastic gauze dressing ♦ warm normal saline solution ♦ moisturizing cream ♦ topical medication (such as micronized silver sulfadiazine cream) ♦ optional: sterile cotton-tipped applicators

Preparation

- Assemble the equipment on the dressing cart.

Key steps

- Explain the procedure to the patient, and provide privacy.
- Administer an analgesic, as ordered, 20 to 30 minutes before beginning the procedure. Alternatively, give an I.V. analgesic immediately before the procedure.
- Wash your hands.
- Put on the sterile gown and the clean mask, cap, and gloves.
- Gently lift off all outer dressings. Soak the middle dressings with warm saline solution. Remove these carefully and slowly to avoid disturbing the graft site. Leave the Xeroflo intact to avoid dislodging the graft.
- Remove and discard the clean gloves, wash your hands, and put on the sterile gloves.
- Assess the condition of the graft. If you see purulent drainage, notify the practitioner.
- Remove the Xeroflo with sterile forceps, and clean the area gently. If necessary, soak

Caring for a donor graft site

Autografts are usually taken from another area of the patient's body with a dermatome, an instrument that cuts uniform, split-thickness skin portions—typically, about 0.013 to 0.05 cm thick. Autografting makes the donor site a partial-thickness wound, which may bleed, drain, and cause pain.

This site needs scrupulous care to prevent infection, which could convert the site to a full-thickness wound. Depending on the graft's thickness, tissue may be obtained from the donor site again in as few as 10 days.

Usually, Xeroflo gauze is applied postoperatively. The outer gauze dressing can be taken off on the first postoperative day; the Xeroflo will protect the new epithelial proliferation.

Care for the donor site as you care for the autograft, using dressing changes at the initial stages to prevent infection and promote healing. Follow these guidelines.

Dressing the wound

- Wash your hands, and put on sterile gloves.
- Remove the outer gauze dressings within 24 hours. Inspect the Xeroflo for signs of infection; then leave it open to the air to speed drying and healing.
- Leave small amounts of fluid accumulation alone. Using sterile technique, larger amounts may be aspirated through the dressing with a small-gauge needle and syringe.
- Apply a lanolin-based cream daily to completely healed donor sites to keep skin tissue pliable and to remove crusts.

Postoperative graft care

Both full-thickness and split-thickness skin grafts require compliance with a postoperative activity schedule to prevent complications.

Postoperative timetable	Instructions
1 to 6 days	Strict elevation, above the head
7 days	5 minutes dangling/hour
8 days	10 minutes dangling/hour
9 days	15 minutes dangling/hour
2 to 3 weeks	Physical therapy for range-of-motion exercises
4 to 6 weeks	Partial weight bearing as tolerated, with an assistive device
6 to 8 weeks	Full weight bearing

the Xeroflo with warm saline solution to ease removal.

- Inspect an allograft for signs of rejection, such as infection and delayed healing. Inspect a sheet graft frequently for blebs. Notify the practitioner for evacuation if necessary. (See *Evacuating fluid from a sheet graft.*)
- Apply topical medication if ordered.
- Place fresh Xeroflo over the site to promote wound healing and prevent infection. Use sterile scissors to cut the appropriate size. Cover this with 4″ × 4″ gauze and elastic gauze dressing.
- Clean completely healed areas, and apply a moisturizing cream to them to keep the skin pliable and to retard scarring.

Special considerations

DO'S & DON'TS

To avoid dislodging the graft, hydrotherapy is usually discontinued, as ordered, 3 to 4 days after grafting. Avoid using a blood pressure cuff over the graft. Don't tug or pull dressings during dressing changes. Keep the patient from lying on the graft.

- If the graft dislodges, apply sterile skin compresses to keep the area moist until the surgeon reapplies the graft. If the graft affects an arm or a leg, elevate the affected extremity to reduce postoperative edema. Check for bleeding and signs of neurovascular impairment—increasing pain, numbness or tingling, coolness, and pallor.

Complications

- Hematoma causing graft failure
- Traumatic injury, infection, an inadequate graft bed, rejection, or compromised nutritional status

Patient teaching

- Teach the patient how to apply moisturizing cream.
- Stress the importance of using a sunscreen with a sun protection factor of 20 or higher and containing titanium dioxide or oxybenzone on all grafted areas to avoid sunburn and discoloration.

Evacuating fluid from a sheet graft

When small pockets of fluid (called *blebs*) accumulate beneath a sheet graft, the fluid will be evacuated using a sterile scalpel and cotton-tipped applicators. First, the center of the bleb is perforated with the scalpel.

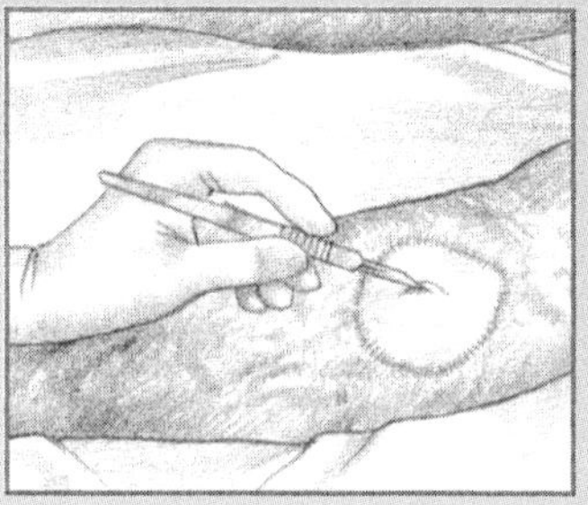

Then the fluid is gently expressed with the cotton-tipped applicators.

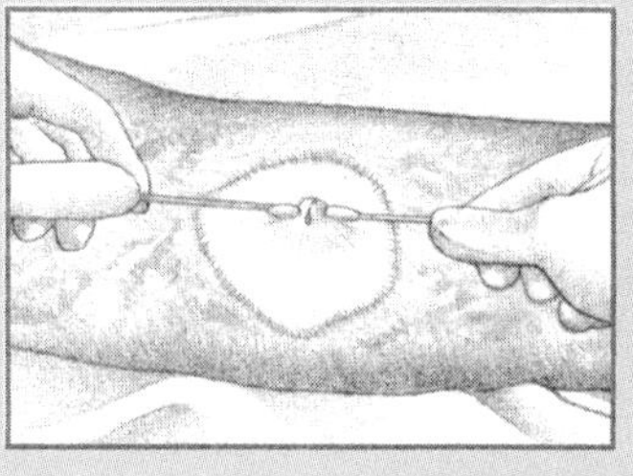

The fluid is never expressed by rolling the bleb to the edge of the graft. This disturbs healing in other areas.

Documentation

Record the time and date of all dressing changes. Document all medications used, and note the patient's response to the medications. Describe the condition of the graft, and note signs of infection or rejection. Record additional treatment, and note the patient's reaction to the graft.

Skin preparation, preoperative

Preoperative skin preparation reduces the risk of infection at the incision site during surgery. It doesn't duplicate or replace full sterile preparation that immediately precedes surgery. The area of preparation always exceeds that of the expected incision, to help minimize microorganisms in the adjacent areas and allow surgical draping without contamination.

The procedure may involve a bath, shower, or local scrub with an antiseptic detergent solution.

Equipment

Antiseptic soap solution ♦ tap water ♦ bath blanket ♦ two clean basins ♦ linen-saver pad ♦ adjustable light ♦ scissors ♦ liquid soap ♦ cotton-tipped applicators ♦ acetone or nail polish remover ♦ orangewood stick ♦ trash bag ♦ towel ♦ gloves ♦ 4″ × 4″ gauze pads ♦ optional: electric clippers

Preparation

- Using warm tap water, dilute the antiseptic soap solution in one basin for washing.
- Pour plain warm water into the second basin for rinsing.

Key steps

- Check the practitioner's order.
- Explain the procedure to the patient, and provide privacy.
- Wash your hands and put on gloves.
- Put the patient in a comfortable position, and drape him with the bath blanket.
- Expose the preparation area, which commonly extends 12″ (30.5 cm) in each direction from the expected incision site.
- To ensure privacy and avoid chilling, expose only one small area at a time while performing skin preparation.
- Position a linen-saver pad beneath the patient.
- Adjust the light to illuminate the preparation area.
- Assess skin condition in the preparation area, and report any rash, abrasion, or laceration to the practitioner.
- A break in the skin increases the risk of infection and could cause cancellation of the planned surgery.
- Have the patient remove all jewelry on or near the operative site.
- Begin removing hair from the preparation area by clipping long hairs with scissors.
- Perform the procedure as near to the time of surgery as possible.
- Proceed with a 10-minute scrub.
- Wash the area with a gauze pad dipped in the antiseptic soap.
- Using a circular motion, start at the expected incision site and work outward, pulling loose skin taut.
- Apply light friction while washing to improve the antiseptic effect.
- Carefully clean skin folds and crevices; scrub the perineal area last if it's part of the preparation area.
- Replace the gauze pad as necessary.
- Use cotton-tipped applicators to clean the umbilicus if needed.
- Dry the area with a clean towel, and remove the linen-saver pad.
- Use an orangewood stick to clean under nails.
- Remove nail polish with remover to see nail bed color to determine adequate oxygenation.
- Place a probe on the patient's fingernail to measure oxygen saturation.
- Give the patient special instructions for care of the prepared area, and remind the patient to keep the area clean for surgery.
- Make sure the patient is comfortable.
- Properly dispose of solutions and the trash bag.
- Dispose of soiled equipment.

Special considerations

- Never shave eyebrows to avoid unsightly regrowth.
- If required, prepare the patient's scalp, put hair in a plastic or paper bag, and store it with the patient's possessions.

Complications

- Rashes
- Nicks

- Lacerations and abrasions (most common) increasing the risk of postoperative infection

Documentation
Record the date, time, and area of preparation. Note the skin's condition before and after preparation. Document complications. Record the patient's tolerance of the procedure. Prepare an incident report if required for nicks, lacerations, or abrasions.

Skin staple and clip removal

Skin staples or clips may be used instead of standard sutures to close lacerations or surgical wounds. Because they can secure a wound more quickly than sutures, they may substitute for surface sutures when cosmetic results aren't a prime consideration, such as in an abdominal closure. When properly placed, staples and clips distribute tension evenly along the suture line with minimal tissue trauma and compression, facilitating healing and minimizing scarring. Because staples and clips are made from surgical stainless steel, tissue reaction to them is minimal. Usually, physicians remove skin staples and clips, but some facilities permit qualified nurses to perform this procedure.

Skin staples and clips are contraindicated when wound location requires cosmetically superior results or when the incision site makes it impossible to maintain at least a 5-mm distance between the staple and underlying bone, vessels, or internal organs.

Equipment
Waterproof trash bag ♦ adjustable light ♦ clean gloves, if needed ♦ sterile gloves ♦ sterile gauze pads ♦ sterile staple or clip extractor ♦ antiseptic cleaning agent ♦ sterile cotton-tipped applicators ♦ compound benzoin tincture or other skin protectant ♦ optional: butterfly adhesive strips or Steri-Strips

Prepackaged, sterile, and disposable staple or clip extractors are available.

Preparation
- Assemble all equipment in the patient's room.
- Check the expiration date on each sterile package, and inspect for tears.
- Open the waterproof trash bag, and place it near the patient's bed.
- Position the bag to avoid reaching across the sterile field or the wound when disposing of soiled articles. Form a cuff by turning down the top of the bag to provide a wide opening, then preventing contamination of instruments or gloves by touching the bag's edge.

Key steps
- If your facility allows you to remove skin staples and clips, check the practitioner's order to confirm the exact timing and details for this procedure.
- Check for patient allergies, especially to adhesive tape and povidone-iodine or other topical solutions or medications.
- Explain the procedure to the patient. Tell him that he may feel a slight pulling or tickling sensation but little discomfort during staple removal. Reassure him that because his incision is healing properly, removing the supporting staples or clips won't weaken the incision line.
- Provide privacy, and place the patient in a comfortable position that doesn't place undue tension on the incision. Because some patients experience nausea or dizziness during the procedure, have the patient recline if possible. Adjust the light to shine directly on the incision.
- Wash your hands thoroughly.
- If the patient's wound has a dressing, put on clean gloves and carefully remove it. Discard the dressing and the gloves in the waterproof trash bag.
- Assess the patient's incision. Notify the practitioner of gaping, drainage, inflammation, and other signs of infection.
- Establish a sterile work area with all the equipment and supplies you'll need for removing staples or clips and for cleaning and dressing the incision. Open the package containing the sterile staple or clip extractor, maintaining asepsis. Put on sterile gloves.

Removing a staple

Position the extractor's lower jaws beneath the span of the first staple (as shown below).

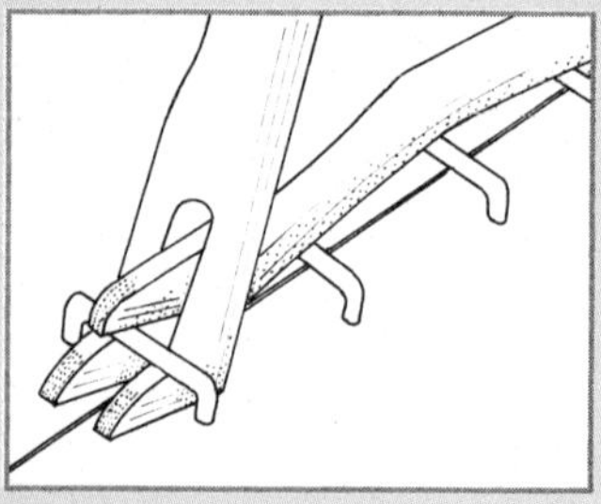

Squeeze the handles until they're completely closed; then lift the staple away from the skin (as shown below). The extractor changes the shape of the staple and pulls the prongs out of the intradermal tissue.

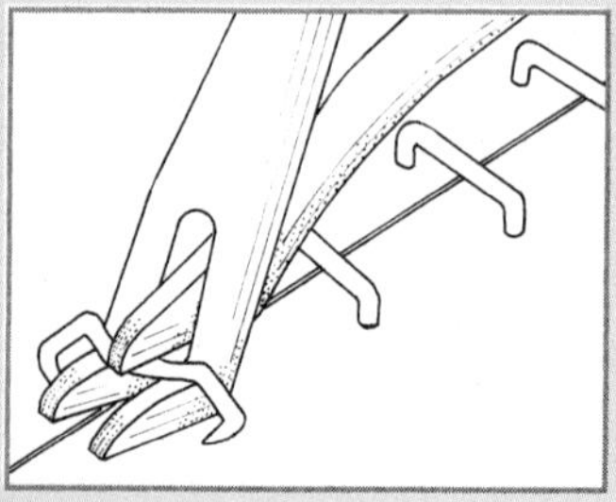

- Wipe the incision gently with sterile gauze pads soaked in an antiseptic cleaning agent or with sterile cotton-tipped applicators to remove surface encrustations.
- Pick up the sterile staple or clip extractor. Then, starting at one end of the incision, remove the staple or clip. (See *Removing a staple*.) Hold the extractor over the trash bag, and release the handle to discard the staple or clip.
- Repeat the procedure for each staple or clip until all are removed.
- Apply a sterile gauze dressing, if needed, to prevent infection and irritation from clothing. Then discard your gloves.
- Make sure the patient is comfortable. According to the practitioner's preference, inform the patient that he may shower in 1 or 2 days if the incision is dry and healing well.
- Properly dispose of solutions and the trash bag, and clean or dispose of soiled equipment and supplies according to facility policy.

Special considerations

- Carefully check the practitioner's order for the time and extent of staple or clip removal. The practitioner may want you to remove only alternate staples or clips initially and to leave the others in place for an additional day or two to support the incision.
- When removing a staple or clip, place the extractor's jaws carefully between the patient's skin and the staple or clip to avoid patient discomfort. If extraction is difficult, notify the practitioner; staples or clips placed too deeply within the skin or left in place too long may resist removal.
- If the wound dehisces after staples or clips are removed, apply butterfly adhesive strips or Steri-Strips to approximate and support the edges, and call the practitioner immediately to repair the wound. (See *Types of adhesive skin closures*.)
- You may also apply butterfly adhesive strips or Steri-Strips after removing staples or clips even if the wound is healing normally to give added support to the incision and prevent lateral tension from forming a wide scar. Use a small amount of compound benzoin tincture or other skin protectant to ensure adherence. Leave the strips in place for 3 to 5 days.

Complications

- None known

Patient teaching

- If the patient is being discharged, teach him how to remove the dressing and care for the wound.
- Instruct him to call the practitioner immediately if he observes wound discharge or any other abnormal change. Tell him that the redness surrounding the incision should gradually disappear and that after a few weeks, only a thin line will be visible.

Types of adhesive skin closures

Steri-Strips are used as a primary means of keeping a wound closed after suture removal. They're made of thin strips of sterile, nonwoven, porous fabric tape.

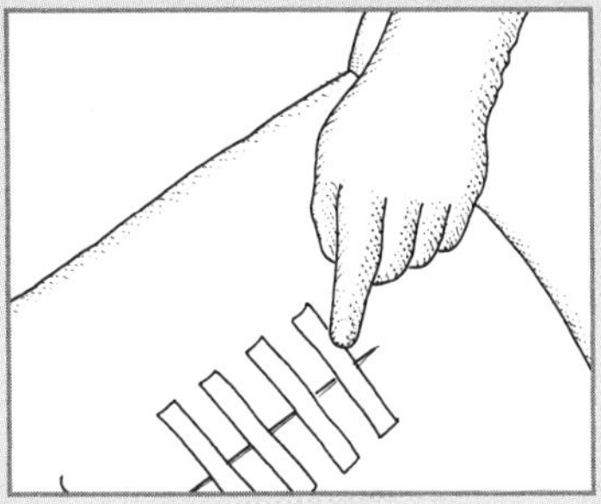

Butterfly closures consist of sterile, waterproof adhesive strips. A narrow, nonadhesive "bridge" connects the two expanded adhesive portions. These strips are used to close small wounds and assist healing after suture removal.

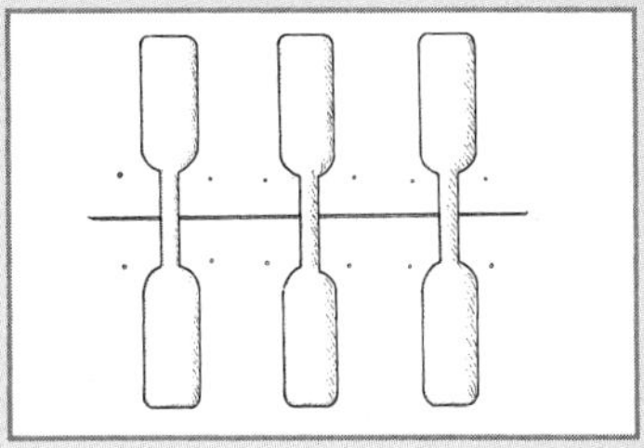

Documentation

Record the date and time of staple or clip removal, number of staples or clips removed, appearance of the incision, dressings or butterfly strips applied, signs of wound complications, and the patient's tolerance of the procedure.

Skull tong care

Applying skeletal traction with skull tongs immobilizes the cervical spine after a fracture or dislocation, invasion by a tumor or infection, or surgery. Three types of skull tongs are commonly used: Crutchfield, Gardner-Wells, and Vinke. (See *Types of skull tongs,* page 464.) Crutchfield tongs are applied by incising the skin with a scalpel, drilling a hole in the exposed skull, and inserting the pins on the tongs into the hole. Gardner-Wells tongs and Vinke tongs are applied less invasively. Gardner-Wells tongs have spring-loaded pins attached to the tongs. These pins are advanced gently into the scalp. Then the tongs are tightened to secure the apparatus.

When any tong device is in place, traction is created by extending a rope from the center of the tongs over a pulley and attaching weights to it. With the help of X-ray monitoring, the weights are adjusted to establish reduction, if necessary, and to maintain alignment. Meticulous pin-site care (three times per day to prevent infection) and frequent observation of the traction apparatus are required to make sure it's working properly.

Equipment

Three medicine cups ♦ one bottle each of ordered cleaning solution, normal saline solution, and povidone-iodine solution ♦ sterile, cotton-tipped applicators ♦ sandbags or cervical collar (hard or soft) ♦ fine mesh gauze strips ♦ 4″ × 4″ gauze pads ♦ sterile gloves ♦ sterile basin ♦ sterile scissors ♦ hair clippers ♦ optional: turning frame, antibacterial ointment

Preparation

- Bring the equipment to the patient's room.
- Place the medicine cups on the bedside table. Fill one cup with a small amount of cleaning solution, one with normal saline solution, and one with povidone-iodine solution.
- Then set out the cotton-tipped applicators.
- Keep the sandbags or cervical collar handy for emergency immobilization of the head and neck if the pins in the tongs should slip.

Types of skull tongs

Skull (or cervical) tongs consist of a stainless steel body with a pin at the end of each arm. Each pin is about 5" (12.5 cm) in diameter and has a sharp tip.

On Crutchfield tongs, the pins are placed about 5" (12.5 cm) apart in line with the long axis of the cervical spine.

On Gardner-Wells tongs, the pins are farther apart. They're inserted slightly above the patient's ears.

On Vinke tongs, the pins are placed at the parietal bones, near the widest transverse diameter of the skull, about 1" (2.5 cm) above the helix.

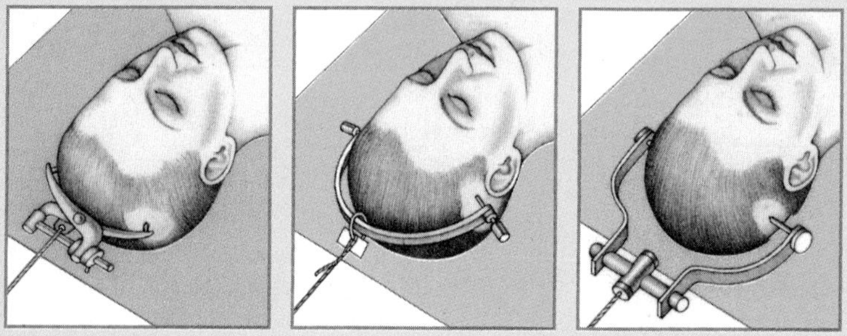

Key steps

- Explain the procedure to the patient, and wash your hands. Tell him that he'll also feel some muscular discomfort in the injured area.
- Before providing care, observe each pin site carefully for signs of infection, such as loose pins, swelling or redness, or purulent drainage. Use hair clippers to trim the patient's hair around the pin sites, when necessary, to facilitate assessment.
- Put on gloves, and gently wipe each pin site with a cotton-tipped applicator dipped in cleaning solution to loosen and remove crusty drainage. Repeat with a fresh applicator, as needed, for thorough cleaning. Use a separate applicator for each site to avoid cross-contamination. Next, wipe each site with normal saline solution to remove excess cleaning solution. Finally, wipe with povidone-iodine solution to provide asepsis at the site and prevent infection.
- After providing care, discard all pin-site cleaning materials.
- If the pin sites are infected, apply a povidone-iodine wrap as ordered. First, obtain strips of fine mesh gauze, or cut a 4" × 4" gauze pad into strips (using sterile scissors and wearing sterile gloves). Soak the strips in a sterile basin of povidone-iodine solution or normal saline solution as ordered, and squeeze out the excess solution. Wrap one strip securely around each pin site. Leave the strip in place to dry until you provide care again. Removing the dried strip aids in debridement and helps clear the infection.
- Check the traction apparatus—rope, weights, and pulleys—at the start of each shift, every 4 hours, and as necessary (for example, after position changes). Make sure the rope hangs freely and that the weights never rest on the floor or become caught under the bed.

Special considerations

- Occasionally, the practitioner may prefer an antibacterial ointment for pin-site care instead of povidone-iodine solution. To remove old ointment, wrap a cotton-tipped applicator with a 4" × 4" gauze pad, moisten it with cleaning solution, and gently clean each site. Keep a box of sterile gauze pads handy at the patient's bedside.

- Watch for signs and symptoms of loose pins, such as persistent pain or tenderness at pin sites, redness, and drainage. The patient may also report feeling or hearing the pins move.

DEVICE SAFETY

If you suspect a pin has loosened or slipped, don't turn the patient until the practitioner examines the skull tongs and fixes them as needed.

- If the pins pull out, immobilize the patient's head and neck with sandbags, or apply a cervical collar. Then carefully remove the traction weights. Apply manual traction to the patient's head by placing your hands on each side of the mandible and pulling very gently while maintaining proper alignment. After you stabilize the alignment, have someone send for the practitioner immediately. Remain calm and reassure the patient. When traction is reestablished, take neurologic vital signs.

ALERT

Never add or subtract weights to the traction apparatus without an order from the practitioner. Doing so can cause neurologic impairment.

- Take neurologic vital signs at the beginning of each shift, every 4 hours, and as necessary (for example, after turning or transporting the patient). Carefully assess the function of cranial nerves, which may be impaired by pin placement. Note any asymmetry, deviation, or atrophy. Review the patient's chart to determine baseline neurologic vital signs on admission to the facility and immediately after the tongs were applied.
- Monitor respirations closely, and keep suction equipment handy. Remember, injury to the cervical spine may affect respiration. Therefore, be alert for signs of respiratory distress, such as unequal chest expansion and an irregular or altered respiratory rate or pattern.
- Patients with skull tongs may be placed on a turning frame to facilitate turning without disrupting vertebral alignment. Establish a turning schedule for the patient (usually a supine position for 2 hours and then a prone position for 1 hour) to help prevent complications of immobility.

Complications

- Infection, excessive tractive force, or osteoporosis causing the skull pins to slip or pull out (Because this interrupts traction, the patient must receive immediate attention to prevent further injury.)

Patient teaching

- Inform the patient that pin sites usually feel tender for several days after the tongs are applied.

Documentation

Record the date, time, and type of pin-site care and the patient's response to the procedure in your notes. Describe signs of infection. Also, note whether weights were added or removed. Record neurologic vital signs, the patient's respiratory status, and the turning schedule on the Kardex.

Spiritual care

Religious beliefs can profoundly influence a patient's recovery rate, attitude toward treatment, and overall response to hospitalization. In certain religious groups, beliefs can preclude diagnostic tests and therapeutic treatments, require dietary restrictions, and prohibit organ donation and artificial prolongation of life. (See *Beliefs and practices of selected religions,* pages 466 to 468.)

Consequently, effective patient care requires identification, recognition of, and respect for the patient's religious beliefs. Data about a patient's spiritual beliefs are obtained from the patient's history, a thorough nursing history, and close attention to his nonverbal cues or seemingly casual remarks that express his spiritual concerns. The nurse should never assume that a patient follows all the practices of his stated religion.

Respecting a patient's beliefs may require the nurse to set aside her own beliefs to help the patient follow his. This aids in cooperation and improved response to

(Text continues on page 468.)

Beliefs and practices of selected religions

A patient's religious beliefs can affect his attitudes toward illness and traditional medicine. By trying to accommodate the patient's religious beliefs and practices in your care plan, you can increase his willingness to learn and comply with treatment regimens. Because religious beliefs may vary within particular sects, individual practices may differ from those described here.

Religion	Birth and death rituals	Dietary restrictions	Practices in health crisis
Adventist	None (baptism of adults only)	Alcohol, coffee, tea, opioids, stimulants; in many groups, meat prohibited also	Communion and baptism performed. Some members believe in divine healing, anointing with oil, and prayer. Some regard Saturday as the Sabbath.
Baptist	At birth, none (baptism of believers only); before death, counseling by clergy member and prayer	Alcohol; in some groups, coffee and tea prohibited also	Some believe in healing by laying on of hands. Resistance to medical therapy occasionally approved.
Christian Science	At birth, none; before death, counseling by a Christian Science practitioner	Alcohol, coffee, and tobacco prohibited	Many members refuse all treatment, including drugs, biopsies, physical examination, and blood transfusions and permit vaccination only when required by law. Alteration of thoughts is believed to cure illness. Hypnotism and psychotherapy are prohibited. (Christian Scientist nurses and nursing homes honor these beliefs.)
Church of Christ	None (baptism at age 8 or older)	Alcohol discouraged	Communion, anointing with oil, laying on of hands, and counseling performed by a minister.
Eastern Orthodox	At birth, baptism and confirmation; before death, last rites (For members of the Russian Orthodox Church, arms are crossed after death, fingers set in cross, and unembalmed	For members of the Russian Orthodox Church and usually the Greek Orthodox Church, no meat or dairy products on Wednesday, Friday, and during Lent	Anointing of the sick. For members of the Russian Orthodox Church, cross necklace is replaced immediately after surgery and shaving of male patients is prohibited except in preparation for surgery. For members of the Greek Orthodox Church,

Beliefs and practices of selected religions *(continued)*

Religion	Birth and death rituals	Dietary restrictions	Practices in health crisis
Eastern Orthodox *(continued)*	body clothed in natural fiber.)		communion and Sacrament of Holy Unction.
Episcopal	At birth, baptism; before death, occasional last rites	For some members, abstention from meat on Friday, fasting before communion (which may be daily)	Communion, prayer, and counseling performed by a minister.
Jehovah's Witnesses	None	Abstention from foods to which blood has been added	Typically, no blood transfusions are permitted; a court order may be required for emergency transfusion.
Judaism	Ritual circumcision on eighth day after birth; burial of dead fetus; ritual washing of dead; burial (including organs and other body tissues) occurs as soon as possible; no autopsy or embalming	For Orthodox and Conservative Jews, kosher dietary laws (for example, pork and shellfish prohibited); for Reform Jews, usually no restrictions	Donation or transplantation of organs requires rabbinical consultation. For Orthodox and Conservative Jews, medical procedures may be prohibited on the Sabbath—from sundown Friday to sundown Saturday—and specific holidays.
Lutheran	Baptism usually performed 6 to 8 weeks after birth	None	Communion, prayer, and counseling performed by a minister.
Jesus Christ of Latter Day Saints (Mormon)	At birth, none (baptism at age 8 or older); before death, baptism and gospel preaching	Alcohol, tobacco, tea, and coffee prohibited; meat intake limited	Belief in divine healing through the laying on of hands; communion on Sunday; some members may refuse medical treatment. Many wear a special undergarment.
Islam	If spontaneous abortion occurs before 130 days, fetus treated as discarded tissue; after 130 days, as a human	Pork prohibited; daylight fasting during ninth month of Islamic calendar	Faith healing for the patient's morale only; conservative members reject medical therapy.

(continued)

Beliefs and practices of selected religions *(continued)*

Religion	Birth and death rituals	Dietary restrictions	Practices in health crisis
Islam *(continued)*	being; before death, confession of sins with family present; after death, only relatives or friends may touch the body		
Orthodox Presbyterian	Infant baptism; scripture reading and prayer before death	None	Communion, prayer, and counseling performed by a minister.
Pentecostal Assembly of God, Foursquare Church	None (baptism only after age of accountability)	Abstention from alcohol, tobacco, meat slaughtered by strangling, any food to which blood has been added, and sometimes pork	Divine healing through prayer, anointing with oil, and laying on of hands.
Roman Catholicism	Infant baptism, including baptism of aborted fetus without sign of clinical death (tissue necrosis); before death, anointing of the sick	Fasting or abstention from meat on Ash Wednesday and on Fridays during Lent; this practice usually waived for the hospitalized	Burial of major amputated limb (sometimes) in consecrated ground; donation or transplantation of organs allowed if the benefit to recipient outweighs the donor's potential harm. Sacrament of the Sick also performed when patients are ill, not just before death. Sometimes performed shortly after admission.
United Methodist	Baptism of children and adults	None	Communion before surgery or similar crisis; donation of body parts encouraged.

treatment and expected outcomes for the patient. Providing spiritual care may require contacting an appropriate member of the clergy in the facility or community, gathering equipment needed to help the pastor perform rites and administer sacraments, and preparing him for a pastoral visit.

Equipment

Clean towels (one or two) ♦ teaspoon or 1-oz (29.6-ml) medicine cup (for baptism) if appropriate ♦ container of water (for emergency baptism) if appropriate ♦ other supplies specific to the patient's religious affiliation

Some health care facilities, particularly those with a religious affiliation, provide baptismal trays. The clergy member may bring holy water, holy oil, or other religious articles to minister to the patient.

Preparation

- For baptism, cover a small table with a clean towel. Fold a second towel, and place it on the table, along with the teaspoon or medicine cup.
- For communion and anointing, cover the bedside stand with a clean towel.

Key steps

- Check the patient's admission record to determine his religious affiliation. Remember that some patients may claim no religious beliefs. However, even an agnostic may wish to speak with a clergy member, so watch and listen carefully for subtle expressions of this desire.
- Remember that a patient may feel acutely distressed because of his inability to participate in religious observances. Help such a patient verbalize his beliefs to relieve stress. Listen to him, and let him express his concerns, but carefully refrain from imposing your beliefs on him to avoid conflict and further stress. If the patient requests, arrange a visit by an appropriate member of the clergy. Consult this clergy member if you need more information about the patient's beliefs.
- Evaluate the patient's behavior for signs of loneliness, anxiety, or fear—emotions that may signal his need for spiritual counsel. Commonly patients experience these feelings at night when they feel especially alone. Stay alert for comments or behaviors that indicate a need to verbalize those feelings.
- If your patient faces the possibility of abortion, amputation, transfusion, or other medical procedures with important religious implications, try to discover the spiritual attitude. Also, try to determine your patient's attitude toward the importance of laying on of hands, confession, communion, observance of holy days (such as the Sabbath), and restrictions in diet or physical appearance. Helping the patient continue his normal religious practices during hospitalization can help reduce stress.
- If the patient is pregnant, find out her beliefs concerning infant baptism and circumcision, and comply with them after delivery.
- If a neonate is in critical condition, call an appropriate clergy member immediately. To perform an emergency baptism, the minister or priest pours a small amount of water into a teaspoon or a medicine cup and sprinkles a few drops over the infant's head while saying, "(Name of child), I baptize you in the name of the Father, the Son, and the Holy Spirit. Amen." In an extreme emergency, you can perform a Roman Catholic baptism, using a container of available water. If you do so, be sure to notify the priest because this sacrament must be administered only once.
- If a Jewish woman delivers a male infant prematurely or by cesarean birth, ask her whether she plans to observe the rite of circumcision (bris), a significant ceremony performed on the eighth day after birth. (Because a patient who delivers a healthy, full-term baby vaginally is usually discharged quickly, this ceremony is normally performed outside the facility.) For a bris, ensure privacy and, if requested, sterilize the instruments.
- If the patient requests communion, prepare him for it before the clergy member arrives. First, place him in Fowler's or semi-Fowler's position if his condition permits. Otherwise, allow him to remain in a supine position. Tuck a clean towel under his chin, and straighten the bed linens.
- If a terminally ill patient requests the Sacrament of the Sick (Last Rites) or special treatment of his body after death, call an appropriate clergy member. For the Roman Catholic patient, call a Roman Catholic priest to administer the sacrament, even if the patient is unresponsive or comatose. To prepare the patient for this sacrament, uncover his arms and fold back the top linens to expose his feet. After the clergy member anoints the patient's forehead, eyes, nose, mouth, hands, and feet, straighten and retuck the bed linens.

Special considerations

- Handle the patient's religious articles carefully to avoid damage or loss. Become familiar with religious resources in your facility. Some facilities employ one or more clergy members who counsel patients and staff and link patients to other pastoral resources.
- If the patient tries to convert you to his personal beliefs, tell him that you respect his beliefs but are content with your own. Similarly, avoid attempts to convert the patient to your personal beliefs.

Complications

- None known

Documentation

Complete a baptismal form, and attach it to the patient's record; send a copy of the form to the appropriate clergy member. Record the rites of circumcision and last rites in your notes. Also record last rites in red on the Kardex so it won't be repeated unnecessarily.

Splint application

By immobilizing the site of an injury, a splint alleviates pain and allows the injury to heal in proper alignment. It also minimizes possible complications, such as excessive bleeding into tissues, restricted blood flow caused by bone pressing against vessels, and possible paralysis from an unstable spinal cord injury. In cases of multiple serious injuries, a splint or spine board allows caretakers to move the patient without risking further damage to bones, muscles, nerves, blood vessels, and skin.

A splint can be applied to immobilize a simple or compound fracture, a dislocation, or a subluxation. (See *Types of splints.*) During an emergency, any injury suspected of being a fracture, dislocation, or subluxation should be splinted. No contraindications exist for rigid splints; don't use traction splints for upper extremity injuries and open fractures.

Equipment

Rigid splint, Velcro support splint, spine board, or traction splint ♦ bindings ♦ padding ♦ sandbags or rolled towels or clothing ♦ optional: roller gauze, cloth strips, sterile or clean compress, ice bag

Several commercial splints are widely available. In an emergency, any long, sturdy object, such as a tree limb, mop handle, or broom—even a magazine—can be used to make a rigid splint for an extremity; a door can be used as a spine board.

An inflatable semirigid splint, called an *air splint,* sometimes can be used to secure an injured extremity. (See *Using an air splint,* page 472.) Velcro straps, 2″ roller gauze, or 2″ cloth strips can be used as bindings. When improvising, avoid using twine or rope, if possible, because they can restrict circulation.

Key steps

- Obtain a complete history of the injury, if possible, and begin a thorough head-to-toe assessment, inspecting for obvious deformities, swelling, or bleeding.
- Ask the patient if he can move the injured area (typically an extremity). Compare it bilaterally with the uninjured extremity, where applicable. Gently palpate the injured area; inspect for swelling, obvious deformities, bleeding, discoloration, and evidence of fracture or dislocation.
- Remove or cut away clothing from the injury site if necessary. Check neurovascular integrity distal to the site. Explain the procedure to the patient to allay his fears.
- If an obvious bone misalignment causes the patient acute distress or severe neurovascular problems, try to align the extremity in its normal anatomic position. Stop, however, if this causes further neurovascular deterioration.

DO'S & DON'TS

Don't try to straighten a dislocation to avoid damaging displaced vessels and nerves. Also, don't attempt reduction of a contaminated bone end because this may cause additional laceration of soft tissues, vessels,

Types of splints

Three kinds of splints are commonly used to help provide support for injured or weakened limbs or to help correct deformities.

A *rigid splint* can be used to immobilize a fracture or dislocation in an extremity, as shown at right. Ideally, two people should apply a rigid splint to an extremity.

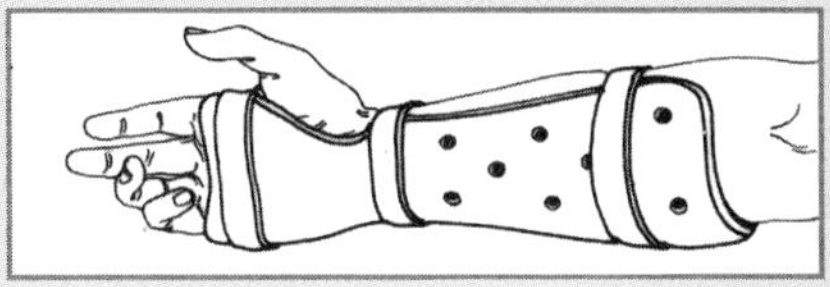

A *traction splint* immobilizes a fracture and exerts a longitudinal pull that reduces muscle spasms, pain, and arterial and neural damage. Used primarily for femoral fractures, a traction splint may also be applied for a fractured hip or tibia. Two trained people should apply a traction splint.

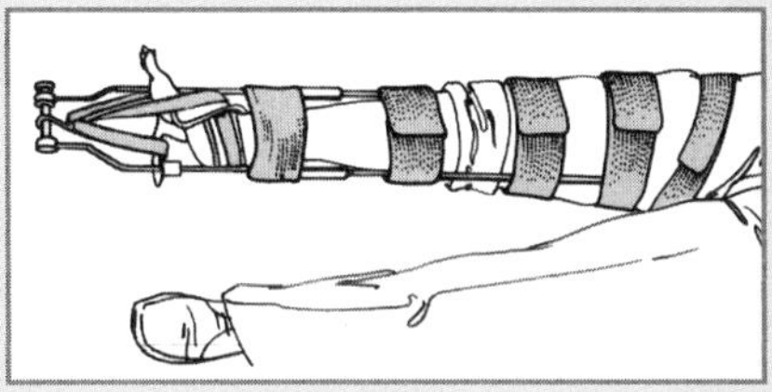

A *spine board*, applied for a suspected spinal fracture, is a rigid splint that supports the injured person's entire body. Three people should apply a spine board.

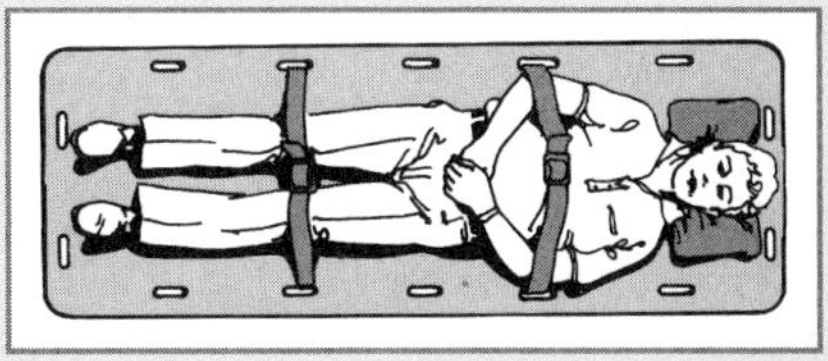

and nerves as well as gross contamination of deep tissues.

- Choose a splint that will immobilize the joints above and below the fracture; pad the splint as necessary to protect bony prominences.

Applying a rigid splint

- Support the injured extremity and apply firm, gentle traction.
- Have an assistant place the splint under, beside, or on top of the extremity, as ordered.
- Tell the assistant to apply the bindings to secure the splint. Don't let them obstruct circulation.

Applying a spine board

- Pad the spine board (or door) carefully, especially the areas that will support the lumbar region and knees, to prevent uneven pressure and discomfort.
- If the patient is lying on his back, place one hand on each side of his head, and apply gentle traction to the head and neck, keeping the head aligned with the body. Have one assistant logroll the patient onto his side while another slides the spine board under the patient. Then instruct the assistants to roll the patient onto the board while you maintain traction and alignment.
- If the patient is prone, logroll him onto the board so he ends up in a supine position.
- To maintain body alignment, use strips of cloth to secure the patient on the spine board; to keep head and neck aligned, place sandbags or rolled towels or clothing on both sides of his head.

Using an air splint

In an emergency, an air splint can be applied to immobilize a fracture or control bleeding, especially from a forearm or lower leg. This compact, comfortable splint is made of double-walled plastic and provides gentle, diffuse pressure over an injured area. The appropriate splint is chosen, wrapped around the affected extremity, secured with Velcro or other strips, and then inflated. The fit should be snug enough to immobilize the extremity without impairing circulation.

An air splint (shown below) may actually control bleeding better than a local pressure bandage. Its clear plastic construction simplifies inspection of the affected site for bleeding, pallor, or cyanosis. An air splint also allows the patient to be moved without further damage to the injured limb.

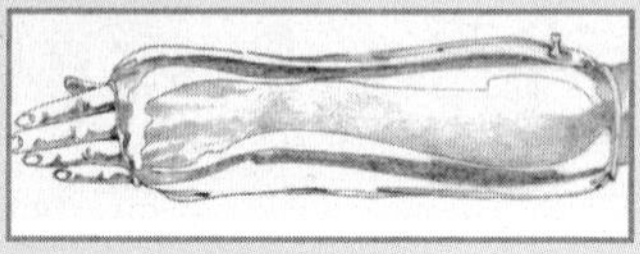

Applying a traction splint

- Place the splint beside the injured leg. (Never use a traction splint on an arm because the major axillary plexus of nerves and blood vessels can't tolerate countertraction.) Adjust the splint to the correct length, and then open and adjust the Velcro straps.
- Have an assistant keep the leg motionless while you pad the ankle and foot and fasten the ankle hitch around them. (You may leave the shoe on.)
- Tell the assistant to lift and support the leg at the injury site as you apply firm, gentle traction.
- While you maintain traction, tell the assistant to slide the splint under the leg, pad the groin to avoid excessive pressure on external genitalia, and gently apply the ischial strap.
- Have the assistant connect the loops of the ankle hitch to the end of the splint.
- Adjust the splint to apply enough traction to secure the leg comfortably in the corrected position.
- After applying traction, fasten the Velcro support splints to secure the leg closely to the splint.

ALERT

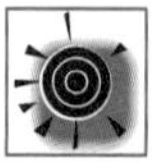

Don't use a traction splint for a severely angulated femur or knee fracture.

Special considerations

- At the scene of an accident, always examine the patient completely for other injuries. Avoid unnecessary movement or manipulation, which might cause additional pain or injury.
- Always consider the possibility of cervical injury in an unconscious patient. If possible, apply the splint before repositioning the patient.
- If the patient requires a rigid splint but one isn't available, use another body part as a splint. To splint a leg in this manner, pad its inner aspect, and secure it to the other leg with roller gauze or cloth strips.
- After applying any type of splint, monitor vital signs frequently because bleeding in fractured bones and surrounding tissues may cause shock. Also monitor the neurovascular status of the fractured limb by assessing skin color and checking for numbness in the fingers or toes. Numbness or paralysis distal to the injury indicates pressure on nerves. (See *Assessing neurovascular status*.)
- Transport the patient to a hospital as soon as possible. Apply ice to the injury. Regardless of the apparent extent of the injury, don't allow the patient to eat or drink anything until the physician evaluates him.
- Indications for removing a splint include evidence of improper application or vascular impairment. Apply gentle traction, and remove the splint carefully under a physician's direct supervision.

ASSESSMENT TIP

Assessing neurovascular status

When assessing an injured extremity, include the following steps and compare your findings bilaterally:

- Inspect the color of fingers or toes.
- To detect edema, note the size of the digits.
- Simultaneously touch the digits of the affected and unaffected extremities and compare temperature.
- Check capillary refill by pressing on the distal tip of one digit until it's white. Then release the pressure, and note how soon the normal color returns. It should return quickly in both the affected and unaffected extremities.
- Check sensation by touching the fingers or toes and asking the patient how they feel. Note reports of any numbness or tingling.
- To check proprioception, tell the patient to close his eyes; then move one digit and ask him which position it's in.
- To test movement, tell the patient to wiggle his toes or move his fingers.
- Palpate the distal pulses to assess vascular patency.

Record your findings for the affected and the unaffected extremities, using standard terminology to avoid ambiguity. Warmth, free movement, rapid capillary refill, and normal color, sensation, and proprioception indicate sound neurovascular status.

Complications

- Fat embolism, indicated by shortness of breath, agitation, and irrational behavior caused by multiple transfers and repeated manipulation of a fracture; usually occurring 24 to 72 hours after injury or manipulation

Documentation

Record the circumstances and cause of the injury. Document the patient's complaints, noting whether the symptoms are localized. Record the patient's neurovascular status before and after applying the splint. Note the type of wound and the amount and type of drainage, if any. Document the time of splint application. If the bone end should slip into surrounding tissue or if transporting causes any change in the degree of dislocation, be sure to note it.

Sputum collection

Secreted by mucous membranes lining the bronchioles, bronchi, and trachea, sputum helps protect the respiratory tract from infection. When expelled from the respiratory tract, sputum carries saliva, nasal and sinus secretions, dead cells, and normal oral bacteria from the respiratory tract. Sputum specimens may be cultured for identification of respiratory pathogens.

The usual method of sputum specimen collection—expectoration—may require ultrasonic nebulization, hydration, or chest percussion and postural drainage. Less common methods include tracheal suctioning and, rarely, bronchoscopy. Tracheal suctioning is contraindicated within 1 hour of eating and in patients with esophageal varices, nausea, facial or basilar skull fractures, laryngospasm, or bronchospasm. It should be performed cautiously in patients with heart disease because it may precipitate arrhythmias.

Equipment

Expectoration

Sterile specimen container with tight-fitting cap ♦ gloves ♦ label ♦ laboratory request form and laboratory biohazard transport bag ♦ aerosol (10% sodium chloride, propylene glycol, acetylcysteine, or sterile or distilled water) as ordered ♦ facial tissues ♦ emesis basin

Tracheal suctioning

#12 to #14 French sterile suction catheter ♦ water-soluble lubricant ♦ laboratory request form and laboratory biohazard transport bag ♦ sterile gloves ♦ mask ♦ goggles ♦ sterile in-line specimen trap (Lukens trap) ♦ normal saline solution ♦ portable suction machine, if wall unit is unavailable ♦ oxygen therapy equipment ♦ optional: nasal airway, to obtain a nasotracheal specimen with suctioning

Commercial suction kits have all equipment except the suction machine and an in-line specimen container.

Preparation

- Equipment and preparation depend on the method of collection.
- Gather the appropriate equipment for the task.

Key steps

- Confirm the patient's identity using two patient identifiers according to facility policy.
- Tell the patient that you'll collect a specimen of sputum (not saliva), and explain the procedure to promote cooperation.
- If possible, collect the specimen early in the morning, before breakfast, to obtain an overnight accumulation of secretions.

Collection by expectoration

- Instruct the patient to sit in a chair or at the edge of the bed. If he can't sit up, place him in high Fowler's position.
- Put on gloves.
- Ask the patient to rinse his mouth with water to reduce specimen contamination. (Avoid mouthwash or toothpaste because they may affect the mobility of organisms in the sputum sample.) Then tell him to cough deeply and expectorate directly into the specimen container. Ask him to produce at least 15 ml of sputum, if possible.
- Cap the container and, if necessary, clean its exterior. Remove and discard your gloves, and wash your hands thoroughly. Label the container with the patient's name and room number, practitioner's name, date and time of collection, and initial diagnosis. Also include on the laboratory request form whether the patient was febrile or taking antibiotics and whether sputum was induced (because such specimens commonly appear watery and may resemble saliva). Send the specimen to the laboratory immediately in a laboratory biohazard transport bag.

Collection by tracheal suctioning

- If the patient can't produce an adequate specimen by coughing, prepare to suction him to obtain the specimen. Explain the suctioning procedure to him, and tell him that he may cough, gag, or feel short of breath during the procedure.
- Check the suction machine to make sure it's functioning properly. Then place the patient in high Fowler's or semi-Fowler's position.
- Administer oxygen to the patient before beginning the procedure.
- Wash your hands thoroughly.
- Put on sterile gloves. Consider one hand sterile and the other hand clean to prevent cross-contamination.
- Connect the suction tubing to the male adapter of the in-line specimen trap. Attach the sterile suction catheter to the rubber tubing of the trap. (See *Attaching a specimen trap to a suction catheter.*)
- Position a mask and goggles over your face. Tell the patient to tilt his head back slightly. Then lubricate the catheter with normal saline solution, and gently pass it through the patient's nostril without suction.
- When the catheter reaches the larynx, the patient will cough. As he does, quickly advance the catheter into the trachea. Tell him to take several deep breaths through his mouth to ease insertion.
- To obtain the specimen, apply suction for 5 to 10 seconds but never longer than 15 seconds because prolonged suction can cause hypoxia. If the procedure must be repeated, let the patient rest for four to six breaths. When collection is completed, discontinue the suction, gently remove the catheter, and administer oxygen.
- Detach the catheter from the in-line trap, gather it up in your dominant hand, and pull the glove cuff inside out and down around the used catheter to enclose it for

Attaching a specimen trap to a suction catheter

Wearing gloves, push the suction tubing onto the male adapter of the in-line trap.

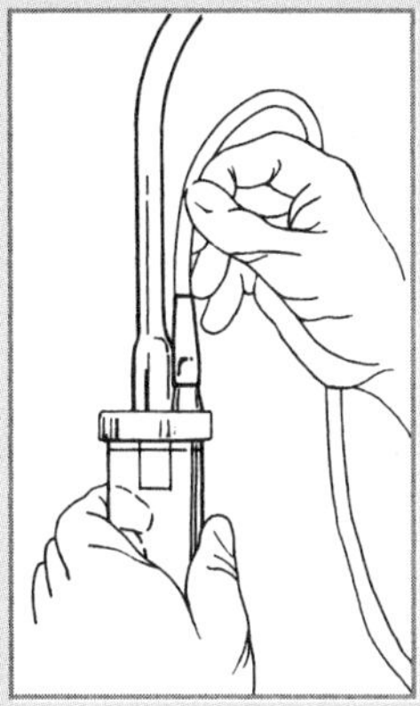

Insert the suction catheter into the rubber tubing of the trap.

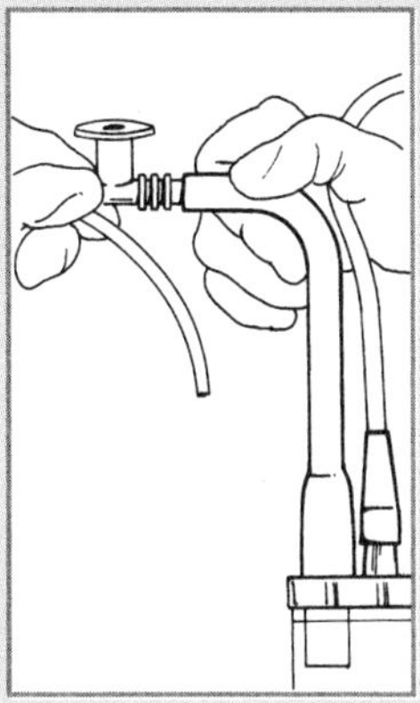

After suctioning, disconnect the in-line trap from the suction tubing and catheter. To seal the container, connect the rubber tubing to the male adapter of the trap.

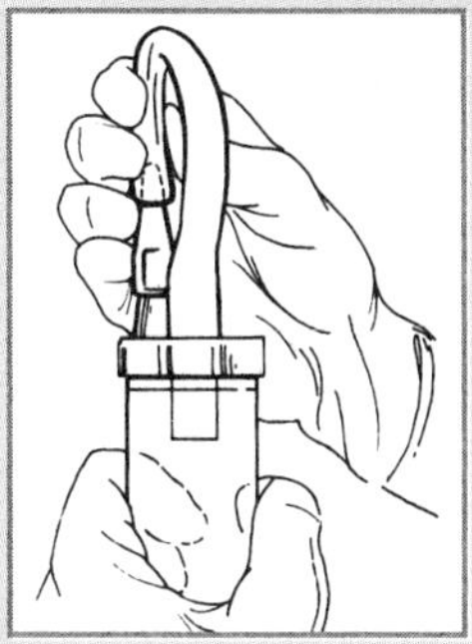

disposal. Remove and discard the other glove and your mask and goggles.

- Detach the trap from the tubing connected to the suction machine. Seal the trap tightly by connecting the rubber tubing to the male adapter of the trap. Examine the specimen to make sure it's actually sputum, not saliva. Label the trap's container as an expectorated specimen, place in a laboratory biohazard transport bag, and send it to the laboratory immediately with a completed laboratory request form.
- Offer the patient a glass of water or mouthwash.

Special considerations

- If you can't obtain a sputum specimen through tracheal suctioning, perform chest percussion to loosen and mobilize secretions, and position the patient for optimal drainage. After 20 to 30 minutes, repeat the tracheal suctioning procedure.
- Before sending the specimen to the laboratory, examine it to make sure it's actually sputum, not saliva, because saliva will produce inaccurate test results.
- Because expectorated sputum is contaminated by normal mouth flora, tracheal suctioning provides a more reliable specimen for diagnosis.

ACTION STAT!

If the patient becomes hypoxic or cyanotic during suctioning, remove the catheter immediately and administer oxygen.

- If the patient has asthma or chronic bronchitis, watch for aggravated bronchospasms with the use of more than a 10% concentration of sodium chloride or acetylcysteine in an aerosol. If he's suspected of having tuberculosis, don't use more than 20% propylene glycol with water when inducing a sputum specimen because a higher concentration inhibits growth of the pathogen and causes erroneous test results. If propylene glycol isn't available, use 10% to 20% acetylcysteine with water or sodium chloride.

Complications

- Arrhythmias during the procedure as a result of coughing, especially when the specimen is obtained by suctioning, in the patient with cardiac disease
- Tracheal trauma or bleeding, vomiting, aspiration, and hypoxemia

Documentation

In your notes, record the collection method used, time and date of collection, how the patient tolerated the procedure, color and consistency of the specimen, and its proper disposition.

Standard precautions

Standard precautions were developed by the Centers for Disease Control and Prevention (CDC) to provide the broadest possible protection against the transmission of infection. The CDC recommends that health care workers handle blood, body fluids (including secretions, excretions, and drainage), tissues, and contact with mucous membranes and broken skin as if they contain infectious agents, regardless of the patient's diagnosis.

Standard precautions encompass much of the isolation precautions previously recommended by the CDC for patients with known or suspected blood-borne pathogens as well as the precautions previously known as body substance isolation. These precautions are to be used in conjunction with the airborne, contact, and droplet precautions.

Standard precautions include wearing gloves for known or anticipated contact with blood, body fluids, tissue, mucous membrane, and nonintact skin. (See *Choosing the right glove*.) If the task or procedure being performed may result in splashing or splattering of blood or body fluids to the face, a mask and goggles or face shield should be worn. If the task or procedure being performed may result in splashing or splattering of blood or body fluids to the body, a fluid-resistant gown or apron should be worn. Additional protective clothing, such as shoe covers, may be appropriate to protect the caregiver's feet in situations that may expose him to large amounts of blood or body fluids (or both) such as care of a trauma patient in the operating room or emergency department.

Equipment

Gloves ♦ masks ♦ goggles, glasses, or face shields ♦ gowns or aprons ♦ resuscitation bag ♦ bags for specimens ♦ Environmental Protection Agency (EPA)–registered tuberculocidal disinfectant or diluted bleach solution (diluted between 1:10 and 1:100, mixed fresh daily), or both, or EPA-registered disinfectant labeled effective against hepatitis B virus (HBV) and human immunodeficiency virus (HIV)

Key steps

- Wash your hands immediately if they become contaminated with blood or body fluids, excretions, secretions, or drainage; wash your hands before and after patient care and after removing gloves. Hand hygiene removes microorganisms from your skin.
- Wear gloves if you will or could come in contact with blood, specimens, tissue, body fluids, secretions or excretions, mucous membranes, broken skin, or contaminated surfaces or objects.
- Change your gloves and wash your hands between patient contacts to avoid cross-contamination.
- Wear a fluid-resistant gown, a mask, goggles and, if necessary, a face shield (for added protection) during procedures, such as surgery, endoscopic procedures, dialysis, assisting with intubation or manipulation of arterial lines, or other procedure with the potential for splashing or splattering body fluids.
- Handle used needles and other sharp instruments carefully. Don't bend, break, reinsert them into their original sheaths, remove needles from syringes, or unnecessarily handle them. Discard them intact immediately after use into a puncture-resistant disposal box. Use tools to pick up broken glass or other sharp objects. These measures reduce the risk of accidental injury or infection.
- Immediately notify your employer's health care provider of needle-stick or other sharp-object injuries, mucosal

Choosing the right glove

Health care workers may develop allergic reactions as a result of their exposure to latex gloves and other products containing natural rubber latex. Patients may also have latex sensitivity. Take the following steps to protect yourself and your patient from allergic reactions to natural rubber latex.

- Use nonlatex (for example, vinyl or synthetic) gloves for activities that aren't likely to involve contact with infectious materials (such as food preparation and routine cleaning).
- Use appropriate barrier protection when handling infectious materials. If you choose latex gloves, use powder-free gloves with reduced protein content.
- After wearing and removing gloves, wash your hands with soap, and dry them thoroughly.
- When wearing latex gloves, don't use oil-based hand creams or lotions (which can cause gloves to deteriorate) unless they've been shown to maintain glove-barrier protection.
- Refer to the material safety data sheet for the appropriate glove to wear when handling chemicals.
- Learn procedures for preventing latex allergy, and learn how to recognize symptoms of latex allergy, such as skin rashes, hives, flushing, itching, asthma, shock, and nasal, eye, or sinus symptoms.
- If you have (or suspect you have) a latex sensitivity, use nonlatex gloves, avoid contact with latex gloves and other latex-containing products, and consult a physician experienced in treating latex allergy.

For latex allergy

If you have a latex allergy, consider these precautions:

- Avoid contact with latex gloves and other products containing latex.
- Avoid areas where you might inhale the powder from latex gloves worn by other workers.
- Tell your employers and your health care providers (physicians, nurses, dentists, and others).
- Wear a medical identification bracelet.
- Follow your physician's instructions for dealing with allergic reactions to latex.

splashes, or contamination of open wounds or nonintact skin with blood or body fluids to allow investigation of the incident and appropriate care and documentation.

- Properly label specimens collected from patients, and place them in plastic bags at the collection site. Attach requisition slips to the outside of the bags.
- Place items—such as nondisposable utensils or instruments—that have come in direct contact with the patient's secretions, excretions, blood, drainage, or body fluids in a single impervious bag or container before removal from the room. Place linens and trash in single bags of sufficient thickness to contain the contents.
- While wearing the appropriate personal protective equipment (PPE), promptly clean blood and body-fluid spills with detergent and water followed by an EPA-registered tuberculocidal disinfectant or diluted bleach solution (diluted between 1:10 and 1:100, mixed daily), or both, or an EPA-registered disinfectant labeled effective against HBV and HIV, provided that the surface hasn't been contaminated with an agent—or volumes of or concentrations of—agents for which higher-level disinfection is recommended.
- Disposable food trays and dishes aren't necessary.
- If you have an exudative lesion, avoid direct patient contact until the condition has resolved and you've been cleared by your employer's health care provider.
- If you have dermatitis or other conditions resulting in broken skin on your hands, avoid situations where you may have contact with blood and body fluids

(even though gloves could be worn) until the condition has resolved and you've been cleared by your employer's health care provider.

Special considerations

- Standard precautions, such as hand hygiene and appropriate use of PPE, should be routine infection-control practices.
- Keep mouthpieces, resuscitation bags, and other ventilation devices nearby to minimize the need for emergency mouth-to-mouth resuscitation, thus reducing the risk of exposure to body fluids.

ALERT

Because you may not always know what organisms may be present in every clinical situation, you must use standard precautions for every contact with blood, body fluids, secretions, excretions, drainage, mucous membranes, and nonintact skin. Use your judgment in individual cases about whether to implement additional isolation precautions, such as airborne, droplet, or contact precautions, or a combination of precautions. What's more, if your work requires you to be exposed to blood, you should receive the HBV vaccine series.

Complications

- Exposure to blood-borne diseases or other infections and the complications they may cause

Documentation

Record special needs for isolation precautions on the nursing care plan and as otherwise indicated by your facility.

Stool collection

Stools are collected to determine the presence of blood, ova and parasites, bile, fat, pathogens, or substances such as ingested drugs. Gross examination of stool characteristics, including color, consistency, and odor, can reveal such conditions as GI bleeding and steatorrhea.

Stool specimens are collected randomly or for specific periods, such as 72 hours. Because stool specimens can't be obtained on demand, proper collection requires careful instructions to the patient to ensure an uncontaminated specimen.

Equipment

Specimen container with lid ♦ gloves ♦ two tongue blades ♦ paper towel or paper bag ♦ bedpan or portable commode ♦ two patient-care reminders (for timed specimens) ♦ laboratory request form and laboratory biohazard transport bag

Key steps

- Explain the procedure to the patient, and his family if necessary, to ensure cooperation and prevent inadvertent disposal of timed stool specimens.

Collecting a random specimen

- Tell the patient to notify you when he has the urge to defecate. Have him defecate into a clean, dry bedpan or commode. Instruct him not to contaminate the specimen with urine or toilet tissue because urine inhibits fecal bacterial growth and toilet tissue contains bismuth, which interferes with test results.
- Put on gloves.
- Using a tongue blade, transfer the most representative stool specimen from the bedpan to the container, and cap the container. If the patient passes blood, mucus, or pus with stools, be sure to include this with the specimen.
- Wrap the tongue blade in a paper towel, and discard it. Remove and discard your gloves, and wash your hands thoroughly to prevent cross-contamination.

Collecting a timed specimen

- Place a patient-care reminder stating SAVE ALL STOOL over the patient's bed and in his bathroom.
- After putting on gloves, collect the first specimen, and include this in the total specimen.
- Obtain the timed specimen as you would a random specimen, but remember to transfer all stools to the specimen container.

- If stools must be obtained with an enema, use only tap water or normal saline solution.
- As ordered, send each specimen to the laboratory immediately with a laboratory request form or, if permitted, refrigerate the specimens collected during the test period, and send them when collection is complete. All specimens must be stored and transported in an approved laboratory biohazard container. Remove and discard your gloves.
- Make sure the patient is comfortable after the procedure and that he has the opportunity to thoroughly clean his hands and perianal area. Perineal care may be necessary for some patients.

Special considerations

- Never place a stool specimen in a refrigerator that contains food or medication to prevent contamination.
- Notify the practitioner if the stool specimen looks unusual.

Complications

- None known

Patient teaching

- If the patient is to collect a specimen at home, instruct him to collect it in a clean container with a tight-fitting lid, to wrap the container in a brown paper bag, and to keep it in the refrigerator (separate from any food items) until it can be transported.

Documentation

Record the time of specimen collection and its transport to the laboratory. Note stool color, odor, and consistency, and unusual characteristics; also note whether the patient had difficulty passing stools.

ST-segment monitoring

A sensitive indicator of myocardial damage, the ST segment is normally flat or isoelectric. A depressed ST segment may result from cardiac glycosides, myocardial ischemia, or a subendocardial infarction. An elevated ST segment suggests myocardial infarction.

Continuous ST-segment monitoring is helpful for patients with acute coronary syndromes and for those who have received thrombolytic therapy or have undergone coronary angioplasty. ST-segment monitoring allows early detection of reocclusion. It's also useful for patients who have had previous episodes of cardiac ischemia without chest pain, those who have difficulty distinguishing between cardiac pain and pain from other sources, and for those who have difficulty communicating. ST-segment monitoring gives the health care provider the ability to identify and reverse ischemia by starting early interventions.

Because ischemia typically occurs in a single area of the heart muscle, some electrocardiogram (ECG) leads can't detect it. Select the most appropriate lead by examining ECG tracings obtained during an ischemic episode. Use the leads that show ischemia for ST-segment monitoring.

Equipment

ECG electrodes ♦ gauze pads ♦ ECG monitor cable ♦ leadwires ♦ alcohol pads ♦ cardiac monitor programmed for ST-segment monitoring ♦ gloves

Preparation

- Plug the cardiac monitor into an electrical outlet, and turn it on to warm up while you prepare the equipment and the patient.

Key steps

- Bring the equipment to the patient's bedside, and explain the procedure to him. Provide privacy. Wash your hands and follow standard precautions. If the patient isn't already on a monitor, turn on the device and attach the cable.
- Select the sites for electrode placement, and prepare the patient's skin for attachment as you would for continuous cardiac monitoring or a 12-lead ECG. Attach the leadwires to the electrodes, and position the electrodes on the patient's skin in the appropriate positions.

Understanding changes in the ST segment

Closely monitoring the ST segment can help detect ischemia or injury before an infarction develops.

ST-segment elevation

An ST segment is considered elevated when it's 1 mm or more above the baseline. An elevated ST segment may indicate myocardial injury.

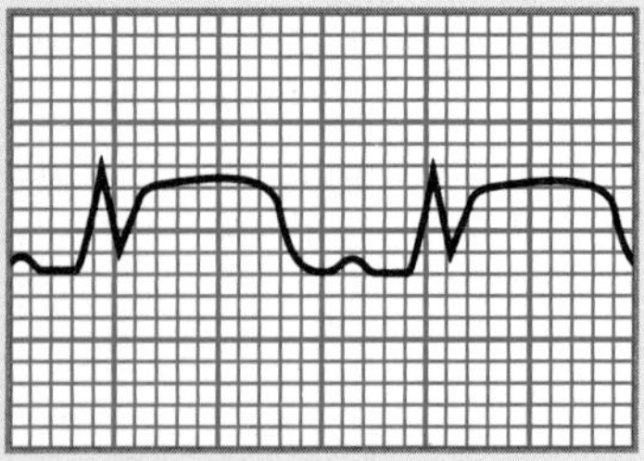

ST-segment depression

An ST segment is considered depressed when it's 0.5 mm or more below the baseline. A depressed ST segment may indicate myocardial ischemia or digoxin toxicity.

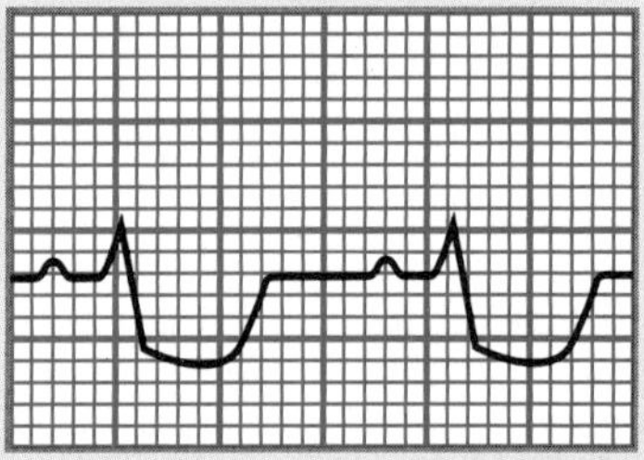

- Activate ST-segment monitoring by pressing the MONITORING PROCEDURES key and then the ST key. Activate individual ST parameters by pressing the ON/OFF parameter key.
- Select the appropriate ECG for each ST channel to be monitored by pressing the PARAMETERS key and then the key labeled ECG.
- Press the key labeled CHANGE LEAD to select the appropriate lead. Repeat this for all 3 channels.
- Adjust the ST-segment measurement points if necessary; adjust baseline for ST segment by pressing the ISO POINT key to move the cursor to the PQ or TP interval.
- Adjust the J point by pressing the key labeled J POINT to move the cursor to the appropriate location.
- Adjust the ST point to 80 msec after the J point. Check your facility's policy for measuring the ST point. Some facilities recommend using 60 msec instead of 80 msec.
- Set the alarm limits for each ST-segment parameter by manipulating the high and low limit keys.
- Press the key labeled STANDARD DISPLAY to return to the display screen.
- Assess the waveform shown on the monitor.

Special considerations

- Be sure to abrade the patient's skin gently to ensure electrode adhesion and promote electrical conductivity.
- If monitoring only one lead, choose the lead most likely to show arrhythmias and ST-segment changes.

ALERT

Always give precedence to the lead that shows arrhythmias.

- Verify limit parameters for the patient with the practitioner. Typically, when a limit is surpassed for more than 1 minute, visual and audible alarms are activated.
- If the patient isn't being monitored continuously, remove the electrodes, clean the skin, and disconnect the leadwires from the electrodes.
- Evaluate the monitor for ST-segment depression or elevation. (See *Understanding changes in the ST segment*.)

Complications
- None known

Documentation
Document the leads being monitored and the ST measurement points in the patient's medical record.

Stump and prosthesis care

Patient care immediately after limb amputation includes wound healing, pain control, reducing edema, and stump shaping and conditioning. Postoperative care of the stump will vary slightly, depending on the amputation site (arm or leg) and the type of dressing applied to the stump (elastic bandage or plaster cast).

After the stump heals, it requires only routine daily care, such as proper hygiene and continued muscle-strengthening exercises. The prosthesis—when in use—also requires daily care. Typically, a plastic prosthesis, the most common type, must be cleaned and lubricated and checked for proper fit. As the patient recovers from the physical and psychological trauma of amputation, he'll need to learn correct procedures for routine daily care of the stump and the prosthesis.

Equipment
Postoperative stump care
Pressure dressing ♦ abdominal (ABD) pad ♦ suction equipment if ordered ♦ overhead trapeze ♦ 1″ adhesive tape, bandage clips or safety pins ♦ sandbags or trochanter roll (for a leg) ♦ elastic stump shrinker or 4″ elastic bandage ♦ tourniquet (optional; as last resort to control bleeding)

Stump and prosthesis care
Mild soap or alcohol pads ♦ stump socks or athletic tube socks ♦ two washcloths ♦ two towels ♦ appropriate lubricating oil

Key steps
- Confirm the patient's identity using two patient identifiers according to facility policy.
- Perform routine postoperative care. Frequently assess the patient's respiratory status and level of consciousness, monitor his vital signs and I.V. infusions, check tube patency, and provide for his comfort and safety.

Monitoring stump drainage
- Because gravity causes fluid to accumulate at the stump, frequently check the amount of blood and drainage on the dressing. Notify the practitioner if accumulations of drainage or blood increase rapidly. If excessive bleeding occurs, notify the practitioner immediately, and apply a pressure dressing or compress the appropriate pressure points. If this doesn't control bleeding, use a tourniquet only as a last resort. Keep a tourniquet available.
- Tape the ABD pad over the moist part of the dressing as necessary. This provides a dry area to help prevent bacterial infection.
- Monitor the suction drainage equipment, and note the amount and type of drainage.

Positioning the extremity
- Elevate the extremity for the first 24 hours to reduce swelling and promote venous return.
- To prevent contractures, position an arm with the elbow extended and the shoulder abducted.
- To correctly position a leg, elevate the foot of the bed slightly, and place sandbags or a trochanter roll against the hip to prevent external rotation.

DO'S & DON'TS

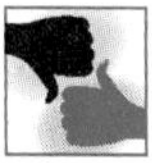

Don't place a pillow under the stump for an extended period because this may lead to the development of contractures.

- After a below-the-knee amputation, maintain knee extension to prevent hamstring muscle contractures.
- After a leg amputation, place the patient on a firm surface in the prone position for at least 2 hours per day, with his legs close together and without pillows under his stomach, hips, knees, or stump, unless this position is contraindicated. This position helps prevent hip flexion, contractures,

and abduction; it also stretches the flexor muscles.

Assisting with prescribed exercises

- After arm amputation, encourage the patient to exercise the remaining arm to prevent muscle contractures. Help the patient perform isometric and range-of-motion (ROM) exercises for both shoulders, as prescribed by the physical therapist, because use of the prosthesis requires both shoulders.
- After leg amputation, stand behind the patient and, if necessary, support him with your hands at his waist during balancing exercises.
- Instruct the patient to exercise the affected and unaffected limbs to maintain muscle tone and increase muscle strength. The patient with a leg amputation may perform push-ups as ordered (in the sitting position, arms at his sides), or pull-ups on the overhead trapeze to strengthen his arms, shoulders, and back in preparation for using crutches.

Wrapping and conditioning the stump

- If the patient doesn't have a rigid cast, apply an elastic stump shrinker to prevent edema and shape the limb in preparation for the prosthesis. Wrap the stump so that it narrows toward the distal end. This helps to ensure comfort when the patient wears the prosthesis.
- If an elastic stump shrinker isn't available, you can wrap the stump in a 4″ elastic bandage. To do this, stretch the bandage to about two-thirds its maximum length as you wrap it diagonally around the stump, with the greatest pressure distally. (Depending on the size of the leg, you may need to use two 4″ bandages.) Secure the bandage with clips, safety pins, or adhesive tape. Make sure that the bandage covers all portions of the stump smoothly because wrinkles or exposed areas encourage skin breakdown. (See *Wrapping a stump*.)
- The use of an immediate postoperative prosthesis has proved effective in decreasing the time until final prosthetic fitting.
- If the patient experiences throbbing after the stump is wrapped, the bandage may be too tight; remove the bandage immediately and reapply it less tightly. Throbbing indicates impaired circulation.
- Check the bandage regularly. Rewrap it when it begins to bunch up at the end (usually about every 12 hours for a moderately active patient) or as necessary.
- After removing the bandage to rewrap it, massage the stump gently, always pushing toward the suture line rather than away from it. This stimulates circulation and prevents scar tissue from adhering to the bone.
- When healing begins, instruct the patient to push the stump against a pillow. Have him progress gradually to pushing against harder surfaces, such as a padded chair and then a hard chair. These conditioning exercises will help the patient adjust to experiencing pressure and sensation in the stump.

DO'S & DON'TS

Avoid applying lotion to the stump because it may clog follicles, increasing the risk of infection. In addition, it's a desired goal of the healing process to toughen the area to tolerate the prosthesis.

Caring for the healed stump

- Bathe the stump but never shave it to prevent infection. If possible, bathe the stump at the end of the day because the warm water may cause swelling, making reapplication of the prosthesis difficult. Don't soak the stump for long periods.
- Rub the stump with alcohol daily to toughen the skin, reducing the risk of skin breakdown. (Avoid using powders or lotions because they can soften or irritate the skin.) Because alcohol may cause severe irritation in some patients, instruct the patient to watch for and report this sign.
- Inspect the stump for redness, swelling, irritation, and calluses. Report any of these to the practitioner. Following the first cast change, many surgeons will have the patient begin partial weight bearing if the wound appears stable.

Wrapping a stump

Proper stump care helps protect the limb, reduces swelling, and prepares the limb for a prosthesis. As you perform the procedure, teach it to the patient.

Start by obtaining two 4″ elastic bandages. Center the end of the first 4″ bandage at the top of the patient's thigh. Unroll the bandage downward over the stump and to the back of the leg (as shown below).

Make three figure-eight turns to adequately cover the ends of the stump. As you wrap, be sure to include the roll of flesh in the groin area. Use enough pressure to ensure that the stump narrows toward the end so that it fits comfortably into the prosthesis.

Use the second 4″ bandage to anchor the first bandage around the waist. For a below-the-knee amputation, use the knee to anchor the bandage in place. Secure the bandage with clips, safety pins, or adhesive tape. Check the stump bandage regularly, and rewrap it if it bunches at the end.

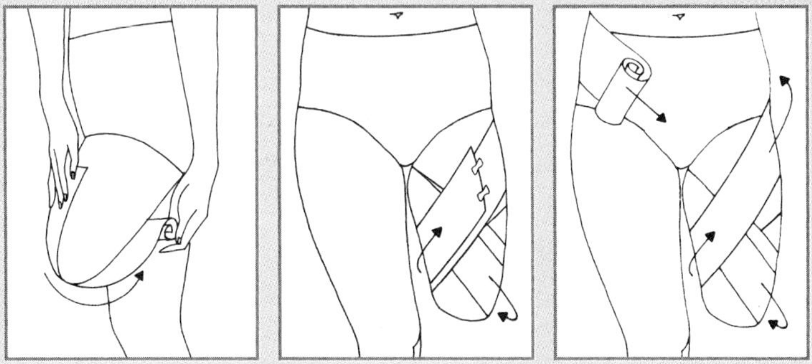

■ Continue muscle-strengthening exercises so that the patient can build the strength he'll need to control the prosthesis.
■ Change and wash the patient's elastic bandages every day to avoid exposing the skin to excessive perspiration, which can be irritating. Wash the elastic bandages in warm water and gentle nondetergent soap; lay them flat on a towel to dry. Machine washing or drying may shrink the elastic bandages. To shape the stump, have the patient wear an elastic bandage 24 hours per day except while bathing.

Caring for the plastic prosthesis

■ Wipe the plastic socket of the prosthesis with a damp cloth and mild soap or alcohol to prevent bacterial accumulation.
■ Wipe the insert (if the prosthesis has one) with a dry cloth.
■ Dry the prosthesis thoroughly; if possible, allow it to dry overnight.
■ Maintain and lubricate the prosthesis as instructed by the manufacturer.
■ Check for malfunctions, and adjust or repair the prosthesis as necessary to prevent further damage.
■ Check the condition of the shoe on a foot prosthesis frequently, and change it as necessary.

Applying the prosthesis

■ Apply a stump sock. Keep the seams away from bony prominences.
■ If the prosthesis has an insert, remove it from the socket, place it over the stump, and insert the stump into the prosthesis.
■ If it has no insert, merely slide the prosthesis over the stump. Secure the prosthe-

Caring for a severed body part

After traumatic amputation, a surgeon may be able to reimplant the severed body part through microsurgery. The chance of successful reimplantation is much greater if the amputated part has received proper care.

If a patient arrives at the hospital with a severed body part, first make sure that bleeding at the amputation site has been controlled. Then follow these guidelines for preserving the body part.

- Put on sterile gloves. Place several sterile gauze pads and an appropriate amount of sterile roller gauze in a sterile basin, and pour sterile normal saline or sterile lactated Ringer's solution over them. *Never* use another solution, and don't try to scrub or debride the part.
- Holding the body part in one gloved hand, carefully pat it dry with sterile gauze. Place saline-soaked gauze pads over the stump, and then wrap the whole body part with saline-soaked roller gauze. Wrap the gauze with a sterile towel if available. Then put this package in a watertight container or bag, and seal it.
- Fill another plastic bag with ice and water, and place the part, still in its watertight container, inside. Seal the outer bag. (Always protect the part from direct contact with ice and—*never* use dry ice—to prevent irreversible tissue damage, which would make the part unsuitable for reimplantation.) Keep the bag ice-cold until the surgeon is ready to perform the reimplantation surgery.
- Label the bag with the patient's name, identification number, identification of the amputated part, the hospital identification number, and the date and time when cooling began.

Note: The body part must be wrapped and cooled quickly. Irreversible tissue damage occurs after only 6 hours at ambient temperature. However, hypothermic management seldom preserves tissues for more than 24 hours.

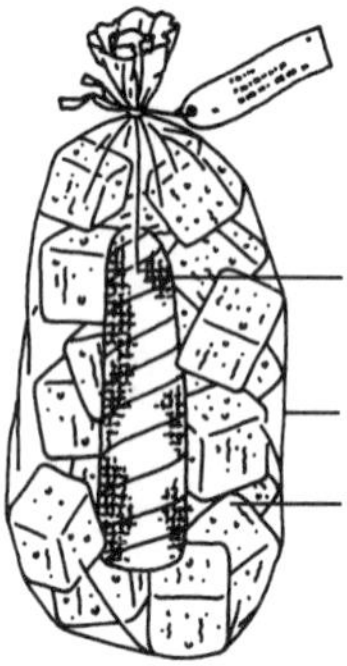

sis onto the stump according to the manufacturer's directions.

Special considerations

- If a patient arrives at the hospital with a traumatic amputation, the amputated part may be saved for possible reimplantation. (See *Caring for a severed body part.*)
- For a below-the-knee amputation, you may substitute an athletic tube sock for a stump sock by cutting off the elastic band. If the patient has a rigid plaster of Paris dressing, perform normal cast care. Check the cast frequently to make sure that it doesn't slip off. If it does, apply an elastic bandage immediately, and notify the practitioner because edema will develop rapidly.

Complications

- Postoperative complications including hemorrhage, stump infection, contractures, and a swollen or flabby stump
- After an amputation complications including skin breakdown or irritation from lack of ventilation; friction from an irritant in the prosthesis; a sebaceous cyst or boil from tight socks; psychological problems, such as denial, depression, or withdrawal; and phantom limb pain caused by stimulation of nerves that once carried sensations from the distal part of the extremity

Patient teaching

- Emphasize to the patient that proper care of his stump can speed healing.
- Tell him to inspect his stump carefully every day, using a mirror, and to continue proper daily stump care.
- Instruct him to call the practitioner if the incision appears to be opening, looks red or swollen, feels warm, is painful to touch, or is seeping drainage.
- Explain to the patient that a 10-lb (4.5-kg) change in body weight will alter his stump size and require a new prosthesis socket to ensure a correct fit.
- Tell the patient to massage the stump toward the suture line to mobilize the scar and prevent its adherence to bone.
- Advise him to avoid exposing the skin around the stump to excessive perspiration, which can be irritating. Tell him to change his elastic bandages or stump socks daily to avoid this.
- Tell the patient that he may experience twitching, spasms, or phantom limb pain as his stump muscles adjust to amputation. Advise him that he can decrease these symptoms with heat, massage, or gentle pressure. If his stump is sensitive to touch, tell him to rub it with a dry washcloth for 4 minutes three times per day.
- Inform the patient that exercising the remaining muscles in an amputated limb must begin the day after surgery. A physical therapist will direct these exercises. For example, arm exercises progress from isometrics to assisted ROM to active ROM. Leg exercises include rising from a chair, balancing on one leg, and ROM exercises of the knees and hips.
- Stress the importance of performing prescribed exercises to help minimize complications, maintain muscle strength and tone, prevent contractures, and promote independence. Stress the importance of positioning to prevent contractures and edema.

Documentation

Record the date, time, and specific procedures of postoperative care, including amount and type of drainage, condition of the dressing, need for dressing reinforcement, and appearance of the suture line and surrounding tissue. Note signs of skin irritation or infection, complications and the interventions taken, the patient's tolerance of exercises, and his psychological reaction to the amputation.

During routine daily care, document the date, time, type of care given, and condition of the skin and suture line, noting signs of irritation, such as redness or tenderness. Record the patient's progress in caring for the stump or prosthesis.

Subcutaneous injection

When injected into the adipose (fatty) tissues beneath the skin, a drug moves into the bloodstream more rapidly than if given by mouth. Subcutaneous (subQ) injection allows slower, more sustained drug administration than I.M. injection; it also causes minimal tissue trauma and carries little risk of striking large blood vessels and nerves.

Absorbed mainly through the capillaries, drugs recommended for subQ injection include nonirritating aqueous solutions and suspensions contained in 0.5 to 2 ml of fluid. Heparin and insulin, for example, are usually administered subQ. (Some patients with diabetes, however, may benefit from an insulin infusion pump.)

Drugs and solutions for subQ injection are injected through a relatively short needle, using meticulous sterile technique. The most common subQ injection sites are the outer aspect of the upper arm, anterior thigh, loose tissue of the lower abdomen, upper hips, buttocks, and upper back. (See *Locating subcutaneous injection sites,* page 486.) Injection is contraindicated in sites that are inflamed, edematous, scarred, or covered by a mole, birthmark, or other lesion. It may also be contraindicated in patients with impaired coagulation mechanisms.

Equipment

Prescribed medication ♦ patient's medication record and chart 25G to 27G ⅝″ or ½″ needle ♦ gloves ♦ 1- or 3-ml syringe

Locating subcutaneous injection sites

Subcutaneous (subQ) injection sites (as indicated by the dotted areas in the illustration below) include the fat pads on the abdomen, upper hips, upper back, and lateral upper arms and thighs. For subQ injections administered repeatedly, such as insulin, rotate sites. Choose one injection site in one area, move to a corresponding injection site in the next area, and so on.

When returning to an area, choose a new site in that area. Preferred injection sites for insulin are the arms, abdomen, thighs, and buttocks. The preferred injection site for heparin is the lower abdominal fat pad, just below the umbilicus.

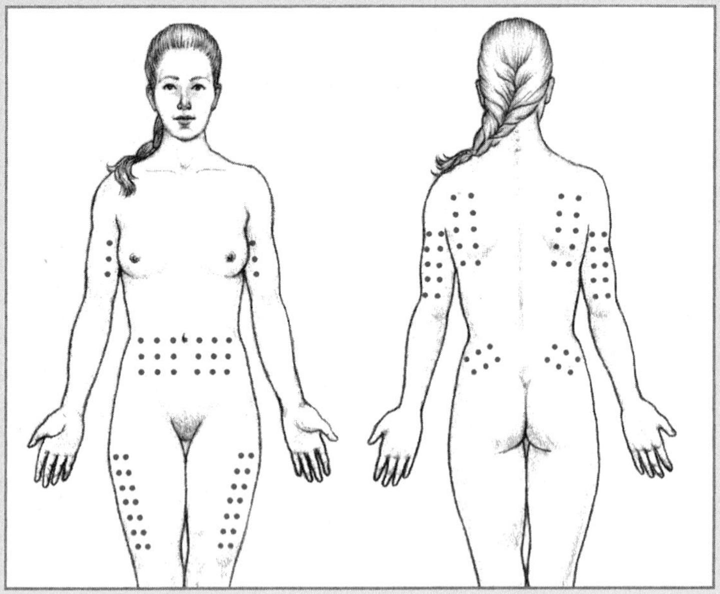

♦ alcohol pads ♦ 2″ × 2″ gauze pad ♦ filter needle ♦ insulin syringe ♦ insulin pump ♦ optional: antiseptic cleaning agent (see *Types of insulin infusion pumps*)

Preparation

- Verify the order on the patient's medication record by checking it against the prescriber's order. Also note whether the patient has any allergies, especially before the first dose.
- Inspect the medication to make sure it isn't abnormally discolored or cloudy and doesn't contain precipitates (unless the manufacturer's instructions allow it).
- Wash your hands. Choose equipment appropriate to the prescribed medication and injection site, and make sure it works properly.
- Check the medication label against the patient's medication record. Read the label again as you draw up the medication for injection.

Single-dose ampules

- Wrap an alcohol pad around the ampule's neck and snap off the top, directing the force away from your body.
- Attach a filter needle to the needle, and withdraw the medication, keeping the needle's bevel tip below the level of the solution.
- Tap the syringe to clear air from it. Cover the needle with the needle sheath.

Types of insulin infusion pumps

A subcutaneous insulin infusion pump provides continuous, long-term insulin therapy for patients with type 1 diabetes mellitus. Complications include infection at the injection site, catheter clogging, and insulin loss from loose reservoir-catheter connections. Insulin pumps work on either an open-loop or a closed-loop system.

Open-loop system

The open-loop pump (shown below) is used most commonly. It infuses insulin but can't respond to changes in the patient's serum glucose levels. These portable, self-contained, programmable insulin pumps are smaller and less obtrusive than ever—about the size of a credit card—and have fewer buttons.

The pump delivers insulin in small (basal) doses every few minutes and large (bolus) doses that the patient sets manually. The system consists of a reservoir containing the insulin syringe, a small pump, an infusion-rate selector that allows insulin release adjustments, a battery, and a plastic catheter with an attached needle leading from the syringe to the subcutaneous injection site. The needle is typically held in place with waterproof tape. The patient can wear the pump on his belt or in his pocket—practically anywhere as long as the infusion line has a clear path to the injection site.

The infusion-rate selector automatically releases about one-half the total daily insulin requirement. The patient releases the remainder in bolus doses before meals and snacks. He must change the syringe daily, and the needle, catheter, and injection site every other day.

Closed-loop system

The self-contained closed-loop system detects and responds to changing serum glucose levels. The typical closed-loop system includes a glucose sensor, a programmable computer, a power supply, a pump, and an insulin reservoir. The computer triggers continuous insulin delivery in appropriate amounts from the reservoir.

Nonneedle catheter system

In the nonneedle delivery system, a tiny plastic catheter is inserted into the skin over a needle using a special insertion device (shown below). The needle is then withdrawn, leaving the catheter in place (shown in inset). This catheter can be placed in the abdomen, thigh, or flank and should be changed every 2 to 3 days.

Close-up of open-loop infusion pump

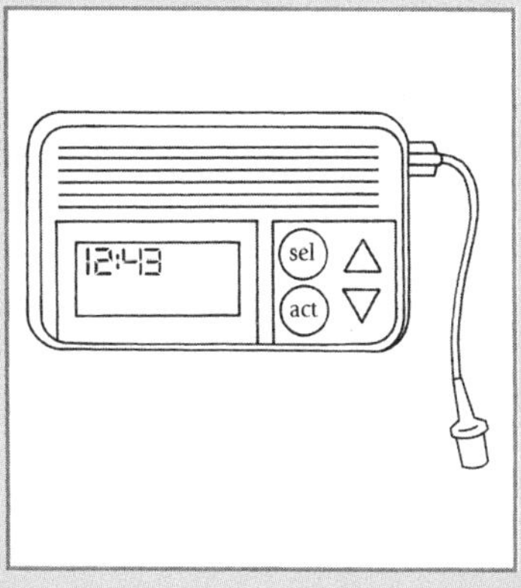

Nonneedle catheter insertion system

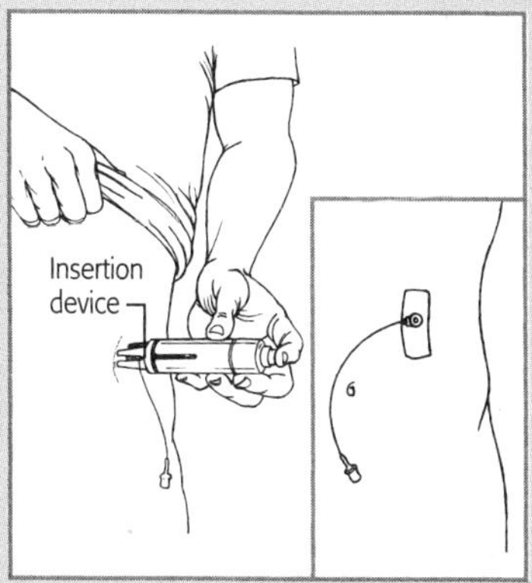

- Before discarding the ampule, check the medication label against the patient's medication record.
- Discard the filter needle and the ampule.
- Attach the appropriate needle to the syringe.

Single-dose or multidose vials

- Reconstitute powdered drugs according to instructions.
- Make sure all crystals have dissolved in the solution.
- Warm the vial by rolling it between your palms to help the drug dissolve faster.
- Clean the vial's rubber stopper with an alcohol pad. Pull the syringe plunger back until the volume of air in the syringe equals the volume of drug to be withdrawn from the vial.
- Without inverting the vial, insert the needle into the vial. Inject the air, invert the vial, and keep the needle's bevel tip below the level of the solution as you withdraw the prescribed amount of medication.
- Cover the needle with the needle sheath. Tap the syringe to clear any air from it.
- Check the medication label against the patient's medication record before discarding the single-dose vial or returning the multidose vial to the shelf.

Key steps

- Confirm the patient's identity using two patient identifiers according to facility policy.
- If your facility uses a bar code scanning system, be sure to scan your ID badge, the patient's ID bracelet, and the medication's bar code.
- Explain the procedure to the patient, and provide privacy.
- Select an appropriate injection site. Rotate sites according to a schedule for repeated injections, using different areas of the body unless contraindicated. (Heparin, for example, should be injected only in the abdomen if possible.)
- Put on gloves.
- Position and drape the patient if necessary.
- Clean the injection site with an alcohol pad, beginning at the center of the site and moving outward in a circular motion. Allow the skin to dry before injecting the drug to avoid a stinging sensation from introducing alcohol into subcutaneous tissues.
- Loosen the protective needle sheath.
- With your nondominant hand, grasp the skin around the injection site firmly to elevate the subcutaneous tissue, forming a 1″ (2.5 cm) fat fold.
- Holding the syringe in your dominant hand, insert the loosened needle sheath between the fourth and fifth fingers of your other hand while still pinching the skin around the injection site. Pull back the syringe with your dominant hand to uncover the needle by grasping the syringe like a pencil. Don't touch the needle.
- Position the needle with its bevel up.
- Tell the patient he'll feel a needle prick.
- Insert the needle quickly in one motion at a 45- or 90-degree angle. (See *Technique for subcutaneous injection*.) Release the patient's skin to avoid injecting the drug into compressed tissue and irritating nerve fibers.
- Pull back the plunger slightly to check for blood return. If none appears, begin injecting the drug slowly. If blood appears on aspiration, withdraw the needle, prepare another syringe, and repeat the procedure.

DO'S & DON'TS

Don't aspirate for blood return when giving insulin or heparin. It isn't necessary with insulin and may cause a hematoma with heparin.

- After injection, remove the needle gently but quickly at the same angle used for insertion.
- Cover the site with an alcohol pad or a 2″ × 2″ gauze pad, and massage the site gently (unless contraindicated, as with heparin and insulin) to distribute the drug and facilitate absorption.
- Remove the alcohol pad, and check the injection site for bleeding and bruising.
- Dispose of injection equipment according to facility policy. To avoid needle-stick injuries, don't resheath the needle.

Special considerations

- When using prefilled syringes, adjust the angle and depth of insertion according to needle length.

Insulin injections

- To establish more consistent blood insulin levels, rotate insulin injection sites within anatomic regions. Preferred insulin injection sites are the arms, abdomen, thighs, and buttocks.
- Make sure the type of insulin, unit dosage, and syringe are correct.
- When combining insulins in a syringe, make sure they're compatible. Regular insulin can be mixed with all other types. Prompt insulin zinc suspension (Semilente insulin) can't be mixed with NPH insulin. Follow facility policy regarding which insulin to draw up first.
- Before drawing up insulin suspension, gently roll and invert the bottle. Don't shake the bottle because this can cause foam or bubbles to develop in the syringe.

Heparin injections

- The preferred site for a heparin injection is the lower abdominal fat pad, 2″ (5 cm) beneath the umbilicus, between the right and left iliac crests. Injecting heparin into this area, which isn't involved in muscle activity, reduces the risk of local capillary bleeding. Always rotate the sites from one side to the other.
- Inject the drug slowly into the fat pad. Leave the needle in place for 10 seconds after injection; then withdraw it.
- Don't administer an injection within 2″ of a scar, a bruise, or the umbilicus.
- Don't aspirate to check for blood return because this can cause bleeding into the tissues at the site.
- Don't rub or massage the site after the injection. Rubbing can cause localized minute hemorrhages or bruises.
- If the patient bruises easily, apply ice to the site for the first 5 minutes after the injection to minimize local hemorrhage, and then apply pressure.

Complications

- Sterile abscesses forming caused by concentrated or irritating solutions
- Lipodystrophy caused by repeated injections in the same site

Patient teaching

- If the patient will be administering subQ injections at home, show him the correct technique and have him do a return demonstration.

Documentation

Record the time and date of the injection, medication and dose administered, injection site and route, and the patient's reaction.

Technique for subcutaneous injection

Before giving the injection, elevate the subcutaneous tissue at the site by grasping it firmly.

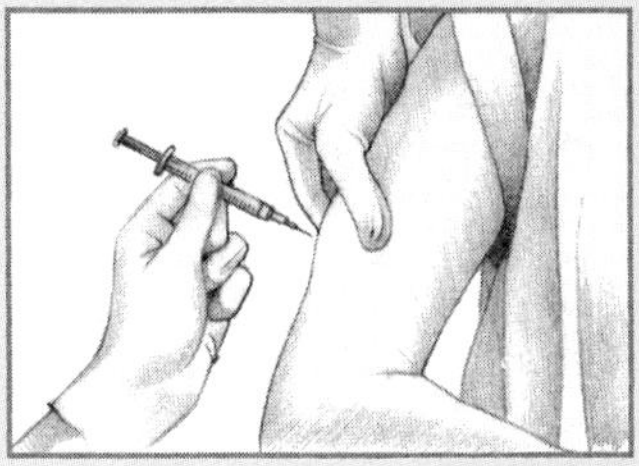

Insert the needle at a 45- or 90-degree angle to the skin surface, depending on needle length and the amount of subcutaneous tissue at the site. Some medications, such as heparin, should always be injected at a 90-degree angle.

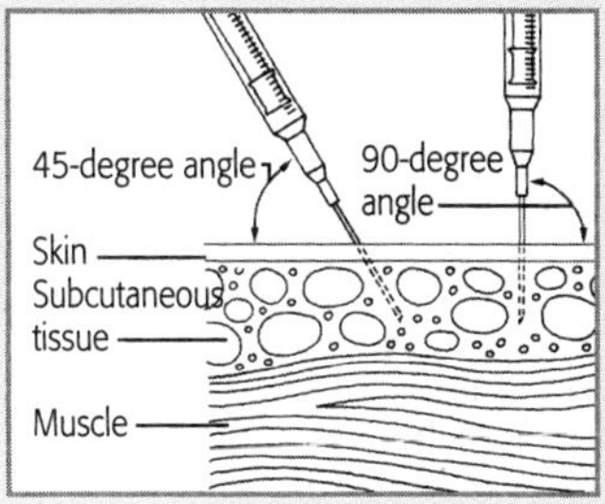

Surgical site verification

Wrong site surgery is a general term referring to a surgical procedure performed on the wrong body part or side of the body, or even on the wrong patient. This error may occur in the operating room or in other settings, such as in ambulatory care or interventional radiology.

Several factors that may contribute to an increased risk of wrong site surgery include inadequate patient assessment, inadequate medical review, inaccurate communication among health care team members, multiple surgeons involved in the procedure, failure to include the patient in the site verification process, and relying solely on the practitioner for surgical site verification.

Because serious consequences can result from wrong site surgery, the nurse must confirm that the correct site has been verified before surgery begins.

Equipment

Surgical consent form ♦ medical record ♦ procedure schedule ♦ hypoallergenic, nonlatex permanent marker

Key steps

- Confirm the patient's identity using two patient identifiers according to facility policy.
- Before the surgical procedure, check the patient's chart for documentation, and compare the information using the medical history and physical examination form, nursing assessment, preprocedure verification checklist, signed surgical consent form with exact procedure site verified, surgical procedure scheduled, and the patient's verbal communication of the correct site.
- After verbally confirming the site with the patient, the surgeon performing the procedure or another member of the surgical team who's fully informed about the patient and the intended procedure marks the site with a permanent marker. The mark needs to be placed so that it's visible after the patient has been prepped and draped.
- Make sure that the surgical team (surgeon, operating room or procedure staff, and anesthesia personnel) identifies the patient and verifies the correct procedure and correct site before beginning the surgery.

Special considerations

- If the patient's condition prevents him from verifying the correct site, the surgeon will identify and mark the site using the medical history and physical examination forms, signed surgical consent form, preprocedure verification checklist, surgical procedure scheduled, X-rays, and other diagnostic imaging studies.

Complications

- None known

Documentation

Complete the preprocedure verification checklist used by your facility, record that the correct site was verified, and note that the patient, a family member, or the surgeon has marked the site with a permanent marker.

Suture removal

The goal of this procedure is to remove skin sutures from a healed wound without damaging newly formed tissue. The timing of suture removal depends on the shape, size, and location of the sutured incision; the absence of inflammation, drainage, and infection; and the patient's general condition. Usually, for a sufficiently healed wound, sutures are removed 7 to 10 days after insertion.

Techniques for removal depend on the method of suturing, but all require sterile procedure to prevent contamination. Although sutures usually are removed by a physician, in many facilities, a nurse may remove them with a physician's order.

Equipment

Waterproof trash bag ♦ adjustable light ♦ clean gloves, if the wound is dressed ♦ sterile gloves ♦ sterile forceps or sterile hemostat ♦ normal saline solution ♦ sterile gauze pads ♦ antiseptic cleaning agent ♦ sterile curve-tipped suture scissors ♦ povidone-iodine pads ♦ optional: adhesive butterfly strips or Steri-Strips and compound benzoin tincture or other skin protectant

Prepackaged, sterile suture-removal trays are available.

Preparation

- Assemble all equipment in the patient's room.
- Check the expiration date on each sterile package, and inspect for tears.
- Open the waterproof trash bag, and place it near the patient's bed. Position the bag properly to avoid reaching across the sterile field or the suture line when disposing of soiled articles.
- Form a cuff by turning down the top of the trash bag to provide a wide opening and prevent contamination of instruments or gloves by touching the bag's edge.

Key steps

- If your facility allows you to remove sutures, check the practitioner's order to confirm the details for this procedure.
- Check for patient allergies, especially to adhesive tape and povidone-iodine or other topical solutions or medications.
- Tell the patient that you're going to remove the stitches from his wound. Assure him that this procedure typically is painless, but that he may feel a tickling sensation as the stitches come out. Reassure him that because his wound is healing properly, removing the stitches won't weaken the incision.
- Provide privacy, and position the patient so he's comfortable without placing undue tension on the suture line. Because some patients experience nausea or dizziness during the procedure, have the patient recline if possible. Adjust the light to have it shine directly on the suture line.
- Wash your hands thoroughly. If the patient's wound has a dressing, put on clean gloves and carefully remove the dressing. Discard the dressing and the gloves in the waterproof trash bag.
- Observe the patient's wound for possible gaping, drainage, inflammation, signs of infection, and embedded sutures. Notify the practitioner if the wound has failed to heal properly. The absence of a healing ridge under the suture line 5 to 7 days after insertion indicates that the line needs continued support and protection during the healing process.
- Establish a sterile work area with all the equipment and supplies you'll need for suture removal and wound care. Open the sterile suture-removal tray, maintaining sterility of the contents, and put on sterile gloves.
- Using sterile technique, clean the suture line to decrease the number of microorganisms present and reduce the risk of infection. The cleaning process should also moisten the sutures sufficiently to ease removal. Soften them further, if needed, with normal saline solution.
- Proceed according to the type of suture you're removing. (See *Methods for removing sutures,* page 492.) Because the visible part of a suture is exposed to skin bacteria and considered contaminated, be sure to cut sutures at the skin surface on one side of the visible part of the suture. Remove the suture by lifting and pulling the visible end off the skin to avoid drawing this contaminated portion back through subcutaneous tissue.
- If ordered, remove every other suture to maintain some support for the incision. Then go back and remove the remaining sutures.
- After removing sutures, wipe the incision gently with gauze pads soaked in an antiseptic cleaning agent or with a povidone-iodine pad. Apply a light sterile gauze dressing, if needed, to prevent infection and irritation from clothing. Then discard your gloves.
- Make sure the patient is comfortable. According to the practitioner's preference, inform the patient that he may shower in 1 or 2 days if the incision is dry and heals well.
- Properly dispose of the solutions and trash bag, and clean or dispose of soiled equipment and supplies according to facility policy.

Methods for removing sutures

Removal techniques depend on the type of sutures to be removed. These illustrations show removal steps for four common suture types. Keep in mind that for all suture types, it's important to grasp and cut sutures in the correct place to avoid pulling the exposed (thus contaminated) suture material through subcutaneous tissue.

Plain interrupted sutures

Using sterile forceps, grasp the knot of the first suture, and raise it off the skin. This will expose a small portion of the suture that was below skin level. Place the rounded tip of sterile curved-tip suture scissors against the skin, and cut through the exposed portion of the suture. Then, still holding the knot with the forceps, pull the cut suture up and out of the skin in a smooth continuous motion to avoid causing the patient pain. Discard the suture. Repeat the process for every other suture, initially; if the wound doesn't gape, you can then remove the remaining sutures as ordered.

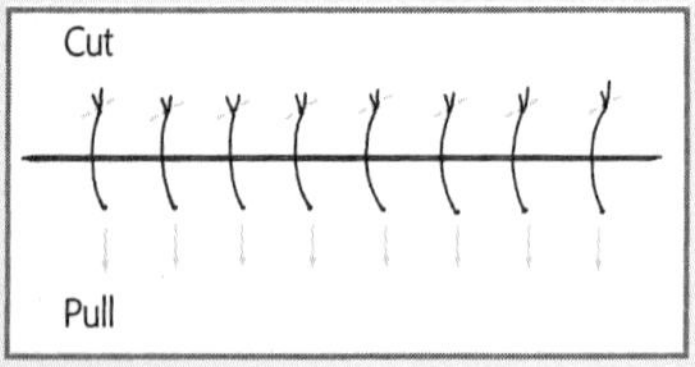

Plain continuous sutures

Cut the first suture on the side opposite the knot. Next, cut the same side of the next suture in line. Then lift the first suture out in the direction of the knot. Proceed along the suture line, grasping each suture where you grasped the knot on the first one.

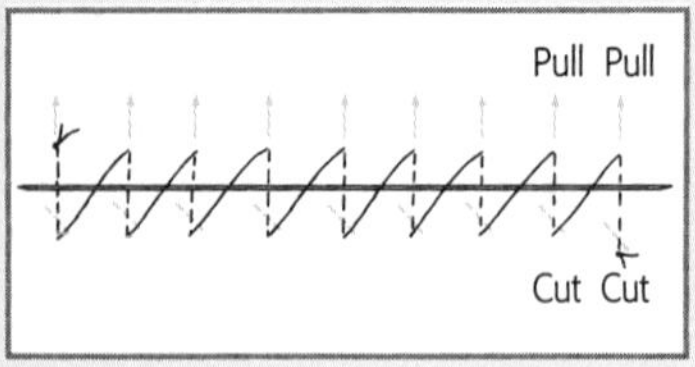

Mattress interrupted sutures

If possible, remove the small, visible portion of the suture opposite the knot by cutting it at each visible end and lifting the small piece away from the skin to prevent pulling it through and contaminating subcutaneous tissue. Then remove the rest of the suture by pulling it out in the direction of the knot. If the visible portion is too small to cut twice, cut it once, and pull the entire suture out in the opposite direction. Repeat these steps for the remaining sutures, and monitor the incision carefully for infection.

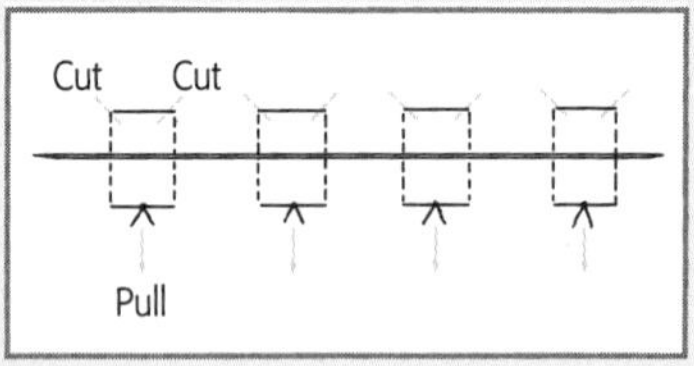

Mattress continuous sutures

Follow the procedure for removing mattress interrupted sutures, first removing the small visible portion of the suture, if possible, to prevent pulling it through and contaminating subcutaneous tissue. Then extract the rest of the suture in the direction of the knot.

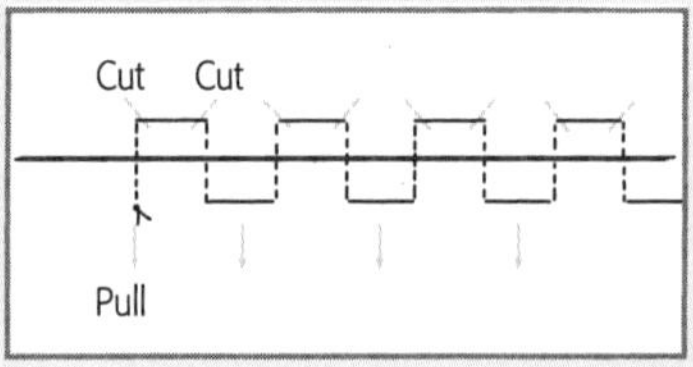

Special considerations

- Be sure to check the practitioner's order for the time of suture removal. Usually, you'll remove sutures on the head and neck 3 to 5 days after insertion; on the chest and abdomen, 5 to 7 days after insertion; and on the lower extremities, 7 to 10 days after insertion.

- If the patient has interrupted sutures or an incompletely healed suture line, remove only those sutures specified by the practitioner. He may want to leave some sutures in place for an additional day or two to support the suture line.
- If the patient has both retention and regular sutures in place, check the practitioner's order for the sequence in which they are to be removed. Because retention sutures link underlying fat and muscle tissue and give added support to the obese or slow-healing patient, they usually remain in place for 14 to 21 days.
- Be particularly careful to clean the suture line before attempting to remove mattress sutures. This decreases the risk of infection when the visible, contaminated part of the stitch is too small to cut twice for sterile removal and must be pulled through tissue. After you have removed mattress sutures this way, monitor the suture line carefully for subsequent infection.
- If the wound dehisces during suture removal, apply butterfly adhesive strips or Steri-Strips to support and approximate the edges, and call the practitioner immediately to repair the wound.
- Apply butterfly adhesive strips or Steri-Strips after any suture removal, if desired, to give added support to the incision line and prevent lateral tension on the wound from forming a wide scar. Use a small amount of compound benzoin tincture or other skin protectant to ensure adherence. Leave the strips in place for 3 to 5 days as ordered.

Complications

- Infection
- Dehiscence

Patient teaching

- If the patient is being discharged, teach him how to remove the dressing and care for the wound.
- Instruct him to call the practitioner immediately if he observes wound discharge or any other abnormal change. Tell him that the redness surrounding the incision should gradually disappear and only a thin line should show after a few weeks.

Documentation

Record the date and time of suture removal, type and number of sutures, appearance of the suture line, signs of wound complications, dressings or butterfly strips applied, and the patient's tolerance of the procedure.

Swab specimens

Correct collection and handling of swab specimens helps the laboratory staff identify pathogens accurately with a minimum of contamination from normal bacterial flora. Collection normally involves sampling inflamed tissues and exudates from the throat, nasopharynx, wounds, eye, ear, or rectum with sterile swabs of cotton or other absorbent material. The type of swab used depends on the part of the body affected. For example, collection of a nasopharyngeal specimen requires a cotton-tipped swab.

After the specimen has been collected, the swab is immediately placed in a sterile tube containing a transport medium and, in the case of sampling for anaerobes, an inert gas. Swab specimens are usually collected to identify pathogens and sometimes to identify asymptomatic carriers of certain easily transmitted disease organisms.

Equipment

Throat specimen

Gloves ♦ tongue blade ♦ penlight ♦ sterile cotton-tipped swab ♦ sterile culture tube with transport medium (or commercial collection kit) ♦ label ♦ laboratory request form and laboratory biohazard transport bag

Nasopharyngeal specimen

Gloves ♦ penlight ♦ sterile, flexible cotton-tipped swab ♦ tongue blade ♦ sterile culture tube with transport medium ♦ label ♦ laboratory request form and laboratory biohazard transport bag ♦ optional: small open-ended Pyrex tube or nasal speculum

Wound specimen

Sterile gloves ♦ sterile forceps ♦ alcohol or povidone-iodine pads ♦ sterile swabs ♦ sterile 10-ml syringe ♦ sterile 21G needle ♦ sterile culture tube with transport medium (or commercial collection kit for aerobic culture) ♦ labels ♦ special anaerobic culture tube containing carbon dioxide or nitrogen ♦ fresh dressings for the wound ♦ laboratory request form and laboratory biohazard transport bag ♦ optional: rubber stopper for needle

Ear specimen

Gloves ♦ normal saline solution ♦ two 2″ × 2″ gauze pads ♦ sterile swabs ♦ sterile culture tube with transport medium ♦ label ♦ 10-ml syringe and 22G 1″ needle (for tympanocentesis) ♦ laboratory request form and laboratory biohazard transport bag

Eye specimen

Sterile gloves ♦ sterile normal saline solution ♦ two 2″ × 2″ gauze pads ♦ sterile swabs ♦ sterile wire culture loop (for corneal scraping) ♦ sterile culture tube with transport medium ♦ label ♦ laboratory request form and laboratory biohazard transport bag

Rectal specimen

Gloves ♦ soap and water ♦ washcloth ♦ sterile swab ♦ normal saline solution ♦ sterile culture tube with transport medium ♦ laboratory request form and laboratory biohazard transport bag

Key steps

- Confirm the patient's identity using two patient identifiers according to facility policy.
- Explain the procedure to the patient to ease his anxiety and ensure cooperation.

Collecting a throat specimen

- Tell the patient that he may gag during the swabbing but that the procedure will probably take less than 1 minute.
- Instruct the patient to sit erect at the edge of the bed or in a chair, facing you. Then wash your hands and put on gloves.
- Ask the patient to tilt his head back. Depress his tongue with the tongue blade, and illuminate his throat with the penlight to check for inflamed areas.
- If the patient starts to gag, withdraw the tongue blade, and tell him to breathe deeply. Once he's relaxed, reinsert the tongue blade but not as deeply as before.
- Using the cotton-tipped swab, wipe the tonsillar areas from side to side, including any inflamed or purulent sites. Make sure you don't touch the tongue, cheeks, or teeth with the swab to avoid contaminating it with oral bacteria.
- Withdraw the swab, and immediately place it in the culture tube. If you're using a commercial kit, crush the ampule of culture medium at the bottom of the tube, and then push the swab into the medium to keep the swab moist.
- Remove and discard your gloves, and wash your hands.
- Label the specimen with the patient's name and identification number, the physician's name, and the date, time, and site of collection.
- On the laboratory request form, indicate whether any organism is strongly suspected, especially *Corynebacterium diphtheriae* (requires two swabs and special growth medium), *Bordetella pertussis* (requires a nasopharyngeal culture and special growth medium), and *Neisseria meningitidis* (requires enriched selective media).
- Place the specimen in a laboratory biohazard transport bag, and send to the laboratory immediately to prevent growth or deterioration of microbes.

Collecting a nasopharyngeal specimen

- Tell the patient that he may gag or feel the urge to sneeze during the swabbing but that the procedure takes less than 1 minute.
- Have the patient sit erect at the edge of the bed or in a chair, facing you. Then wash your hands and put on gloves.
- Ask the patient to blow his nose to clear his nasal passages. Then check his nostrils for patency with a penlight.
- Tell the patient to occlude one nostril first and then the other as he exhales. Lis-

ten for the more patent nostril because you'll insert the swab through it.

- Ask the patient to cough to bring organisms to the nasopharynx for a better specimen.
- While it's still in the package, bend the sterile swab in a curve, and then open the package without contaminating the swab.
- Ask the patient to tilt his head back, and gently pass the swab through the more patent nostril about 3″ to 4″ (7.5 to 10 cm) into the nasopharynx, keeping the swab near the septum and floor of the nose. Rotate the swab quickly and remove it. (See *Obtaining a nasopharyngeal specimen.*)
- Alternatively, depress the patient's tongue with a tongue blade, and pass the bent swab up behind the uvula. Rotate the swab and withdraw it.
- Remove the cap from the culture tube, insert the swab, and break off the contaminated end. Then close the tube tightly.
- Remove and discard your gloves, and wash your hands.
- Label the specimen for culture, complete a laboratory request form, and send the specimen to the laboratory immediately in a laboratory biohazard transport bag. If you're collecting a specimen to isolate a possible virus, check with the laboratory for the recommended collection technique.

Obtaining a nasopharyngeal specimen

After you've passed the swab into the nasopharynx, quickly but gently rotate the swab to collect the specimen. Then remove the swab, taking care not to injure the nasal mucous membrane.

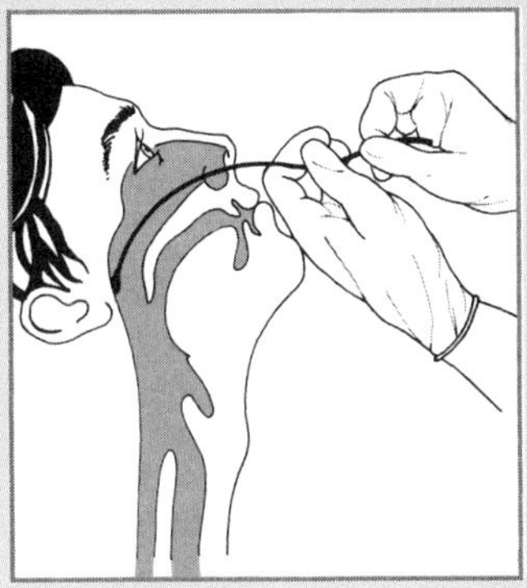

Collecting a wound specimen

- Wash your hands, prepare a sterile field, and put on sterile gloves. With sterile forceps, remove the dressing to expose the wound. Dispose of the soiled dressings properly.
- Clean the area around the wound with an alcohol or a povidone-iodine pad to reduce the risk of contaminating the specimen with skin bacteria. Then allow the area to dry.
- For an aerobic culture, use a sterile cotton-tipped swab to collect as much exudate as possible, or insert the swab deeply into the wound, and gently rotate it. Remove the swab from the wound, and immediately place it in the aerobic culture tube. Send the tube to the laboratory immediately with a completed laboratory request form. Never collect exudate from the skin and then insert the same swab into the wound; this could contaminate the wound with skin bacteria.
- For an anaerobic culture, insert the sterile cotton-tipped swab deeply into the wound, rotate it gently, remove it, and immediately place it in the anaerobic culture tube. (See *Using an anaerobic specimen collector,* page 496.) Or insert a sterile 10-ml syringe, without a needle, into the wound, and aspirate 1 to 5 ml of exudate into the syringe. Then attach the 21G needle to the syringe, and immediately inject the aspirate into the anaerobic culture tube. If an anaerobic culture tube is unavailable, obtain a rubber stopper, attach the needle to the syringe, and gently push all the air out of the syringe by pressing on the plunger. Stick the needle tip into the rubber stopper, remove and discard your gloves, and send the syringe of aspirate to the laboratory immediately with a completed laboratory request form in a laboratory biohazard transport bag.
- Put on sterile gloves.
- Apply a new dressing to the wound.

Using an anaerobic specimen collector

Because most anaerobes die when exposed to oxygen, they must be transported in tubes filled with carbon dioxide or nitrogen. The anaerobic specimen collector shown here includes a rubber-stopper tube filled with carbon dioxide, a small inner tube, and a swab attached to a plastic plunger.

Before specimen collection, the small inner tube containing the swab is held in place with the rubber stopper (as shown below left). After collecting the specimen, quickly replace the swab in the inner tube, and depress the plunger to separate the inner tube from the stopper (as shown below right), forcing it into the larger tube and exposing the specimen to a carbon dioxide–rich environment.

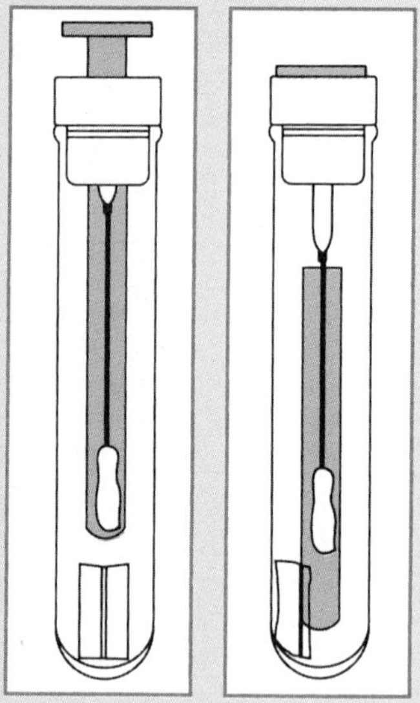

Collecting an ear specimen

- Wash your hands and put on gloves.
- Gently clean excess debris from the patient's ear with normal saline solution and gauze pads.
- Insert the sterile swab into the ear canal, and rotate it gently along the walls of the canal to avoid damaging the eardrum.
- Withdraw the swab, being careful not to touch other surfaces to avoid contaminating the specimen.
- Place the swab in the sterile culture tube with transport medium.
- Remove and discard your gloves, and wash your hands.
- Label the specimen for culture, complete a laboratory request form, and send the specimen to the laboratory immediately in a laboratory biohazard transport bag.

Collecting a middle ear specimen

- Put on gloves, and clean the outer ear with normal saline solution and gauze pads. Remove and discard your gloves. After the physician punctures the eardrum with a needle and aspirates fluid into the syringe, label the container, complete a laboratory request form, and send the specimen to the laboratory immediately in a laboratory biohazard transport bag.

Collecting an eye specimen

- Wash your hands and put on sterile gloves.
- Gently clean excess debris from the outside of the eye with normal saline solution and gauze pads, wiping from the inner to the outer canthus.
- Retract the lower eyelid to expose the conjunctival sac. Gently rub the sterile swab over the conjunctiva, being careful not to touch other surfaces. Hold the swab parallel to the eye, rather than pointed directly at it, to prevent corneal irritation or trauma due to sudden movement. (If a corneal scraping is required, this procedure is performed by a physician, using a wire culture loop.)
- Immediately place the swab or wire loop in the culture tube with transport medium.
- Remove and discard your gloves, and wash your hands.
- Label the specimen for culture, complete a laboratory request form, and send the

specimen to the laboratory immediately in a laboratory biohazard transport bag.

Collecting a rectal specimen

- Wash your hands and put on gloves.
- Clean the area around the patient's anus using a washcloth and soap and water.
- Insert the swab, moistened with normal saline solution or sterile broth medium, through the anus, and advance it about ⅜″ (1 cm) for infants or 2″ (4.2 cm) for adults. While withdrawing the swab, gently rotate it against the walls of the lower rectum to sample a large area of the rectal mucosa.
- Place the swab in a culture tube with transport medium.
- Remove and discard your gloves, and wash your hands.
- Label the specimen for culture, complete a laboratory request form, and send the specimen to the laboratory immediately in a laboratory biohazard transport bag.

Special considerations

- Note recent antibiotic therapy on the laboratory request form.

Wound specimen

- Although you would normally clean the area around a wound to prevent contamination by normal skin flora, don't clean a perineal wound with alcohol because this could irritate sensitive tissues. Also, make sure that antiseptic doesn't enter the wound.

Eye specimen

- Don't use an antiseptic before culturing to avoid irritating the eye and inhibiting growth of organisms in the culture. If the patient is a child or an uncooperative adult, ask a coworker to restrain the patient's head to prevent eye trauma resulting from sudden movement.

Complications

- None known

Documentation

Record the time, date, and site of specimen collection and any recent or current antibiotic therapy. Also note whether the specimen has an unusual appearance or odor.

T

Temperature assessment

Body temperature represents the balance between heat produced by metabolism, muscular activity, and other factors and heat lost through the skin, lungs, and body wastes. A stable temperature pattern promotes proper function of cells, tissues, and organs; a change in this pattern usually signals the onset of illness. Research supports observations that rectal temperature is the most accurate, followed by oral temperature, and then axillary temperature.

Temperature can be measured with an electronic digital or infrared thermometer. (See *Electronic and tympanic thermometers*.) Oral temperature in adults normally ranges from 97° to 99.5° F (36.1° to 37.5° C); rectal temperature is usually 1° F higher; axillary temperature reads 1° to 2° F lower; and tympanic temperature reads 0.5° to 1° F higher.

ALERT

Use caution with rectal thermometers in an infant and a young child to help prevent injury. Don't leave the patient alone until the thermometer has been removed.

Temperature normally fluctuates with rest and activity. Lowest readings typically occur between 4 and 5 a.m.; the highest readings, between 4 and 8 p.m. Other factors that influence temperature include gender, age, emotional conditions, and environment. Women normally have higher temperatures than men, especially during ovulation. Normal temperature is highest in neonates and lowest in elderly persons. Heightened emotions raise temperature; depressed emotions lower it. A hot external environment can raise temperature; a cold environment can lower it.

Equipment

Electronic digital or infrared thermometer or tympanic thermometer ♦ water-soluble lubricant (for rectal temperature) ♦ gloves (for rectal temperature) ♦ facial tissue ♦ disposable thermometer sheath or probe cover ♦ alcohol pad

Preparation

- If you use an electronic digital or infrared thermometer, make sure that it has been recharged.

Key steps

- Confirm the patient's identity using two patient identifiers according to facility policy.
- Explain the procedure to the patient, and wash your hands. If the patient has had hot or cold liquids, chewed gum, or smoked, wait 15 minutes before taking an oral temperature.
- To use a disposable sheath or probe cover, disinfect the thermometer with an alcohol pad. Insert it into the disposable sheath opening, and then twist to tear the seal at the dotted line. Pull it apart.

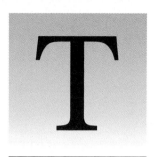

Using an electronic digital thermometer

- Insert the probe into a disposable probe cover. If taking a rectal temperature, lubricate the probe cover to reduce friction and ease insertion. Leave the probe in place until the maximum temperature appears on the digital display.

Using a tympanic thermometer

- Make sure that the lens under the probe is clean and shiny. Attach a disposable probe cover.
- Examine the patient's ears. They should be free from cerumen to obtain an accurate reading.
- Stabilize the patient's head, and then gently pull the ear straight back (for children up to age 1) or up and back (for children age 1 and older to adult) to straighten the external auditory canal. This technique ensures that the probe tip is directed at the tympanic membrane.
- Insert the thermometer until the ear canal is sealed. The thermometer should be inserted toward the tympanic membrane in the same way that an otoscope is inserted. Then press the activation button and hold it for 1 second. The temperature will appear on the display.

DO'S & DON'TS

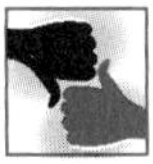

For infants younger than age 3 months, take three temperature readings and use the highest reading.

Taking an oral temperature

- Position the tip of the thermometer under the patient's tongue, as far back as possible on either side of the frenulum linguae. Placing the tip in this area promotes contact with superficial blood vessels and contributes to an accurate reading.
- Instruct the patient to close his lips but to avoid biting down with his teeth.
- Leave an electronic thermometer in place until the maximum temperature is displayed.
- For an electronic thermometer, note the temperature, and then remove and discard the probe cover.

Electronic and tympanic thermometers

You can take an oral, rectal, or axillary temperature with various electronic digital thermometers. A tympanic thermometer may also be available.

Use the oral route for adults who are awake, alert, oriented, and cooperative. For infants, young children, and confused or unconscious patients, you may need to take the temperature rectally.

Tympanic thermometer

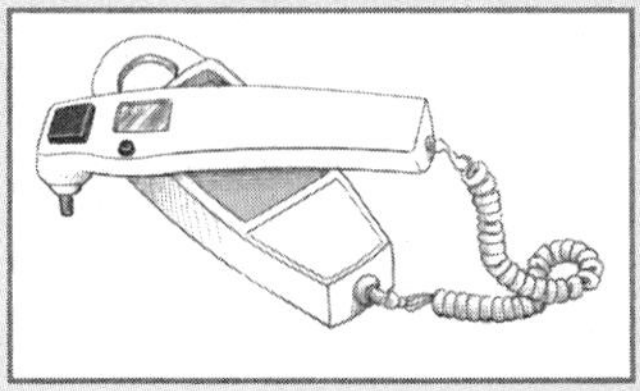

Chemical-dot thermometer

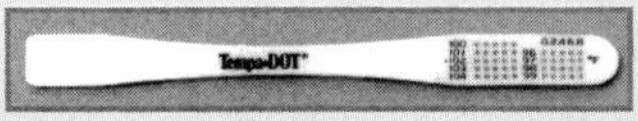

Individual electronic digital thermometer

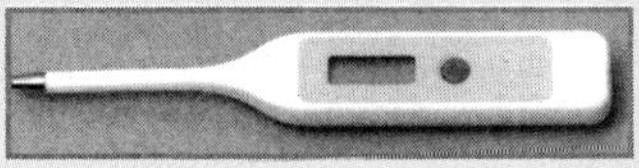

Institutional electronic digital thermometer

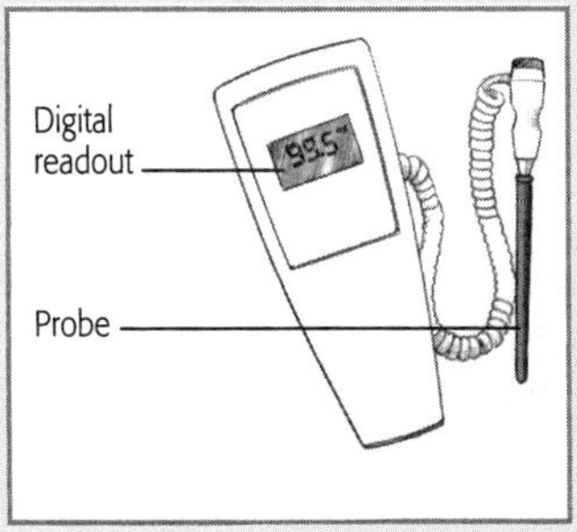

Taking a rectal temperature

- Position the patient on his side with his top leg flexed, and drape him to provide privacy. Then fold back the bed linens to expose the anus.

- Squeeze lubricant onto a facial tissue to prevent contamination of the lubricant supply. Put on gloves.
- Lubricate about ½″ (1.3 cm) of the thermometer tip for an infant, 1″ (2.5 cm) for a child, and 1½″ (3.8 cm) for an adult. Lubrication reduces friction and thus eases insertion. This step may be unnecessary when using disposable rectal sheaths because they're prelubricated.
- Lift the patient's upper buttock, and insert the thermometer about ½″ for an infant or 1½″ for an adult. Gently direct the thermometer along the rectal wall toward the umbilicus. This will avoid perforating the anus or rectum or breaking the thermometer. It also will help ensure an accurate reading because the thermometer will register hemorrhoidal artery temperature instead of fecal temperature.
- Hold the electronic thermometer until the maximum temperature is displayed. Holding the thermometer prevents damage to rectal tissues caused by displacement or loss of the thermometer into the rectum.
- Carefully remove the thermometer, wiping it as necessary. Then wipe the patient's anal area to remove lubricant or stool. Remove and dispose of the rectal sheath. Remove and discard your gloves. Wash your hands.

Taking an axillary temperature

- Position the patient with the axilla exposed.
- Gently pat the axilla dry with a facial tissue because moisture conducts heat. Avoid harsh rubbing, which generates heat.
- Ask the patient to reach across his chest and grasp his opposite shoulder, lifting his elbow.
- Position the thermometer in the center of the axilla, with the tip pointing toward the patient's head.
- Tell him to keep grasping his shoulder and to lower his elbow and hold it against his chest. This promotes skin contact with the thermometer.
- Remove an electronic thermometer when it displays the maximum temperature. Axillary temperature takes longer to register than oral or rectal temperature because the thermometer isn't enclosed in a body cavity.
- Grasp the end of the thermometer and remove it from the axilla.

Special considerations

- Oral measurement is contraindicated in patients who are unconscious, disoriented, or seizure-prone; in young children and infants; and in patients who must breathe through their mouths. Rectal measurement is contraindicated in patients with diarrhea, recent rectal or prostate surgery or injury because it may injure inflamed tissue, or recent myocardial infarction because anal manipulation may stimulate the vagus nerve, causing bradycardia or another rhythm disturbance.
- Use the same thermometer for repeated temperature taking to avoid spurious variations caused by equipment differences.

DO'S & DON'TS

Don't avoid taking an oral temperature when the patient is receiving nasal oxygen because oxygen administration raises oral temperature by only about 0.3° F (0.2° C).

Complications

- None known

Patient teaching

- Teach the patient and his family the correct way to take a temperature.
- Instruct them when to call their practitioner.

Documentation

Record the time, route, and temperature on the patient's chart.

TENS application, use and removal

Transcutaneous electrical nerve stimulation (TENS) is defined as the application of electrical stimulation to the skin for pain relief. It's based on the gate control theory of pain, which proposes that painful impulses pass through a "gate" in the brain. TENS is performed with a portable, battery-powered device that transmits painless electric current to peripheral nerves or directly to a painful area over relatively large nerve fibers. This treatment effectively alters the patient's perception of pain by blocking painful stimuli traveling over smaller fibers.

Used for postoperative patients and those with chronic pain, TENS reduces the need for analgesic drugs and may allow the patient to resume normal activities. Typically, a course of TENS treatments lasts 3 to 5 days. Some conditions, such as phantom limb pain, may require continuous stimulation; other conditions, such as a painful arthritic joint, require shorter periods (3 to 4 hours). (See *Current uses of TENS*.)

TENS is contraindicated for patients with cardiac pacemakers because it can interfere with pacemaker function. The procedure is also contraindicated for pregnant patients because its effect on the fetus is unknown. It's also contraindicated in patients with dementia. TENS should be used cautiously in all patients with cardiac disorders. TENS electrodes shouldn't be placed on the head or neck of patients with vascular disorders or seizure disorders.

Equipment

TENS device ♦ alcohol pads ♦ electrodes ♦ electrode gel ♦ warm water and soap ♦ leadwires ♦ charged battery pack ♦ battery recharger ♦ adhesive patch or hypoallergenic tape

Commercial TENS kits are available. They include the stimulator, leadwires, electrodes, spare battery pack, battery recharger, and sometimes the adhesive patch.

Preparation

- Before beginning the procedure, always test the battery pack to make sure it's fully charged.

Current uses of TENS

Transcutaneous electrical nerve stimulation (TENS) must be prescribed by a physician and is most successful if it's administered and taught to the patient by a therapist skilled in its use. TENS has been used for temporary relief of acute pain, such as postoperative incision pain, and for ongoing relief of chronic pain such as sciatica. Other types of pain that respond to TENS include:

- arthritis
- bone fracture pain
- bursitis
- cancer-related pain
- lower back pain
- musculoskeletal pain
- myofascial pain
- neuralgia and neuropathy
- phantom limb pain
- whiplash.

Key steps

- Confirm the patient's identity using two patient identifiers according to facility policy.
- Wash your hands and follow standard precautions, as appropriate. Provide privacy. If the patient has never seen a TENS unit, show him the device and explain the procedure.

Before TENS treatment

- With an alcohol pad, thoroughly clean and dry the skin where the electrode will be applied.
- Apply electrode gel to the bottom of each electrode.
- Place the ordered number of electrodes on the proper skin area, leaving at least 2″ (5 cm) between them. (See *Positioning TENS electrodes*, page 502.) Secure them with the adhesive patch or hypoallergenic tape. Tape all sides evenly so that the electrodes are firmly attached to the skin.
- Plug the pin connectors into the electrode sockets.

Positioning TENS electrodes

In transcutaneous electrical nerve stimulation (TENS), electrodes placed around peripheral nerves (or an incisional site) transmit mild electrical pulses to the brain. The current is thought to block pain impulses. The patient can influence the level and frequency of his pain relief by adjusting the controls on the device.

Typically, electrode placement varies even though patients may have similar complaints. Electrodes can be placed in several ways:

- to cover the painful area or surround it, as with muscle tenderness or spasm or painful joints
- to "capture" the painful area between electrodes, as with incisional pain.

In peripheral nerve injury, electrodes should be placed proximal to the injury (between the brain and the injury site) to avoid increasing pain. Placing electrodes in a hypersensitive area also increases pain. In an area lacking sensation, electrodes should be placed on adjacent dermatomes.

These illustrations show combinations of electrode placement (solid squares) and areas of nerve stimulation (shaded area) for lower back and leg pain.

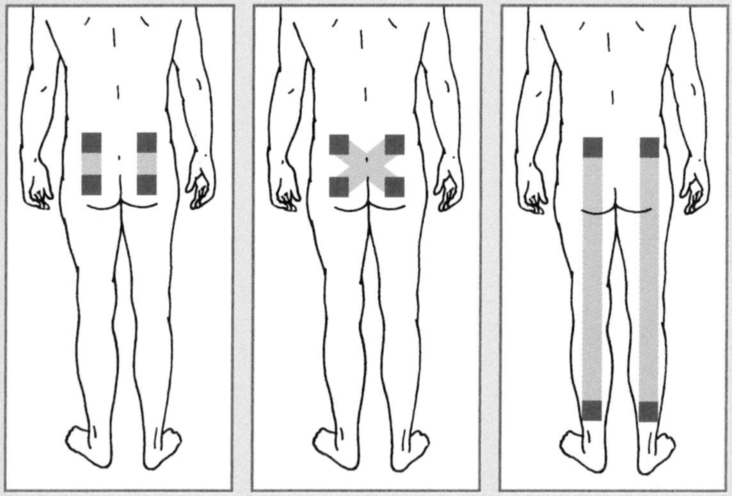

DEVICE SAFETY

To protect the cords, hold the connectors—not the cords themselves—during insertion.

- Turn the channel controls to the OFF position or as recommended in the operator's manual.
- Plug the leadwires into the jacks in the control box.
- Turn the amplitude and rate dials slowly as the manual directs. (The patient should feel a tingling sensation.) Adjust the controls on this device to the prescribed settings or to settings that are most comfortable. Most patients select stimulation frequencies of 60 to 100 Hz.
- Attach the TENS control box to part of the patient's clothing, such as a belt, pocket, or bra.
- To make sure the device is working effectively, monitor the patient for signs of excessive stimulation, such as muscle twitches, and for signs of inadequate stimulation, signaled by the patient's inability to feel any mild tingling sensation.

After TENS treatment

- Turn off the controls, and unplug the electrode leadwires from the control box.
- If another treatment will be given soon, leave the electrodes in place; if not, remove them.
- Clean the electrodes with soap and water, and clean the patient's skin with alcohol pads. (Don't soak the electrodes in alcohol because it will damage the rubber.)
- Remove the battery pack from the unit, and replace it with a charged battery pack.
- Recharge the used battery pack so it's always ready for use.

Special considerations

- If you must move electrodes during the procedure, turn off controls first. Follow the physician's orders regarding electrode placement and control settings. Incorrect placement of the electrodes will result in inappropriate pain control. Setting the controls too high can cause pain; setting them too low will fail to relieve pain.

ALERT

Never place electrodes near the patient's eyes or over nerves that innervate the carotid sinus or laryngeal or pharyngeal muscles to avoid interference with critical nerve function.

- If TENS is used continuously for postoperative pain, remove the electrodes at least daily to check for skin irritation, and provide skin care.

Complications

- None known

Patient teaching

- If appropriate, let the patient study the operator's manual. Teach him how to place the electrodes properly and how to take care of the TENS unit.

Documentation

On the patient's medical record and the nursing care plan, record the electrode sites and the control settings. Document the patient's tolerance of treatment. Also evaluate pain control.

Thoracentesis

Thoracentesis involves the aspiration of fluid or air from the pleural space. It relieves pulmonary compression and respiratory distress by removing accumulated air or fluid that results from injury or such conditions as tuberculosis or cancer. It also provides a specimen of pleural fluid or tissue for analysis and allows instillation of chemotherapeutic agents or other medications into the pleural space. Thoracentesis is contraindicated in patients with bleeding disorders.

Equipment

Prepackaged thoracentesis tray that includes sterile gloves, sterile drapes, 70% isopropyl alcohol or povidone-iodine solution, 1% or 2% lidocaine, 5-ml syringe with 21G and 25G needles for anesthetic injection, 17G thoracentesis needle for aspiration, 50-ml syringe, three-way stopcock and tubing, sterile specimen containers, sterile hemostat, sterile 4" × 4" gauze pads ♦ adhesive tape ♦ sphygmomanometer ♦ gloves ♦ stethoscope ♦ laboratory request slips ♦ drainage bottles ♦ optional: Teflon catheter, biopsy needle, prescribed sedative with 3-ml syringe and 21G needle, and drainage bottles if the physician expects a large amount of drainage

Preparation

- Assemble all equipment at the patient's bedside or in the treatment area.
- Check the expiration date on each sterile package, and inspect for tears.
- Prepare the necessary laboratory request form.
- Make sure the patient has signed an appropriate consent form.
- Note drug allergies, especially to the local anesthetic.
- Have the patient's chest X-rays available.
- Label all medications, medication containers, and other solutions on and off the sterile field.

Key steps

- Confirm the patient's identity using two patient identifiers according to facility policy.
- Explain the procedure to the patient. Inform him that he may feel some discomfort and a sensation of pressure during the needle insertion. Provide privacy and emotional support. Wash your hands.
- Administer the prescribed sedative as ordered.
- Obtain baseline vital signs, and assess respiratory function.
- Position the patient. Make sure he's firmly supported and comfortable. Although the choice of position varies, you'll usually seat the patient on the edge of the bed with his legs supported and his head and folded arms resting on a pillow on the overbed table. Or, have him straddle a chair backward and rest his head and folded arms on the back of the chair. If the patient is unable to sit, turn him on the unaffected side with the arm of the affected side raised above his head. Elevate the head of the bed 30 to 45 degrees if such elevation isn't contraindicated. Proper positioning stretches the chest or back and allows easier access to the intercostal spaces.
- Remind the patient not to cough, breathe deeply, or move suddenly during the procedure to avoid puncture of the visceral pleura or lung. If the patient coughs, the physician will briefly halt the procedure and withdraw the needle slightly to prevent puncture.
- Expose the patient's entire chest or back as appropriate.
- Wash your hands again before touching the sterile equipment. Then, using sterile technique, open the thoracentesis tray and assist the physician as necessary in disinfecting the site.
- If an ampule of local anesthetic isn't included in the sterile tray and a multidose vial of local anesthetic is to be used, assist the physician by wiping the rubber stopper with an alcohol pad and holding the inverted vial while the physician withdraws the anesthetic solution.
- After draping the patient and injecting the anesthetic, the physician attaches a three-way stopcock with tubing to the aspirating needle and turns the stopcock to prevent air from entering the pleural space through the needle.
- Attach the other end of the tubing to the drainage bottle.
- The physician then inserts the needle into the pleural space and attaches a 50-ml syringe to the needle's stopcock. A hemostat may be used to hold the needle in place and prevent pleural tear or lung puncture. As an alternative, the physician may introduce a Teflon catheter into the needle, remove the needle, and attach a stopcock and syringe or drainage tubing to the catheter to reduce the risk of pleural puncture by the needle.
- Support the patient verbally throughout the procedure, and keep him informed of each step. Assess him for signs of anxiety, and provide reassurance as necessary.
- Check vital signs regularly during the procedure. Continually observe the patient for such signs of distress as pallor, vertigo, faintness, weak and rapid pulse, decreased blood pressure, dyspnea, tachypnea, diaphoresis, chest pain, blood-tinged mucus, and excessive coughing. Alert the physician if such signs develop because they may indicate complications, such as hypovolemic shock or tension pneumothorax.
- Put on gloves and assist the physician as necessary in specimen collection, fluid drainage, and dressing the site.
- After the physician withdraws the needle or catheter, apply pressure to the puncture site, using a sterile 4″ × 4″ gauze pad. Then apply a new sterile gauze pad, and secure it with tape.
- Place the patient in a comfortable position, take his vital signs, and assess his respiratory status.
- Label the specimens properly, and send them to the laboratory.
- Discard disposable equipment. Clean nondisposable items, and return them for sterilization.
- Check the patient's vital signs and the dressing for drainage every 15 minutes for 1 hour. Then continue to assess the patient's vital signs and respiratory status as indicated by his condition.

- A chest X-ray is usually done afterward to check for pneumothorax.

Special considerations

- To prevent pulmonary edema and hypovolemic shock after thoracentesis, fluid is removed slowly, and no more than 1,000 ml of fluid is removed during the first 30 minutes. Removing the fluid increases the negative intrapleural pressure, which can lead to edema if the lung doesn't reexpand to fill the space.
- Pleuritic or shoulder pain may indicate pleural irritation by the needle point.
- A chest X-ray is usually ordered after the procedure to detect pneumothorax and evaluate the results of the procedure.

Complications

- Pneumothorax (possibly leading to mediastinal shift and requiring chest tube insertion) occurring if the needle punctures the lung and allows air to enter the pleural cavity
- Pyogenic infection resulting from contamination during the procedure
- Other potential difficulties including pain, cough, anxiety, dry taps, and subcutaneous hematoma

Documentation

Record the date and time of thoracentesis; location of the puncture site; volume and description (color, viscosity, odor) of the fluid withdrawn; specimens sent to the laboratory; vital signs and respiratory assessment before, during, and after the procedure; postprocedural tests such as a chest X-ray; complications and the nursing action taken; and the patient's reaction to the procedure.

Thoracic drainage

Thoracic drainage uses gravity and possibly suction to restore negative pressure and remove any material that collects in the pleural cavity. An underwater seal in the drainage system allows air and fluid to escape from the pleural cavity but doesn't allow air to reenter. The system is a self-contained, disposable system that collects drainage, creates a water seal, and controls suction in a compact, one-piece unit. (See *Disposable drainage system,* page 506.)

Specifically, thoracic drainage may be ordered to remove accumulated air, fluids (blood, pus, chyle, serous fluids, gastric juices), or solids (blood clots) from the pleural cavity; to restore negative pressure in the pleural cavity; or to reexpand a partially or totally collapsed lung.

Equipment

Thoracic drainage system (Pleur-evac, Atrium, Argyle, or Thora-Klex system, which can function as gravity draining systems or be connected to suction to enhance chest drainage) ♦ sterile distilled water (usually 1 L) ♦ adhesive tape ♦ sterile clear plastic tubing ♦ two rubber-tipped Kelly clamps ♦ sterile 50-ml catheter-tip syringe ♦ suction source, if ordered

Preparation

- Check the practitioner's order to determine the type of drainage system to be used and specific procedural details.
- If appropriate, request the drainage system and suction system from the central supply department.
- Collect the appropriate equipment, and take it to the patient's bedside.

Key steps

- Explain the procedure to the patient, and wash your hands.
- Maintain sterile technique throughout the entire procedure and whenever you make changes in the system or alter any of the connections to avoid introducing pathogens into the pleural space.

Setting up a commercially prepared disposable system

- Open the packaged system and place it on the floor in the rack supplied by the manufacturer to avoid accidentally knocking it over or dislodging the components. After the system is prepared, it may be hung from the side of the patient's bed.
- Remove the plastic connector from the short tube that's attached to the water-seal chamber. Using a 50-ml catheter-tip syringe, instill sterile distilled water into the water-seal chamber until it reaches the

Disposable drainage system

A commercially prepared disposable drainage system combines drainage collection, water seal, and suction control in one unit. The system ensures patient safety with positive- and negative-pressure relief valves and has a prominent air-leak indicator.

Pleur-evac system

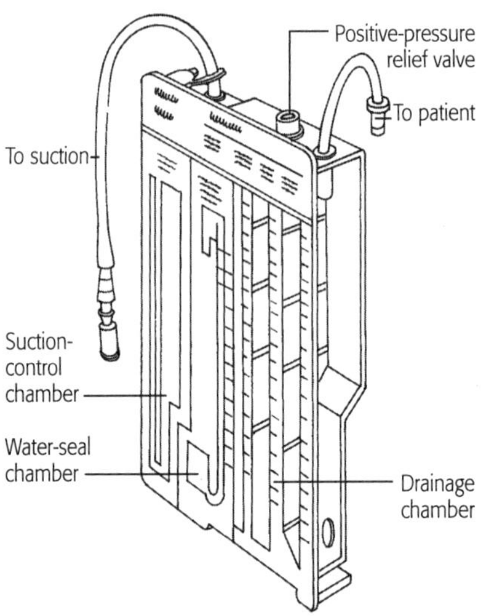

2-cm mark or the mark specified by the manufacturer. The Thora-Klex system is ready to use, but 15 ml of sterile water may be added to help detect air leaks. Replace the plastic connector.

- If suction is ordered, remove the cap (also called the *muffler* or *atmosphere vent cover*) on the suction-control chamber to open the vent. Next, instill sterile distilled water until it reaches the 20-cm mark or the ordered level, and recap the suction-control chamber.
- Using the long tube, connect the patient's chest tube to the closed drainage collection chamber. Secure the connection with tape.
- Connect the short tube on the drainage system to the suction source, and turn on the suction. Gentle bubbling should begin in the suction chamber, indicating that the correct suction level has been reached.

Managing closed-chest underwater seal drainage

- Repeatedly note the character, consistency, and amount of drainage in the drainage collection chamber.
- Mark the drainage level in the drainage collection chamber by noting the time and date at the drainage level on the chamber every 8 hours (or more often if there's a large amount of drainage).
- Check the water level in the water-seal chamber every 8 hours. If necessary, carefully add sterile distilled water until the level reaches the 2-cm mark indicated on the water-seal chamber of the commercial system.
- Check for fluctuation in the water-seal chamber as the patient breathes. Normal fluctuations of 2″ to 4″ (5 to 10 cm) reflect pressure changes in the pleural space during respiration. To check for fluctuation when a suction system is being used, momentarily disconnect the suction system so

the air vent is opened, and observe for fluctuation.

- Check for intermittent bubbling in the water-seal chamber. This occurs normally when the system is removing air from the pleural cavity. If bubbling isn't readily apparent during quiet breathing, have the patient take a deep breath or cough. Absence of bubbling indicates that the pleural space has sealed.
- Check the water level in the suction-control chamber. Detach the chamber or bottle from the suction source; when bubbling ceases, observe the water level. If necessary, add sterile distilled water to bring the level to the –20-cm line or as ordered.
- Check for gentle bubbling in the suction control chamber as this indicates that the proper suction level has been reached. Vigorous bubbling in this chamber increases the rate of water evaporation.
- Periodically check that the air vent in the system is working properly. Occlusion of the air vent results in a buildup of pressure in the system that could cause the patient to develop a tension pneumothorax.
- Coil the system's tubing, and secure it to the edge of the bed. Be sure the tubing remains at the level of the patient. Avoid creating dependent loops, kinks, or pressure on the tubing. Avoid lifting the drainage system above the patient's chest because fluid may flow back into the pleural space.
- Be sure to keep two rubber-tipped clamps at the bedside to clamp the chest tube if the commercially prepared system cracks or to locate an air leak in the system.
- Encourage the patient to cough frequently and breathe deeply to help drain the pleural space and expand the lungs.
- Tell him to sit upright for optimal lung expansion and to splint the insertion site while coughing to minimize pain.
- Check the rate and quality of the patient's respirations, and auscultate his lungs periodically to assess air exchange in the affected lung. Diminished or absent breath sounds may indicate that the lung hasn't reexpanded.
- Tell the patient to report breathing difficulty immediately.

ACTION STAT!

Notify the practitioner immediately if the patient develops cyanosis, rapid or shallow breathing, subcutaneous emphysema, chest pain, or excessive bleeding.

- Some facilities permit milking of tubing when clots are visible. This is a controversial procedure because it creates increased intrapleural pressure, so be sure to check your facility's policy. If permitted, gently milk the tubing in the direction of the drainage chamber when clots are visible.
- Check the chest tube dressing at least every 8 hours. Palpate the area surrounding the dressing for crepitus or subcutaneous emphysema, which indicates that air is leaking into the subcutaneous tissue surrounding the insertion site. Change the dressing if necessary or according to facility policy.
- Encourage active or passive range-of-motion (ROM) exercises for the patient's arm or the affected side if he has been splinting the arm. Usually, the thoracotomy patient will splint his arm to decrease his discomfort.
- Give ordered pain medication as needed for comfort and to help with deep-breathing, coughing, and ROM exercises.
- Remind the ambulatory patient to keep the drainage system below chest level and to be careful not to disconnect the tubing to maintain the water seal. With a suction system, the patient must stay within range of the length of tubing attached to a wall outlet or portable pump.

Special considerations

- Instruct staff and visitors to avoid touching the equipment to prevent complications from separated connections.
- If excessive continuous bubbling is present in the water-seal chamber, especially if suction is being used, rule out a leak in the drainage system. Try to locate the leak by clamping the tube momentarily at various points along its length. Begin clamping at the tube's proximal end, and work down toward the drainage system, paying special attention to the seal around the connections. If a connection is loose, push it back

together and tape it securely. The bubbling will stop when a clamp is placed between the air leak and the water seal. If you clamp along the tube's entire length and the bubbling doesn't stop, the drainage unit may be cracked and need replacement.

- If the commercially prepared drainage collection chamber fills, replace it. To do this, double-clamp the tube close to the insertion site (use two clamps facing in opposite directions), exchange the system, remove the clamps, and retape the connection.

ALERT

Never leave the tubes clamped for more than a minute to prevent a tension pneumothorax, which may occur when clamping stops air and fluid from escaping.

- If the commercially prepared system cracks, clamp the chest tube momentarily with the two rubber-tipped clamps at the bedside (placed there at the time of tube insertion). Place the clamps close to each other near the insertion site; they should face in opposite directions to provide a more complete seal. Observe the patient for altered respirations while the tube is clamped. Then replace the damaged equipment. (Prepare the new unit before clamping the tube.)

Complications

- Tension pneumothorax resulting from excessive accumulation of air, drainage, or both and eventually exerting pressure on the heart and aorta, causing a precipitous fall in cardiac output

Documentation

Record the date and time thoracic drainage began, type of system used, amount of suction applied to the pleural cavity, presence or absence of bubbling or fluctuation in the water-seal chamber, initial amount and type of drainage, and the patient's respiratory status.

At the end of each shift record the frequency of system inspection; how frequently chest tubes were milked; amount, color, and consistency of drainage; presence or absence of bubbling or fluctuation in the water-seal chamber; the patient's respiratory status; condition of the chest dressings; pain medication, if given; and complications and the nursing action taken.

Tilt table

The tilt table, a padded table or bed-length board that can be raised gradually from a horizontal to a vertical position, can help prevent the complications of prolonged bed rest. Used for the patient with a spinal cord injury, brain damage, orthostatic hypotension, or any other condition that prevents free standing, the tilt table increases tolerance of the upright position, conditions the cardiovascular system, stretches muscles, and helps prevent contractures, bone demineralization, and urinary calculus formation.

Equipment

Tilt table with footboard and restraining straps ♦ sphygmomanometer ♦ stethoscope ♦ antiembolism stockings or elastic bandages ♦ optional: abdominal binder

Preparation

- Common types of tilt tables include the electric table, which moves at a slow, steady rate; the manual table, which is raised by a handle; and the spring-assisted table, which is raised by a pedal.
- Familiarize yourself with operating instructions for the model you'll be using.

Key steps

- Explain the use and benefits of the tilt table to the patient.
- Apply antiembolism stockings to restrict vessel walls and help prevent blood pooling and edema. If necessary, apply an abdominal binder to avoid pooling of blood in the splanchnic region, which contributes to insufficient cerebral circulation and orthostatic hypotension.
- Make sure the tilt table is locked in the horizontal position. Then summon assistance and transfer the patient to the table,

placing him in the supine position with his feet flat against the footboard.

- If the patient can't bear weight on one leg, place a wooden block between the footboard and the weight-bearing foot, permitting the non-weight-bearing leg to dangle freely.
- Fasten the safety straps, then take the patient's blood pressure and pulse rate.
- Tilt the table slowly in 15- to 30-degree increments, evaluating the patient constantly. Take his blood pressure every 3 to 5 minutes because movement from the supine to the upright position decreases systolic pressure. Be alert for signs and symptoms of insufficient cerebral circulation, including dizziness, nausea, pallor, diaphoresis, tachycardia, or a change in mental status. If the patient experiences any of these signs or symptoms, or hypotension or seizures, return the table immediately to the horizontal position.
- If the patient tolerates the position shift, continue to tilt the table until reaching the desired angle, usually between 45 degrees and 80 degrees. A 60-degree tilt gives the patient the physiologic effects and sensations of standing upright.
- Gradually return the patient to the horizontal position, and check his vital signs. Then obtain assistance and transfer the patient onto the stretcher for transport back to his room.

Special considerations

- Let the patient's response determine the angle of tilt and duration of elevation, but avoid a prolonged upright positioning because it may lead to venous stasis.

ALERT

Never leave the patient unattended on the tilt table because marked physiologic changes, such as hypotension or severe headache, can occur suddenly.

Complications

- Sudden hypotension, severe headache, and other dramatic physiologic changes

Documentation

Record the angle and duration of elevation; changes in the patient's pulse rate, blood pressure, and physical and mental status; and his response to treatment.

Topical skin medication application

Topical drugs are applied directly to the skin surface. They include lotions, pastes, ointments, creams, powders, shampoos, patches, and aerosol sprays. Topical medications are absorbed through the epidermal layer into the dermis. The extent of absorption depends on the vascularity of the region.

Nitroglycerin, fentanyl, nicotine, and certain supplemental hormone replacements are used for systemic effects. Most other topical medications are used for local effects. Ointments have a fatty base, which is an ideal vehicle for such drugs as antimicrobials and antiseptics. Typically, topical medications should be applied two to three times per day to achieve their therapeutic effect.

Equipment

Patient's medication record and chart ♦ prescribed medication ♦ gloves ♦ sterile tongue blades ♦ 4″ × 4″ sterile gauze pads ♦ transparent semipermeable dressing ♦ adhesive tape ♦ solvent (such as cottonseed oil)

Key steps

- Verify the order on the patient's medication record by checking it against the prescriber's order on the chart.
- Make sure the label on the medication agrees with the medication order. Read the label again before you open the container and as you remove the medication from the container. Check the expiration date.
- Confirm the patient's identity using two patient identifiers according to facility policy.
- If your facility uses a bar code scanning system, be sure to scan your ID badge, the patient's ID bracelet, and the medication's bar code.

- Provide privacy.
- Explain the procedure thoroughly to the patient because he may have to apply the medication by himself after discharge.
- Wash your hands to prevent cross-contamination, and glove your dominant hand. Use gloves on both hands if exposure to body fluids is likely.
- Help the patient assume a comfortable position that provides access to the area to be treated.
- Expose the area to be treated. Make sure the skin or mucous membrane is intact (unless the medication has been ordered to treat a skin lesion such as an ulcer). Applying medication to broken or abraded skin may cause unwanted systemic absorption and result in further irritation.
- If necessary, clean the skin of debris, including crusts, epidermal scales, and old medication. You may have to change the glove if it becomes soiled.

Applying paste, cream, or ointment

- Open the container. Place the lid or cap upside down to prevent contamination of the inside surface.
- Remove a tongue blade from its sterile wrapper, and cover one end with medication from the tube or jar. Then transfer the medication from the tongue blade to your gloved hand.
- Apply the medication to the affected area with long, smooth strokes that follow the direction of hair growth. This technique avoids forcing medication into hair follicles, which can cause irritation and lead to folliculitis. Avoid excessive pressure when applying the medication because it could abrade the skin.
- To prevent contamination of the medication, use a new tongue blade each time you remove medication from the container.

Removing ointment

- Wash your hands and put on gloves. Then rub solvent on them and apply it liberally to the ointment-treated area in the direction of hair growth. Alternatively, saturate a sterile gauze pad with the solvent and use the pad to gently remove the ointment. Remove excess oil by gently wiping the area with a sterile gauze pad. Don't rub too hard to remove the medication because you could irritate the skin.

Applying other topical medications

- To apply shampoos, follow package directions. (See *Using medicated shampoos.*)
- To apply aerosol sprays, shake the container, if indicated, to completely mix the medication. Hold the container 6″ to 12″ (15 to 30 cm) from the skin, or follow the manufacturer's recommendation. Spray a thin film of the medication evenly over the treatment area.
- To apply powders, dry the skin surface, making sure to spread skin folds where moisture collects. Then apply a thin layer of powder over the treatment area.
- To protect applied medications and prevent them from soiling the patient's clothes, tape an appropriate amount of sterile gauze pad or a transparent semipermeable dressing over the treated area. With certain medications (such as topical steroids), semipermeable dressings may be contraindicated. Check medication information and cautions. If you're applying a topical medication to the patient's hands or feet, cover the site with white cotton gloves for the hands or terry cloth scuffs for the feet.
- In children, topical medications (such as steroids) should be covered loosely only with a diaper. Don't use plastic pants.
- Assess the patient's skin for signs of irritation, allergic reaction, or breakdown.

Special considerations

- Never apply medication without first removing previous applications to prevent skin irritation from an accumulation of medication.
- Be sure to wear gloves to prevent absorption by your own skin. If the patient has an infectious skin condition, use sterile gloves and dispose of old dressings according to facility policy.
- Don't apply ointments to mucous membranes as liberally as you would to the skin because mucous membranes are usually moist and absorb ointment more quickly

Using medicated shampoos

Medicated shampoos include keratolytic and cytostatic agents, coal tar preparations, and lindane (gamma benzene hexachloride) solutions. They can be used to treat such conditions as dandruff, psoriasis, and head lice. However, they're contraindicated in patients with broken or abraded skin.

Because application instructions may vary among brands, check the label on the shampoo before starting the procedure to ensure use of the correct amount. Keep the shampoo away from the patient's eyes. If any shampoo should accidentally get in his eyes, irrigate them promptly with water. Likewise, keep the shampoo from running into the patient's mouth. Selenium sulfide, used in cytostatic agents, is extremely toxic if ingested.

To apply a medicated shampoo, follow these steps:

- Prepare the patient for shampoo treatment by explaining the procedure.
- Shake the bottle of shampoo well to mix the solution evenly.
- Wet the patient's hair thoroughly and wring out excess water.
- Apply the proper amount of shampoo, as directed on the label.
- Work the shampoo into a lather, adding water as necessary. Part the hair and work the shampoo into the scalp, taking care not to use your fingernails.
- Leave the shampoo on the scalp and hair for as long as instructed (usually 5 to 10 minutes). Then rinse the hair thoroughly.
- Towel-dry the patient's hair.
- After the hair is dry, comb or brush it. Use a fine-tooth comb to remove nits if necessary.

than the skin does. Also don't apply too much ointment to any skin area because it might cause irritation and discomfort, stain clothing and bedding, and make removal difficult.

- Never apply ointment to the eyelids or ear canal unless ordered. The ointment might congeal and occlude the tear duct or ear canal.
- Inspect the treated area frequently for adverse effects such as signs of an allergic reaction.

Complications

- Skin irritation, a rash, or an allergic reaction

Patient teaching

- Instruct the patient on how to use the medication at home. If possible, have the patient give a return demonstration.

Documentation

Record the medication applied; time, date, and site of application; and condition of the patient's skin at the time of application. Note the patient's tolerance and subsequent effects of the medication, if any.

Total parenteral nutrition

When the patient can't meet his nutritional needs by oral or enteral feedings, he may require I.V. nutritional support, or parenteral nutrition. The patient's diagnosis, history, and prognosis determine the need for parenteral nutrition. Generally, this treatment is prescribed for the patient who can't absorb nutrients though the GI tract for more than 10 days. More specific indications include:

- debilitating illness lasting longer than 2 weeks
- loss of 10% or more of pre-illness weight
- serum albumin level below 3.5 g/dl
- excessive nitrogen loss from wound infection, fistulas, or abscesses
- renal or hepatic failure
- a nonfunctioning GI tract for 5 to 7 days in a severely catabolic patient.

Other reasons for initiating parenteral nutrition include massive small-bowel resection, bone marrow transplantation, high-dose chemotherapy or radiation therapy, and major surgery.

Infants with congenital or acquired disorders may need parenteral nutrition to promote growth and development. Specific disorders that may require parenteral nutrition include tracheoesophageal fistula, gastroschisis, duodenal atresia, cystic fibrosis, meconium ileus, diaphragmatic hernia, volvulus, malrotation of the gut, and annular pancreas.

Parenteral nutrition shouldn't be given to patients with a normally functioning GI tract, and it has limited value for well-nourished patients whose GI tract will resume normal function within 10 days. It may also be inappropriate for patients with a poor prognosis or if the risks of parenteral nutrition outweigh the benefits.

Parenteral nutrition may be given through a peripheral or central venous (CV) line. Depending on the solution, it may be used to boost the patient's calorie intake, to supply full calorie needs, or to surpass the patient's calorie requirements. Infusion-specific filtration and an electronic infusion device should be used to administer parenteral nutrition.

The type of parenteral solution prescribed depends on the patient's condition and metabolic needs and the administration route. The solution usually contains protein, carbohydrates, electrolytes, vitamins, and trace minerals. A lipid emulsion provides the necessary fat. (See *Types of parenteral nutrition*, pages 514 and 515.)

Nutritional solutions containing concentrations exceeding 10% dextrose, 5% protein, or both, such as TPN, should be given through a CV line with the distal tip in the superior vena cava or right atrium. Because TPN is in a lipid emulsion, it should be filtered through a 1.2-micron filter. Peripheral parenteral nutrition (PPN) has a concentration of 10% dextrose and 5% protein or less and can be given through a peripheral line. The maximum administration period for PPN should be 7 to 10 days, unless supplemental oral or enteral feeding is also provided.

The most common delivery route for TPN is through a CV catheter into the superior vena cava. The catheter may also be placed through the infraclavicular approach or, less commonly, through the supraclavicular, internal jugular, or antecubital fossa approach.

Equipment

Bag or bottle of prescribed parenteral nutrition solution ♦ sterile I.V. tubing with attached extension tubing ♦ 0.22-micron filter (or 1.2-micron filter if solution contains lipids or albumin) ♦ reflux valve ♦ time tape ♦ alcohol pads ♦ electronic infusion pump ♦ portable glucose monitor ♦ scale ♦ intake and output record ♦ sterile gloves ♦ optional: mask

Preparation

- Make sure that the solution, the patient, and the equipment are ready.
- Remove the solution from the refrigerator at least 1 hour before use to avoid pain, hypothermia, venous spasm, and venous constriction, which can result from delivery of a chilled solution.
- Check the solution against the practitioner's order for the correct patient name, expiration date, and formula components.
- Observe the container for cracks and the solution for cloudiness, turbidity, and particles. If present, return the solution to the pharmacy.
- When you're ready to administer the solution, explain the procedure to the patient.
- Check the name on the solution container against the name on the patient's wristband. Confirm the patient's identity using two patient identifiers according to facility policy.
- Then put on gloves and, if specified by facility policy, a mask. Throughout the procedure, use strict sterile technique.
- In sequence, connect the pump tubing, the micron filter with attached extension tubing (if the tubing doesn't contain an in-line filter), and the reflux valve. Insert the filter as close to the catheter site as possible. If the tubing doesn't have luer-lock connections, tape all connections to prevent accidental separation, which could

lead to air embolism, exsanguination, and sepsis.

- Next, squeeze the I.V. drip chamber and, holding the drip chamber upright, insert the tubing spike into the I.V. bag or bottle. Then release the drip chamber. Squeezing the drip chamber before spiking an I.V. bottle prevents accidental dripping of the parenteral nutrition solution. An I.V. bag, however, shouldn't drip.
- Next, prime the tubing. Invert the filter at the distal end of the tubing, and open the roller clamp. Let the solution fill the tubing and the filter. Gently tap it to dislodge air bubbles trapped in the Y-ports.
- If indicated, attach a time tape to the parenteral nutrition container for accurate measurement of fluid intake.
- Record the date and time you hung the fluid, and initial the parenteral nutrition solution container.
- Next, attach the setup to the infusion pump, and prepare it according to the manufacturer's instructions.
- Remove and discard your gloves.
- With the patient in the supine position, flush the catheter with normal saline solution, according to facility policy.
- Then put on gloves, and clean the catheter injection cap with an alcohol pad.

Key steps

- If you're attaching the container of parenteral nutrition solution to a CV line, clamp the CV line before disconnecting it to prevent air from entering the catheter. If a clamp isn't available, ask the patient to perform Valsalva's maneuver just as you change the tubing, if possible. Or, if the patient is being mechanically ventilated, change the I.V. tubing immediately after the machine delivers a breath at peak inspiration. Both of these measures increase intrathoracic pressure and prevent air embolism.
- Using sterile technique, attach the tubing to the designated luer-lock port. After connecting the tubing, remove the clamp, if applicable.
- Set the infusion pump at the ordered flow rate, and start the infusion. Check to make sure that the catheter junction is secure.
- Tag the tubing with the date and time of change.

Starting the infusion

- Because parenteral nutrition solution usually contains a large amount of glucose, you may need to start the infusion slowly to allow the patient's pancreatic beta cells time to increase their output of insulin. Depending on the patient's tolerance, parenteral nutrition is usually initiated at a rate of 40 to 50 ml/hour and then advanced by 25 ml/hour every 6 hours (as tolerated) until the desired infusion rate is achieved. However, when the glucose concentration is low, as occurs in most PPN formulas, you can initiate the rate necessary to infuse the complete 24-hour volume and discontinue the solution without tapering.
- You may allow a parenteral nutrition solution container to hang for 24 hours.

Changing solutions

- Prepare the new solution and I.V. tubing as described earlier. Put on gloves. Remove the protective caps from the solution containers, and wipe the tops of the containers with alcohol pads.
- Turn off the infusion pump and close the flow clamps. Using strict sterile technique, remove the spike from the solution container that's hanging and insert it into the new container.
- Hang the new container and tubing alongside the old. Turn on the infusion pump, set the flow rate, and open the flow clamp completely.
- If you're attaching the solution to a peripheral line, examine the skin above the insertion site for redness and warmth and assess for pain. If you suspect phlebitis, remove the existing I.V. line and start a line in a different vein. Also, insert a new line if the I.V. catheter has been in place for 72 hours or more to reduce the risk of phlebitis and infiltration.
- Turn off the infusion pump and close the flow clamp on the old tubing. Disconnect the tubing from the catheter hub, and connect the new tubing. Open the flow clamp on the new container to a moderately slow rate.

Types of parenteral nutrition

Type	Solution components/liter	Uses
Total parenteral nutrition (TPN) by way of central venous (CV) line	▪ $D_{15}W$ to $D_{25}W$ (1 L dextrose 25% = 850 nonprotein calories) ▪ Crystalline amino acids 2.5% to 8.5% ▪ Electrolytes, vitamins, trace elements, and insulin, as ordered ▪ Lipid emulsion 10% to 20% (usually infused as a separate solution)	▪ 2 weeks or more ▪ For patients with large calorie and nutrient needs ▪ Provides calories, restores nitrogen balance, and replaces essential vitamins, electrolytes, minerals, and trace elements ▪ Promotes tissue synthesis, wound healing, and normal metabolic function ▪ Allows bowel rest and healing; reduces activity in the gallbladder, pancreas, and small intestine ▪ Improves tolerance of surgery
Total nutrient admixture	▪ 1 day's nutrients are contained in a single, 3-L bag (also called 3:1 solution) ▪ Combines lipid emulsion with other parenteral solution components	▪ 2 weeks or more ▪ For relatively stable patients because solution components can be adjusted just once daily ▪ For other uses, see TPN (above)
Peripheral parenteral nutrition (PPN)	▪ D_5W to $D_{10}W$ ▪ Crystalline amino acids 2.5% to 5% ▪ Electrolytes, minerals, vitamins, and trace elements, as ordered ▪ Lipid emulsion 10% or 20% (1 L of dextrose 10% and amino acids 3.5% infused at the same time as 1 L of lipid emulsion = 1,440 nonprotein calories) ▪ Heparin or hydrocortisone, as ordered	▪ 2 weeks or less ▪ Provides up to 2,000 calories/day ▪ Maintains adequate nutritional status in patients who can tolerate relatively high fluid volume, in those who usually resume bowel function and oral feedings after a few days, and in those who are susceptible to infections associated with the CV catheter

▪ Remove the old tubing from the infusion pump, and insert the new tubing according to the manufacturer's instructions. Then turn on the infusion pump, set it to the desired flow rate, and open the flow clamp completely. Remove the old equipment and dispose of it properly.

Special considerations

Basic solution
- Nutritionally complete
- Requires minor surgical procedure for CV line insertion (can be done at bedside by physician)
- Highly hypertonic solution
- May cause metabolic complications (glucose intolerance, electrolyte imbalance, essential fatty acid deficiency)

I.V. lipid emulsion
- May not be used effectively in severely stressed patients (especially burn patients)
- May interfere with immune mechanisms; in patients suffering respiratory compromise, reduces carbon dioxide buildup
- Given by way of CV line; irritates peripheral vein in long-term use

- See TPN (above)
- Reduces need to handle bag, reducing risk of contamination
- Decreases nursing time and reduces need for infusion sets and electronic devices, lowering facility costs, increasing patient mobility, and allowing easier adjustment to home care
- Has limited use because not all types and amounts of components are compatible
- Precludes use of certain infusion pumps because they can't accurately deliver large volumes of solution; precludes use of standard I.V. tubing filters because a 0.22-micron filter blocks lipid and albumin molecules

Basic solution
- Nutritionally complete for short time
- Can't be used in nutritionally depleted patients
- Can't be used in volume-restricted patients because PPN requires large fluid volume
- Doesn't cause weight gain
- Avoids insertion and care of CV line but requires adequate venous access; site must be changed every 72 hours
- Delivers less hypertonic solutions than CV line TPN
- May cause phlebitis and increases risk of metabolic complications
- Less chance of metabolic complications than with CV line TPN

I.V. lipid emulsion
- As effective as dextrose for calorie source
- Diminishes phlebitis if infused at same time as basic nutrient solution
- Irritates vein in long-term use
- Reduces carbon dioxide buildup when pulmonary compromise is present

Special considerations

- Always infuse a parenteral nutrition solution at a constant rate without interruption to avoid blood glucose fluctuations. If the infusion slows, consult the practitioner before changing the infusion rate.
- Monitor the patient's vital signs every 4 hours or more often if necessary. Watch

for an increased temperature, an early sign of catheter-related sepsis.

- Check the patient's blood glucose every 6 hours. He may require supplementary insulin, which the pharmacist may add directly to the solution. The patient may require additional subcutaneous doses.
- Because most patients receiving PPN are in a protein-wasted state, the therapy causes marked changes in fluid and electrolyte status and in levels of glucose, amino acids, minerals, and vitamins. Therefore, record daily intake and output accurately. Specify the volume and type of each fluid, and calculate the daily calorie intake.
- Monitor the results of routine laboratory tests, and report abnormal findings to the practitioner to allow for appropriate changes in the parenteral nutrition solution. Such tests typically include measurement of serum electrolyte, calcium, blood urea nitrogen, creatinine, and blood glucose levels at least three times weekly; serum magnesium and phosphorus levels twice weekly; liver function studies, complete blood count and differential, and serum albumin and transferrin levels weekly; and urine nitrogen balance and creatinine-height index studies weekly. A serum zinc level is obtained at the start of parenteral nutrition therapy. The practitioner may also order serum prealbumin, total lymphocyte count, amino acid levels, fatty acid-phospholipid fraction, skin testing, and expired gas analysis.
- Physically assess the patient daily. If ordered, measure arm circumference and skin-fold thickness over the triceps. Weigh him at the same time each morning after he voids; he should be weighed in similar clothing and on the same scale. Suspect fluid imbalance if he gains more than 1 lb (0.5 kg) daily.
- Change the dressing over the catheter according to your facility's policy or whenever the dressing becomes wet, soiled, or nonocclusive. Always use strict sterile technique. When performing dressing changes, watch for signs of phlebitis and catheter retraction from the vein. Measure the catheter length from the insertion site to the hub for verification.
- Change the tubing and filters every 24 hours or according to facility policy.
- Closely monitor the catheter site for swelling, which may indicate infiltration. Extravasation of parenteral nutrition solution can lead to tissue necrosis. (See *Correcting parenteral nutrition problems.*)
- Use caution when using the parenteral nutrition line for other functions.

DO'S & DON'TS

Don't use a single-lumen CV catheter to infuse blood or blood products, to give a bolus injection, to administer simultaneous I.V. solutions, to measure CV pressure, or to draw blood for laboratory tests.

- Provide regular mouth care. Also provide emotional support. Keep in mind that patients commonly associate eating with positive feelings and become disturbed when they can't eat.
- Teach the patient the potential adverse effects and complications of parenteral nutrition. Encourage the patient to inspect his mouth regularly for signs of parotitis, glossitis, and oral lesions. Tell him that he may have fewer bowel movements while receiving parenteral nutrition therapy. Encourage him to remain physically active to help his body use the nutrients more fully.

Complications

- Catheter-related sepsis
- Thrombosis or sepsis due to malpositioned subclavian or jugular vein catheter (rare)
- Air embolism (a potentially fatal complication) occurring during I.V. tubing changes if tubing is inadvertently disconnected; also resulting from undetected hairline cracks in tubing
- Necrosis and then sloughing of the epidermis and dermis due to extravasation of parenteral nutrition solution

Patient teaching

- Meet with the patient before discharge to be sure that he knows how to perform the administration procedure and how to handle complications.

Correcting parenteral nutrition problems

This chart outlines common complications of parenteral nutrition along with their signs and symptoms and appropriate interventions.

Complications	Signs and symptoms	Interventions
Metabolic problems		
Hepatic dysfunction	Elevated serum aspartate aminotransferase, alkaline phosphatase, and bilirubin levels	Reduce total calorie and dextrose intake, making up lost calories by administering lipid emulsion. Change to cyclical infusion. Use specific hepatic formulations only if patient has encephalopathy.
Hypercapnia	Heightened oxygen consumption, increased carbon dioxide production, and measured respiratory quotient of 1 or greater	Reduce total calorie and dextrose intake and balance dextrose and fat calories.
Hyperglycemia	Fatigue, restlessness, confusion, anxiety, weakness, polyuria, dehydration, elevated serum glucose level and, in severe hyperglycemia, delirium or coma	Restrict dextrose intake by decreasing either infusion rate or dextrose concentration. Compensate for calorie loss by administering lipid emulsion. Begin insulin therapy.
Hyperosmolarity	Confusion, lethargy, seizures, hyperosmolar hyperglycemic nonketotic syndrome, hyperglycemia, dehydration, and glycosuria	Discontinue dextrose infusion. Administer insulin and half-normal saline solution with 10 to 20 mEq/L of potassium to rehydrate patient.
Hypocalcemia	Polyuria, dehydration, and elevated blood and urine glucose levels	Increase calcium supplements.
Hypoglycemia	Sweating, shaking, and irritability after infusion has stopped	Increase dextrose intake or decrease exogenous insulin intake.
Hypokalemia	Muscle weakness, paralysis, paresthesia, and arrhythmias	Increase potassium supplements.
Hypomagnesemia	Tingling around mouth, paresthesia in fingers, mental changes, and hyperreflexia	Increase magnesium supplements.

(continued)

Correcting parenteral nutrition problems *(continued)*

Complications	Signs and symptoms	Interventions
Hypophosphatemia	Irritability, weakness, paresthesia, coma, and respiratory arrest	Increase phosphate supplements.
Metabolic acidosis	Elevated serum chloride level and reduced serum bicarbonate level	Increase acetate and decrease chloride in parenteral nutrition solution.
Metabolic alkalosis	Reduced serum chloride level and elevated serum bicarbonate level	Decrease acetate and increase chloride in parenteral nutrition solution.
Zinc deficiency	Dermatitis, alopecia, apathy, depression, taste changes, confusion, poor wound healing, and diarrhea	Increase zinc supplements.
Mechanical problems		
Clotted I.V. catheter	Interrupted flow rate and resistance to flushing and blood withdrawal	Attempt to aspirate clot. If unsuccessful, instill a thrombolytic agent, such as alteplase, to clear catheter lumen, as ordered.
Cracked or broken tubing	Fluid leaking from tubing	Apply a padded hemostat above break to prevent air from entering line.
Dislodged catheter	Catheter out of vein	Apply pressure to site with a sterile gauze pad.
Too-rapid infusion	Nausea, headache, and lethargy	Adjust infusion rate and, if applicable, check infusion pump.
Other problems		
Air embolism	Apprehension, chest pain, tachycardia, hypotension, cyanosis, seizures, loss of consciousness, and cardiac arrest	Clamp catheter. Place patient in a steep, left lateral Trendelenburg position. Administer oxygen, as ordered. If cardiac arrest occurs, begin cardiopulmonary resuscitation. When catheter is removed, cover insertion site with dressing for 24 to 48 hours.
Extravasation	Swelling and pain around insertion site	Stop infusion. Assess patient for cardiopulmonary abnormalities; chest X-ray may be required.

Correcting parenteral nutrition problems *(continued)*

Complications	Signs and symptoms	Interventions
Phlebitis	Pain, tenderness, redness, and warmth at insertion site	Apply gentle heat to area, and elevate insertion site, if possible.
Pneumothorax and hydrothorax	Dyspnea, chest pain, cyanosis, and decreased breath sounds	Assist with chest tube insertion and maintain chest tube suctioning, as ordered.
Septicemia	Red and swollen catheter site, chills, fever, and leukocytosis	Remove catheter and culture tip. Obtain blood culture if patient has fever. Give appropriate antibiotics.
Venous thrombosis	Erythema and edema at insertion site; ipsilateral swelling of arm, neck, face, and upper chest; pain at insertion site and along vein; malaise; fever; and tachycardia	Notify practitioner and remove catheter promptly. Administer heparin, if ordered. Venous flow studies may be ordered.

- Teach the patient about potential adverse effects and complications.

Documentation

Document the times of the dressing, filter, and solution changes; the condition of the catheter insertion site; your observations of the patient's condition; and complications and interventions. (See *Documenting TPN*.)

Documenting TPN

If a patient is receiving total parenteral nutrition (TPN), be sure to record:

- central line type and location
- insertion site condition
- volume and rate of the solution infused
- your observations of any adverse reactions and your interventions
- when you discontinued a central or peripheral I.V. line for TPN
- date and time and the type of dressing applied after TPN was discontinued
- administration site appearance.

Tracheal suction

Tracheal suction involves the removal of secretions from the trachea or bronchi by means of a catheter inserted through the mouth or nose, tracheal stoma, a tracheostomy tube, or an endotracheal (ET) tube. In addition to removing secretions, tracheal suctioning also stimulates the cough reflex. This procedure helps maintain a patent airway to promote optimal exchange of oxygen and carbon dioxide and to prevent pneumonia that results from pooling of secretions. Performed as frequently as the patient's condition warrants, tracheal suction calls for strict aseptic technique.

Tracheal suction is only one component of bronchial hygiene. Encourage the patient to clear his airways by coughing and teach him proper cough techniques. Also encourage adequate hydration to facilitate the removal of secretions. Perform suctioning only when necessary and when other methods of removing secretions haven't been effective. Suctioning shouldn't be performed as a routine procedure. Assess the patient for clinical signs that suctioning is necessary, such as coarse breath sounds on auscultation, noisy respirations, prolonged expiratory breath sounds, and increased or decreased heart rate, respiratory rate, or blood pressure.

Equipment

Oxygen source (mechanical ventilator, wall or portable unit, and handheld resuscitation bag with a mask, 15-mm adapter, or a positive end-expiratory pressure valve, if indicated) ♦ wall or portable suction apparatus ♦ collection container ♦ connecting tube ♦ suction catheter kit, or a sterile suction catheter, one sterile glove, one clean glove, and a disposable sterile solution container ♦ 1-L bottle of sterile water or normal saline solution ♦ sterile water-soluble lubricant (for nasal insertion) ♦ syringe for deflating cuff of ET or tracheostomy tube ♦ waterproof trash bag ♦ goggles and face mask or face shield ♦ optional: sterile towel

Preparation

- Choose a sterile suction catheter of the appropriate size. The diameter should be no larger than half the inside diameter of the tracheostomy or ET tube to minimize hypoxia during suctioning. (A #12 or #14 French catheter may be used for an 8-mm or larger tube.)
- Place the suction apparatus on the patient's overbed table or bedside stand. Position the table or stand on your preferred side of the bed to facilitate suctioning.
- Attach the collection container to the suction unit and the connecting tube to the collection container.
- Label and date the normal saline solution or sterile water.
- Open the waterproof trash bag.

Key steps

- Confirm the patient's identity using two patient identifiers according to facility policy.
- Before suctioning, determine whether your facility requires an order and obtain one, if necessary.
- Assess the patient's vital signs, breath sounds, and general appearance to establish a baseline for comparison after suctioning. Review the patient's ABG values and oxygen saturation levels if they're available. Evaluate the patient's ability to cough and deep-breathe because this will help move secretions up the tracheobronchial tree. If you'll be performing nasotracheal suctioning, check the patient's history for a deviated septum, nasal polyps, nasal obstruction, nasal trauma, epistaxis, or mucosal swelling.
- Wash your hands. Explain the procedure to the patient. Tell him that suctioning usually causes transient coughing or gagging but that coughing is helpful for removing secretions. Continue to reassure the patient throughout the procedure to minimize anxiety, promote relaxation, and decrease oxygen demand.
- Unless contraindicated, place the patient in semi-Fowler's or high Fowler's position to promote lung expansion and productive coughing.
- Remove the top from the normal saline solution or water bottle.
- Put on the face mask and goggles.
- Open the package containing the sterile solution container.
- Using strict aseptic technique, open the suction catheter kit, and put on the gloves. If using individual supplies, open the suction catheter and the gloves, placing the nonsterile glove on your nondominant hand and the sterile glove on your dominant hand.
- Using your nondominant (nonsterile) hand, pour the normal saline solution or sterile water into the solution container.
- Place a small amount of sterile water-soluble lubricant on the sterile area. Lubricant may be used to facilitate passage of the catheter during nasotracheal suctioning.

■ Place a sterile towel over the patient's chest, if desired, to provide an additional sterile area.
■ Using your dominant (sterile) hand, remove the catheter from its wrapper. Keep it coiled so it can't touch a nonsterile object. Using your other hand to manipulate the connecting tubing, attach the catheter to the tubing (as shown below).

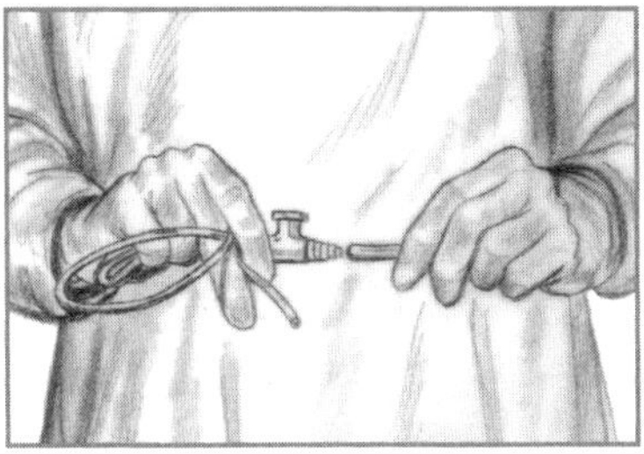

■ Using your nondominant hand, set the suction pressure according to facility policy. Typically, pressure may be set between 100 and 150 mm Hg. Higher pressures don't enhance secretion removal and may cause traumatic injury. Occlude the suction port to assess suction pressure (as shown below).

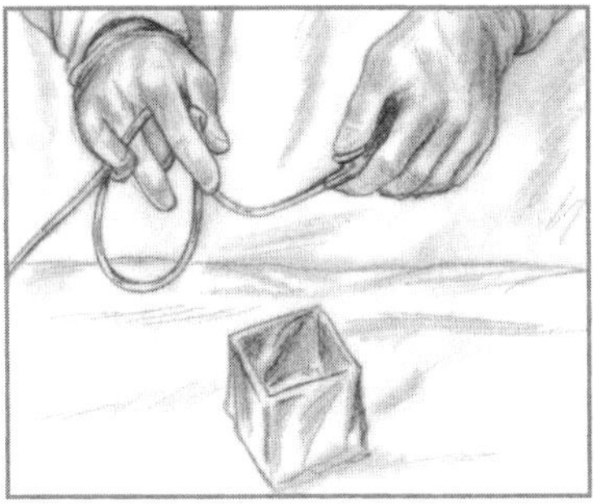

■ Dip the catheter tip in the saline solution to lubricate the outside of the catheter and reduce tissue trauma during insertion.
■ With the catheter tip in the sterile solution, occlude the control valve with the thumb of your nondominant hand. Suction a small amount of solution through the catheter (as shown top of next column) to lubricate the inside of the catheter, thus facilitating passage of secretions through it.

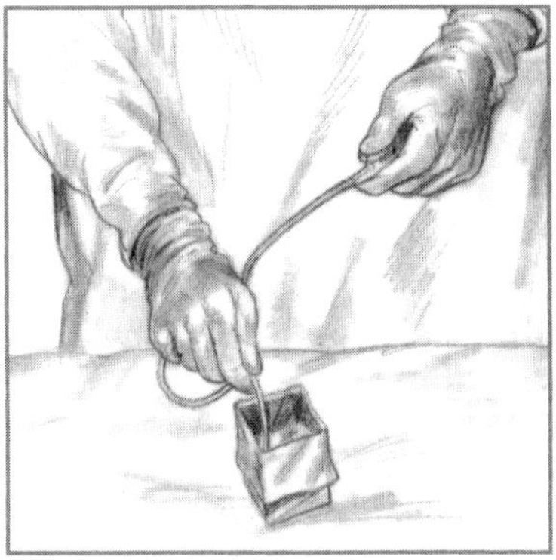

■ For nasal insertion of the catheter, lubricate the tip of the catheter with the sterile, water-soluble lubricant to reduce tissue trauma during insertion.
■ If the patient isn't intubated, instruct him to take three to six deep breaths to help minimize or prevent hypoxia during suctioning.
■ If the patient isn't intubated but is receiving oxygen, evaluate his need for preoxygenation. If indicated, instruct the patient to take three to six deep breaths while using his supplemental oxygen. (If needed, the patient may continue to receive supplemental oxygen during suctioning by leaving his nasal cannula in one nostril or by keeping the oxygen mask over his mouth.)
■ If the patient is being mechanically ventilated, preoxygenate him to minimize hypoxia after suctioning. Use the ventilator rather than a handheld resuscitation bag to hyperoxygenate and hyperinflate the lungs before suctioning. Be aware that providing hyperoxygenation on some ventilators requires a washout time of up to 2 minutes to ensure a higher oxygen concentration to travel through the tubing and reach the patient. Newer models may be able to provide increased oxygen concentrations to the patient in less time.
■ To preoxygenate using the ventilator, first adjust the fraction of inspired oxygen (FIO_2) and tidal volume according to your facility's policy and the patient's needs. Next, use the sigh mode to deliver three to six breaths. If you have an assistant for the procedure, the assistant can manage the

Closed tracheal suctioning

The closed tracheal suction system can ease removal of secretions and reduce patient complications. Consisting of a sterile suction catheter in a clear plastic sleeve, (as shown below) the system permits the patient to remain connected to the ventilator during suctioning.

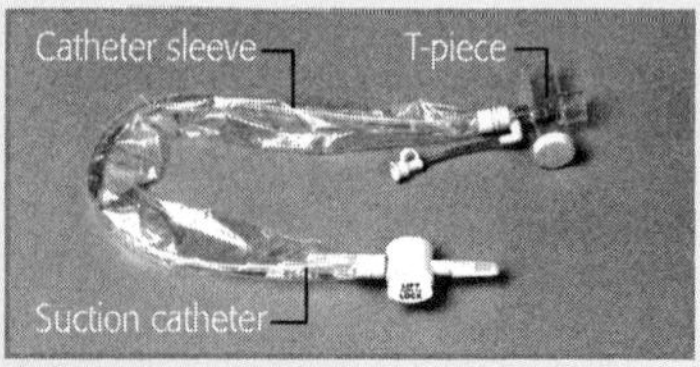

With this system, the patient can maintain the tidal volume, oxygen concentration, and positive end-expiratory pressure (PEEP) delivered by the ventilator while being suctioned. In turn, this reduces the occurrence of suction-induced hypoxemia.

Because the catheter remains in a protective sleeve, another advantage of this system is a reduced risk of infection, even when the same catheter is used many times. The caregiver doesn't need to touch the catheter and the ventilator circuit remains closed.

A closed tracheal suction device allows the patient to remain connected to the ventilator during suctioning. As a result, the patient may continue to be oxygenated and receive PEEP while being suctioned. In patients receiving intermittent mandatory mechanical ventilation, closed tracheal suctioning may reduce arterial desaturation and eliminate the need for preoxygenation.

On the negative side, closed tracheal suctioning has been found to produce increased negative airway pressure when certain ventilatory modes are used, increasing the risk of atelectasis and hypoxemia.

Implementation

To perform the procedure, gather the closed suction system that consists of a control valve, a T-piece to connect the artificial airway to the ventilator breathing circuit, and a catheter sleeve that encloses the catheter and has connections at each end for the control valve and the T-piece. Then follow these steps:

- Wash your hands.
- Remove the closed suction system from its wrapping. Attach the control valve to the connecting tubing.
- Depress the thumb suction control valve, and keep it depressed while setting the suction pressure to the desired level.
- Connect the T-piece to the ventilator breathing circuit; make sure that the irrigation port is closed. Then connect the T-piece to the patient's endotracheal or tracheostomy tube (as shown below).

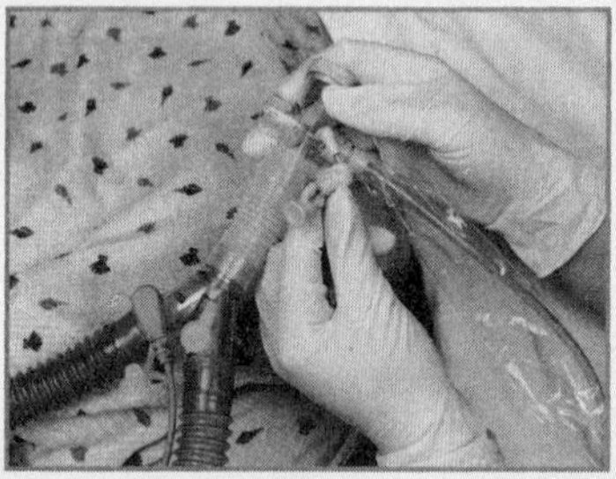

- Hyperoxygenate and hyperinflate the patient using the ventilator.

patient's oxygen needs while you perform suctioning.

Nasotracheal insertion in the nonintubated patient

- Disconnect the oxygen from the patient, if applicable.
- Using your nondominant hand, raise the tip of the patient's nose to straighten the passageway and facilitate catheter insertion.
- Insert the catheter into the patient's nostril while gently rolling it between your fingers to help it advance through the turbinates.

■ Put on clean gloves. Steadying the T-piece, use the thumb and index finger of the other hand to advance the catheter through the tube and into the patient's tracheobronchial tree (as shown below). It may be necessary to gently retract the

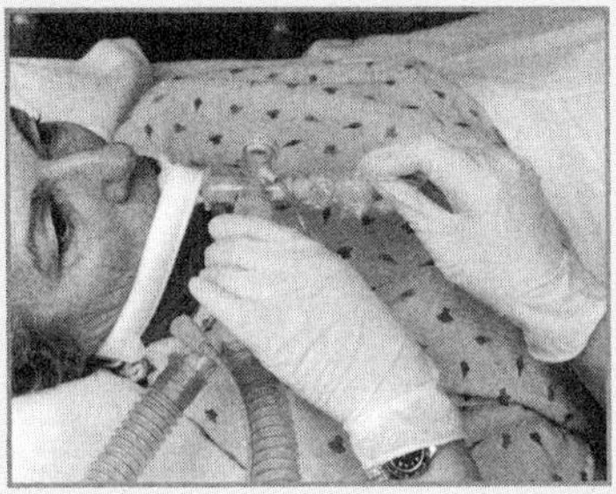

catheter sleeve as you advance the catheter.

■ While continuing to hold the T-piece and control valve, apply intermittent suction and withdraw the catheter until it reaches its fully extended length in the sleeve. Repeat the procedure only if necessary.

■ After you've finished suctioning, flush the catheter by maintaining suction while slowly introducing normal saline solution or sterile water into the irrigation port.

■ Place the thumb control valve in the OFF position.

■ Dispose of and replace the suction equipment and supplies according to facility policy.

■ Remove your gloves and wash your hands.

■ Change the closed suction system every 24 hours to minimize the risk of infection.

■ As the patient inhales, quickly advance the catheter as far as possible. To avoid oxygen loss and tissue trauma, don't apply suction during insertion.

■ If the patient coughs as the catheter passes through the larynx, briefly hold the catheter still and then resume advancement when the patient inhales.

Insertion in the intubated patient

■ If you're using a closed system, see *Closed tracheal suctioning*.

■ Using your nonsterile hand, disconnect the patient from the ventilator.

■ Using your sterile hand, gently insert the suction catheter into the artificial airway (as shown below). Advance the catheter, without applying suction, until you meet resistance. If the patient coughs, pause briefly and then resume advancement.

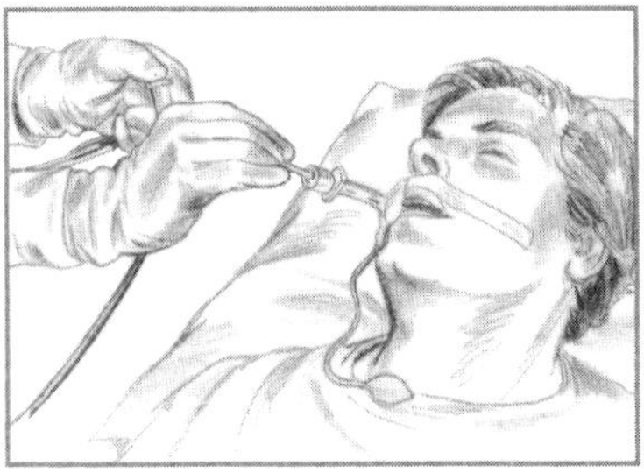

Suctioning the patient

■ After inserting the catheter, apply suction intermittently by removing and replacing the thumb of your nondominant hand over the control valve. Simultaneously use your dominant hand to withdraw the catheter as you roll it between your thumb and forefinger. This rotating motion prevents the catheter from pulling tissue into the tube as it exits, thus avoiding tissue trauma.

■ Never suction more than 10 to 15 seconds at a time to prevent hypoxia. Don't pass the catheter more than twice to reduce trauma to the tracheal mucosa.

■ If the patient is intubated, use your nondominant hand to stabilize the tip of the ET tube as you withdraw the catheter to prevent mucous membrane irritation or accidental extubation.

■ If applicable, resume oxygen delivery by reconnecting the source of oxygen or ventilation, and hyperoxygenating the patient's lungs before continuing to prevent or relieve hypoxia.

■ Observe the patient, and allow him to rest for a few minutes before the next suctioning. The timing of each suctioning and the length of each rest period depend on his tolerance of the procedure and the absence of complications. To enhance secretion removal, encourage the patient to cough between suctioning attempts.

- Observe the secretions. If they're thick, clear the catheter periodically by dipping the tip in the saline solution and applying suction. Normally, sputum is watery and tends to be sticky. Tenacious or thick sputum usually indicates dehydration. Watch for color variations. White or translucent color is normal; yellow indicates pus; green indicates retained secretions or Pseudomonas infection; brown usually indicates old blood; red indicates fresh blood; and a "red currant jelly" appearance indicates Klebsiella infection. When sputum contains blood, note whether it's streaked or well mixed. Also indicate how often blood appears.
- Monitor the patient's heart rate and rhythm. If the patient is being monitored, observe for arrhythmias. Should they occur, stop suctioning and ventilate the patient.

After suctioning

- After suctioning, hyperoxygenate the patient being maintained on a ventilator by using the ventilator's sigh mode, as described above.
- Readjust the FIO_2 and, for ventilated patients, the tidal volume to the ordered settings.
- After suctioning the lower airway, assess the patient's need for upper airway suctioning. If the cuff of the ET or tracheostomy tube is inflated, suction the upper airway before deflating the cuff with a syringe. (See "Oronasopharyngeal suction," page 339, and "Endotracheal tube care," page 166.) Always change the catheter and sterile glove before resuctioning the lower airway to avoid introducing microorganisms into the lower airway.
- Discard the gloves and catheter in the waterproof trash bag. Clear the connecting tubing by aspirating the remaining saline solution or water. Discard and replace suction equipment and supplies according to facility policy. Wash your hands.
- Auscultate the lungs bilaterally and take the patient's vital signs, if indicated, to assess the procedure's effectiveness. Note his skin color, breathing pattern, and respiratory rate.

Special considerations

- Raising the patient's nose into the sniffing position helps align the larynx and pharynx and may facilitate passing the catheter during nasotracheal suctioning. If the patient's condition permits, have an assistant extend the patient's head and neck above his shoulders. The patient's lower jaw may need to be moved up and forward. If the patient is responsive, ask him to stick out his tongue so he can't swallow the catheter during insertion.
- During suctioning, the catheter typically is advanced as far as the mainstem bronchi. However, because of tracheobronchial anatomy, the catheter tends to enter the right mainstem bronchi instead of the left. Using an angled catheter, such as a catheter coudé, may help you guide the catheter into the left mainstem bronchus. Rotating the patient's head to the right seems to have a limited effect.
- In addition to the closed tracheal method, oxygen insufflation offers a new approach to suctioning. This method uses a double-lumen catheter that allows oxygen insufflation during the suctioning procedure.

DEVICE SAFETY

Don't allow the collection container on the suction machine to become more than three-quarters full to keep from damaging the machine.

Complications

- Hypoxemia and dyspnea from oxygen being removed along with secretions
- Altered respiratory patterns due to anxiety and pain
- Cardiac arrhythmias resulting from hypoxia and stimulation of the vagus nerve in the tracheobronchial tree
- Tracheal or bronchial trauma resulting from traumatic or prolonged suctioning
- Hypoxemia, arrhythmias, hypertension, or hypotension in the patients with com-

Tracheal suctioning at home

If a patient can't mobilize secretions effectively by coughing, he may have to perform tracheal suctioning at home using either clean or aseptic technique. Most patients use clean technique, which consists of thorough hand washing and possibly wearing a clean glove. However, a patient with poor hand-washing technique, recurrent respiratory infections or a compromised immune system or one who has had recent surgery, may need to use aseptic technique.

Clean technique

Because the cost of disposable catheters can be prohibitive, many patients reuse disposable catheters, but the practice remains controversial. If the catheter has thick secretions adhering to it, the patient may clean it with Control III, a quaternary compound.

An alternative to disposable catheters is to use nondisposable, red rubber catheters. These catheters contain latex, so use with caution. Consult your facility's policy regarding the care and cleaning of suction catheters in the home setting.

Supplies needed

The supplies needed vary with the technique used. If the patient will be using clean technique, he'll need suction catheter kits (or clean gloves, suction catheters, and a basin) and distilled water. If he'll be using sterile technique, everything must be sterile: suction catheters, gloves, basin, and water (or normal saline solution).

The type of suction machine necessary will depend on the patient's needs. You'll need to evaluate the amount of suction the machine provides, how easy it is to clean, the volume of the collection bottles, how much it costs, and whether the machine has an overflow safety device to prevent secretions from entering the compressor. You'll also need to determine whether the patient needs a machine that operates on batteries and, if so, how long the batteries will last and whether and how they can be recharged.

Nursing goals

Before discharge, the patient and his family should demonstrate the suctioning procedure. They also need to recognize the indications for suctioning, the signs and symptoms of infection, the importance of adequate hydration, and when to use adjunct therapy, such as aerosol therapy, chest physiotherapy, oxygen therapy, or a handheld resuscitation bag. At discharge, arrange for a home health care provider and a durable medical equipment vendor to follow up with the patient.

promised cardiovascular or pulmonary status
- Bleeding from suctioning in patients with a history of nasopharyngeal bleeding, those who are taking anticoagulants, those who have recently had a tracheostomy, and those who have a blood disease
- Further increased intracranial pressure (ICP) in patients with current increased ICP
- Laryngospasm or bronchospasm (rare complications) during suctioning

Patient teaching

- Patients who can't mobilize secretions effectively may need to perform tracheal suctioning after discharge. (See *Tracheal suctioning at home*.)

Documentation

Record the date and time of the procedure; technique used; reason for suctioning; amount, color, consistency, and odor (if any) of secretions; any complications and interventions taken; and the patient's subjective response to the procedure. Chart preprocedure and postprocedure breath sounds and vital signs.

Tracheostomy care

Whether a tracheotomy is performed in an emergency or after careful preparation, as a permanent measure or as temporary therapy, the goals are the same: to ensure airway patency by keeping the tube free from mucus buildup, to maintain mucous membrane and skin integrity, and to prevent infection.

The patient may have one of three types of tracheostomy tube—uncuffed, cuffed, or fenestrated. Tube selection depends on the patient's condition and the physician's preference. An uncuffed tube, which may be plastic or metal, allows air to flow freely around the tracheostomy tube and through the larynx, reducing the risk of tracheal damage. Uncuffed tubes may be used for a permanent tracheostomy. A cuffed tube, made of plastic, is disposable. It's used for patients on mechanical ventilation and patients at risk for aspiration. A plastic fenestrated tube permits speech through the upper airway when the external opening is capped and the cuff is deflated. It also allows for easy removal of the inner cannula for cleaning. However, a fenestrated tube may become occluded.

If the patient is on a ventilator, a tube with an inflated cuff must be used to seal the space between the trachea and the tube so that air moves through the tube to the lungs. The patient who's breathing normally on his own may need the cuff inflated when he takes nutrition orally.

Tracheostomy care should be performed using aseptic technique until the stoma has healed to prevent infection. For recently performed tracheotomies—less than 7 days postoperatively—or unhealed tracheostomies, the site should be assessed at least every 4 hours and the stoma should be cleaned and re-dressed every 8 hours. Tracheostomy care should be performed at least every shift on a healed tracheostomy. Sterile gloves should be worn for all manipulations at the tracheostomy site. After the stoma has healed, clean gloves may be substituted for sterile ones.

Provide safety measures for the patient, such as admitting him to a room close to the nurses' station, keeping an emergency tracheostomy tray on the unit, and a label at the nurses' station near the call unit if the patient can't speak.

Keep with the patient at all times (especially when traveling for tests) an emergency replacement tracheostomy tube of the present size and one size smaller, a curved hemostat or tracheal dilator/obturator for the current tube, and a large-bore suction catheter and suction machine. Make sure that the areas the patient may travel to (such as X-ray) have working suction equipment.

Equipment

Aseptic stoma and outer-cannula care

Waterproof trash bag ♦ two sterile solution containers ♦ normal saline solution ♦ hydrogen peroxide ♦ sterile cotton-tipped applicators ♦ sterile 4″ × 4″ gauze pads ♦ sterile gloves ♦ prepackaged sterile tracheostomy dressing (or 4″ × 4″ gauze pad) ♦ equipment and supplies for suctioning and mouth care ♦ water-soluble lubricant or topical antibiotic cream ♦ materials as needed for cuff procedures and changing tracheostomy ties (see below)

Aseptic inner-cannula care

All of the preceding equipment plus a prepackaged commercial tracheostomy care set, or sterile forceps ♦ sterile nylon brush ♦ sterile 6″ (15-cm) pipe cleaners ♦ clean gloves ♦ a third sterile solution container ♦ disposable temporary inner cannula (for a patient on a ventilator)

Changing tracheostomy ties

30″ (76-cm) length of tracheostomy twill tape ♦ bandage scissors ♦ sterile gloves ♦ hemostat

Emergency tracheostomy tube replacement

Sterile tracheal dilator or sterile hemostat ♦ sterile obturator that fits the tracheostomy tube in use ♦ two extra sterile tracheostomy tubes and obturators in the appropriate size ♦ suction equipment and supplies

Keep these supplies in full view in the patient's room at all times for easy access in case of an emergency. Consider taping an emergency sterile tracheostomy tube in a sterile wrapper to the head of the bed for easy access in an emergency.

Cuff procedures

5- or 10-ml syringe ♦ padded hemostat ♦ stethoscope

Preparation

- Wash your hands, and assemble all equipment and supplies in the patient's room. Check the expiration date on each sterile package and inspect the package for tears.
- Open the waterproof trash bag, and place it next to you so that you can avoid reaching across the sterile field or the patient's stoma when discarding soiled items.
- Establish a sterile field near the patient's bed (usually on the overbed table), and place equipment and supplies on it.
- Pour sterile normal saline solution, hydrogen peroxide, or a mixture of equal parts of both solutions into one of the sterile solution containers, and then pour normal saline solution into the second sterile container for rinsing.
- For inner-cannula care, you may use a third sterile solution container to hold the gauze pads and cotton-tipped applicators saturated with cleaning solution.
- If you're replacing the disposable inner cannula, open the package containing the new inner cannula while maintaining sterile technique.
- Obtain or prepare new tracheostomy ties, if indicated.

Key steps

- Confirm the patient's identity using two patient identifiers according to facility policy.
- Assess the patient's condition to determine his need for care.
- Explain the procedure to the patient even if he's unresponsive. Provide privacy.
- Place the patient in semi-Fowler's position (unless it's contraindicated) to decrease abdominal pressure on the diaphragm and promote lung expansion.
- Remove any humidification or ventilation device.
- If the patient is being mechanically ventilated, administer hyperoxygenation and hyperinflation using the ventilator settings. If he's breathing on his own, evaluate the need for preoxygenation and instruct him to take deep breaths.
- Using sterile technique, suction the entire length of the tracheostomy tube to clear the airway of any secretions that may hinder oxygenation. (See "Tracheal suction," page 519.)
- Reconnect the patient to the humidifier or ventilator, if necessary.

Cleaning a stoma and outer cannula

- Put on sterile gloves.
- With your dominant hand, saturate a sterile gauze pad or cotton-tipped applicator with the cleaning solution. Squeeze out the excess liquid to prevent accidental aspiration. Wipe the patient's neck under the tracheostomy tube flanges and twill tapes.
- Saturate a second pad or applicator, and wipe until the skin surrounding the tracheostomy is cleaned. Use additional pads or cotton-tipped applicators to clean the stoma site and the tube's flanges. Wipe only once with each pad or applicator, and then discard it to prevent contamination of a clean area with a soiled pad or applicator.
- Rinse debris and peroxide (if used) with one or more sterile 4″ × 4″ gauze pads dampened in normal saline solution. Dry the area thoroughly with additional sterile gauze pads, and then apply a new sterile tracheostomy dressing.
- Remove and discard your gloves.

Cleaning a nondisposable inner cannula

- Put on sterile gloves.
- Using your nondominant hand, remove and discard the patient's tracheostomy dressing. With the same hand, disconnect the ventilator or humidification device, and unlock the tracheostomy tube's inner cannula by rotating it counterclockwise. Place the inner cannula in the container with hydrogen peroxide.

- Working quickly, use your dominant hand to scrub the cannula with the sterile nylon brush. If the brush doesn't slide easily into the cannula, use a sterile pipe cleaner.
- Immerse the cannula in the container of normal saline solution, and agitate it for about 10 seconds to rinse it thoroughly because hydrogen peroxide can irritate the tracheal mucosa.
- Inspect the cannula for cleanliness. Repeat the cleaning process, if necessary. If it's clean, tap it gently against the inside edge of the sterile container to remove excess liquid and prevent aspiration. Don't dry the outer surface because a thin film of moisture acts as a lubricant during insertion.
- Reinsert the inner cannula into the patient's tracheostomy tube. Lock it in place and then gently pull on it to make sure that it's positioned securely. Reconnect the mechanical ventilator. Apply a new sterile tracheostomy dressing.
- If the patient can't tolerate being disconnected from the ventilator for the time it takes to clean the inner cannula, replace the existing inner cannula with a clean one and reattach the mechanical ventilator. Then clean the cannula just removed from the patient, and store it in a sterile container for use the next time.

Caring for a disposable inner cannula

- Put on clean gloves.
- Using your dominant hand, remove the patient's inner cannula. After evaluating the secretions in the cannula, discard it properly.
- Pick up the new inner cannula, touching only the outer locking portion. Insert the cannula into the tracheostomy and, following the manufacturer's instructions, lock it securely.

Changing tracheostomy ties

- Change the ties as necessary and when soiled after the first change by the physician.
- Obtain assistance from another nurse or a respiratory therapist because of the risk of accidental tube expulsion during this procedure. Patient movement or coughing can dislodge the tube.
- Wash your hands thoroughly, and put on sterile gloves.
- If you aren't using commercially packaged tracheostomy ties, prepare new ties from a 30″ (76-cm) length of twill tape by folding one end back 1″ (2.5 cm) on itself. With the bandage scissors, cut a ½″ (1.3-cm) slit down the center of the tape from the folded edge.
- Prepare the other end of the tape the same way.
- Hold both ends together and, using scissors, cut the resulting circle of tape so that one piece is approximately 10″ (25 cm) long and the other is about 20″ (51 cm) long.
- Assist the patient into semi-Fowler's position, if possible.
- After your assistant puts on gloves, instruct her to hold the tracheostomy tube in place to prevent its expulsion during replacement of the ties. If you must perform the procedure without assistance, fasten the clean ties in place before removing the old ties to prevent tube expulsion.
- With the assistant's gloved fingers holding the tracheostomy tube in place, cut the soiled tracheostomy ties and discard them. If using scissors, be careful not to cut the tube of the pilot balloon.
- Thread the slit end of one new tie a short distance through the eye of one tracheostomy tube flange from the underside; use the hemostat, if needed, to pull the tie through. Thread the other end of the tie completely through the slit end, and pull it taut so it loops firmly through the flange. This avoids knots that can cause throat discomfort, tissue irritation, pressure, and necrosis at the patient's throat.
- Fasten the second tie to the opposite flange in the same manner.
- Instruct the patient to flex his neck while you bring the ties around to the side, and tie them together with a square knot. Flexion produces the same neck circumference as coughing and helps prevent an overly tight tie. Instruct your assistant to place one finger under the tapes as you tie them to ensure that they're tight enough to avoid slippage but loose enough to prevent

choking or jugular vein constriction. Placing the closure on the side allows easy access and prevents pressure necrosis at the back of the neck when the patient is recumbent.

- After securing the ties, cut off the excess tape with the scissors and instruct your assistant to release the tracheostomy tube.
- Make sure that the patient is comfortable and can reach the call button easily.
- Check tracheostomy-tie tension frequently on patients with traumatic injury, radical neck dissection, or cardiac failure because neck diameter can increase from swelling and cause constriction; also check neonatal or restless patients frequently because ties can loosen and cause tube dislodgment.

Concluding tracheostomy care

- Replace any humidification device.
- Provide oral care as needed because the oral cavity can become dry and malodorous or develop sores from encrusted secretions.
- Observe soiled dressings and any suctioned secretions for amount, color, consistency, and odor.
- Properly clean or dispose of all equipment, supplies, solutions, and trash, according to facility policy.
- Remove and discard your gloves.
- Make sure that all necessary supplies are readily available at the bedside.
- Repeat the procedure at least once every 8 hours or as needed. Change the dressing as often as necessary regardless of whether you also perform the entire cleaning procedure because a wet dressing with exudate or secretions predisposes the patient to skin excoriation, breakdown, and infection.

Deflating and inflating a tracheostomy cuff

- Read the cuff manufacturer's instructions because cuff types and procedures vary widely. (See *Comparing tracheostomy tubes,* page 530.)
- Assess the patient's condition, explain the procedure to him, and reassure him. Wash your hands thoroughly.
- Help the patient into semi-Fowler's position, if he's able.
- Suction the oropharyngeal cavity to prevent pooled secretions from descending into the trachea after cuff deflation.
- Release the padded hemostat clamping the cuff inflation tubing, if a hemostat is present.
- Insert a 5- or 10-ml syringe into the cuff pilot balloon, and very slowly withdraw all air from the cuff. Leave the syringe attached to the tubing for later reinflation of the cuff. Slow deflation allows positive lung pressure to push secretions upward from the bronchi. Cuff deflation may also stimulate the patient's cough reflex, producing additional secretions.
- Remove any ventilation device. Suction the lower airway through any existing tube to remove all secretions. Reconnect the ventilation device to the patient.
- While the cuff is deflated, observe the patient for adequate ventilation, and suction as necessary. If the patient has difficulty breathing, reinflate the cuff immediately by depressing the syringe plunger very slowly. Use a stethoscope to listen over the trachea for the air leak, and then inject the least amount of air necessary to achieve an adequate tracheal seal.
- When inflating the cuff, you may use the minimal-leak technique or the minimal occlusive volume technique to help gauge the proper inflation point.
- Be careful not to exceed 20 mm Hg. If pressure exceeds 20 mm Hg, notify the practitioner because you may need to change to a larger-size tube, use higher inflation pressures, or permit a larger air leak. The patient may also have a fistula if more air is needed to inflate the cuff. The recommended cuff pressure is about 18 mm Hg.
- After you've inflated the cuff, if the tubing doesn't have a one-way valve at the end, clamp the inflation line with a padded hemostat (to protect the tubing) and remove the syringe.
- Check for a minimal-leak cuff seal. Place your stethoscope over the trachea and listen while injecting air with a syringe into the pilot balloon until you no longer hear an air leak. Then slowly remove air until

Comparing tracheostomy tubes

Made of plastic or metal, tracheostomy tubes come in uncuffed, cuffed, and fenestrated varieties. Tube selection depends on the patient's condition and the physician's preference. This chart lists the advantages and disadvantages of some commonly used tubes.

Type	Advantages	Disadvantages
Uncuffed (plastic or metal) 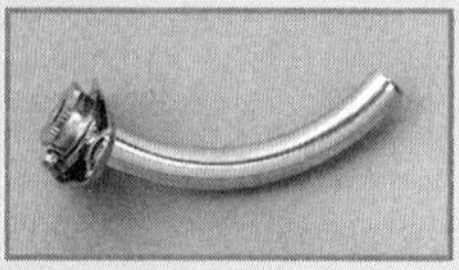	▪ Permits air to flow freely around the tracheostomy tube and through the larynx ▪ Reduces the risk of tracheal damage ▪ Is a safer choice for children	▪ Increases the risk of aspiration in adults ▪ May require adapter for mechanical ventilation
Cuffed (plastic) 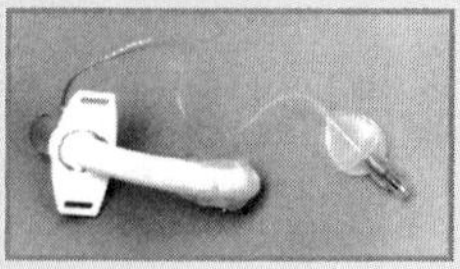	▪ Is disposable ▪ Stops the cuff and the tube from separating accidentally inside the trachea because the cuff is bonded to the tube ▪ Doesn't require periodic deflating to lower pressure because the cuff pressure is low and evenly distributed against the tracheal wall ▪ Reduces the risk of tracheal damage	▪ May cost more than other tubes
Fenestrated (plastic) 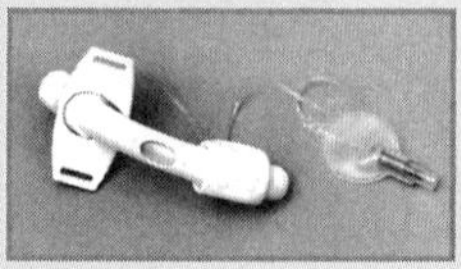	▪ Permits speech through the upper airway when the external opening is capped and the cuff is deflated ▪ Allows breathing by mechanical ventilation with the inner cannula in place and the cuff inflated ▪ Allows easy removal of the inner cannula for cleaning	▪ May have possible occlusion of the fenestrations ▪ May allow the inner cannula to dislodge

you hear a slight hiss at the end of inspiration. You shouldn't feel air coming from the patient's mouth, nose, or tracheostomy site, and a conscious patient shouldn't be able to speak.

▪ Stay alert for air leaks from the cuff itself. Suspect a leak if injection of air fails to inflate the cuff or increase cuff pressure, if you're unable to inject the amount of air you withdrew, if the patient can speak, if ventilation fails to maintain adequate respiratory movement with pressures or volumes previously considered adequate, or if air escapes during the ventilator's inspiratory cycle.

▪ Note the exact amount of air used to inflate the cuff to detect tracheal malacia if more air is consistently needed.

▪ Make sure that the patient is comfortable and can easily reach the call button and communication aids.

- Properly clean or dispose of all equipment, supplies, and trash according to facility policy.
- Replenish any used supplies, and make sure that all necessary emergency supplies are at the bedside.

Special considerations

- Keep appropriate equipment at the patient's bedside for immediate use in an emergency.
- Consult the practitioner about first-aid measures you can use for your tracheostomy patient should an emergency occur. Follow facility policy regarding procedure if a tracheostomy tube is expelled or if the outer cannula becomes blocked. If the patient's breathing is obstructed—for example, when the tube is blocked with mucus that can't be removed by suctioning or by withdrawing the inner cannula—call the appropriate code, and provide manual resuscitation with a handheld resuscitation bag or reconnect the patient to the ventilator. Don't remove the tracheostomy tube entirely because this may allow the airway to close completely. Use extreme caution when attempting to reinsert an expelled tracheostomy tube because of the risk of tracheal trauma, perforation, compression, and asphyxiation. Reassure the patient until the physician arrives (usually 1 minute or less in this type of code or emergency).
- Refrain from changing tracheostomy ties unnecessarily during the immediate postoperative period before the stoma track is well formed (usually 4 days) to avoid accidental dislodgment and expulsion of the tube. Unless secretions or drainage is a problem, ties can be changed once per day.
- Refrain from changing a single-cannula tracheostomy tube or the outer cannula of a double-cannula tube. Because of the risk of tracheal complications, the physician usually changes the cannula, with the frequency of change depending on the patient's condition.
- If the patient's neck or stoma is excoriated or infected, apply a water-soluble lubricant or topical antibiotic cream as ordered. Remember not to use a powder or an oil-based substance on or around a stoma because aspiration can cause infection and abscess.
- Replace all equipment, including solutions, regularly according to facility policy to reduce the risk of nosocomial infections.

Complications

- Hemorrhage at the operative site, causing drowning; bleeding or edema in tracheal tissue, causing airway obstruction; aspiration of secretions; introduction of air into the pleural cavity, causing pneumothorax; hypoxia or acidosis, triggering cardiac arrest; and introduction of air into surrounding tissues, causing subcutaneous emphysema (occurring within the first 48 hours after tracheostomy tube insertion)
- Tracheal stenosis, tracheomalacia, and fistula formation (late complications)
- Skin excoriation and infections due to secretions collecting under dressings and twill tape
- Occlusion of the cannula opening and obstruction of the airway due to hardened mucus or a slipped cuff
- Stimulation of the cough reflex if the tube becomes displaced and the tip rests on the carina; also causing blood vessel erosion and hemorrhage
- Tracheal erosion and necrosis due to the presence of the tube or cuff pressure

Patient teaching

- Teach the patient how to change and clean the tube.
- If the patient is being discharged with suction equipment (a few patients are), make sure that he and his family feel knowledgeable and comfortable about using the equipment.
- Make appropriate referrals for home care.

Documentation

Record the date, time, and type of the procedure; the amount, consistency, color, and odor of secretions; stoma and skin condition; the patient's respiratory status before, during, and after the procedure; change of the tracheostomy tube by the physician; duration of any cuff deflation; amount of any cuff inflation; and cuff pressure readings and specific body position. Note any complications and interventions taken, any patient or family teaching and their comprehension and progress, and the patient's tolerance of the treatment.

Tracheotomy

A tracheotomy involves the surgical creation of an external opening—called a *tracheostomy*—into the trachea and insertion of an indwelling tube to maintain the airway's patency. If all other attempts to establish an airway have failed, a physician may perform a tracheotomy at the patient's bedside. This procedure may be necessary when an airway obstruction results from laryngeal edema, foreign body obstruction, or a tumor. An emergency tracheotomy may also be performed when endotracheal intubation is contraindicated.

Use of a cuffed tracheostomy tube provides and maintains a patent airway, prevents the unconscious or paralyzed patient from aspirating food or secretions, allows removal of tracheobronchial secretions from the patient unable to cough, replaces an endotracheal tube, and permits the use of positive-pressure ventilation.

When laryngectomy accompanies a tracheostomy, the physician may insert a laryngectomy tube—a shorter version of a tracheostomy tube. In addition, the patient's trachea is sutured to the skin surface. Consequently, with a laryngectomy, accidental tube expulsion doesn't precipitate immediate closure of the tracheal opening. When healing occurs, the patient has a permanent neck stoma through which respiration takes place.

Although tracheostomy tubes come in plastic and metal, plastic tubes are commonly used in emergencies because they have a universal adapter for respiratory support equipment, such as a mechanical ventilator, and a cuff to allow positive-pressure ventilation.

Equipment

Tracheostomy tube of the proper size (usually #13 to #38 French or #00 to #9 Jackson) with obturator ♦ tracheostomy tape ♦ sterile tracheal dilator ♦ vein retractor ♦ sutures and needles ♦ 4″ × 4″ gauze pads ♦ sterile drapes, gloves, mask, and gown ♦ sterile bowls ♦ stethoscope ♦ sterile tracheostomy ♦ dressing ♦ pillow ♦ tracheostomy ties ♦ suction apparatus ♦ alcohol pad ♦ povidone-iodine solution ♦ sterile water ♦ 5-ml syringe with 22G needle ♦ local anesthetic such as lidocaine ♦ oxygen therapy device ♦ oxygen source ♦ emergency equipment to be kept at bedside, including suctioning equipment, sterile obturator, sterile tracheostomy tube, sterile inner cannula, sterile tracheostomy tube and inner cannula one size smaller than tubes in use, sterile tracheal dilator or sterile hemostats

Many hospitals use prepackaged sterile tracheotomy trays.

Preparation

- Have one person stay with the patient while another obtains the necessary equipment.
- Wash your hands; then, maintaining sterile technique, open the tray and the packages containing the solution.
- Take the tracheostomy tube from its container, and place it on the sterile field.
- If necessary, set up the suction equipment, and make sure it works.
- When the physician opens the sterile bowls, pour in the appropriate solution.

Key steps

- Explain the procedure to the patient even if he's unresponsive.
- Assess his condition and provide privacy. Maintain ventilation until the tracheotomy is performed.
- Wipe the top of the local anesthetic vial with an alcohol pad. Invert the vial so that the physician can withdraw the anesthetic using the 22G needle attached to the 5-ml syringe.
- Before the physician begins, place a pillow under the patient's shoulders and neck and hyperextend his neck.
- The physician will put on a sterile gown, gloves, and mask.
- Help the physician with the tube insertion as needed. (See *Assisting with a tracheotomy.*)

Assisting with a tracheotomy

To perform a tracheotomy, the physician will first clean the area from the chin to the nipples with povidone-iodine solution. Next, he'll place sterile drapes on the patient and locate the area for the incision—usually 1 to 2 cm below the cricoid cartilage. Then he'll inject a local anesthetic.

He'll make a horizontal or vertical incision in the skin. (A vertical incision helps avoid arteries, veins, and nerves on the lateral borders of the trachea.) Then he'll dissect subcutaneous fat and muscle and move the muscle aside with vein retractors to locate the tracheal rings. He'll make an incision between the second and third tracheal rings (as shown above right) and use hemostats to control bleeding.

He'll inject a local anesthetic into the tracheal lumen to suppress the cough reflex, and then he'll create a stoma in the trachea. When this is done, carefully apply suction to remove blood and secretions that may obstruct the airway or be aspirated into the lungs. Next, the physician will insert the tracheostomy tube and obturator into the stoma (as shown middle right). After inserting the tube, he'll remove the obturator.

Apply a sterile tracheostomy dressing, and anchor the tube with tracheostomy ties (as shown below right). Check for air movement through the tube and auscultate the lungs to ensure proper placement.

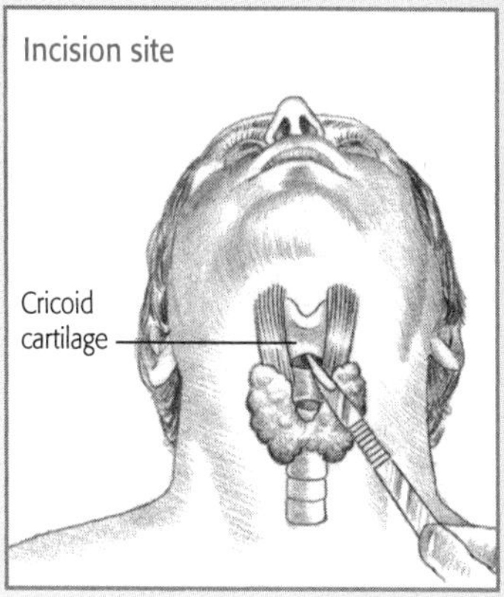

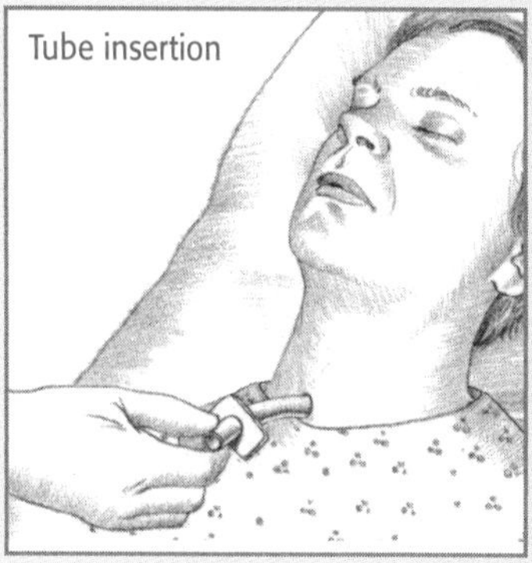

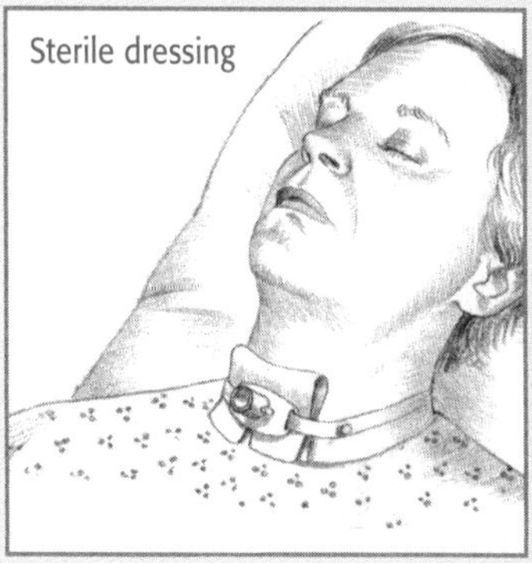

An alternative approach

In another approach, the physician inserts the tracheostomy tube percutaneously at the bedside. Using either a series of dilators or a pair of forceps, he creates a stoma for tube insertion. Unlike the surgical technique, this method dilates rather than cuts the tissue structures.

After the skin is prepared and anesthetized, the physician makes a 1-cm midline incision. When the stoma reaches the desired size, the physician inserts the tracheostomy tube. When the tube is in place, inflate the cuff, secure the tube, and check the patient's breath sounds. Next, obtain a portable chest X-ray.

- When the tube is in position, attach it to the appropriate oxygen therapy device.
- Inject air into the distal cuff port to inflate the cuff.
- The physician will suture the corners of the incision and secure the tracheostomy tube with tape.
- Put on sterile gloves.
- Apply the sterile tracheostomy dressing under the tracheostomy tube flange. Place the tracheostomy ties through the openings of the tube flanges, and tie them on the side of the patient's neck. This allows easy access and prevents pressure necrosis at the back of the neck.
- Clean or dispose of the used equipment according to policy. Replenish all supplies as needed.
- Make sure a chest X-ray is ordered to confirm tube placement.

Special considerations

- Assess the patient's vital signs and respiratory status every 15 minutes for 1 hour, then every 30 minutes for 2 hours, and then every 2 hours until his condition is stable.
- Monitor the patient carefully for signs of infection. Ideally, the tracheotomy should be performed using sterile technique as described. But, in an emergency, this may not be possible.
- Make sure the following equipment is always at the patient's bedside:
  - suctioning equipment because the patient may need his airway cleared at any time
  - the sterile obturator used to insert the tracheostomy tube in case the tube is expelled
  - a sterile tracheostomy tube and obturator (the same size as the one used) in case the tube must be replaced quickly
  - a spare, sterile inner cannula that can be used if the cannula is expelled
  - a sterile tracheostomy tube and obturator one size smaller than the one used, which may be needed if the tube is expelled and the trachea begins to close
  - a sterile tracheal dilator or sterile hemostats to maintain an open airway before inserting a new tracheostomy tube.
- Review emergency first-aid measures, and always follow facility policy concerning an expelled or blocked tracheostomy tube. When a blocked tube can't be cleared by suctioning or withdrawing the inner cannula, policy may require you to stay with the patient while someone else calls the practitioner or the appropriate code. You should continue trying to ventilate the patient with whatever method works—for example, a handheld resuscitation bag. Don't remove the tracheostomy tube entirely; doing so may close the airway completely.
- Use extreme caution if you try to reinsert an expelled tracheostomy tube to avoid tracheal trauma, perforation, compression, and asphyxiation.

Complications

- Airway obstruction (from improper tube placement), hemorrhage, edema, a perforated esophagus, subcutaneous or mediastinal emphysema, aspiration of secretions, tracheal necrosis (from cuff pressure), infection, or lacerations of arteries, veins, or nerves

Documentation

Record the reason for the procedure, the date and time it took place, and the patient's respiratory status before and after the procedure. Include any complications that occurred during the procedure, the amount of cuff pressure, and the respiratory therapy initiated after the procedure. Also, note the patient's response to respiratory therapy.

Transabdominal tube feeding and care

To access the stomach, duodenum, or jejunum, the physician may place a tube through the patient's abdominal wall. This may be done surgically or percutaneously. A gastrostomy or jejunostomy tube is usually inserted during intra-abdominal surgery. The tube may be used for feeding during the immediate postoperative period or it may provide long-term enteral access, depending on the type of surgery. Typically, the physician will suture the tube in place to prevent gastric contents from leaking.

In contrast, a percutaneous endoscopic gastrostomy (PEG) or jejunostomy (PEJ) tube can be inserted endoscopically without the need for laparotomy or general anesthesia. Typically, the insertion is done in the endoscopy suite or at the patient's bedside. A PEG or PEJ tube may be used for nutrition, drainage, and decompression. Contraindications to endoscopic placement include obstruction (such as an esophageal stricture or duodenal blockage), previous gastric surgery, morbid obesity, and ascites. These conditions would necessitate surgical placement.

With either type of tube placement, feedings may begin after 24 hours (or when peristalsis resumes).

After a time, the tube may need replacement, and the physician may recommend a similar tube, such as an indwelling urinary catheter or a mushroom catheter, or a gastrostomy button—a skin-level feeding tube.

Nursing care includes providing skin care at the tube site, maintaining the feeding tube, administering feeding, monitoring the patient's response to feeding, adjusting the feeding schedule, and preparing the patient for self-care after discharge.

Equipment

Feeding

Feeding formula ♦ large-bulb or catheter-tip syringe ♦ 120 ml of water ♦ 4″ × 4″ gauze pads ♦ soap ♦ skin protectant ♦ hypoallergenic tape ♦ gravity-drip administration bags ♦ mouthwash, toothpaste, or mild salt solution ♦ stethoscope ♦ gloves ♦ optional: enteral infusion pump

Decompression

Suction apparatus with tubing ♦ straight drainage collection set

Preparation

- Always check the expiration date on commercially prepared feeding formulas.
- If the formula has been prepared by the dietitian or pharmacist, check the preparation time and date.
- Discard any opened formula that's more than 1 day old.
- Commercially prepared administration sets and enteral pumps allow continuous formula administration.
- Place the desired amount of formula into the gavage container and purge air from the tubing.
- To avoid contamination, hang only a 4- to 6-hour supply of formula at a time.

Key steps

- Provide privacy, and wash your hands.
- Confirm the patient's identity using two patient identifiers according to facility policy.
- Explain the procedure to the patient. Tell him, for example, that feedings usually start at a slow rate and increase as tolerated. After he tolerates continuous feedings, he may progress to intermittent feedings, as ordered.
- Assess for bowel sounds with a stethoscope before feeding, and monitor for abdominal distention.
- Ask the patient to sit, or assist him into semi-Fowler's position, for the entire feeding. This helps to prevent esophageal reflux and pulmonary aspiration of the formula. For an intermittent feeding, have him maintain this position throughout the feeding and for 1 hour afterward.
- Put on gloves. Before starting the feeding, measure residual gastric contents. Attach the syringe to the feeding tube and aspirate. If the contents measure more than twice the amount infused, hold the feeding and recheck in 1 hour. If residual contents remain too high, notify the practitioner. Chances are the formula isn't being absorbed properly. Keep in mind that residual contents will be minimal with PEJ tube feedings.
- Allow 30 ml of water to flow into the feeding tube to establish patency.
- Be sure to administer formula at room temperature. Cold formula may cause cramping.

Intermittent feedings

- Allow gravity to help the formula flow over 30 to 45 minutes. Faster infusions may cause bloating, cramps, or diarrhea.

- Begin intermittent feeding with a low volume (200 ml) daily. According to the patient's tolerance, increase the volume per feeding, as needed, to reach the desired calorie intake.
- When the feeding finishes, flush the feeding tube with 30 to 60 ml of water to maintain patency and provide hydration.
- Cap the tube to prevent leakage.
- Rinse the feeding administration set thoroughly with hot water to avoid contaminating subsequent feedings. Allow it to dry between feedings.

Continuous feedings

- Measure residual gastric contents every 4 hours.
- To administer the feeding with a pump, set up the equipment according to the manufacturer's guidelines, and fill the feeding bag. To administer the feeding by gravity, fill the container with formula and purge air from the tubing.
- Monitor the gravity drip rate or pump infusion rate frequently to ensure accurate delivery of formula.
- Flush the feeding tube with 30 to 60 ml of water every 4 hours to maintain patency and to provide hydration.
- Monitor intake and output to anticipate and detect fluid or electrolyte imbalances.

Decompression

- To decompress the stomach, connect the PEG port to the suction device with tubing or straight gravity drainage tubing. Jejunostomy feeding may be given simultaneously via the PEJ port of the dual-lumen tube.

Tube exit site care

- Provide daily skin care.
- Gently remove the dressing by hand. Never cut away the dressing over the catheter because you might cut the tube or the sutures holding the tube in place.
- At least daily and as needed, clean the skin around the tube's exit site using a 4″ × 4″ gauze pad soaked in the prescribed cleaning solution. When healed, wash the skin around the exit site daily with soap. Rinse the area with water and pat dry. Apply skin protectant if necessary.
- Anchor a gastrostomy or jejunostomy tube to the skin with hypoallergenic tape to prevent peristaltic migration of the tube. This also prevents tension on the suture anchoring the tube in place.
- Coil the tube, if necessary, and tape it to the abdomen to prevent pulling and contamination of the tube. PEG and PEJ tubes have toggle-bolt-like internal and external bumpers that make tape anchors unnecessary. (See *Caring for a PEG or PEJ site*.)

Special considerations

- If the patient vomits or complains of nausea, feeling too full, or regurgitation, stop the feeding immediately and assess his condition. Flush the feeding tube and attempt to restart the feeding again in 1 hour (measure residual gastric contents first). You may have to decrease the volume or rate of feedings. If the patient develops dumping syndrome, which includes nausea, vomiting, cramps, pallor, and diarrhea, the feedings may have been given too quickly.
- Provide mouth care frequently. Brush all surfaces of the teeth, gums, and tongue at least twice daily using mouthwash, toothpaste, or mild salt solution.
- You can administer most tablets and pills through the tube by crushing them and diluting as necessary. (However, don't crush enteric-coated or sustained-release drugs, which lose their effectiveness when crushed.) Medications should be in liquid form for administration.
- Control diarrhea resulting from dumping syndrome by using continuous pump or gravity-drip infusions, diluting the feeding formula, or adding antidiarrheal medications.

Complications

- GI or other systemic problems, mechanical malfunction, and metabolic disturbances
- Cramping, nausea, vomiting, bloating, and diarrhea related to medication, too-rapid infusion rate, formula contamination, osmolarity, or temperature (too cold or too warm); fat malabsorption; or intestinal atrophy from malnutrition

Caring for a PEG or PEJ site

The exit site of a percutaneous endoscopic gastrostomy (PEG) tube or percutaneous endoscopic jejunostomy (PEJ) tube requires routine observation and care. Follow these care guidelines:

■ Change the dressing daily while the tube is in place.

■ After removing the dressing, carefully slide the tube's outer bumper away from the skin (as shown below) ½" (1.3 cm).

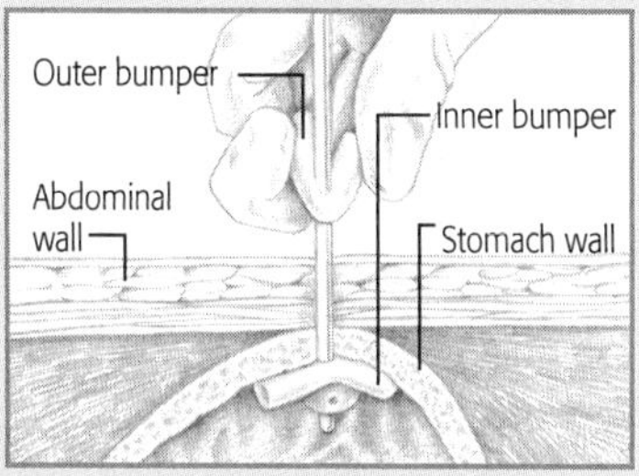

■ Examine the skin around the tube. Look for redness and other signs of infection or erosion.

■ Gently depress the skin surrounding the tube and inspect for drainage (as shown top of next column). Expect minimal wound drainage initially after implantation. This should subside in about 1 week.

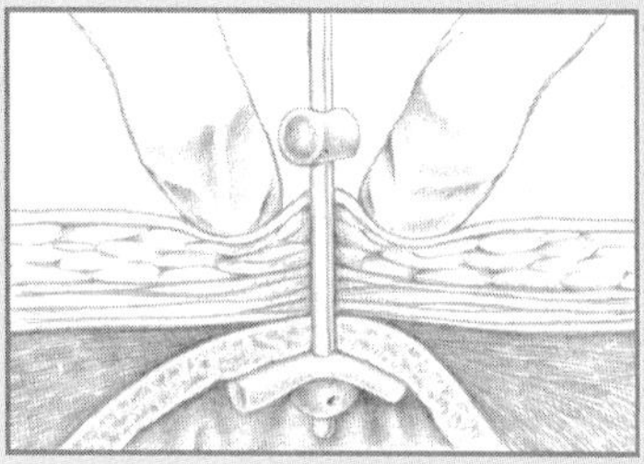

■ Inspect the tube for wear and tear. (A tube that wears out will need replacement.)

■ Clean the site with the prescribed cleaning solution. Then apply antiseptic ointment over the exit site, according to facility guidelines.

■ Rotate the outer bumper 90 degrees to avoid repeating the same tension on the same skin area, and slide the outer bumper back over the exit site.

■ If leakage appears at the PEG site, or if the patient risks dislodging the tube, apply a sterile gauze dressing over the site. Don't put sterile gauze underneath the outer bumper. Loosening the anchor this way allows the feeding tube free play, which could lead to wound abscess.

■ Write the date and time of the dressing change on the tape.

■ Constipation resulting from inadequate hydration or insufficient exercise

■ Systemic problems caused by pulmonary aspiration, infection at the tube exit site, or contaminated formula

■ PEG or PEJ tube migration if the external bumper loosens; occlusion resulting from incompletely crushed and liquefied medication particles or inadequate tube flushing; and ruptured or cracked tube from age, drying, or frequent manipulation

■ Vitamin and mineral deficiencies, glucose tolerance, and fluid and electrolyte imbalances following bouts of diarrhea or constipation

Patient teaching

■ Instruct the patient and family members or other caregivers in all aspects of enteral feedings, including tube maintenance and site care.

■ Specify signs and symptoms to report to the practitioner, define emergency situations, and review actions to take.

■ When the tube needs replacement, advise the patient that the physician may insert a replacement gastrostomy button or a latex, indwelling, or mushroom catheter after removing the initial feeding tube. The procedure may be done in the physician's office or the hospital's endoscopy suite.

■ As the patient's tolerance to tube feeding improves, he may wish to try syringe feed-

Syringe feeding instructions

If your patient is required to feed himself by syringe when he returns home, you'll need to teach him how to do so before he's discharged. Here are some points to emphasize.

Initial instructions

First, show the patient how to clamp the feeding tube, remove the syringe's bulb or plunger, and place the tip of the syringe into the feeding tube (as shown below). Then have him instill between 30 and 60 ml of water into the feeding tube.

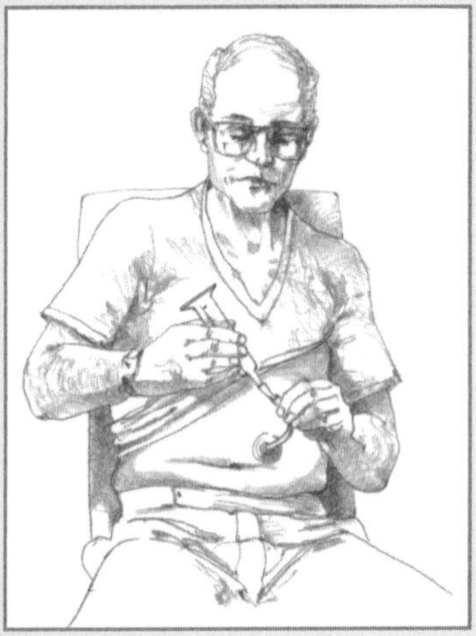

Next, tell him to pour the feeding solution into the syringe and begin the feeding (as shown top of next column). As the solution flows into the stomach, show him how to tilt the syringe to allow air bubbles to escape. Describe the discomfort that air bubbles may cause.

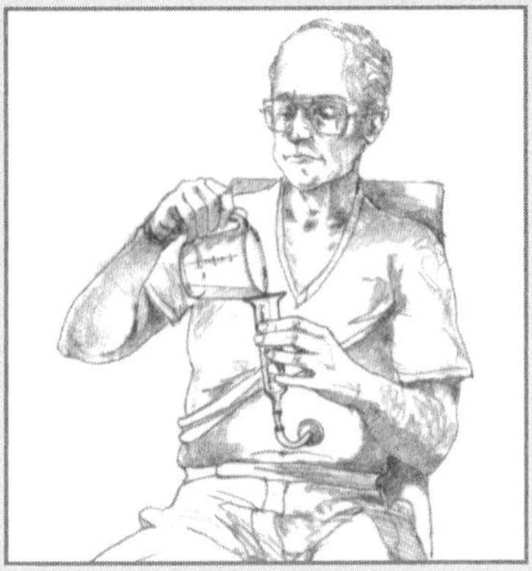

Tips for free flow

When about one-fourth of the feeding solution remains, direct the patient to refill the syringe. Caution him to avoid letting the syringe empty completely.

Demonstrate how to increase and decrease the solution's flow rate by raising or lowering the syringe. Explain also that he may need to dilute a thick solution to promote free flow.

Finishing up

Inform the patient that the feeding infusion process should take about 15 minutes or more. If the process takes less than 15 minutes, dumping syndrome may result.

Show the patient the steps needed to finish the feeding, including how to flush the tube with water, clamp the tube, and clean the equipment for later use. Naturally, if he's using disposable gear, urge him to discard it properly. Review how to store unused feeding solution as appropriate.

ings rather than intermittent feedings. If appropriate, teach him how to feed himself by this method. (See *Syringe feeding instructions*.)

Documentation

On the intake and output record, note the date, time, and amount of each feeding and the water volume instilled. Maintain total volumes for nutrients and water separately to allow calculation of nutrient intake. In your notes, document the type of formula, the infusion method and rate, the patient's tolerance of the procedure and formula, and the amount of residual gastric contents. Record complications and abdominal assessment findings. Note patient-teaching topics covered, and note the patient's progress in self-care.

Transcranial Doppler monitoring

Transcranial Doppler ultrasonography is a noninvasive method of monitoring blood flow in the intracranial vessels, specifically the circle of Willis. This procedure is used in the intensive care unit to monitor patients who have experienced cerebrovascular disorders, such as stroke, head trauma, or subarachnoid hemorrhage. It can help detect intracranial stenosis, vasospasm, and arteriovenous malformations as well as assess collateral pathways. Because it has the advantage of monitoring a continuous waveform, it can be used in intraoperative monitoring of cerebral circulation.

The transcranial Doppler unit transmits pulses of low-frequency ultrasound, which are then reflected back to the transducer by the red blood cells moving in the vessel being monitored. This information is then processed by the instrument into an audible signal and a velocity waveform, which is displayed on the monitor. The displayed waveform is actually a moving graph of blood flow velocities with TIME displayed along the horizontal axis, VELOCITY displayed along the vertical axis, and AMPLITUDE represented by various colors or intensities within the waveform. The heart's contractions speed up the movement of blood cells during systole and slow it down during diastole, resulting in a waveform that varies in velocity over the cardiac cycle.

Transcranial Doppler monitoring provides instantaneous, real-time information about cerebral blood flow and is noninvasive and painless for the patient. The unit itself is portable and easy to use. The method's disadvantage is the reliance on the ability of the ultrasound waves to penetrate thin areas of the cranium; this is difficult if the patient has thickening of the temporal bone, which increases with age.

The transcranial Doppler unit should always be used with its power set at the lowest level needed to provide an adequate waveform. This procedure requires specialized training to ensure accurate vessel identification and correct interpretation of the signals.

Equipment

Transcranial Doppler unit ♦ transducer with an attachment system ♦ terry cloth headband ♦ ultrasonic coupling gel ♦ marker

Key steps

- Confirm the patient's identity using two patient identifiers according to facility policy.
- Explain the procedure to the patient, and answer any questions he has as thoroughly as possible. Place him in the proper position—usually the supine position.
- Turn the Doppler unit on and observe as it performs a self-test. The screen should show six parameters: PEAK (CM/S), MEAN (CM/S), DEPTH (M/M), DELTA (%), EMBOLI (AGR), and PI+.
- Enter the patient's name and identification number in the appropriate place on the Doppler unit. Depending on the unit you're using, you may need to enter additional information, such as the patient's diagnosis or the practitioner's name.
- Indicate the vessel that you wish to monitor (usually the right or left middle cerebral artery [MCA]). You'll also need to set the approximate depth of the vessel within the skull (50 mm for the MCA).
- Use the keypad to increase the power level to 100% to initially locate the signal. You can later decrease the level as needed, depending on the thickness of the patient's skull.
- Examine the temporal region of the patient's head, and mentally identify the three windows of the transtemporal access route: posterior, middle, and anterior (as shown top of next page).

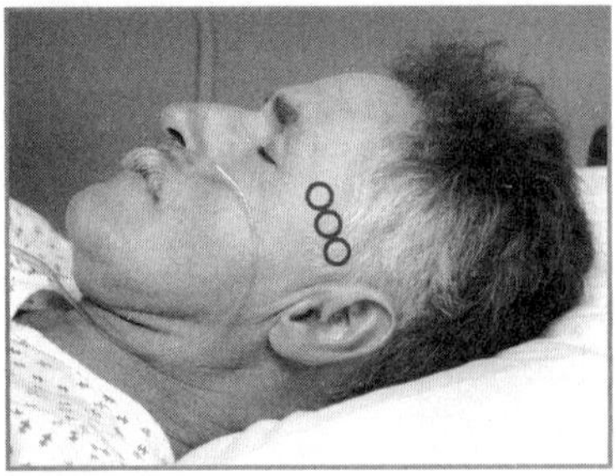

- Apply a generous amount of ultrasonic gel at the level of the temporal bone between the tragus of the ear and the end of the eyebrow, over the area of the three windows.
- Place the transducer on the posterior window. Angle the transducer slightly in an anterior direction, and slowly move it in a narrow circle. This movement is commonly called the *flashlighting technique*. As you hold the transducer at an angle and perform flashlighting, also begin to very slowly move the transducer forward across the temporal area. As you do this, listen for the audible signal with the highest pitch. This sound corresponds to the highest velocity signal, which corresponds to the signal of the vessel you're assessing. You can also use headphones to help you better evaluate the audible signal and provide patient privacy.
- After you've located the highest-pitched signal, use a marker to draw a circle around the transducer head on the patient's temple (as shown below). Note the angle of the transducer so that you can duplicate it after the transducer attachment system is in place.

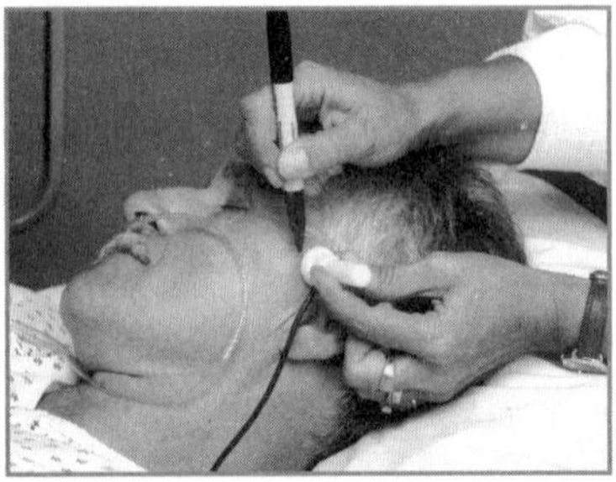

- Place the transducer system on the patient. To do this, first place the plate of the transducer attachment system over the patient's temporal area; match the circular opening in the plate exactly with the circle drawn on the patient's head. Holding the plate in place, encircle the patient's head with the straps attached to the system. Finally, tighten the straps so that the transducer attachment system will stay in place on the patient's head.
- Fill the circular opening in the plate with the ultrasonic gel.
- Place the transducer in the gel-filled opening in the attachment system plate. Using the plastic screws provided, loosely secure the two plates together. This will hold the transducer in place but allow it to rotate for the best angle.
- Adjust the position and angle of the transducer until you again hear the highest-pitched audible signal. When you hear this signal, look at the waveform on the monitor screen. You should see a clear waveform with a bright white line (called an envelope) at the upper edge of the waveform. The envelope exactly follows the contours of the waveform itself.
- If the envelope doesn't follow the waveform's contours, adjust the GAIN setting. If the signal is wrapping around the screen, use the SCALE key to increase the scale and the BASELINE key to drop the baseline.
- When you've determined that you have the strongest, highest-pitched signal and the best waveform, lock the transducer in place by tightening the plastic screws (as shown below). The tightened plates will hold the transducer at the angle you've chosen. Disconnect the transducer handle.

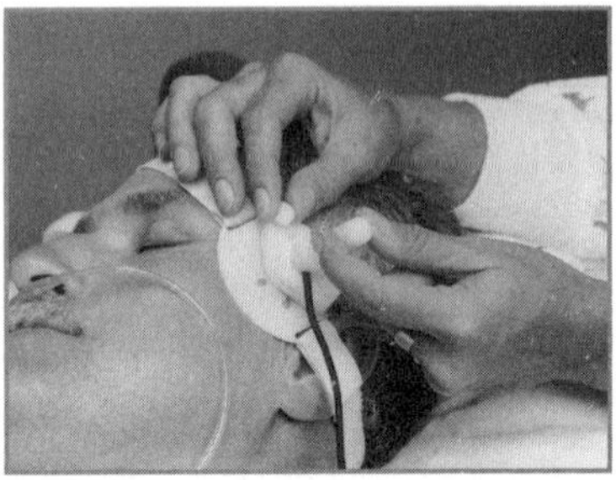

Comparing velocity waveforms

A normal transcranial Doppler signal is usually characterized by mean velocities that fall within the normal reported values. Additional information can be gathered by evaluating the shape of the velocity waveform.

Effect of significant proximal vessel obstruction

A delayed systolic upstroke can be seen in a waveform when significant proximal vessel obstruction is present.

Normal

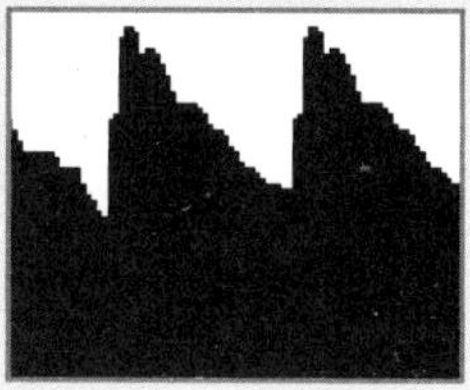

Proximal vessel obstruction

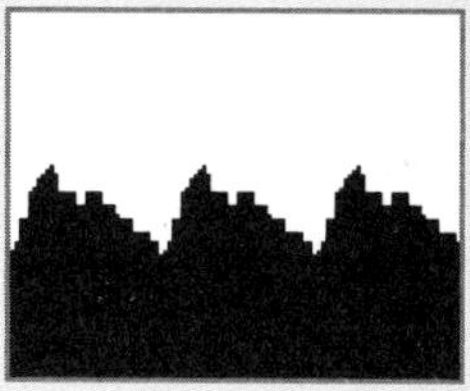

Effect of increased cerebrovascular resistance

Changes in cerebrovascular resistance, as occur with increased intracranial pressure, cause a decrease in diastolic flow.

Normal

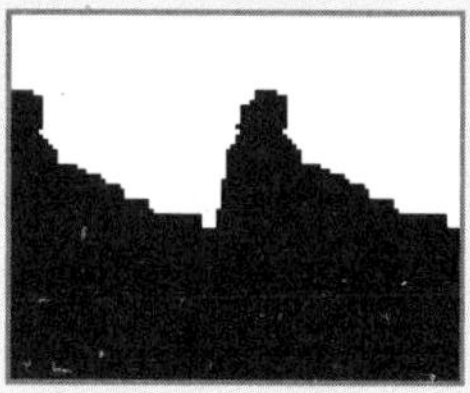

Increased resistance

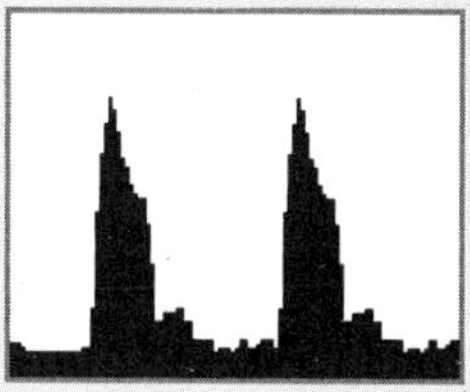

- Place a wide terry cloth headband over the transducer attachment system, and secure it around the patient's head to provide additional stability for the transducer.
- Look at the monitor screen. You should be able to see a waveform and read the numeric values of the peak, mean velocities, and pulsatility index (PI+) above the displayed waveform. The shape of the waveform reveals more information. (See *Comparing velocity waveforms*.)

Special considerations

- Velocity changes in the transcranial Doppler signal correlate with changes in cerebral blood flow. The parameter that most clearly reflects this change is the mean velocity. First, establish a baseline for the mean velocity. As the patient's velocity increases or decreases, the value (%) will change negatively or positively from the baseline.
- Emboli appear as high-intensity transients occurring randomly during the cardiac cycle. Emboli make a distinctive "clicking," "chirping," or "plunking" sound. You can set up an emboli counter to count either the total number of emboli aggregates or the rate of embolic events per minute.
- Various screens can be stored on the system's hard drive and can be recalled or printed.
- Before using the transcranial Doppler system, be sure to remove turban head dressings or thick dressings over the test site.

Complications

- None known

Documentation

Record the date and the time that the monitoring began, and note which artery is being monitored. Document any patient teaching as well as the patient's tolerance of the procedure.

Transdermal drug administration

Through an adhesive patch or a measured dose of ointment applied to the skin, transdermal drugs deliver constant, controlled medication directly into the bloodstream for a prolonged systemic effect.

Medications available in transdermal form include nitroglycerin, used to control angina; scopolamine, used to treat motion sickness; estradiol, used for postmenopausal hormone replacement; clonidine, used to treat hypertension; nicotine, used for smoking cessation; and fentanyl, an opioid analgesic used to control chronic pain. Nitroglycerin ointment dilates coronary vessels for up to 4 hours; a nitroglycerin disk or pad can produce the same effect for as long as 24 hours. A scopolamine patch can relieve motion sickness for as long as 72 hours, transdermal estradiol lasts for up to 1 week, clonidine and nicotine patches last for 24 hours, and a fentanyl patch can last for up to 72 hours.

Contraindications for transdermal drug application include skin allergies or skin reactions to the drug. Transdermal drugs shouldn't be applied to broken or irritated skin because they would increase irritation, or to scarred or callused skin, which might impair absorption.

Equipment

Patient's medication record and chart ♦ gloves ♦ prescribed medication (patch or ointment) ♦ application strip or measuring paper (for nitroglycerin ointment) ♦ adhesive tape ♦ plastic wrap (optional for nitroglycerin ointment) or semipermeable dressing

Key steps

- Verify the order on the patient's medication record by checking it against the prescriber's order.
- Wash your hands and put on gloves.
- Check the label on the medication to make sure you'll be giving the correct drug in the correct dose. Note the expiration date.
- Confirm the patient's identity using two patient identifiers according to facility policy.
- If your facility uses a bar code scanning system, be sure to scan your ID badge, the patient's ID bracelet, and the medication's bar code.
- Explain the procedure to the patient and provide privacy.
- Remove previously applied medication.

Applying transdermal ointment

- Place the prescribed amount of ointment on the application strip or measuring paper, taking care not to get any on your skin. (See *Applying nitroglycerin ointment.*)
- Apply the strip to a dry, hairless area of the body. Don't rub the ointment into the skin.
- Tape the strip and ointment to the skin.
- If desired, cover the application strip with the plastic wrap, and tape the wrap in place.

Applying a transdermal patch

- Open the package and remove the patch.
- Without touching the adhesive surface, remove the clear plastic backing.
- Apply the patch to a dry, hairless area—behind the ear, for example, as with scopolamine.
- Write the date, time, and your initials on the dressing.

After applying transdermal medications

- Store the medication as ordered.
- Instruct the patient to keep the area around the patch or ointment as dry as possible.

Special considerations

- Reapply daily transdermal medications at the same time every day to ensure a continuous effect, but alternate the application sites to avoid skin irritation. Before reapplying nitroglycerin ointment, remove the plastic wrap, application strip, and any remaining ointment from the patient's skin at the previous site.
- When applying a scopolamine or fentanyl patch, instruct the patient not to

Applying nitroglycerin ointment

Unlike most topical medications, nitroglycerin ointment is used for its transdermal systemic effect. It's used to dilate the veins and arteries, thus improving cardiac perfusion in a patient with cardiac ischemia or angina pectoris.

To apply nitroglycerin ointment, start by taking the patient's baseline blood pressure so that you can compare it with later readings. Remove any previously applied nitroglycerin ointment. Gather your equipment. Nitroglycerin ointment, which is prescribed by the inch, comes with a rectangular piece of ruled paper to be used in applying the medication. Squeeze the prescribed amount of ointment onto the ruled paper (as shown below). Put on gloves, if desired, to avoid contact with the medication.

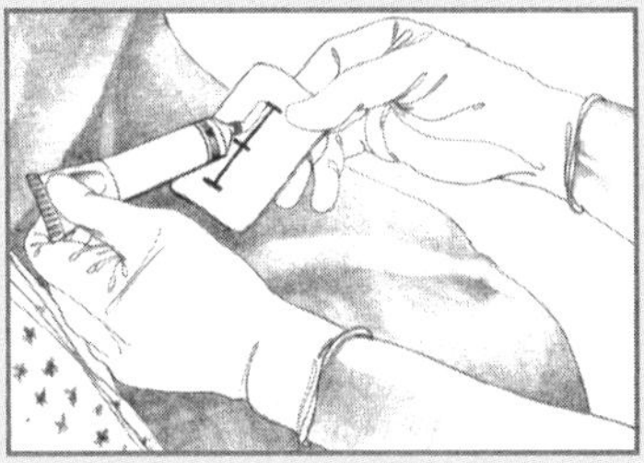

After measuring the correct amount of ointment, tape the paper—drug side down—directly to the skin (as shown below). (Some facilities require you to use the paper to apply the medication to the patient's skin, usually on the chest or arm. Spread a thin layer of the ointment over a 3" [7.6-cm] area.) For increased absorption, the practitioner may request that you cover the site with plastic wrap or a transparent semipermeable dressing.

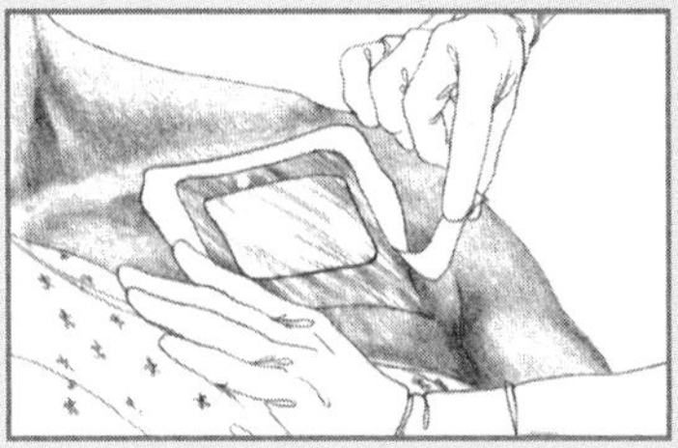

After 5 minutes, record the patient's blood pressure. If it has dropped significantly and he has a headache (from vasodilation of blood vessels in his head), notify the practitioner immediately. He may reduce the dose. If the patient's blood pressure has dropped but he has no symptoms, instruct him to lie still until it returns to normal.

drive or operate machinery until his response to the drug has been determined.
- Warn a patient using a clonidine patch to check with his practitioner before taking an over-the-counter cough preparation because such drugs may counteract clonidine's effects.

Complications

- Skin irritation, such as pruritus and a rash
- Headaches and, in elderly patients, orthostatic hypotension caused by transdermal nitroglycerin medications
- Dry mouth and drowsiness caused by scopolamine
- Increased risk of endometrial cancer, thromboembolic disease, and birth defects caused by transdermal estradiol
- Severe rebound hypertension, especially if withdrawn suddenly, caused by clonidine

Patient teaching

- Explain the procedure to the patient who will be applying transdermal drugs at home.

Documentation

Record the type of medication; date, time, and site of application; and dose. Also note any adverse effects and the patient's response.

Transducer system setup

The exact type of transducer system used depends on the patient's needs and the physician's preference. Some systems monitor pressure continuously, whereas others monitor pressure intermittently. Single-pressure transducers monitor only one type of pressure—for example, pulmonary artery pressure (PAP). Multiple-pressure transducers can monitor two or more types of pressure, such as PAP and central venous pressure.

Equipment

Bag of heparin flush solution (usually 500 ml normal saline solution with 500 or 1,000 units heparin) ♦ pressure cuff ♦ medication-added label ♦ preassembled disposable pressure tubing with flush device and disposable transducer ♦ monitor and monitor cable ♦ I.V. pole with transducer mount ♦ carpenter's level

Preparation

- Turn on the monitor before gathering the equipment to give it sufficient time to warm up.
- Gather the equipment you'll need.
- Wash your hands.

Key steps

- To set up and zero a single-pressure transducer system, perform the following steps.

Setting up the system

- Follow facility policy on adding heparin to the flush solution. If your patient has a history of bleeding or clotting problems, use heparin with caution. Add the ordered amount of heparin to the solution—usually, 1 to 2 units of heparin/ml of solution—and then label the bag.
- Put the pressure module into the monitor, if necessary, and connect the transducer cable to the monitor.
- Remove the preassembled pressure tubing from the package. If necessary, connect the pressure tubing to the transducer. Tighten all tubing connections.
- Position all stopcocks so the flush solution flows through the entire system. Then roll the tubing's flow regulator to the OFF position.
- Spike the flush solution bag with the tubing, invert the bag, open the roller clamp, and squeeze all the air through the drip chamber. Next, compress the tubing's drip chamber, filling it no more than halfway with the flush solution.
- Place the flush solution bag into the pressure infuser bag. To do this, hang the pressure infuser bag on the I.V. pole, and then position the flush solution bag inside the pressure infuser bag.
- Open the tubing's flow regulator, uncoil the tube if you haven't already done so, and remove the protective cap at the end of the pressure tubing. Squeeze the continuous flush device slowly to prime the entire system, including the stopcock ports, with the flush solution.
- As the solution nears the disposable transducer, hold the transducer at a 45-degree angle (as shown below). This forces the solution to flow upward to the transducer. In doing so, the solution forces any air out of the system.

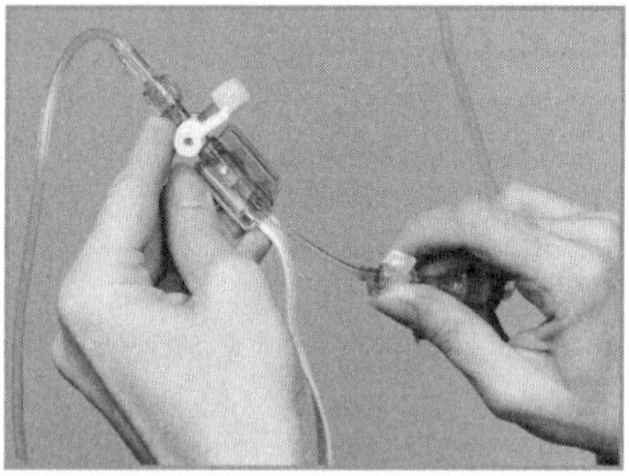

- When the solution nears a stopcock, open the stopcock to air, allowing the solution to flow into the stopcock (as shown top of next page). When the stopcock fills, close it to air and turn it open to the remainder of the tubing. Do this for each stopcock.

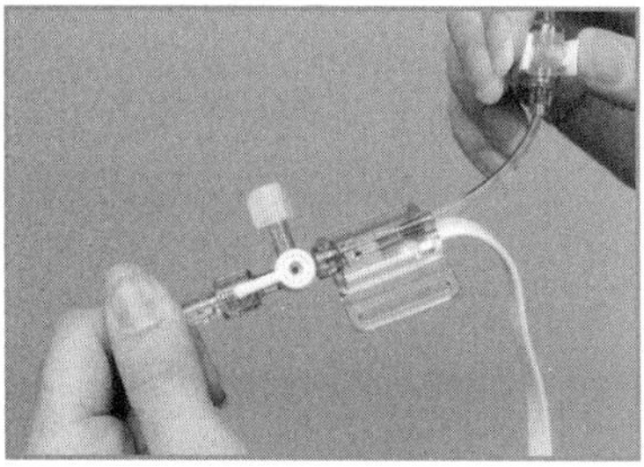

■ After you've completely primed the system, replace the protective cap at the end of the tubing.
■ Inflate the pressure infuser bag to 300 mm Hg. This bag keeps the pressure in the arterial line higher than the patient's systolic pressure, preventing blood backflow into the tubing and ensuring a continuous flow rate. When you inflate the pressure bag, take care that the drip chamber doesn't completely fill with fluid. Afterward, flush the system again to remove all air bubbles.
■ Replace the vented caps on the stopcocks with sterile nonvented caps. If you're going to mount the transducer on an I.V. pole, insert the device into its holder.

Zeroing the system

■ Now you're ready for a preliminary zeroing of the transducer. To ensure accuracy, position the patient and the transducer on the same level each time you zero the transducer or record a pressure. Typically, the patient lies flat in bed, if he can tolerate that position.
■ Next, use the carpenter's level to position the air-reference stopcock or the air-fluid interface of the transducer level with the phlebostatic axis (midway between the posterior chest and the sternum at the fourth intercostal space, midaxillary line). Alternatively, you may level the air-reference stopcock or the air-fluid interface to the same position as the catheter tip.
■ After leveling the transducer, turn the stopcock next to the transducer off to the patient and open to air. Remove the cap to the stopcock port. Place the cap inside an opened sterile gauze package to prevent contamination.
■ Now zero the transducer. To do so, follow the manufacturer's directions for zeroing.
■ When you've finished zeroing, turn the stopcock on the transducer so that it's closed to air and open to the patient. This is the monitoring position. Replace the cap on the stopcock. You're then ready to attach the single-pressure transducer to the patient's catheter. Now you've assembled a single-pressure transducer system. The photograph below shows how the system will look.

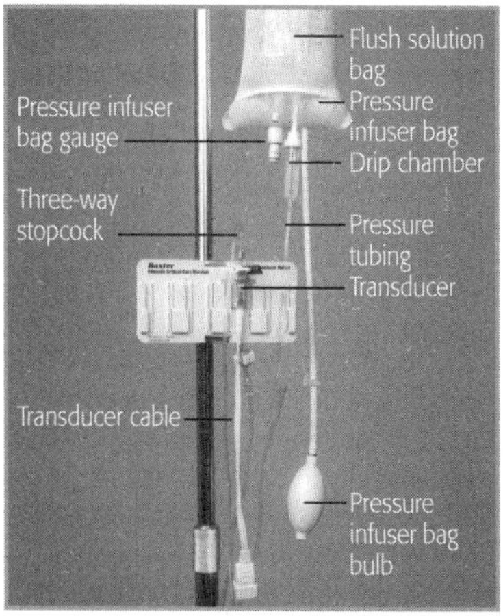

Special considerations

■ You may use any of several methods to set up a multiple-pressure transducer system. The easiest way is to add to the single-pressure system. You'll also need another bag of heparin flush solution in a second pressure infuser bag. Then you'll prime the tubing, mount the second transducer, and connect an additional cable to the monitor. Finally, you'll zero the second transducer.
■ Alternatively, your facility may use a Y-type tubing setup with two attached pressure transducers. This method requires only one bag of heparin flush solution. To set up the system, proceed as you would for a single transducer, with this exception: First, prime one branch of the Y-type tubing and then the other. Next, attach two cables to the monitor in the modules for each pressure that you'll be measuring. Finally, zero each transducer.

Complications

- None known

Documentation

Document the patient's position for zeroing so that other health care team members can replicate the placement.

Transfer from bed to stretcher

Transfer from bed to stretcher, one of the most common transfers, can require the help of one or more coworkers, depending on the patient's size and condition and the primary nurse's physical abilities. Techniques for achieving this transfer include the straight lift, carry lift, lift sheet, and sliding board. The nurse should always remember to maintain good body mechanics—a wide base of support and bent knees—when transferring a patient, to reduce the risk of injury to the patient and herself. To reduce the risk of injury to the patient during transfer, the nurse should make sure that the patient maintains proper body alignment—back straight, head in neutral position, and extremities in a functional position.

In the straight (or patient-assisted) lift—used to move a child, a very light patient, or a patient who can assist transfer—the transfer team members place their hands and arms under the patient's buttocks and, if necessary, his shoulders. Other patients may require a four-person straight lift, detailed below. In the carry lift, team members roll the patient onto their upper arms and hold him against their chests. In the lift sheet transfer, they place a sheet under the patient and lift or slide him onto the stretcher. In the sliding board transfer, two team members slide him onto the stretcher.

Equipment

Stretcher ♦ sliding board or lift sheet, if necessary

Preparation

- Adjust the bed to the same height as the stretcher.

Key steps

- Tell the patient that you're going to move him from the bed to the stretcher, and place him in the supine position.
- Ask team members to remove watches and rings to avoid scratching the patient during transfer.

Four-person straight lift

- Place the stretcher parallel to the bed, and lock the wheels of both to ensure the patient's safety.
- Stand at the center of the stretcher, and have another team member stand at the patient's head. The two other team members should stand next to the bed, on the other side—one at the center and the other at the patient's feet.
- Slide your arms, palms up, beneath the patient, while the other team members do the same. In this position, you and the team member directly opposite support the patient's buttocks and hips; the team member at the head of the bed supports the patient's head and shoulders; the one at the foot supports the patient's legs and feet.
- On a count of three, the team members lift the patient several inches, move him onto the stretcher, and slide their arms out from under him. Keep movements smooth to minimize patient discomfort and avoid muscle strain by team members.

Four-person carry lift

- Place the stretcher perpendicular to the bed, with the head of the stretcher at the foot of the bed. Lock the bed and stretcher wheels to ensure the patient's safety.
- Raise the bed to a comfortable working height.
- Line up all four team members on the same side of the bed as the stretcher, with the tallest member at the patient's head and the shortest at his feet. The member at the patient's head is the leader of the team and gives the lift signals.
- Tell the team members to flex their knees and slide their hands, palms up, under the patient until he rests securely on their upper arms. Make sure that the patient is adequately supported at the head and shoulders, buttocks and hips, and legs and feet.

■ On a count of three, the team members straighten their knees and roll the patient onto his side, against their chests. This positioning reduces strain on the lifters and allows them to hold the patient for several minutes, if necessary.
■ Together, the team members step back, with the member supporting the feet moving the farthest. The team members move forward to the stretcher's edge and, on a count of three, lower the patient onto the stretcher by bending at the knees and sliding their arms out from under the patient.

Four-person lift sheet transfer

■ Position the bed, stretcher, and team members for the straight lift. Then instruct the team to hold the edges of the sheet under the patient, grasping them close to the patient to obtain a firm grip, provide stability, and spare the patient undue feelings of instability.
■ On a count of three, the team members lift or slide the patient onto the stretcher in a smooth, continuous motion to avoid muscle strain and minimize patient discomfort.

Sliding-board transfer

■ Place the stretcher parallel to the bed, and lock the wheels of both to ensure the patient's safety.
■ Stand next to the bed, and instruct a coworker to stand next to the stretcher.
■ Reach over the patient and pull the far side of the bedsheet toward you to turn the patient slightly on his side. Your coworker then places the sliding board beneath the patient, making sure the board bridges the gap between the stretcher and the bed.
■ Ease the patient onto the sliding board and release the sheet. Your coworker then grasps the near side of the sheet at the patient's hips and shoulders and pulls him onto the stretcher in a smooth, continuous motion. She then reaches over the patient, grasps the far side of the sheet, and logrolls him toward her.
■ Remove the sliding board as your coworker returns the patient to the supine position.

After all transfers

■ Position the patient comfortably on the stretcher, apply safety straps, and raise and secure the side rails.

Special considerations

■ When transferring a helpless or markedly obese patient from the bed to a stretcher, begin by lifting and moving him (in increments) to the edge of the bed. Then rest for a few seconds, repositioning the patient if necessary, and lift him onto the stretcher. If the patient can bear weight on his arms or legs, two or three coworkers can perform this transfer: One can support the buttocks and guide the patient, another can stabilize the stretcher by leaning over it and guiding the patient into position, and a third can transfer any attached equipment. If a team member isn't available to guide equipment, move I.V. lines and other tubing first to make sure that they're out of the way and not in danger of pulling loose, or disconnect tubes if possible. If the patient is light, three coworkers can perform the carry lift; however, no matter how many team members are present, someone must stabilize the patient's head if he can't support it himself, has cervical instability or injury, or has undergone surgery.
■ Depending on the patient's size and condition, a lift sheet transfer can require two to seven people.

Complications

■ None known

Documentation

Record the time and, if necessary, the type of transfer in your notes. Complete other required forms.

Transfer from bed to wheelchair

For the patient with diminished or absent lower-body sensation or one-sided weakness, immobility, or injury, transfer from the bed to a wheelchair may require partial support to full assistance—initially by at least two health care team members. Subsequent transfer of the patient with generalized weakness may be performed by one nurse.

After transfer, proper positioning and body alignment helps prevent excessive pressure on bony prominences, which predisposes the patient to skin breakdown.

Equipment

Wheelchair with locks (or sturdy chair) ♦ pajama bottoms (or robe) ♦ shoes or slippers with nonslip soles ♦ watch with a second hand ♦ stethoscope ♦ sphygmomanometer ♦ optional: transfer board if appropriate (see *Teaching use of a transfer board*)

Key steps

- Explain the procedure to the patient and demonstrate his role.
- Place the wheelchair parallel to the bed, facing the foot of the bed, and lock its wheels. Make sure that the bed wheels are also locked. Raise the footrests to avoid interfering with the transfer.
- Check pulse rate and blood pressure with the patient in a supine position to obtain a baseline. Then help him put on the pajama bottoms and slippers or shoes with nonslip soles to prevent falls.
- Raise the head of the bed and allow the patient to rest briefly to adjust to posture changes. Then bring him to the dangling position. Recheck his pulse rate and blood pressure if you suspect cardiovascular instability.

DO'S & DON'TS

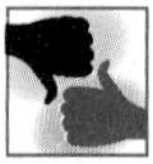

Don't proceed until the patient's pulse rate and blood pressure are stabilized to prevent falls.

- Tell the patient to move toward the edge of the bed and, if possible, to place his feet flat on the floor. Stand in front of the patient, blocking his toes with your feet and his knees with yours to prevent his knees from buckling.
- Flex your knees slightly, place your arms around the patient's back above the waist but below the level of the axilla, and tell him to place his hands on the edge of the bed. Avoid bending at your waist to prevent back strain.
- Ask the patient to push himself off the bed and to support as much of his own weight as possible. At the same time, straighten your knees and hips, raising the patient as you straighten your body.
- Supporting the patient as needed, pivot toward the wheelchair, keeping your knees next to his. Tell the patient to grasp the farthest armrest of the wheelchair with his closest hand.
- Help the patient lower himself into the wheelchair by flexing your hips and knees, but not your back. Instruct him to reach back and grasp the other wheelchair armrest as he sits to avoid abrupt contact with the seat. Fasten the seat belt to prevent falls and, if necessary, check his pulse rate and blood pressure to assess cardiovascular stability. If the pulse rate is 20 beats or more above baseline, stay with the patient and monitor him closely until it returns to normal because he's experiencing orthostatic hypotension.
- If the patient can't position himself correctly, help him move his buttocks against the back of the chair so that the ischial tuberosities, not the sacrum, provide the base of support.
- Place the patient's feet flat on the footrests, pointed straight ahead. Then position the knees and hips with the correct amount of flexion and in appropriate alignment. If appropriate, use elevating leg rests to flex the patient's hips at more than 90 degrees; this position relieves pressure on the popliteal space and places more weight on the ischial tuberosities.
- Position the patient's arms on the wheelchair's armrests with shoulders abducted, elbows slightly flexed, forearms pronated, and wrists and hands in the neutral position. If necessary, support or elevate the patient's hands and forearms with a pillow to prevent dependent edema.

Special considerations

- If the patient starts to fall during transfer, ease him to the closest surface—bed, floor, or chair. Never stretch to finish the transfer. Doing so can cause loss of balance,

Teaching use of a transfer board

For the patient who can't stand, a transfer board allows safe transfer from his bed to a wheelchair. To perform this transfer, take the following steps.

- First, explain and demonstrate the procedure. Eventually, the patient may become proficient enough to transfer himself independently or with some supervision.
- Help the patient put on pajama bottoms or a robe and shoes or slippers.
- Place the wheelchair angled slightly and facing the foot of the bed. Lock the wheels, and remove the armrest closest to the patient. Make sure that the bed is flat, and adjust its height so that it's level with the wheelchair seat.
- Assist the patient to a sitting position on the edge of the bed, with his feet resting on the floor. Make sure that the front edge of the wheelchair seat is aligned with the back of the patient's knees, as shown below left.
- Ask the patient to lean away from the wheelchair while you slide one end of the transfer board under him.
- Now place the other end of the transfer board on the wheelchair seat, and help the patient return to the upright position.
- Stand in front of the patient to prevent him from sliding forward. Tell him to push down with both arms, lifting the buttocks up and onto the transfer board. The patient then repeats this maneuver, edging along the board, until he's seated in the wheelchair. If the patient can't use his arms to assist with the transfer, stand in front of him, put your arms around him, and—if he's able—have him put his arms around you. Gradually slide him across the board until he's safely in the chair, as shown below right.
- When the patient is in the wheelchair, fasten a seat belt, if necessary.
- Then remove the transfer board, replace the wheelchair armrest, and reposition the patient in the wheelchair.

Positioning the transfer board

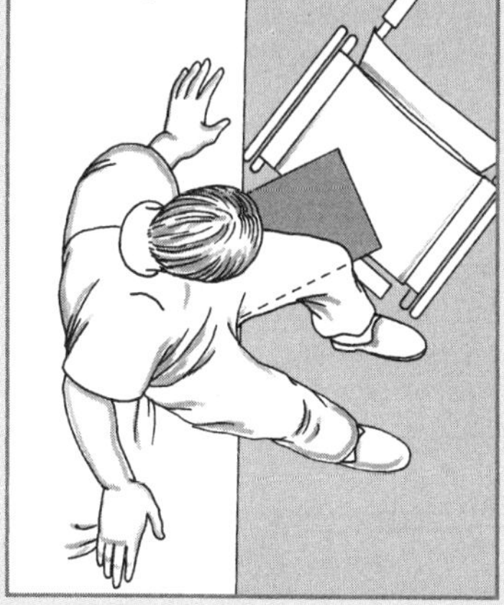

Assisting the patient

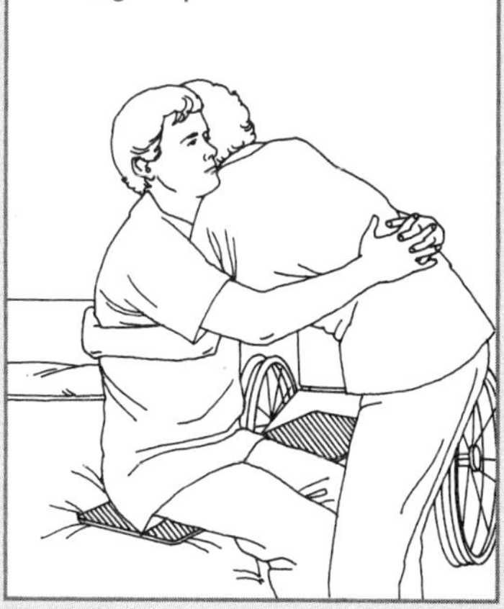

falls, muscle strain, and other injuries to you and to the patient.

- If the patient has one-sided weakness, follow the preceding steps, but place the wheelchair on the patient's unaffected side. Instruct the patient to pivot and bear as much weight as possible on the unaffected side. Support the affected side because the patient will tend to lean to this side. Use pillows to support the hemiplegic patient's affected side to prevent slumping in the wheelchair.

Complications

- None known

Patient teaching

- Teach the patient and his family the appropriate transfer techniques, as needed.

Documentation

Record the time of transfer and the extent of assistance in your notes, and note how the patient tolerated the activity.

Transfer with hydraulic lift

Using a hydraulic lift to raise the immobile patient from the supine to the sitting position permits a safe, comfortable transfer between the bed and a chair. It's indicated for the obese or immobile patient for whom manual transfer poses the potential for nurse or patient injury.

Although one person can operate most hydraulic lift models, it's better to have two staff members present during transfer to stabilize and support the patient. To reduce the risk of harm to a patient, it's important to maintain the patient's body alignment during transfer. (See *Using a hydraulic lift*.)

Equipment

Hydraulic lift, with sling, chains or straps, and hooks ♦ chair or wheelchair

Preparation

- Because hydraulic lift models may vary in weight capacity, check the manufacturer's specifications before attempting patient transfer.
- Make sure that the bed and wheelchair wheels are locked before beginning the transfer.

Key steps

- Explain the procedure to the patient, and reassure him that the hydraulic lift can safely support his weight and won't tip over.
- Ensure the patient's privacy. If the patient has an I.V. line or urinary drainage bag, move it first. Arrange tubing securely to prevent dangling during transfer. If the tubing of the urinary drainage bag isn't long enough to permit the transfer, clamp the tubing and drainage bag and place it on the patient's abdomen during transfer. After the transfer, replace the drainage bag in a dependent position and unclamp the tubing.
- Make sure that the side rail opposite you is raised and secure. Then roll the patient toward you, onto his side, and raise the side rail. Walk to the opposite side of the bed and lower the side rail.
- Place the sling under the patient's buttocks with its lower edge below the greater trochanter. Then fanfold the far side of the sling against the back and buttocks.
- Roll the patient toward you onto the sling, and raise the side rail. Then lower the opposite side rail.
- Slide your hands under the patient and pull the sling from beneath him, smoothing out all wrinkles. Then roll the patient onto his back and center him on the sling.
- Place the appropriate chair next to the head of the bed, facing the foot.
- Lower the side rail next to the chair, and raise the bed only until the base of the lift can extend under the bed. To avoid alarming and endangering the patient, don't raise the bed completely.
- Set the lift's adjustable base to its widest position to ensure optimal stability. Then move the lift so that its arm lies perpendicular to the bed, directly over the patient.
- Connect one end of the chains (or straps) to the side arms on the lift; connect the other, hooked end to the sling. Face the hooks away from the patient to prevent them from slipping and to avoid the risk of their pointed edges injuring the patient. The patient may place his arms inside or outside the chains (or straps) or he may grasp them when the slack is gone to avoid injury.
- Tighten the turnscrew on the lift. Then depending on the type of lift you're using, pump the handle or turn it clockwise until the patient has assumed a sitting position and his buttocks clear the bed surface by 1" or 2" (2.5 or 5 cm). Momentarily suspend the patient above the bed until he

Using a hydraulic lift

After placing the patient in a supine position in the center of the sling, position the hydraulic lift above him, as shown here. Then attach the chains to the hooks on the sling.

Turn the lift handle clockwise to raise the patient to the sitting position. If he's positioned properly, continue to raise him until he's suspended just above the bed.

After positioning the patient above the wheelchair, turn the lift handle counterclockwise to lower him onto the seat. When the chains become slack, stop turning and unhook the sling from the lift.

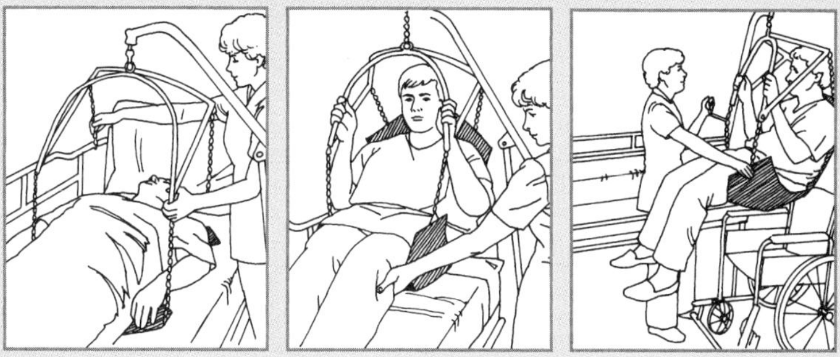

feels secure in the lift and sees that it can bear his weight.

- Steady the patient as you move the lift or, preferably, have another coworker guide the patient's body while you move the lift. Depending on the type of lift you're using, the arm should now rest in front or to one side of the chair.
- Release the turnscrew. Then depress the handle or turn it counterclockwise to lower the patient into the chair. While lowering the patient, push gently on his knees to maintain the correct sitting posture. After lowering the patient into the chair, fasten the seat belt to ensure his safety.
- Remove the hooks or straps from the sling, but leave the sling in place under the patient so you'll be able to transfer him back to the bed from the chair. Then move the lift away from the patient.
- To return the patient to bed, reverse the procedure.

Special considerations

- If the patient has an altered center of gravity (caused by a halo vest or a lower-extremity cast, for example), obtain help from a coworker before transferring him with a hydraulic lift.

Complications

- None known

Patient teaching

- If the patient will require the use of a hydraulic lift for transfers after discharge, teach his family how to use this device correctly and allow them to practice with supervision.

Documentation

Record the time of transfer in your notes, and note how the patient tolerated the activity.

Transfusion of blood and blood products

Whole blood transfusion replenishes the volume and the oxygen-carrying capacity of the circulatory system by increasing the mass of circulating red cells. Transfusion of packed red blood cells (RBCs), from which 80% of the plasma has been removed, restores only the oxygen-carrying capacity. After plasma is removed, the resulting component has a hematocrit of 65% to 80% and a usual volume of 250 to 300 ml.

Each unit of whole blood or RBCs contains enough hemoglobin to raise the hemoglobin concentration in an average-sized adult 1 g/dl. Both types of transfusion treat decreased hemoglobin level and hematocrit. Whole blood is usually used only when decreased levels result from hemorrhage; packed RBCs are used when such depressed levels accompany normal blood volume to avoid possible fluid and circulatory overload. (See *Transfusing blood and selected components,* pages 554 to 557.) Whole blood and packed RBCs contain cellular debris, requiring in-line filtration during administration.

Before starting the transfusion, positive patient identification, the therapy's appropriateness, blood compatibility, practitioner's order, and signed consent form should be verified by the nurse. In addition to confirming patient identity with the appropriate blood or blood component identification numbers, the patient's identity must also be verified using two patient identifiers, aside from the patient's room number, according to facility policy.

Blood and blood components should be filtered and transfused through an appropriate blood administration set. Straight-line and Y-type blood administration sets are commonly used. Although filters come in mesh and microaggregate types, the latter type is preferred, especially when transfusing multiple units of blood. Highly effective leukocyte removal filters are available for use when transfusing blood and packed RBCs. The use of these filters can postpone sensitization to transfusion therapy.

Administer packed RBCs with a Y-type set. Using a straight-line set forces you to piggyback the tubing so you can stop the transfusion if necessary but still keep the vein open. Piggybacking increases the chance of harmful microorganisms entering the tubing as you're connecting the blood line to the established line.

Single units of whole blood or blood components should be transfused within a 4-hour period. The start of the transfusion should begin within 30 minutes from the time the blood is released from the blood bank. No medications should be added to the blood other than normal saline solution. Patients should also be monitored 15 minutes after the start of therapy and at 15- to 30-minute intervals throughout the transfusion.

Multiple-lead tubing minimizes the risk of contamination, especially when transfusing multiple units of blood (a straight-line set would require multiple piggybacking). A Y-type set gives you the option of adding normal saline solution to packed cells—decreasing their viscosity—if the patient can tolerate the added fluid volume.

Equipment

Blood recipient set (170- to 260-micron filter and tubing with drip chamber for blood, or combined set) ♦ I.V. pole ♦ gloves ♦ gown ♦ face shield ♦ multiple-lead tubing ♦ whole blood or packed RBCs ♦ 250 ml of normal saline solution ♦ venipuncture equipment, if necessary (should include 20G or larger catheter) ♦ optional: ice bag, warm compresses

Preparation

- Avoid obtaining either whole blood or packed RBCs until you're ready to begin the transfusion.
- Prepare the equipment when you're ready to start the infusion.
- If the patient doesn't have an I.V. line in place, perform a venipuncture, using a 20G or larger-diameter catheter. Avoid using an existing line if the needle or catheter lumen is smaller than 20G. Central venous access devices may also be used for transfusion therapy.

Key steps

- Confirm the patient's identity using two patient identifiers according to facility policy.
- Explain the procedure to the patient. Explain possible signs and symptoms of a transfusion reaction (chills, rash, fever, flank or back pain, dizziness, or blood in

urine) and to report these possible signs and symptoms to the nurse.

- Make sure that the patient has signed an informed consent form before transfusion therapy is initiated.
- Obtain whole blood or packed RBCs from the blood bank within 30 minutes of the transfusion start time. Check the expiration date on the blood bag, and observe for abnormal color, RBC clumping, gas bubbles, and extraneous material. Return outdated or abnormal blood to the blood bank.
- Record the patient's baseline vital signs.
- Compare the patient's confirmed identity with that on the blood bag label. Check the blood bag identification number, ABO blood group, and Rh compatibility. Also, compare the patient's blood bank identification number, if present, with the number on the blood bag. Identification of blood and blood products is performed at the patient's bedside by two licensed professionals, according to facility policy.
- Put on gloves, a gown, and a face shield.
- Using a blood administration set, close all the clamps on the set. Then insert the spike of the line you're using for the normal saline solution into the bag of saline solution. Next, open the port on the blood bag, and insert the spike of the line you're using to administer the blood or cellular component into the port. Hang the bag of normal saline solution and blood or cellular component on the I.V. pole, open the clamp on the line of saline solution, and squeeze the drip chamber until it's half full. Then remove the adapter cover at the tip of the blood administration set, open the main flow clamp, and prime the tubing with saline solution.
- If you're administering packed RBCs with a blood administration set, you can add normal saline solution to the bag to dilute the cells by closing the clamp between the patient and the drip chamber and opening the clamp from the blood. Then lower the blood bag below the saline container and let 30 to 50 ml of normal saline solution flow into the packed cells. Finally, close the clamp to the blood bag, rehang the bag, rotate it gently to mix the cells and normal saline solution, and close the clamp to the saline container.
- If you're administering whole blood, gently invert the bag several times to mix the cells.
- Attach the prepared blood administration set to the venipuncture device, and flush it with normal saline solution. Then close the clamp to the saline solution, and open the clamp between the blood bag and the patient. Adjust the flow rate to no greater than 5 ml/minute for the first 15 minutes of the transfusion to observe for a possible transfusion reaction.
- Remain with the patient and watch for signs of a transfusion reaction. If such signs develop, stop the transfusion and record his vital signs. Infuse saline solution at a moderately slow infusion rate, and notify the practitioner at once. If no signs of a reaction appear within 15 minutes, you'll need to adjust the flow clamp to the ordered infusion rate. The rate of infusion should be as rapid as the patient's circulatory system can tolerate.
- It's undesirable for RBC preparations to remain at room temperature for more than 4 hours. If the infusion rate must be so slow that the entire unit can't be infused within 4 hours, notify the blood bank so they can divide the unit and keep one portion refrigerated until it's time to administer it.
- After completing the transfusion, you'll need to put on gloves and remove and discard the used infusion equipment. Then remember to reconnect the original I.V. fluid, if necessary, or discontinue the I.V. infusion.
- Return the empty blood bag to the blood bank, if facility policy dictates, and discard the tubing and filter.
- Record the patient's vital signs.

Special considerations

- Although some microaggregate filters can be used for up to 10 units of blood, always replace the filter and tubing if more than 1 hour elapses between transfusions. When administering multiple units of blood under pressure, use a blood warmer to avoid hypothermia. Blood components may be warmed to no more than 107.6° F (42° C).

(Text continues on page 556.)

Transfusing blood and selected components

Blood component	Indications
Whole blood ▪ Complete blood with no additional processing after collection (except testing)	▪ Symptomatic chronic anemia ▪ Prevention of morbidity from anemia in patients at greatest risk for tissue hypoxia ▪ Active bleeding with signs and symptoms of hypovolemia ▪ Preoperative hemoglobin < 9 g/dl with possibility of major blood loss ▪ Sickle cell disease (red cell exchange)
Packed red blood cells (RBCs) ▪ Same as whole blood except most of the plasma removed	▪ Symptomatic chronic anemia ▪ Prevention of morbidity from anemia in patients at greatest risk for tissue hypoxia ▪ Active bleeding with signs and symptoms of hypovolemia ▪ Preoperative hemoglobin < 9 g/dl with possibility of major blood loss ▪ Sickle cell disease (red cell exchange)
Platelets ▪ Platelet sediment from whole blood	▪ Bleeding due to critically decreased circulating platelet counts or functionally abnormal platelets ▪ Prevention of bleeding due to thrombocytopenia ▪ Platelet count < 50,000/ml before surgery or a major invasive procedure
Fresh frozen plasma (FFP) ▪ Uncoagulated plasma separated from RBCs and rich in clotting factors	▪ Bleeding ▪ Coagulation factor deficiencies ▪ Warfarin reversal ▪ Thrombotic thrombocytopenic purpura
Cryoprecipitate ▪ Insoluble plasma portion of FFP containing fibrinogen, Factor VIII:c, Factor VIII:vWF, Factor XIII, and fibronectin	▪ Bleeding associated with hypofibrinogenemia or dysfibrinogenemia ▪ Significant factor XIII deficiency (prophylactic or treatment)

ABO and Rh compatibility	Nursing considerations
▪ ABO identical: –Type A receives type A –Type B receives type B –Type AB receives type AB –Type O receives type O ▪ Rh match necessary	▪ Keep in mind that whole blood is seldom administered. ▪ Use a blood administration set to infuse blood within 4 hours. ▪ Administer only with 0.9% normal saline solution. ▪ Closely monitor patient volume status during administration for risk of volume overload.
▪ ABO compatibility: –Type A receives type A or O –Type B receives type B or O –Type AB receives type AB or O –Type O receives type O ▪ Rh match necessary	▪ Use a blood administration set to infuse blood within 4 hours. ▪ Administer only with 0.9% normal saline solution. ▪ Keep in mind that an RBC transfusion isn't appropriate for anemias treatable by nutritional or drug therapies.
▪ ABO identical when possible ▪ Rh-negative recipients should receive Rh-negative platelets when possible	▪ Use a filtered component drip administration set to infuse. ▪ If ordered, administer prophylactic pretransfusion medications, such as antihistamines or acetaminophen, to reduce chills, fever, and allergic reactions. ▪ Use single-donor platelets if the patient has a need for repeated transfusions due to risk of allergic reaction to foreign leukocyte antigens that may be present on leukocytes and platelets. ▪ Keep in mind that platelets shouldn't be used to treat autoimmune thrombocytopenia or thrombocytopenic purpura unless patient has a life-threatening hemorrhage.
▪ ABO compatibility required ▪ Rh match not required	▪ Use a blood administration set to infuse rapidly. ▪ Monitor the patient for signs of hypocalcemia because the citric acid in FFP may bind to calcium. ▪ Remember that FFP must be infused within 24 hours of being thawed.
▪ ABO compatibility preferred but not necessary ▪ Rh match not required	▪ Use a blood administration set to infuse. ▪ Add 0.9% normal saline solution to each bag of cryoprecipitate as necessary to facilitate transfusion. ▪ Keep in mind that cryoprecipitate must be administered within 6 hours of thawing. ▪ Before administering, check laboratory studies to confirm a deficiency of one of the specific clotting factors present in cryoprecipitate.

(continued)

Transfusing blood and selected components *(continued)*

Blood component	Indications
Factor VIII concentrate ▪ Recombinant genetically engineered product, derivative obtained from plasma	▪ Hemophilia A ▪ von Willebrand's disease
Albumin 5% (buffered saline); Albumin 25% (salt poor) ▪ A small plasma protein prepared by fractionating pooled plasma	▪ Volume lost due to burns, trauma, surgery, or infection ▪ Hypoproteinemia (with or without edema)
Immune globulin ▪ Processed human plasma from multiple donors that contains 95% immunoglobulin (IgG), < 2.5% IgA, and a fraction of IgM	▪ Primary and secondary immune deficiencies ▪ Kawasaki syndrome ▪ Idiopathic thrombocytopenia purpura ▪ Neurologic disorders (Guillain-Barré syndrome, dermatomyositis, myasthenia gravis)

- For rapid blood replacement, you may need to use a pressure bag. Be aware that excessive pressure may develop, leading to broken blood vessels and extravasation, with hematoma and hemolysis of the infusing RBCs.
- If the transfusion stops, take these steps as needed:
  - Check that the I.V. container is at least 3′ (1 m) above the insertion device.
  - Make sure that the flow clamp is open and that the blood completely covers the filter. If it doesn't, squeeze the drip chamber until it does.
  - Gently rock the bag back and forth, agitating blood cells that may have settled.
  - Untape the dressing over the I.V. site to check needle placement. Reposition the needle if necessary.
  - Flush the line with saline solution and restart the transfusion. Using a Y-type set, close the flow clamp to the patient and lower the blood bag. Next, open the saline clamp and allow some saline solution to flow into the blood bag. Rehang the blood bag, open the flow clamp to the patient, and reset the flow rate.
  - If a hematoma develops at the I.V. site, immediately stop the infusion. Remove the I.V. cannula. Notify the practitioner and expect to place ice on the site intermittently for 8 hours; then apply warm compresses. Follow facility policy.
  - If the blood bag empties before the next one arrives, administer normal saline solution slowly. If you're using a Y-type set, close the blood-line clamp, open the saline clamp, and let the saline run slowly until the new blood arrives.

ABO and Rh compatibility	Nursing considerations
▪ Not required	▪ Be aware that patients with hemophilia A or von Willebrand's disease should be treated with cryoprecipitate only when appropriate factor VIII concentrates are not available.
▪ Not required	▪ Administer by I.V. injection using a filter needle or use the administration set supplied by the manufacturer.
▪ Not required	▪ Use the administration set supplied by the manufacturer and set rate based on patient's condition and response. ▪ Keep in mind that albumin isn't to be used to treat severe anemia. ▪ Administer cautiously in patients with cardiac and pulmonary disease because heart failure may result in volume overload.
	▪ Reconstitute the lyophilized powder with 0.9% sodium chloride injection, 5% dextrose, or sterile water. ▪ Administer at the minimal concentration available and at the slowest practical rate.

Decrease the flow rate or clamp the line before attaching the new unit of blood.

- Know that measures to prevent disease transmission include laboratory testing of blood products and careful screening of potential donors, neither of which is guaranteed.

Complications

- Infectious disease that's transmitted during a transfusion and undetected until days, weeks, or even months later, when it produces signs and symptoms
- Hepatitis C, accounting for most post-transfusion hepatitis cases
- Human immunodeficiency virus (HIV)
- Cytomegalovirus
- Transfusion-related syphilis
- Circulatory overload and hemolytic, allergic, febrile, and pyogenic reactions resulting from any transfusion
- Coagulation disturbances, citrate intoxication, hyperkalemia, acid-base imbalance, loss of 2, 3-diphosphoglycerate, ammonia intoxication, and hypothermia resulting from massive transfusion

Documentation

Record the date and time of the transfusion, the type and amount of transfusion product, the patient's vital signs, your check of all identification data, and the patient's response. Document any transfusion reaction and treatment. (See *Documenting blood transfusions,* page 558.)

Documenting blood transfusions

Whether you administer blood or blood components, you must use proper identification and crossmatching procedures.

After matching the patient's name, medical record number, blood group (or type) and Rh factor (the patient's and the donor's), the crossmatched data, and the blood bank identification number with the label on the blood bag, you'll need to clearly record that you did so. The blood or blood component must be identified and documented properly by two health care professionals as well.

On the transfusion record, document:

- date and time the transfusion was started and completed
- name of the health care professional who verified the information
- catheter type and gauge
- total amount of the transfusion
- patient's vital signs before and after the transfusion
- any infusion device used
- flow rate and if blood warming unit was used.

If the patient receives his own blood, document on the intake and output records:

- amount of autologous blood retrieved
- amount of autologous blood infused
- laboratory data during and after the autotransfusion
- patient's pretransfusion and posttransfusion vital signs.

Pay particular attention to:

- patient's coagulation profile
- hemoglobin level, hematocrit, and arterial blood gas and calcium levels.

Transfusion reaction management

A transfusion reaction typically stems from a major antigen-antibody reaction and can result from a single or massive transfusion of blood or blood products. Although many reactions occur during transfusion or within 96 hours afterward, infectious diseases transmitted during a transfusion may go undetected until days, weeks, or months later, when signs and symptoms appear.

A transfusion reaction requires immediate recognition and prompt nursing action to prevent further complications and, possibly, death—particularly if the patient is unconscious or so heavily sedated that he can't report the common symptoms. (See *Managing transfusion reactions.*)

Equipment

Normal saline solution ♦ I.V. administration set ♦ sterile urine specimen container ♦ needle, syringe, and tubes for blood samples ♦ transfusion reaction report form ♦ optional: oxygen, epinephrine, hypothermia blanket, leukocyte removal filter

Key steps

- As soon as you suspect an adverse reaction, stop the transfusion and start the saline infusion (using a new I.V. administration set) at a keep-vein-open rate to maintain venous access.

Do's & don'ts

Don't discard the blood bag or administration set.

- Notify the practitioner.
- Monitor the patient's vital signs every 15 minutes or as indicated by the severity and type of reaction.
- Compare the labels on all blood containers with corresponding patient identification forms to verify that the transfusion was the correct blood or blood product.
- Notify the blood bank of a possible transfusion reaction and collect blood samples, as ordered. Immediately send the samples, all transfusion containers (even if empty), and the administration set to the blood bank. The blood bank will test these materials to further evaluate the reaction.

(Text continues on page 562.)

Managing transfusion reactions

A patient receiving a transfusion of processed blood products risks possible complications, such as hemosiderosis and hypothermia. This chart describes *endogenous reactions,* those caused by an antigen-antibody reaction in the recipient, and exogenous reactions, those caused by external factors in administered blood.

Reaction and causes	Signs and symptoms	Nursing interventions
Endogenous		
Allergic ▪ Allergen in donor blood ▪ Donor blood hypersensitive to certain drugs	▪ Anaphylaxis (chills, facial swelling, laryngeal edema, pruritus, urticaria, wheezing), fever, nausea and vomiting	▪ Administer antihistamines, as prescribed. ▪ Monitor patient for anaphylactic reaction, and administer epinephrine and corticosteroids if indicated. **Prevention** ▪ As prescribed, premedicate patient with diphenhydramine (Benadryl) before subsequent transfusion. ▪ Observe patient closely for first 30 minutes of transfusion.
Bacterial contamination ▪ Organisms that can survive cold, such as *Pseudomonas* or *Staphylococcus*	▪ Chills, fever, vomiting, abdominal cramping, diarrhea, shock, signs of renal failure	▪ Provide broad-spectrum antibiotics, corticosteroids, or epinephrine, as prescribed. **Prevention** ▪ Maintain strict blood-storage control. ▪ Change blood administration set and filter every 4 hours or after every two units. ▪ Infuse each unit of blood over 2 to 4 hours; stop infusion if time span exceeds 4 hours. ▪ Maintain sterile technique when administering blood products. ▪ Inspect blood before transfusion for air, clots, and dark purple color.
Febrile ▪ Bacterial lipopolysaccharides ▪ Antileukocyte-recipient antibodies directed against donor white blood cells	▪ Fever up to 104° F (40° C), chills, headache, facial flushing, palpitations, cough, chest tightness, increased pulse rate, flank pain	▪ Relieve symptoms with an antipyretic or antihistamine, as ordered. ▪ If patient requires further transfusions, use frozen red blood cells (RBCs), add a special leukocyte removal filter to blood line, or premedicate him with acetaminophen, as ordered, before starting another transfusion.

(continued)

Managing transfusion reactions *(continued)*

Reaction and causes	Signs and symptoms	Nursing interventions
Endogenous (*continued*)		
Febrile *(continued)*		**Prevention** ■ Premedicate patient with an antipyretic, an antihistamine and, possibly, a steroid. ■ Use leukocyte-poor or washed RBCs. Use a leukocyte removal filter specific to blood component.
Hemolytic ■ ABO or Rh incompatibility ■ Intradonor incompatibility ■ Improper crossmatching ■ Improperly stored blood	■ Chest pain, dyspnea, facial flushing, fever, chills, shaking, hypotension, flank pain, hemoglobinuria, oliguria, bloody oozing at infusion site or surgical incision site, burning sensation along vein receiving blood, shock, renal failure	■ Monitor blood pressure. ■ Manage shock with I.V. fluids, oxygen, epinephrine, a diuretic, and a vasopressor, as ordered. ■ Obtain posttransfusion-reaction blood samples and urine specimens for analysis. ■ Observe for signs of hemorrhage resulting from disseminated intravascular coagulation. **Prevention** ■ Before transfusion, check donor and recipient blood types to ensure blood compatibility. ■ Transfuse blood slowly for first 30 minutes of transfusion.
Plasma protein incompatibility ■ Immunoglobulin (Ig) A incompatibility	■ Abdominal pain, diarrhea, dyspnea, chills, fever, flushing, hypotension	■ Administer oxygen, fluids, epinephrine or, possibly, a steroid, as ordered. **Prevention** ■ Transfuse only IgA-deficient blood or well-washed RBCs.
Exogenous		
Bleeding tendencies ■ Low platelet count in stored blood, causing thrombocytopenia	■ Abnormal bleeding and oozing from a cut, a break in the skin surface, or the gums; abnormal bruising and petechiae	■ Administer platelets, fresh frozen plasma (FFP), or cryoprecipitate, as ordered. ■ Monitor platelet count. **Prevention** ■ Use only fresh blood (less than 7 days old) when possible.

Managing transfusion reactions *(continued)*

Reaction and causes	Signs and symptoms	Nursing interventions
Exogenous (*continued*)		
Circulatory overload ▪ May result from infusing whole blood too rapidly	▪ Increased plasma volume, back pain, chest tightness, chills, fever, dyspnea, flushed feeling, headache, hypertension, increased central venous and jugular vein pressure	▪ Monitor blood pressure. ▪ Administer diuretics, as ordered. **Prevention** ▪ Transfuse blood slowly. ▪ Don't exceed two units in 4 hours; fewer for elderly patients, infants, or patients with cardiac conditions.
Elevated blood ammonia level ▪ Increased ammonia level in stored donor blood	▪ Confusion, forgetfulness, lethargy	▪ Monitor ammonia level in blood. ▪ Decrease amount of protein in patient's diet. ▪ If indicated, give neomycin or lactulose (Cholac). **Prevention** ▪ Use only RBCs, FFP, or fresh blood, especially if patient has hepatic disease.
Hemosiderosis ▪ Increased level of hemosiderin (iron-containing pigment) from RBC destruction, especially after many transfusions	▪ Iron plasma level exceeding 200 mg/dl	▪ Perform phlebotomy to remove excess iron. **Prevention** ▪ Administer blood only when absolutely necessary.
Hypocalcemia ▪ Citrate toxicity occurs when citrate-treated blood is infused rapidly (Citrate binds with calcium, causing a calcium deficiency, or normal citrate metabolism becomes impeded by hepatic disease.)	▪ Arrhythmias, hypotension, muscle cramps, nausea and vomiting, seizures, tingling in fingers	▪ Slow or stop transfusion, depending on patient's reaction. Expect a more severe reaction in hypothermic patients or patients with elevated potassium level. **Prevention** ▪ Infuse blood slowly.
Hypothermia ▪ Rapid infusion of large amounts of cold blood, which decreases body temperature	▪ Chills; shaking; hypotension; arrhythmias, especially bradycardia; cardiac arrest, if core temperature falls below 86° F (30° C)	▪ Stop transfusion. ▪ Warm patient with blankets. ▪ Obtain an electrocardiogram (ECG). **Prevention** ▪ Warm blood to 95° to 98° F (35° to 36.7° C) especially before massive transfusions.

(continued)

Managing transfusion reactions *(continued)*

Reaction and causes	Signs and symptoms	Nursing interventions
Exogenous *(continued)*		
Increased oxygen affinity for hemoglobin ▪ Decreased level of 2,3-diphosphoglycerate in stored blood, causing an increase in oxygen's hemoglobin affinity (When this occurs, oxygen stays in patient's bloodstream and isn't released into body tissues.)	▪ Depressed respiratory rate, especially in patients with chronic lung disease	▪ Monitor arterial blood gas levels, and provide respiratory support, as needed. **Prevention** ▪ Use only RBCs or fresh blood, if possible.
Potassium intoxication ▪ An abnormally high level of potassium in stored plasma caused by RBC hemolysis	▪ Diarrhea, intestinal colic, flaccidity, muscle twitching, oliguria, renal failure, bradycardia progressing to cardiac arrest, ECG changes with tall, peaked T waves	▪ Obtain an ECG. ▪ Administer sodium polystyrene sulfonate (Kayexalate) orally or by enema. **Prevention** ▪ Use fresh blood when administering massive transfusions.

▪ Collect the first posttransfusion urine specimen, mark the collection slip "Possible transfusion reaction," and send it to the laboratory immediately. The laboratory tests this urine specimen for the presence of hemoglobin, which indicates a hemolytic reaction.
▪ Closely monitor intake and output. Note evidence of oliguria or anuria because hemoglobin deposition in the renal tubules can cause renal damage.
▪ If prescribed, administer oxygen, epinephrine, or other drugs, and apply a hypothermia blanket to reduce fever.
▪ Make the patient as comfortable as possible, and provide reassurance as necessary.

Special considerations

▪ Treat all transfusion reactions as serious until proven otherwise. If the practitioner anticipates a transfusion reaction, such as one that may occur in a leukemia patient, he may order prophylactic treatment with antihistamines or antipyretics to precede blood administration.
▪ To avoid a possible febrile reaction, the practitioner may order the blood washed to remove as many leukocytes as possible, or a leukocyte removal filter may be used during the transfusion.

Complications

▪ None known

Documentation

Record the time and date of the transfusion reaction, the type and amount of infused blood or blood products, the clinical signs of the transfusion reaction in order of occurrence, the patient's vital signs, specimens sent to the laboratory for analysis, treatment given, and the patient's response to treatment. If required by facility policy, complete the transfusion reaction form.

Tube feeding

Tube feeding is the delivery of a liquid feeding formula directly to the stomach (known as gastric gavage), duodenum, or jejunum. Gastric gavage typically is indicated for the patient who can't eat normally because of dysphagia, or oral or esophageal obstruction or injury. Gastric feedings may also be given to an unconscious or intubated patient, or to a patient recovering from GI tract surgery who can't ingest food orally.

Nutrition support should be initiated after 1 to 2 weeks without nutrient intake. Enteral feeding is preferable to parenteral therapy provided there are no contraindications, access can be safely attained, and oral intake isn't possible. For short-term (less than 30-day) feeding, nasogastric (NG) or nasoenteric tubes are preferable to gastrostomy or jejunostomy tubes. Tube feeding is contraindicated in patients who have no bowel sounds or a suspected intestinal obstruction.

Duodenal or jejunal feedings decrease the risk of aspiration because the formula bypasses the pylorus. Jejunal feedings result in reduced pancreatic stimulation; thus, patients may require an elemental diet. Patients usually receive gastric feedings on an intermittent schedule. For duodenal or jejunal feedings, however, most patients seem to better tolerate a continuous slow drip.

Liquid nutrient solutions come in various formulas for administration through an NG tube, a small-bore feeding tube, gastrostomy or jejunostomy tube, percutaneous endoscopic gastrostomy or jejunostomy tube, or gastrostomy feeding button. (See "Transabdominal tube feeding and care," page 534, and "Gastrostomy feeding button care," page 221.)

Equipment

Gastric feedings

Feeding formula ♦ graduated container ♦ bulb syringe ♦ 120 ml of water ♦ gavage bag with tubing and flow regulator clamp ♦ towel or linen-saver pad ♦ 60-ml syringe ♦ pH test strip ♦ optional: infusion controller and tubing set (for continuous administration), adapter to connect gavage tubing to feeding tube

Duodenal or jejunal feedings

Feeding formula ♦ enteral administration set containing a gavage container, drip chamber, roller clamp or flow regulator, and tube connector ♦ I.V. pole ♦ 60-ml syringe with adapter tip ♦ water ♦ optional: pump administration set (for an enteral infusion pump), Y-connector

Nasal and oral care

Cotton-tipped applicators ♦ water-soluble lubricant ♦ sponge-tipped swabs ♦ petroleum jelly

A bulb syringe or large catheter-tip syringe may be substituted for a gavage bag after the patient demonstrates tolerance for a gravity drip infusion. The practitioner may order an infusion pump to ensure accurate delivery of the prescribed formula.

Preparation

- Be sure to refrigerate formulas prepared in the dietary department or pharmacy. Refrigerate commercial formulas only after opening them.
- Check the dates on all formula containers and discard expired commercial formulas. Use powdered formulas within 24 hours of mixing.
- Always shake the container well to mix the solution thoroughly.
- Allow the formula to warm to room temperature before administration. Cold formula can increase the chance of diarrhea.
- Never warm formula over direct heat or in a microwave because heat may curdle the formula or change its chemical composition, and hot formula may injure the patient.
- Pour 60 ml of water into the graduated container. After closing the flow clamp on the administration set, pour the appropriate amount of formula into the gavage bag.
- Hang no more than a 4- to 6-hour supply at one time to prevent bacterial growth.
- Open the flow clamp on the administration set to remove air from the lines. This keeps air from entering the patient's stomach and causing distention and discomfort.

Key steps

- Confirm the patient's identity using two patient identifiers according to facility policy.
- Provide privacy, and wash your hands.
- Inform the patient that he'll receive nourishment through the tube, and explain the procedure to him. If possible, give him a schedule of subsequent feedings.
- If the patient has a nasal or oral tube, cover his chest with a towel or linen-saver pad to protect him and the bed linens from spills.
- Assess the patient's abdomen for bowel sounds and distention.

Delivering a gastric feeding

- To limit the risk of aspiration and reflux, raise the head of the patient's bed 30 to 45 degrees during feeding and for 1 hour after feeding. Use intermittent or continuous feeding regimens rather than the rapid bolus method.
- Check placement of the feeding tube to make sure it hasn't slipped out since the last feeding.

ALERT

Never administer a tube feeding until you're sure the tube is properly positioned in the patient's stomach. Administering a feeding through a misplaced tube can cause formula to enter the patient's lungs.

- To check tube patency and position, remove the cap or plug from the feeding tube, and use the syringe to aspirate stomach contents. Examine the aspirate and place a small amount on the pH test strip. The probability of gastric placement is increased if the aspirate has a gastric fluid appearance (grassy-green, clear and colorless with mucus shreds, or brown) and has a pH of less than or equal to 5.0.
- If there's no gastric secretion return, the tube may be in the esophagus. You'll need to advance the tube and recheck placement before proceeding.
- To assess gastric emptying, aspirate and measure residual gastric contents. Hold feedings if residual volume is greater than the predetermined amount specified in the practitioner's order (usually 50 to 100 ml). Reinstill any aspirate obtained.
- Connect the gavage bag tubing to the feeding tube. Depending on the type of tube used, you may need to use an adapter to connect the two.
- If you're using a bulb or catheter-tip syringe, remove the bulb or plunger and attach the syringe to the pinched-off feeding tube to prevent excess air from entering the patient's stomach, causing distention. If you're using an infusion controller, thread the tube from the formula container through the controller according to the manufacturer's directions. Blue food dye can be added to food to quickly identify aspiration. Purge the tubing of air and attach it to the feeding tube.
- Open the regulator clamp on the gavage bag tubing and adjust the flow rate appropriately. When using a bulb syringe, fill the syringe with formula and release the feeding tube to allow formula to flow through it. The height at which you hold the syringe will determine flow rate. When the syringe is three-quarters empty, pour more formula into it.
- To prevent air from entering the tube and the patient's stomach, never allow the syringe to empty completely. If you're using an infusion controller, set the flow rate according to the manufacturer's directions. Always administer a tube feeding slowly—typically 200 to 350 ml over 15 to 30 minutes, depending on the patient's tolerance and the practitioner's order—to prevent sudden stomach distention, which can cause nausea, vomiting, cramps, and diarrhea.
- After administering the appropriate amount of formula, flush the tubing by adding about 60 ml of water to the gavage bag or bulb syringe, or manually flush it using a barrel syringe. This maintains the tube's patency by removing excess formula, which could occlude the tube.
- If you're administering a continuous feeding, flush the feeding tube every 4 hours to help prevent tube occlusion. Monitor gastric emptying every 4 hours.
- To discontinue gastric feeding (depending on the equipment you're using), close

the regulator clamp on the gavage bag tubing, disconnect the syringe from the feeding tube, or turn off the infusion controller.

- Cover the end of the feeding tube with its plug or cap to prevent leakage and contamination of the tube.
- Leave the patient in semi-Fowler's or high Fowler's position for at least 1 hour.
- Rinse all reusable equipment with warm water.
- Dry it and store it in a convenient place for the next feeding. Change equipment every 24 hours or according to facility policy.

Delivering a duodenal or jejunal feeding

- Elevate the head of the bed and place the patient in low Fowler's position.
- Open the enteral administration set and hang the gavage container on the I.V. pole.
- If you're using a nasoduodenal tube, measure its length to check tube placement. Remember that you may not get any residual when you aspirate the tube.
- Open the flow clamp and regulate the flow to the desired rate. To regulate the rate using a volumetric infusion pump, follow the manufacturer's directions for setting up the equipment. Most patients receive small amounts initially, with volumes increasing gradually when tolerance is established.
- Flush the tube every 4 hours with water to maintain patency and provide hydration. A needle catheter jejunostomy tube may require flushing every 2 hours to prevent formula buildup inside the tube. A Y-connector may be useful for frequent flushing. Attach the continuous feeding to the main port, and use the side port for flushes.
- Change equipment every 24 hours or according to facility policy.

Special considerations

- If the feeding solution doesn't initially flow through a bulb syringe, attach the bulb and squeeze it gently to start the flow. Then remove the bulb. Never use the bulb to force the formula through the tube.
- If the patient becomes nauseated or vomits, stop the feeding immediately. The patient may vomit if the stomach becomes distended from overfeeding or delayed gastric emptying.
- To reduce oropharyngeal discomfort from the tube, allow the patient to brush his teeth or care for his dentures regularly, and encourage frequent gargling. If the patient is unconscious, administer oral care with wet sponge-tipped swabs every 4 hours. Use petroleum jelly on dry, cracked lips. Dry mucous membranes may indicate dehydration, which requires increased fluid intake. Clean the patient's nostrils with cotton-tipped applicators, apply lubricant along the mucosa, and assess the skin for signs of breakdown.
- During continuous feedings, assess the patient frequently for abdominal distention. Flush the tubing by adding about 50 ml of water to the gavage bag or bulb syringe. This maintains the tube's patency by removing excess formula, which could occlude the tube.
- If the patient develops diarrhea, administer small, frequent, less concentrated feedings, or administer bolus feedings over a longer time. Make sure the formula isn't cold and that proper storage and sanitation practices have been followed. The loose stools associated with tube feedings make extra perineal and skin care necessary. Changing to a formula with more fiber may eliminate liquid stools.
- If the patient becomes constipated, the practitioner may increase the fruit, vegetable, or sugar content of the formula. Assess the patient's hydration status because dehydration may produce constipation. Increase fluid intake as necessary. If the condition persists, administer an appropriate drug or enema, as ordered.
- Drugs can be administered through the feeding tube. Except for enteric-coated drugs or timed-release medications, crush tablets or open and dilute capsules in water before administering them. Be sure to flush the tubing afterward to ensure full instillation of medication. Keep in mind that some drugs may change the osmolarity of the feeding formula and cause diarrhea.

- Small-bore feeding tubes may kink, making instillation impossible. If you suspect this problem, try changing the patient's position, or withdraw the tube a few inches and restart. Never use a guide wire to reposition the tube.
- Constantly monitor the flow rate of a blended or high-residue formula to determine if the formula is clogging the tubing as it settles. To prevent such clogging, squeeze the bag frequently to agitate the solution.
- Collect blood samples as ordered. Glycosuria, hyperglycemia, and diuresis can indicate an excessive carbohydrate level, leading to hyperosmotic dehydration, which can be fatal. Monitor blood glucose levels to assess glucose tolerance. (A patient with a serum glucose level of less than 200 mg/dl is considered stable.) Monitor serum electrolytes, blood urea nitrogen, serum glucose, serum osmolality, and other pertinent findings to determine the patient's response to therapy and assess his hydration status.
- Check the flow rate hourly to ensure correct infusion. (With an improvised administration set, use a time tape to record the rate because it's difficult to get precise readings from an irrigation container or enema bag.)
- For duodenal or jejunal feeding, most patients tolerate a continuous drip better than bolus feedings. Bolus feedings can cause such complications as hyperglycemia and diarrhea.
- Until the patient acquires a tolerance for the formula, you may need to dilute it to one-half or three-quarters strength to start, and increase it gradually. A patient under stress or receiving steroids may experience a pseudodiabetic state. Assess him frequently to determine the need for insulin.
- If possible, use smaller-lumen tubes to prevent irritation and erosion of mucosa. Check your facility's policy regarding the frequency of changing feeding tubes to prevent complications.

Complications

- Erosion of esophageal, tracheal, nasal, and oropharyngeal mucosa resulting if tubes are left in place for a long time
- Bloating and retention from frequent or large-volume feedings using the gastric route
- Metabolic disturbances causing dehydration, diarrhea, and vomiting
- Cramping and abdominal distention usually indicating intolerance
- Clogging of the feeding tube when using the duodenal or jejunal route; also causing metabolic, fluid, and electrolyte abnormalities including hyperglycemia, hyperosmolar dehydration, coma, edema, hypernatremia, and essential fatty acid deficiency
- Dumping syndrome, in which a large amount of hyperosmotic solution in the duodenum causes excessive diffusion of fluid through the semipermeable membrane and results in diarrhea; in the patient with low serum albumin levels; these symptoms resulting from low oncotic pressure in the duodenal mucosa

Patient teaching

- Teach the patient about the infusion control device to maintain accuracy, use of syringe or bag and tubing, care of the tube and insertion site, and forumla mixing.
- Tell the patient that the formula may be mixed in an electric blender according to the package directions.
- Tell the patient that formula not used within 24 hours must be discarded. If the formula must hang for more than 8 hours, advise him to use a gavage or pump administration set with an ice pouch to decrease the incidence of bacterial growth.
- Instruct the patient to use a new bag daily.
- Teach family members signs and symptoms to report to the practitioner or home care nurse as well as measures to take in an emergency.

Documentation

On the intake and output sheet, record the date, volume of formula, and volume of water. In your notes, include abdominal assessment (including tube exit site, if appropriate), amount of residual gastric contents, verification of tube placement, tube patency, and amount, type, and time of feeding. Document the patient's tolerance to the feeding, including nausea, vomiting, cramping, diarrhea, and distention. Note the result of blood and urine tests, hydration status, and any drugs given through the tube. Include the date and time of administration set changes, oral and nasal hygiene, and results of specimen collections.

U

Ultraviolet light therapy

Light therapy is a viable alternative for a variety of conditions, such as psoriasis, eczema, vitiligo, mycosis fungoides, and other dermatoses. Typically, patients require anywhere from 20 to 30 treatments to see results, depending on the severity of their condition.

Ultraviolet (UV) light causes profound biological changes, including UV light-induced immune suppression and temporary suppression of epidermal basal cell division followed by a later increase in cell turnover. Emitted by the sun, the UV spectrum is subdivided into three bands—A, B, and C—each of which affects the skin differently. Ultraviolet A (UVA) radiation (with a relatively long wavelength of 320 to 400 nm) rapidly darkens preformed melanin pigment, may augment ultraviolet B (UVB) in causing sunburn and skin aging, and may induce phototoxicity in the presence of some drugs. UVB radiation (with a wavelength of 280 to 320 nm) causes sunburn and erythema. Ultraviolet C (UVC) radiation (with a wavelength of 200 to 280 m) is usually absorbed by the earth's ozone layer and doesn't reach the ground. However, UVC kills bacteria and is used in operating room germicidal lamps.

The drug methoxsalen, a psoralen agent, creates artificial sensitivity to UVA by binding with the deoxyribonucleic acid in epidermal basal cells. Treating skin with a photosensitizing agent, such as methoxsalen, and UVA is called psoralen plus UVA (PUVA) therapy (or photochemotherapy). Administered before a UV light treatment, methoxsalen photosensitizes the skin to enhance therapeutic effect. Other drugs used in photochemotherapy in combination with PUVA include acitretin (Soriatane), an oral vitamin A derivative, and methotrexate. Topical preparations, such as crude coal tar, may be used in combination with UVB (known as the Goeckerman treatment).

Contraindications to PUVA and UVB therapy include a history of photosensitivity diseases, skin cancer, arsenic ingestion, or cataracts or cataract surgery; current use of photosensitivity-inducing drugs; and previous skin irradiation (which can induce skin cancer). UV light therapy is also contraindicated in patients who have undergone previous ionizing chemotherapy and patients who are using photosensitizing or immunosuppressant drugs. PUVA is contraindicated in pregnant women.

UV light therapy requires a team approach to be safe and effective. Implementing the treatment plan requires knowledge, skills, and expertise of the entire health care team.

Equipment

UVA radiation

Fluorescent black-light lamp ♦ high-intensity UVA fluorescent bulbs ♦ goggles

UVB radiation

Fluorescent sunlamp or hot quartz lamp ♦ sunlamp bulbs ♦ goggles

UV treatments

Oral or topical phototherapeutic medications, if necessary ♦ body-sized light chamber or smaller light box ♦ dark, polarized goggles ♦ sunscreen, if necessary ♦ hospital gown ♦ towels

Preparation

■ The patient can undergo UV light therapy in the hospital, physician's office, or at home. Typically set into a reflective cabinet, the light source consists of a bank of high-intensity fluorescent bulbs. (At home, the patient may use a small fluorescent sunlamp.)

■ Check the practitioner's orders to confirm the light treatment type and dose. For PUVA, the initial dose is based on the patient's skin type and is increased according to the treatment protocol and as tolerated. (See *Comparing skin types*.)

■ The practitioner calculates the UVB dose based on skin type estimation or by determining a minimal erythema dose—the smallest amount of UV light needed to produce mild erythema.

Comparing skin types

Skin type	Sunburn and tanning history
I	Always burns; never tans; sensitive ("Celtic" skin)
II	Burns easily; tans minimally
III	Burns moderately; tans gradually to light brown (average Caucasian skin)
IV	Burns minimally; always tans well to moderately brown (olive skin)
V	Rarely burns; tans profusely to dark (brown skin)
VI	Never burns; deeply pigmented; not sensitive (black skin)

Key steps

■ Inform the patient that UV light treatments produce a mild sunburn that helps to reduce or resolve skin lesions.

■ Review the patient's health history for contraindications to UV light therapy. Ask whether he's currently taking photosensitizing drugs, such as anticonvulsants, certain antihypertensives, phenothiazines, salicylates, sulfonamides, tetracyclines, tretinoin, and various cancer drugs.

■ If the patient is to have PUVA therapy, make sure he takes methoxsalen (with food) 1½ hours before treatment.

■ To begin therapy, instruct the patient to disrobe and put on a hospital gown. Have him remove the gown or expose just the treatment area after he's in the phototherapy unit. Make sure he wears goggles to protect his eyes and a sunscreen, towels, or the hospital gown to protect vulnerable skin areas. All male patients receiving PUVA must wear protection over the groin area.

■ If the patient is having local UVB treatment, position him at the correct distance from the light source. For instance, for facial treatment with a sunlamp, position the patient's face about 12″ (30.5 cm) from the lamp. For body treatment, position the patient's body about 30″ (76 cm) from either the sunlamp or the hot quartz lamp.

■ During therapy, make sure the patient wears goggles at all times. If you're observing him through light-chamber windows, you should wear goggles as well. If the patient must stand for the treatment, ask him to report dizziness to ensure his safety.

■ After delivering the prescribed UVB dose, help the patient out of the unit, and instruct him to shield exposed areas of skin from sunlight for 8 hours after therapy.

Special considerations

■ Overexposure to UV light (sunburn) can result from prolonged treatment and an inadequate distance between the patient and light sources. It can also result from the use of photosensitizing drugs or from overly sensitive skin.

Skin care guidelines

A patient receiving ultraviolet (UV) light treatments must know how to protect his skin from injury. Provide the patient with the following skin care tips:

- Encourage the patient to use emollients and drink plenty of fluids to combat dry skin and maintain adequate hydration. Warn him to avoid hot baths or showers and to use soap sparingly. Heat and soap promote dry skin.
- Instruct the patient to notify his practitioner before taking medication, including aspirin, to prevent heightened photosensitivity.
- If the patient is receiving psoralen plus UVA therapy, review his methoxsalen dosage schedule. Explain that deviating from it could result in burns or ineffective treatment. Urge him to wear appropriate sunglasses outdoors for at least 24 hours after taking methoxsalen. Recommend yearly eye examinations to detect cataract formation.
- If the patient uses a sunlamp at home, advise him to let the lamp warm for 5 minutes before treatment. Stress the importance of exposing his skin to the light for the exact amount of time that the practitioner has prescribed. Instruct the patient to protect his eyes with goggles and to use a dependable timer or have someone else time his therapy. Above all, urge him never to use the sunlamp when he's tired to avoid falling asleep under the lamp and sustaining a burn.
- Teach the patient first aid for localized burning: Tell him to apply cool water soaks for 20 minutes or until skin temperature cools. For more extensive burns, recommend tepid tap water baths after notifying the practitioner about the burn. After the patient bathes, suggest using an oil-in-water moisturizing lotion (not a petroleum-jelly-based product, which can trap radiant heat).
- Tell the patient to limit natural light exposure, to use a sunscreen when he's outdoors, and to notify his practitioner immediately if he discovers unusual skin lesions.
- Advise the patient to avoid harsh soaps and chemicals, such as paints and solvents, and to discuss ways to manage physical and psychological stress, which may exacerbate skin disorders.

- Prevent eye damage by using gray or green polarized lenses during UVB therapy or UV-opaque sunglasses during PUVA therapy. The patient undergoing PUVA therapy should wear these glasses for 24 hours after treatment because methoxsalen can cause photosensitivity.
- Before giving methoxsalen or etretinate, check to ensure that baseline liver function studies have been done. Keep in mind that both drugs are hepatotoxic agents and are never given together. Liver function and blood lipid studies are required before treatment with acitretin and at regular intervals during treatment. Liver function studies and a complete blood count are required before and during methotrexate treatment.
- If the practitioner prescribes tar preparations with UVB treatment, watch for signs of sensitivity, such as erythema, pruritus, and eczematous reactions. If you apply carbonis detergens to the patient's skin before UV light therapy, be sure to remove it completely with mineral oil just before treatment begins to let the light penetrate the skin.

Complications

- Erythema with UVB therapy (Minimal erythema without discomfort is acceptable, but treatments are suspended if marked edema, swelling, or blistering occurs.)
- Erythema, nausea, and pruritus with PUVA therapy
- Long-term adverse effects including premature aging (xerosis, wrinkles, and mottled skin), lentigines, telangiectasia, increased risk of skin cancer, and ocular damage if eye protection isn't used

Patient teaching

- Tell the patient to look for marked erythema, blistering, peeling, or other signs of overexposure 4 to 6 hours after UVB therapy and 24 to 48 hours after UVA therapy. In either case, the erythema should disappear within another 24 hours. Tell him that mild dryness and desquamation will occur in 1 to 2 days. Teach him appropriate skin care measures. (See *Skin care guidelines*.) Advise him to notify the practitioner if overexposure occurs. Typically, the practitioner recommends stopping treatment for a few days and then starting over at a lower exposure level.
- Teach the patient to minimize UV light effects by using emollients, sunscreens, and cover-ups.

Documentation

Record the date and time of initial and subsequent treatments, the UV wavelength used, and the name and dose of any oral or topical medications given. Record the exact duration of therapy, the distance between the light source and the skin, and the patient's tolerance. Note safety measures used such as eye protection. Describe the patient's skin condition before and after treatment. Note improvements and adverse reactions, such as increased pruritus, oozing, and scaling.

Urinary diversion stoma care

Urinary diversions provide an alternative route for urine flow when a disorder, such as an invasive bladder tumor, impedes normal drainage. A permanent urinary diversion is indicated in any condition that requires a total cystectomy. In conditions requiring temporary urinary drainage or diversion, a suprapubic or urethral catheter is usually inserted to divert the flow of urine temporarily. The catheter remains in place until the incision heals.

Urinary diversions may also be indicated for patients with neurogenic bladder, congenital anomaly, traumatic injury to the lower urinary tract, or severe chronic urinary tract infection. Ileal conduit and continent urinary diversion are the two types of permanent urinary diversions with stomas. (See *Types of permanent urinary diversion,* page 572.) These procedures usually require the patient to wear a urine-collection appliance and to care for the stoma created during surgery. Evaluation by the wound ostomy continence nurse will facilitate site selection and postoperative stoma care.

Equipment

Soap and warm water ♦ waste receptacle (such as an impervious or wax-coated bag) ♦ linen-saver pad ♦ hypoallergenic paper tape ♦ povidone-iodine pads ♦ urine collection container ♦ rubber catheter (usually #14 or #16 French) ♦ ruler ♦ scissors ♦ urine-collection appliance (with or without antireflux valve) ♦ graduated cylinder ♦ cottonless gauze pads (some rolled, some flat) ♦ washcloth ♦ skin barrier in liquid, paste, wafer, or sheet form ♦ stoma covering (nonadherent gauze pad or panty liner) ♦ two pairs of gloves ♦ optional: adhesive solvent, irrigating syringe, tampon, hair dryer, electric razor, regular gauze pads, vinegar, deodorant tablets

Commercially packaged stoma care kits are available. In place of soap and water, you can use adhesive remover pads, if available, or cotton gauze saturated with adhesive solvent.

Some appliances come with a semipermeable skin barrier (impermeable to liquid but permeable to vapor and oxygen, which is essential for maintaining skin integrity). Wafer-type barriers may offer more protection against irritation than adhesive appliances. For example, a carbon-zinc barrier is economical and easy to apply. Its putty-like consistency allows it to be rolled between the palms to form a "washer" that can encircle the base of the stoma. This barrier can withstand enzymes, acids, and other damaging discharge material. All semipermeable barriers are easily removed along with the adhesive, causing less damage to the skin.

Preparation

- Assemble all the equipment on the patient's overbed table.

Types of permanent urinary diversion

Two types of urinary diversions—the ileal conduit and the continent urinary diversion—are described here. Another type of continent urinary diversion (not pictured here) is "hooked" back to the urethra, obviating the need for a stoma.

Ileal conduit

A segment of the ileum is excised, and the two ends of the ileum that result from excision of the segment are sutured closed. Then the ureters are dissected from the bladder and anastomosed to the ileal segment. One end of the ileal segment is closed with sutures; the opposite end is brought through the abdominal wall, thereby forming a stoma.

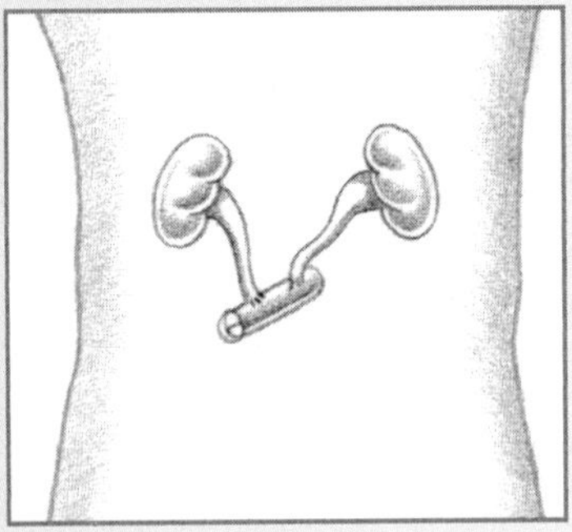

Continent urinary diversion

A tube is formed from part of the ascending colon and ileum. One end of the tube is brought to the skin to form the stoma. At the internal end of this tube, a nipple valve is constructed so urine won't drain out unless a catheter is inserted through the stoma into the newly formed bladder pouch. The urethral neck is sutured closed.

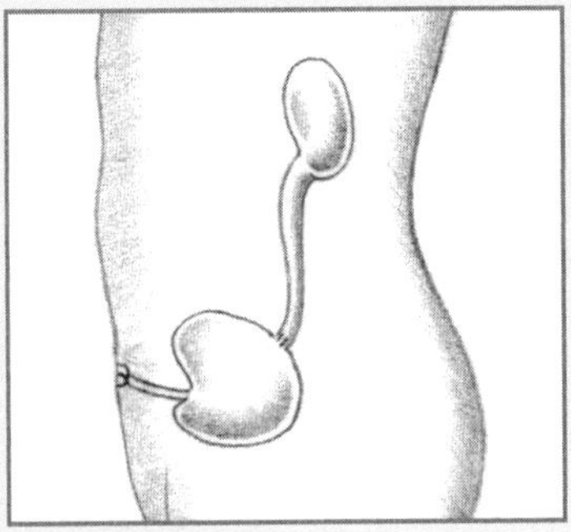

- Tape the waste receptacle to the table for ready access. Provide privacy for the patient, and wash your hands.
- Measure the diameter of the stoma with a ruler. Cut the opening of the appliance with the scissors—it shouldn't be more than ⅛" (0.3 cm) larger than the diameter of the stoma.
- Moisten the faceplate of the appliance with a small amount of solvent or water to prepare it for adhesion.
- Performing these preliminary steps at the bedside allows you to demonstrate the procedure and show the patient that it isn't difficult, which will help him to relax.

Key steps

- Wash your hands again. Explain the procedure to the patient as you go along, and offer constant reinforcement and reassurance to counteract negative reactions that may be elicited by stoma care.
- Place the bed in low Fowler's position so the patient's abdomen is flat. This position eliminates skin folds that could cause the appliance to slip or irritate the skin and allows the patient to observe or participate.
- Put on the gloves and place the linen-saver pad under the patient's side, near the stoma. Open the drain valve of the appliance being replaced to empty the urine into the graduated cylinder. Then, to remove the appliance, apply soap and water or adhesive solvent as you gently push the skin back from the pouch. If the appliance is disposable, discard it into the waste receptacle. If it's reusable, clean it with soap and lukewarm water and let it air-dry.

ALERT

To avoid irritating the patient's stoma, avoid touching it with adhesive solvent. If adhesive remains on the skin, gently rub it off with a dry gauze pad. Discard used gauze pads in the waste receptacle.

- To prevent a constant flow of urine onto the skin while you're changing the appliance, wick the urine with an absorbent, lint-free material. (See *Wicking urine from a stoma.*)
- Use water to carefully wash off any crystal deposits that may have formed around the stoma. If urine has stagnated and has a strong odor, use soap to wash it off. Be sure to rinse thoroughly to remove any oily residue that could cause the appliance to slip.
- Follow your facility's skin care policy to treat any minor skin problems.
- Dry the peristomal area thoroughly with a gauze pad because moisture will keep the appliance from sticking. Use a hair dryer if you wish. Remove any hair from the area with scissors or an electric razor to prevent hair follicles from becoming irritated when the pouch is removed, which can cause folliculitis.
- Inspect the stoma to see if it's healing properly and to detect complications. Check the color and the appearance of the suture line, and examine any moisture or effluent. Inspect the peristomal skin for redness, irritation, and intactness.
- Apply the skin barrier. If you apply a wafer or sheet, cut it to fit over the stoma. Remove any protective backing and set the barrier aside with the adhesive side up. If you apply a liquid barrier (such as Skin-Prep), saturate a gauze pad with it and coat the peristomal skin. Move in concentric circles outward from the stoma until you've covered an area 2″ (5 cm) larger than the wafer. Let the skin dry for several minutes—it should feel tacky. Gently press the wafer around the stoma, sticky side down, smoothing from the stoma outward.
- If you're using a barrier paste, open the tube, squeeze out a small amount, and then discard it. Then squeeze a ribbon of paste directly onto the peristomal skin about ½″ (1.3 cm) from the stoma, making a complete circle. Make several more concentric circles outward. Dip your fingers into lukewarm water, and smooth the paste until the skin is completely covered from the edge of the stoma to 3″ to 4″ (7.5 to 10 cm) outward. The paste should be ¼″ to ½″ (0.6 to 1.3 cm) thick. Then discard the gloves, wash your hands, and put on new gloves.
- Remove the material used for wicking urine, and place it in the waste receptacle.
- Next, place the appliance over the stoma, leaving only a small amount (⅜″ to ¾″ [1 to 2 cm]) of skin exposed.
- Secure the faceplate of the appliance to the skin with paper tape, if recommended. To do this, place a piece of tape lengthwise on each edge of the faceplate so that the tape overlaps onto the skin.
- Dispose of the used materials appropriately.

Wicking urine from a stoma

Use a piece of rolled, cottonless gauze or a tampon to wick urine from a stoma. Working by capillary action, wicking absorbs urine while you prepare the patient's skin to hold a urine-collection appliance.

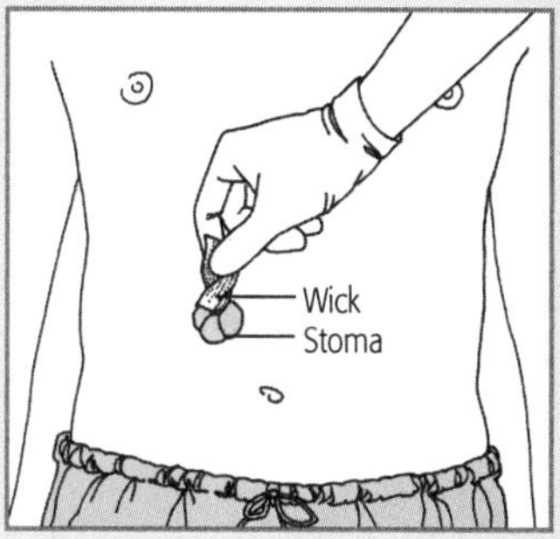

Special considerations

- If the patient has a continent urinary diversion, make sure you know how to meet his special needs. (See *Caring for the patient with a continent urinary diversion,* page 574.)

Caring for the patient with a continent urinary diversion

In this procedure, an alternative to the traditional ileal conduit, a pouch created from the ascending colon and terminal ileum serves as a new bladder, which empties through a stoma. To drain urine continuously, several drains are inserted into this reconstructed bladder and left in place for 3 to 6 weeks until the new stoma heals. The patient will be discharged from the hospital with the drains in place. He'll return to have them removed and to learn to catheterize his stoma.

First hospitalization

- Immediately after surgery, monitor intake and output from each drain. Be alert for decreased output, which may indicate that urine flow is obstructed.
- Watch for common postoperative complications, such as infection or bleeding. Also watch for signs of urinary leakage, which include increased abdominal distention, and urine appearing around the drains or midline incision.
- Irrigate the drains as ordered.
- Clean the area around the drains daily—first with povidone-iodine solution and then with sterile water. Apply a dry, sterile dressing to the area. Use precut 4" x 4" drain dressings around the drain to absorb leakage.
- To increase the patient's mobility and comfort, connect the drains to a leg bag.

Second hospitalization or outpatient

- After the patient's drains are removed, teach him how to catheterize the stoma. Begin by gathering the following equipment on a clean towel rubber catheter (usually #14 or #16 French), water-soluble lubricant, washcloth, stoma covering (nonadherent gauze pad or panty liner), hypoallergenic adhesive tape, and an irrigating solution (optional).
- Apply water-soluble lubricant to the catheter tip to facilitate insertion.
- Remove and discard the stoma cover. Using the washcloth, clean the stoma and the area around it, starting at the stoma and working outward in a circular motion.
- Hold the urine-collection container under the catheter; then slowly insert the catheter into the stoma. Urine should begin to flow into the container. If it doesn't, gently rotate the catheter or redirect its angle. If the catheter drains slowly, it may be plugged with mucus. Irrigate it with sterile saline solution or sterile water to clear it. When the flow stops, pinch the catheter closed and remove it.

Home care

- Teach the patient how to care for the drains and their insertion sites during the 3 to 6 weeks he'll be at home before their removal, and teach him how to attach them to a leg bag. Also teach him how to recognize the signs of infection and obstruction.
- After the drains are removed, teach the patient how to empty the pouch, and establish a schedule. Initially, he should catheterize the stoma and empty the pouch every 2 to 3 hours. Later, he should catheterize every 4 hours while awake and also irrigate the pouch each morning and evening, if ordered. Instruct him to empty the pouch whenever he feels a sensation of fullness.
- Tell the patient that the catheters are reusable, but only after they've been cleaned. He should clean the catheter thoroughly with warm, soapy water, rinse it thoroughly, and hang it to dry over a clean towel. He should store cleaned and dried catheters in plastic bags. Tell him he can reuse catheters for up to 1 month before discarding them. However, he should immediately discard any catheter that becomes discolored or cracked.

Complications

- Bleeding caused by an ill-fitting appliance because intestinal mucosa is delicate; occurring especially with an ileal conduit, the most common type of urinary diversion stoma, because a segment of the intestine forms the conduit
- Peristomal skin becoming reddened or excoriated from too-frequent changing or improper placement of the appliance, poor skin care, or allergic reaction to the appliance or adhesive
- Constant leakage around the appliance resulting from improper placement of the appliance or from poor skin turgor

Patient teaching

- The patient's attitude toward his urinary diversion stoma plays a big part in determining how well he'll adjust to it. To encourage a positive attitude, help him get used to the idea of caring for his stoma and the appliance as though they are natural extensions of himself. When teaching him to perform the procedure, give him written instructions and provide positive reinforcement after he completes each step. Suggest that he perform the procedure in the morning when urine flows most slowly.
- Help the patient choose between disposable and reusable appliances by telling him the advantages and disadvantages of each. Emphasize the importance of correct placement and of a well-fitted appliance to prevent seepage of urine onto the skin. When positioned correctly, most appliances remain in place for at least 3 days and for as long as 5 days if no leakage occurs. After 5 days, the appliance should be changed.
- Because urine flows constantly, it accumulates quickly, becoming even heavier than stools. To prevent the weight of the urine from loosening the seal around the stoma and separating the appliance from the skin, tell the patient to empty the appliance through the drain valve when it is one-third to one-half full.
- Instruct the patient to connect his appliance to a urine-collection container before he goes to sleep. The continuous flow of urine into the container during the night prevents the urine from accumulating and stagnating in the appliance.
- Teach the patient sanitary and dietary measures that can protect the peristomal skin and control the odor that commonly results from alkaline urine, infection, or poor hygiene. Reusable appliances should be washed with soap and lukewarm water, then air-dried thoroughly to prevent brittleness. Soaking the appliance in vinegar and water or placing deodorant tablets in it can further dissipate stubborn odors. An acid-ash diet that includes ascorbic acid and cranberry juice may raise urine acidity, thereby reducing bacterial action and fermentation (the underlying causes of odor). Generous fluid intake also helps to reduce odors by diluting the urine.
- Inform the patient about support services provided by ostomy clubs and the American Cancer Society. Members of these organizations routinely visit hospitals and other health care facilities to explain ostomy care and the types of appliances available and to help patients learn to function normally with a stoma.

Documentation

Record the appearance and color of the stoma and whether it's inverted, flush with the skin, or protruding. If it protrudes, note by how much it protrudes above the skin. (The normal range is ½″ to ¾″ [1.5 to 2 cm].) Record the appearance and condition of the peristomal skin, noting any redness or irritation or complaints by the patient of itching or burning.

Urine collection

A random urine specimen, usually collected as part of the physical examination or at various times during hospitalization, permits laboratory screening for urinary and systemic disorders as well as for drug use. A clean-catch midstream specimen is replacing random collection because it provides a virtually uncontaminated specimen without the need for catheterization.

When the patient can void voluntarily, a midstream specimen is commonly collected for culture and sensitivity testing. To protect the patient's rights, the nurse should assess the patient's level of understanding for the purpose of the test and the method of collection. This allows for clarification of any misunderstanding and promotes patient cooperation. Reference to the medical record for indications of infection will explain the purpose of the specimen procedure to the patient.

Specimens should always be covered and refrigerated. Covering the specimen prevents carbon dioxide from diffusing into the air, which could result in the urine becoming alkaline and fostering bacterial growth. If a sample isn't refrigerated for over 2 hours, it should be discarded. If the patient is menstruating, the nurse should make a note of this on the laboratory request form.

An indwelling catheter specimen—obtained either by clamping the drainage tube and emptying the accumulated urine into a container or by aspirating a specimen with a syringe—requires sterile collection technique to prevent catheter contamination and urinary tract infection. This method is contraindicated after genitourinary surgery.

Equipment

Random specimen

Bedpan or urinal with cover, if necessary ♦ gloves ♦ graduated container ♦ specimen container with lid ♦ label ♦ laboratory request form

Clean-catch midstream specimen

Soap and water ♦ gloves ♦ graduated container ♦ three sterile 2″ × 2″ gauze pads ♦ povidone-iodine solution ♦ sterile specimen container with lid ♦ label ♦ bedpan or urinal, if necessary ♦ laboratory request form

Commercial clean-catch kits containing antiseptic towelettes, sterile specimen container with lid and label, and instructions for use in several languages are widely used.

Indwelling catheter specimen

Gloves ♦ alcohol pad ♦ 10-ml syringe ♦ 21G or 22G 1½″ needle ♦ tube clamp ♦ sterile specimen container with lid ♦ label ♦ laboratory request form

Key steps

- Confirm the patient's identity using two patient identifiers according to facility policy.
- Tell the patient that you need a urine specimen for laboratory analysis. Explain the procedure to him and his family, if necessary, to promote cooperation and prevent accidental disposal of specimens.

Collecting a random specimen

- Provide privacy. Instruct the patient on bed rest to void into a clean bedpan or urinal, or ask the ambulatory patient to void into either one in the bathroom.
- Put on gloves.
- Pour at least 120 ml of urine into the specimen container, and cap the container securely. If the patient's urine output must be measured and recorded, pour the remaining urine into the graduated container. Otherwise, discard the remaining urine. If you inadvertently spill urine on the outside of the container, clean and dry it to prevent cross-contamination.
- After you label the sample container with the patient's name and room number and the date and time of collection, attach the request form and send it to the laboratory immediately. Delayed transport of the specimen may alter test results.
- Clean the graduated container and urinal or bedpan, and return them to their proper storage. Discard disposable items.
- Wash your hands thoroughly to prevent cross-contamination. Offer the patient a washcloth and soap and water to wash his hands.

Collecting a clean-catch midstream specimen

- Because the goal is a virtually uncontaminated specimen, explain the procedure to the patient carefully. Provide illustrations to emphasize the correct collection technique, if possible.
- Tell the male patient to remove all clothing from the waist down and to stand in front of the toilet as for urination; tell the female patient to sit far back on the toilet

seat and spread her legs. Then have the patient clean the periurethral area (tip of the penis or labial folds, vulva, and urethral meatus) with soap and water and then wipe the area three times, each time with a fresh 2″ × 2″ gauze pad soaked in povidone-iodine solution, or with the wipes provided in a commercial kit. For the uncircumcised male patient, emphasize the need to retract his foreskin to effectively clean the meatus and to keep it retracted during voiding.

■ Instruct the female patient to separate her labial folds with her thumb and forefinger. Tell her to wipe down one side with the first pad and discard it, to wipe the other side with the second pad and discard it and, finally, to wipe down the center over the urinary meatus with the third pad and discard it. Stress the importance of cleaning from front to back to avoid contaminating the genital area with fecal matter. Tell her to straddle the bedpan or toilet to allow labial spreading. She should continue to keep her labia separated while voiding.

■ Instruct the patient to begin voiding into the bedpan, urinal, or toilet. Then without stopping the urine stream, the patient should move the collection container into the stream, collecting about 30 to 50 ml at the midstream portion of the voiding. He can then finish voiding into the bedpan, urinal, or toilet.

■ Put on gloves before discarding the first and last portions of the voiding, and measure the remaining urine in a graduated container for intake and output records, if necessary. Be sure to include the amount in the specimen container when recording the total amount voided.

■ Take the sterile container from the patient, and cap it securely. Avoid touching the inside of the container or the lid. If the outside of the container is soiled, clean it and wipe it dry. Remove gloves and discard them properly.

■ Wash your hands thoroughly. Tell the patient to wash his hands also.

■ Label the container with the patient's name and room number, name of test, type of specimen, collection time, and suspected diagnosis, if known. If a urine culture has been ordered, note current antibiotic therapy on the laboratory request form. Send the container to the laboratory immediately, or place it on ice to prevent specimen deterioration and altered test results.

Aspirating a urine specimen

If the patient has an indwelling urinary catheter in place, clamp the tube distal to the aspiration port for about 30 minutes. Wipe the port with an alcohol pad, and insert a needle and a 20- or 30-ml syringe into the port perpendicular to the tube. Aspirate the required amount of urine, and expel it into the specimen container. Remove the clamp on the drainage tube.

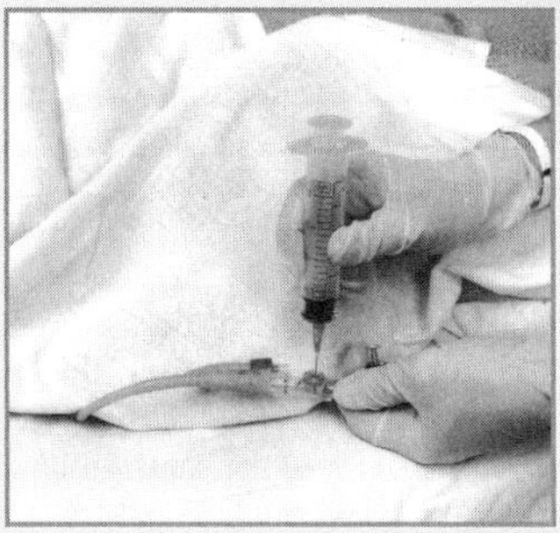

Collecting an indwelling catheter specimen

■ About 30 minutes before collecting the specimen, clamp the drainage tube to allow urine to accumulate.

■ Put on gloves. If the drainage tube has a built-in sampling port, wipe the port with an alcohol pad. Uncap the needle on the syringe, and insert the needle into the sampling port at a 90-degree angle to the tubing. Aspirate the specimen into the syringe. (See *Aspirating a urine specimen*.)

Special considerations

■ If the drainage tube doesn't have a sampling port and the catheter is made of rubber, obtain the specimen from the catheter.

Other types of catheters will leak after you withdraw the needle. To withdraw the specimen from a rubber catheter, wipe it with an alcohol pad just above where it connects to the drainage tube. Insert the needle into the rubber catheter at a 45-degree angle and withdraw the specimen. Never insert the needle into the shaft of the catheter because this may puncture the lumen leading to the catheter balloon.

- Transfer the specimen to a sterile container, label it, and send it to the laboratory immediately or place it on ice. If a urine culture is to be performed, be sure to list current antibiotic therapy on the laboratory request form.
- If the catheter isn't made of rubber or has no sampling port, wipe the area where the catheter joins the drainage tube with an alcohol pad. Disconnect the catheter, and allow urine to drain into the sterile specimen container. Avoid touching the inside of the sterile container with the catheter, and don't touch anything with the catheter drainage tube to avoid contamination. When you have collected the specimen, wipe both connection sites with an alcohol pad and join them. Cap the specimen container, label it, and send it to the laboratory immediately or place it on ice.

ALERT

Make sure that you unclamp the drainage tube after collecting the specimen to prevent urine backflow, which may cause bladder distention and infection.

Complications

- None known

Documentation

Record the times of specimen collection and transport to the laboratory. Specify the test as well as the appearance, odor, color, and any unusual characteristics of the specimen. If necessary, record the urine volume on the intake and output record.

Urine collection, timed

Because hormones, proteins, and electrolytes are excreted in small, variable amounts in urine, specimens for measuring these substances must typically be collected over an extended period to yield quantities of diagnostic value.

A 24-hour specimen is used most commonly because it provides an average excretion rate for substances eliminated during this period. Timed specimens may also be collected for shorter periods, such as 2 or 12 hours, depending on the specific information needed.

A timed urine specimen may also be collected after administering a challenge dose of a chemical—insulin, for example—to detect various renal disorders.

Equipment

Large collection bottle with a cap or stopper, or a commercial plastic container ♦ preservative, if necessary ♦ gloves ♦ bedpan or urinal if patient doesn't have an indwelling catheter ♦ graduated container if patient is on intake and output measurement ♦ ice-filled container if a refrigerator isn't available ♦ label ♦ laboratory request form and laboratory biohazard transport container ♦ four patient-care reminders

Check with the laboratory to find out which preservatives may need to be added to the specimen or whether a dark collection bottle is required.

Key steps

- Confirm the patient's identity using two patient identifiers according to facility policy.
- Explain the procedure to the patient and his family, as necessary, to enlist their cooperation and prevent accidental disposal of urine during the collection period. Emphasize that failure to collect even one specimen during the collection period invalidates the test and requires that it begin again.
- Place patient-care reminders over the patient's bed, in his bathroom, and on the urinal or indwelling catheter collection

bag. Include the date and the collection interval.

- Instruct the patient to save all urine during the collection period, to notify you after each voiding, and to avoid contaminating the urine with stool or toilet tissue. Explain any dietary or drug restrictions, and make sure he understands and is willing to comply with them.

2-hour collection

- If possible, instruct the patient to drink two to four 8-oz (473 to 946 ml) glasses of water about 30 minutes before collection begins. After 30 minutes, tell him to void. Put on gloves and discard this specimen so the patient starts the collection period with an empty bladder.
- If ordered, administer a challenge dose of medication (such as glucose solution or corticotropin), and record the time.
- If possible, offer the patient a glass of water at least every hour during the collection period to stimulate urine production. After each voiding, put on gloves and add the specimen to the collection bottle.
- Instruct the patient to void about 15 minutes before the end of the collection period, if possible, and add this specimen to the collection bottle.
- At the end of the collection period, remove and discard your gloves and send the appropriately labeled collection bottle to the laboratory immediately in an approved laboratory biohazard transport container, along with a properly completed laboratory request form.

12- and 24-hour collection

- Put on gloves and ask the patient to void. Then discard this urine so the patient starts the collection period with an empty bladder. Record the time.
- After putting on gloves and pouring the first urine specimen into the collection bottle, add the required preservative. Then refrigerate the bottle or keep it on ice until the next voiding, as appropriate.
- Collect all urine voided during the prescribed period. Just before the collection period ends, ask the patient to void again, if possible. Add this last specimen to the collection bottle, pack it in ice to inhibit deterioration of the specimen, and remove and discard your gloves. Label the collection bottle, place it in an approved laboratory biohazard transport container, and send it to the laboratory with a properly completed laboratory request form.

Special considerations

- Keep the patient well hydrated before and during the test to ensure adequate urine flow.
- Before collection of a timed specimen, make sure the laboratory will be open when the collection period ends to help ensure prompt, accurate results. Never store a specimen in a refrigerator that contains food or medication to avoid contamination. If the patient has an indwelling catheter in place, put the collection bag in an ice-filled container at his bedside.
- Instruct the patient to avoid exercise and ingestion of coffee, tea, or any drugs (unless directed otherwise by the practitioner) before the test to avoid altering test results.
- If you accidentally discard a specimen during the collection period, you'll need to restart the collection. This may result in an additional day of hospitalization, which may cause the patient personal and financial hardship. Therefore, emphasize the need to save all the patient's urine during the collection period to everyone involved in his care as well as to his family and other visitors.

Complications

- None known

Patient teaching

- If the patient must continue collecting urine at home, provide written instructions for the appropriate method. Tell him that he can keep the collection bottle in a brown bag in his refrigerator at home, separate from other refrigerator contents.

Documentation

Record the date and intervals of specimen collection and when the collection bottle was sent to the laboratory.

Urine glucose and ketone tests

Reagent strip tests are used to monitor urine glucose and ketone levels and to screen for diabetes. Urine glucose tests are less accurate than blood glucose tests and are used less frequently because of the increasing convenience of blood self-testing. Urine ketone tests monitor fat metabolism, help diagnose carbohydrate deprivation and diabetic ketoacidosis, and help distinguish between diabetic and nondiabetic coma.

Glucose oxidase tests (such as Diastix, Tes-Tape, and Clinistix strips) produce color changes when patches of reagents implanted in handheld plastic strips react with glucose in the patient's urine; urine ketone strip tests (such as Keto-Diastix and Ketostix) are similar. All test results are read by comparing color changes with a standardized reference chart.

Equipment

Specimen container ♦ gloves ♦ glucose or ketone test strip ♦ reference color chart

DO'S & DON'TS

Wear gloves as barrier protection when performing all urine tests.

Key steps

- Confirm the patient's identity using two patient identifiers according to facility policy.
- Explain the test to the patient, and if he's a newly diagnosed diabetic, teach him how to perform the test himself. Check his history for medications that may interfere with test results.
- Before each test, instruct the patient not to contaminate the urine specimen with stool or toilet tissue.
- Test urine specimen immediately after the patient voids.

Glucose oxidase strip testing

- Explain the test to the patient and, if he's diagnosed with diabetes, teach him to perform it himself. Check his history for medications that may interfere with test results. Put on gloves before collecting a specimen for the test, and remove them to record test results.
- Instruct the patient to void. Ask him to drink a glass of water, if possible, and collect a second-voided specimen after 30 to 45 minutes.
- If you're using a Clinistix strip, dip the reagent end of the strip into the urine for 2 seconds. Remove excess urine by tapping the strip against the specimen container's rim, wait for exactly 10 seconds, and then compare its color with the color chart on the test strip container. Ignore color changes that occur after 10 seconds. Record the result.
- If you're using a Diastix strip, dip the reagent end of the strip into the urine for 2 seconds. Tap off excess urine from the strip, wait for exactly 30 seconds, and then compare the strip's color with the color chart on the test strip container. Ignore color changes that occur after 30 seconds. Record the result.
- If you're using a Tes-Tape strip, pull about 1½" (3.8 cm) of the reagent strip from the dispenser, and dip one end about ¼" (0.6 cm) into the specimen for 2 seconds. Tap off excess urine from the strip, wait exactly 60 seconds, and then compare the darkest part of the tape with the color chart on the dispenser. If the test result exceeds 0.5%, wait an additional 60 seconds and make a final comparison. Record the result.

Ketone strip testing

- Explain the test to the patient and, if he has diabetes or if he's to perform the test at home, teach him to perform it himself.
- Put on gloves and collect a second-voided midstream specimen.
- If you're using a Ketostix strip, dip the reagent end of the strip into the specimen and remove it immediately. Wait exactly 15 seconds, and then compare the color of the strip with the color chart on the test strip container. Ignore color changes that occur after 15 seconds. Remove and discard your gloves, and record the test result.

■ If you're using a Keto-Diastix strip, dip the reagent end of the strip into the specimen and remove it immediately. Tap off excess urine from the strip, and hold the strip horizontally to prevent mixing of chemicals between the two reagent squares. Wait exactly 15 seconds, and then compare the color of the ketone part of the strip with the color chart on the test strip container. After 30 seconds, compare the color of the glucose part of the strip with the color chart. Remove and discard gloves, and record the test results.

Special considerations

■ Keep reagent tablets and strips in a cool, dry place at a temperature below 86° F (30° C), but don't refrigerate them.
■ Keep the container tightly closed. Don't use discolored or outdated tablets or strips.

Complications

■ None known

Patient teaching

■ If the patient has diabetes, teach him how to perform the test at home.

Documentation

Record the test results according to the information on the reagent containers, or use a flowchart designed to record this information. If you're teaching a patient how to perform the test, keep a record of his progress.

Urine pH

The pH of urine—its alkalinity or acidity—reflects the kidneys' ability to maintain a normal hydrogen ion concentration in plasma and extracellular fluids. The normal hydrogen ion concentration in urine varies, ranging from pH 4.6 to 8.0, but it usually averages around pH 6.0.

The simplest procedure for testing the pH of urine consists of dipping a reagent strip (such as Combistix) into a fresh specimen of the patient's urine and comparing the resultant color change with a standardized color chart.

An alkaline pH (above 7.0), resulting from a diet low in meat but high in vegetables, dairy products, and citrus fruits, causes turbidity and the formation of phosphate, carbonate, and amorphous crystals. Alkaline urine may also result from urinary tract infection and from metabolic or respiratory alkalosis.

An acid pH (below 7.0), resulting from a high-protein diet, also causes turbidity as well as the formation of oxalate, cystine, amorphous urate, and uric acid crystals. Acid urine may also result from renal tuberculosis, phenylketonuria, alkaptonuria, pyrexia, diarrhea, starvation, and all forms of acidosis.

Measuring urine pH can also help monitor some medications, such as methenamine, that are active only at certain pH levels.

Equipment

Clean-catch kit ♦ urine specimen container ♦ gloves ♦ reagent strips

The reagent strip has a pH indicator as part of a battery of indicators.

Key steps

■ Confirm the patient's identity using two patient identifiers according to facility policy.
■ Wash your hands thoroughly and put on gloves.
■ Provide patient with a specimen container, and instruct him to collect a clean-catch midstream specimen. (See "Urine collection," page 575.) Dip the reagent strip into the urine, remove it, and tap off the excess urine from the strip.
■ Hold the strip horizontally to avoid mixing reagents from adjacent test areas on the strip. Then compare the color on the strip with the standardized color chart on the strip package. This comparison can be made up to 60 seconds after immersing the strip. Note the results promptly as the reagent strip may continue to change color.
■ Discard the urine specimen. If you're monitoring the patient's intake and output, measure the amount of urine discarded.

- Remove and discard your gloves, and wash your hands thoroughly to prevent cross-contamination.

Special considerations

- Use only a fresh urine specimen because bacterial growth at room temperature changes urine pH.
- Avoid letting a drop of urine run off the reagent strip onto adjacent reagent spots on the strip because the other reagents can change the pH result.
- Be aware that urine collected at night is usually more acidic than urine collected during the day.

Complications

- None known

Documentation

Record the test results, time of voiding, and amount voided.

Urine specific gravity

The kidneys maintain homeostasis by varying urine output and urine concentration of dissolved salts. Urine specific gravity measures the concentration of urine solutes, which reflects the kidneys' capacity to concentrate urine. The capacity to concentrate urine is among the first functions lost when renal tubular damage occurs.

Urine specific gravity is determined by comparing the weight of a urine specimen with that of an equivalent volume of distilled water, which is 1.000. Because urine contains dissolved salts and other substances, it's heavier than 1.000. Urine specific gravity ranges from 1.003 (very dilute) to 1.035 (highly concentrated); normal values range from 1.010 to 1.025. Specific gravity is commonly measured with a urinometer (a specially calibrated hydrometer designed to float in a cylinder of urine). The more concentrated the urine, the higher the urinometer floats—and the higher the specific gravity. Specific gravity may also be measured by a refractometer, which measures the refraction of light as it passes through a urine specimen, or a reagent strip test.

Elevated specific gravity reflects an increased concentration of urine solutes, which occurs in conditions that cause renal hypoperfusion, and may indicate heart failure, dehydration, hepatic disorders, or nephrosis. Low specific gravity reflects failure to reabsorb water and concentrate urine; it may indicate hypercalcemia, hypokalemia, alkalosis, acute renal failure, pyelonephritis, glomerulonephritis, or diabetes insipidus.

Although urine specific gravity is commonly measured with a random urine specimen, more accurate measurement is possible with a controlled specimen collected after fluids are withheld for 12 to 24 hours.

Equipment

Calibrated urinometer and cylinder, refractometer, or reagent strips (Multistix) ♦ gloves ♦ graduated specimen container

Key steps

- Explain the procedure to the patient, and tell him when you'll need the specimen. Explain why you're withholding fluids and for how long to ensure his cooperation.

Measuring with a urinometer

- Put on gloves and collect a random urine specimen. Let the specimen reach room temperature (71.6° F [22° C]) before testing because this is the temperature at which most urinometers are calibrated.
- Fill the cylinder about three-fourths full of urine. Then gently spin the urinometer and drop it into the cylinder.
- When the urinometer stops bobbing, read the specific gravity from the calibrated scale marked directly on the stem of the urinometer. Make sure the instrument floats freely and doesn't touch the sides of the cylinder. Read the scale at the lowest point of the meniscus to ensure an accurate reading. (See *Using a urinometer*.)
- Discard the urine, and rinse the cylinder and urinometer in cool water. Warm water coagulates proteins in urine, making them stick to the instrument.
- Remove your gloves and wash your hands thoroughly to prevent cross-contamination.

Measuring with a refractometer

- Put on gloves and collect a random or controlled urine specimen.
- Place a single drop of urine on the refractometer slide.
- Turn on the light and look through the eyepiece to see the specific gravity indicated on a scale. (Some instruments have a digital display.)

Measuring with a reagent strip

- Put on gloves and obtain a random or controlled urine specimen.
- Dip the reagent end of the test strip into the specimen for 2 seconds.
- Tap the strip on the rim of the specimen container to remove excess urine, and compare the resultant color change with the color chart supplied with the kit.

Special considerations

- Test the urinometer in distilled water at room temperature to ensure that its calibration is 1.000.
- If necessary, correct the urinometer reading for temperature effects; add 0.001 to your observed reading for every 5.4° F (3° C) above the calibration temperature of 71.6° F (22° C); subtract 0.001 for every 5.4° F below 71.6° F.

Complications

- None known

Documentation

Record the specific gravity, volume, color, odor, and appearance of the collected urine specimen.

Using a urinometer

With the urinometer floating in a cylinder of urine, position your eye at a level even with the bottom of the meniscus and read the specific gravity from the scale printed on the urinometer.

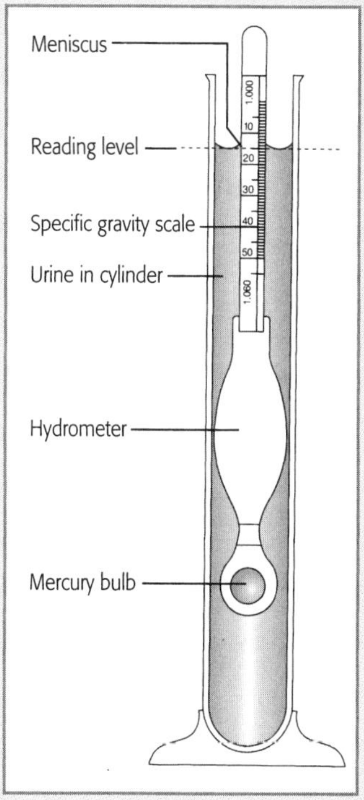

V

Vacuum-assisted closure therapy

Vacuum-assisted closure (VAC) therapy, also known as *negative pressure wound therapy,* is used to enhance delayed or impaired wound healing. The VAC device applies localized subatmospheric pressure to draw the edges of the wound toward the center. It's applied after a special dressing is placed in the wound or over a graft or flap; this wound packing removes fluids from the wound and stimulates growth of healthy granulation tissue. (See *Understanding vacuum-assisted closure therapy*.)

VAC therapy is indicated for acute and traumatic wounds, pressure ulcers, and chronic open wounds, such as diabetic ulcers, meshed grafts, and skin flaps. It's contraindicated for fistulas that involve organs or body cavities, necrotic tissue with eschar, untreated osteomyelitis, and malignant wounds. This therapy should be used cautiously in patients with active bleeding, in those taking anticoagulants, and when achieving wound hemostasis has been difficult.

Equipment

Waterproof trash bag ♦ goggles ♦ gown, if indicated ♦ emesis basin ♦ normal saline solution ♦ clean gloves ♦ sterile gloves ♦ sterile scissors ♦ linen-saver pad ♦ 30-ml piston syringe with 19G catheter ♦ reticulated foam ♦ fenestrated tubing ♦ evacuation tubing ♦ skin protectant wipe ♦ transparent occlusive air-permeable drape ♦ evacuation canister ♦ vacuum unit

Preparation

- Assemble the VAC device at the bedside according to manufacturer's instructions.
- Set negative pressure according to the practitioner's order (25 to 200 mm Hg).

Key steps

- Check the practitioner's order, and assess the patient's condition.
- Explain the procedure to the patient, provide privacy, and wash your hands. Put on goggles—and a gown, if necessary—to protect yourself from wound drainage and contamination.
- Place a linen-saver pad under the patient to catch any spills and avoid linen changes. Position the patient to allow maximum wound exposure. Place the emesis basin under the wound to collect any drainage.
- Put on clean gloves. Remove the soiled dressing and discard it in the waterproof trash bag. Attach the 19G catheter to the 30-ml piston syringe and irrigate the wound three times using the normal saline solution.
- Clean the area around the wound with normal saline solution; wipe intact skin with a skin protectant wipe and allow it to dry well. Remove and discard your gloves.
- Put on sterile gloves. Using sterile scissors, cut the foam to the shape and measurement of the wound. More than one piece of foam may be necessary if the first piece is cut too small.
- Carefully place the foam in the wound. Next, place the fenestrated tubing into the center of the foam. The fenestrated tubing, embedded into the foam, delivers negative pressure to the wound.

Understanding vacuum-assisted closure therapy

Vacuum-assisted closure (VAC) therapy, also called *negative pressure wound therapy,* is an option to consider when a wound fails to heal in a timely manner. VAC therapy encourages healing by applying localized subatmospheric pressure at the site of the wound. This reduces edema and bacterial colonization and stimulates the formation of granulation tissue.

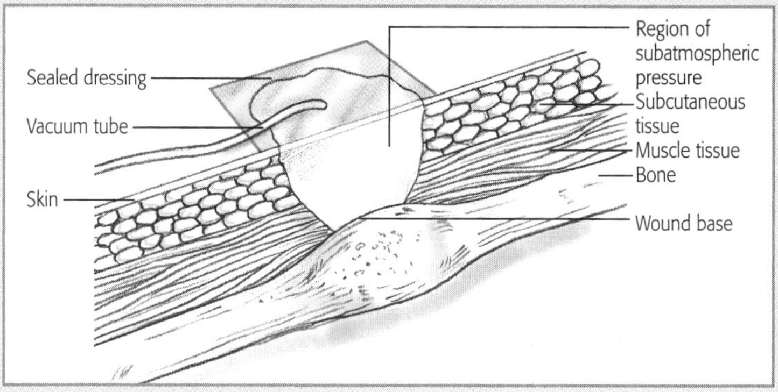

- Place the transparent occlusive air permeable drape over the foam, enclosing both the foam and the tubing. Remove and discard your gloves.
- Connect the free end of the fenestrated tubing to the evacuation tubing connected to the evacuation canister.
- Turn on the vacuum unit.
- Make sure the patient is comfortable.
- Properly dispose of drainage, solution, linen-saver pad, and trash bag, and clean or dispose of soiled equipment and supplies according to facility policy and Centers for Disease Control and Prevention guidelines.

Special considerations

- Change the dressing every 48 hours. Try to coordinate dressing change with the practitioner's visit so he can inspect the wound.
- Measure the amount of drainage every shift.
- Adjust the negative pressure setting according to the practitioner's orders.

Device safety

Audible and visual alarms alert you if the unit is tipped greater than 45 degrees, the canister is full, the dressing has an air leak, or the canister becomes dislodged.

Complications

- Temporary increased pain and risk of infection due to care and cleaning of wounds

Documentation

Document the frequency and duration of therapy, the amount of negative pressure applied, the size and condition of the wound, and the patient's response to treatment.

Vagal maneuvers

When a patient suffers sinus, atrial, or junctional tachyarrhythmias, vagal maneuvers—*Valsalva's maneuver* and *carotid sinus massage*—can slow his heart rate. These maneuvers work by stimulating nerve endings, which respond as they would to an increase in blood pressure. They send this message to the brain stem, which in turn stimulates the autonomic nervous system to increase vagal tone and decrease the heart rate.

In Valsalva's maneuver, the patient holds his breath and bears down, raising his intrathoracic pressure. When this pressure increase is transmitted to the heart and great vessels, venous return, stroke volume, and systolic blood pressure decrease. Within seconds, the baroreceptors respond to these changes by increasing the heart rate and causing peripheral vasoconstriction.

When the patient exhales at the end of the maneuver, his blood pressure rises to its previous level. This increase, combined with the peripheral vasoconstriction caused by bearing down, stimulates the vagus nerve, decreasing the heart rate.

ALERT

Valsalva's maneuver is contraindicated in patients with increased intracranial pressure. It shouldn't be taught to patients who aren't alert or cooperative.

In carotid sinus massage, manual pressure applied to the left or right carotid sinus slows the heart rate. This method is used both to diagnose and treat tachyarrhythmias. The patient's response to carotid sinus massage depends on the type of arrhythmia. If he has sinus tachycardia, his heart rate will slow gradually during the procedure and speed up again after it. If he has atrial tachycardia, the arrhythmia may stop and the heart rate may remain slow because the procedure increases atrioventricular (AV) block. With atrial fibrillation or flutter, the ventricular rate may not change; AV block may even worsen. With paroxysmal atrial tachycardia, reversion to sinus rhythm occurs only 20% of the time. Nonparoxysmal tachycardia and ventricular tachycardia won't respond.

Vagal maneuvers are contraindicated in patients with severe coronary artery disease, acute myocardial infarction, or hypovolemia. Carotid sinus massage is contraindicated in patients with cardiac glycoside toxicity or cerebrovascular disease and for patients who have had carotid surgery.

Although usually performed by a physician, vagal maneuvers may also be done by a specially trained nurse under a physician's supervision.

Equipment

Crash cart with emergency medications and airway equipment ♦ electrocardiogram (ECG) monitor and electrodes ♦ I.V. catheter and tubing ♦ tourniquet ♦ dextrose 5% in water (D_5W) ♦ clippers if needed, cardiotonic drugs (optional)

Key steps

- Confirm the patient's identity using two patient identifiers according to facility policy.
- Explain the procedure to the patient to ease his fears and promote cooperation. Ask him to let you know if he feels light-headed.
- Place the patient in a supine position. Insert an I.V. line, if necessary. Then administer D_5W at a keep-vein-open rate, as ordered. This line will be used if emergency drugs become necessary.
- Prepare the patient's skin, including shaving if necessary, and attach ECG electrodes. Adjust the size of the ECG complexes on the monitor so that you can see the arrhythmia clearly.

Valsalva's maneuver

- Ask the patient to take a deep breath and bear down, as if he were trying to defecate. If he doesn't feel light-headed or dizzy, and if no new arrhythmias occur, have him hold his breath and bear down for 10 seconds.
- If he does feel dizzy or light-headed, or if you see a new arrhythmia on the monitor—asystole for more than 6 seconds, frequent premature ventricular contractions (PVCs), or ventricular tachycardia or ventricular fibrillation—allow him to exhale and stop bearing down.
- After 10 seconds, ask him to exhale and breathe quietly. If the maneuver was suc-

Performing carotid sinus massage

Before applying manual pressure to the patient's right carotid sinus, locate the bifurcation of the carotid artery on the right side of the neck. Turn the patient's head slightly to the left and hyperextend the neck. This brings the carotid artery closer to the skin and moves the sternocleidomastoid muscle away from the carotid artery.

Then, using a circular motion, gently massage the right carotid sinus between your fingers and the transverse processes of the spine for 3 to 5 seconds. Don't massage for more than 5 seconds to avoid risking life-threatening complications.

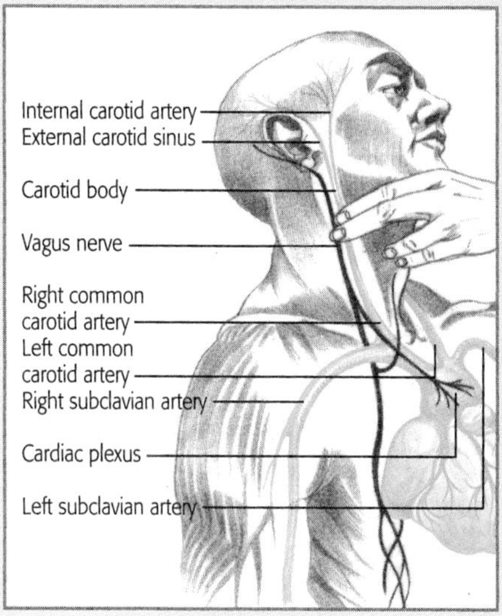

cessful, the monitor will show his heart rate slowing before he exhales.

Carotid sinus massage

- Begin by obtaining a rhythm strip, using the lead that shows the strongest P waves.
- Auscultate both carotid sinuses. If you detect bruits, inform the physician and don't perform carotid sinus massage. If you don't detect bruits, proceed as ordered. (See *Performing carotid sinus massage*.)
- Monitor the ECG throughout the procedure. Stop massaging when the ventricular rate slows sufficiently to permit diagnosis of the rhythm. Or, stop as soon as any evidence of a rhythm change appears. Have the crash cart handy to give emergency treatment if a dangerous arrhythmia occurs.
- If the procedure has no effect within 5 seconds, stop massaging the right carotid sinus and begin to massage the left. If this also fails, administer cardiotonic drugs, as ordered.

Special considerations

- Remember that a brief period of asystole—from 3 to 6 seconds—and several PVCs may precede conversion to normal sinus rhythm.
- If the vagal maneuver succeeded in slowing the patient's heart rate and converting the arrhythmia, continue monitoring him for several hours.

Complications

- Rapid drop in arterial pressure in elderly patients, patients receiving cardiac glycosides, and patients with heart block, hypertension, coronary artery disease, diabetes mellitus, or hyperkalemia (see *Adverse effects of vagal maneuvers*, page 588)

Documentation

Record the date and time of the procedure, who performed it, and why it was necessary. Note the patient's response, any complications, and the interventions taken. If possible, obtain a rhythm strip before, during, and after the procedure.

Adverse effects of vagal maneuvers

Valsalva's maneuver and carotid sinus massage are useful for slowing the heart rate. However, they can cause complications, some of which are life-threatening.

Valsalva's maneuver

Valsalva's maneuver can cause bradycardia, accompanied by a decrease in cardiac output, possibly leading to syncope. The bradycardia will usually pass quickly, but if it doesn't or if it advances to complete heart block or asystole, begin basic life support (BLS) followed—if necessary—by advanced cardiac life support (ACLS).

Valsalva's maneuver can mobilize venous thrombi and cause bleeding. Monitor the patient for signs and symptoms of vascular occlusion, including neurologic changes, chest discomfort, and dyspnea. Report such problems at once, and prepare the patient for diagnostic testing or transfer him to the intensive care unit (ICU), as ordered.

Carotid sinus massage

Because carotid sinus massage can cause ventricular fibrillation, ventricular tachycardia, and standstill as well as worsening atrioventricular block that leads to junctional or ventricular escape rhythms, you'll need to monitor the patient's electrocardiogram (ECG) closely. If his ECG indicates complete heart block or asystole, start BLS at once, followed by ACLS. If emergency medications don't convert the complete heart block, the patient may need a temporary pacemaker.

Carotid sinus massage can cause cerebral damage from inadequate tissue perfusion, especially in elderly patients. It can also cause a stroke, either from decreased perfusion caused by total carotid artery blockage or from migrating endothelial plaque loosened by carotid sinus compression. Watch the patient carefully during and after the procedure for changes in his neurologic status. If you note any, tell the practitioner at once and prepare the patient for further diagnostic tests or transfer him to the ICU, as ordered.

Vaginal medication insertion

Vaginal medications include suppositories, creams, gels, and ointments. These medications can be inserted as a topical treatment for infection (particularly Trichomonas vaginalis and monilial vaginitis) or inflammation or as a contraceptive. Suppositories melt when they contact the vaginal mucosa, and their medication diffuses topically (as effectively as creams, gels, and ointments).

Vaginal medications usually come with a disposable applicator that enables placement of medication in the anterior and posterior fornices. Vaginal administration is most effective when the patient can remain lying down afterward to retain the medication.

Equipment

Patient's medication record and chart ♦ prescribed medication and applicator, if necessary ♦ water-soluble lubricant ♦ gloves ♦ small sanitary pad

Key steps

- If possible, plan to insert vaginal medications at bedtime, when the patient is recumbent.
- Verify the order on the patient's medication record by checking it against the prescriber's order.
- Confirm the patient's identity using two patient identifiers according to facility policy.
- If your facility uses a bar code scanning system, be sure to scan your ID badge, the patient's ID bracelet, and the medication's bar code.
- Wash your hands, explain the procedure to the patient, and provide privacy.

- Ask the patient to void.
- Ask the patient if she would rather insert the medication herself. If so, provide appropriate instructions. If not, proceed with the following steps.
- Help her into the lithotomy position.
- Expose only the perineum.

Inserting a suppository

- Remove the suppository from the wrapper, and lubricate it with water-soluble lubricant.
- Put on gloves and expose the vagina.
- With an applicator or the forefinger of your free hand, insert the suppository about 2″ (5 cm) into the vagina. (See *How to insert a vaginal suppository.*)

Inserting ointments, creams, or gels

- Insert the plunger into the applicator. Then attach the applicator to the tube of medication.
- Gently squeeze the tube to fill the applicator with the prescribed amount of medication. Detach the applicator from the tube, and lubricate the applicator.
- Put on gloves and expose the vagina.
- Insert the applicator as you would a small suppository, and administer the medication by depressing the plunger on the applicator.

After vaginal insertion

- Remove and discard your gloves.
- Wash the applicator with soap and warm water and store it, unless it's disposable. If the applicator can be used again, label it so that it will be used only for the same patient.
- To prevent the medication from soiling the patient's clothing and bedding, provide a sanitary pad.
- Help the patient return to a comfortable position, and advise her to remain in bed as much as possible for the next several hours.
- Wash your hands thoroughly.

Special considerations

- Refrigerate vaginal suppositories that melt at room temperature.

How to insert a vaginal suppository

If the suppository is small, place it in the tip of an applicator. Then lubricate the applicator, hold it by the cylinder, and insert it into the vagina. To ensure the patient's comfort, direct the applicator down initially, toward the spine, and then up and back, toward the cervix (as shown below).

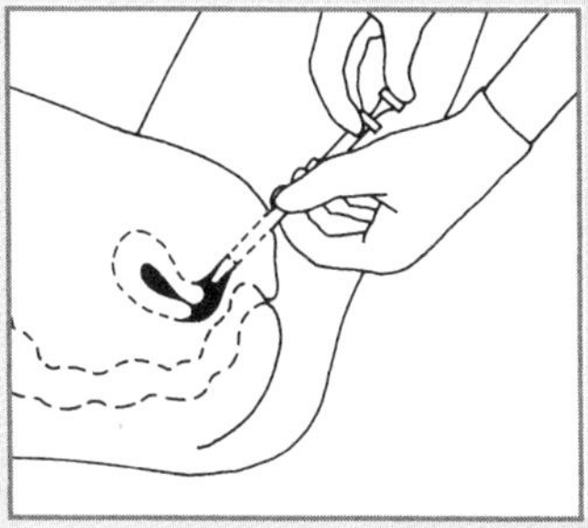

When the suppository reaches the distal end of the vagina, depress the plunger. Remove the applicator while the plunger is still depressed.

Complications

- Local irritation

Patient teaching

- If possible, teach the patient how to insert the vaginal medication because she may have to administer it herself after discharge. Give her a patient-teaching sheet if one is available.
- Instruct the patient not to wear a tampon after inserting vaginal medication because it would absorb the medication and decrease its effectiveness.
- Instruct the patient to avoid sexual intercourse during treatment.

Documentation

Record the medication administered as well as time and date. Note adverse effects and any other pertinent information.

Vascular access port maintenance

Surgically implanted under local anesthesia by a physician, a vascular access device consists of a silicone catheter attached to a reservoir, which is covered with a self-sealing silicone rubber septum. It's most commonly used for patients who require I.V. therapy for at least 6 months. The most common type of vascular access device is a vascular access port (VAP). (See *Understanding VAPs*.)

The VAP reservoir can be made of titanium (as with implanted infusion ports), stainless steel, or molded plastic. The type selected depends on the patient's needs.

Implanted in a pocket under the skin, the attached indwelling catheter tunnels through the subcutaneous tissue into a vein and the catheter is advanced so that the catheter tip lies in a central vein—for example, the subclavian vein. A VAP can also be used for arterial access or be implanted into the epidural space, peritoneum, or pericardial or pleural cavity.

Sterile technique must be maintained when accessing the VAP. Correct needle placement is verified by aspiration of blood and should be done before administering medications or I.V. solutions. The noncoring needle used to access the port should be changed every 7 days. Hemodynamic monitoring and venipuncture shouldn't be performed on the extremity containing the implanted device.

Typically, VAPs deliver intermittent infusions. Most commonly used for chemotherapy, a VAP can also deliver I.V. fluids, medications, and blood. It can also be used to obtain blood samples.

VAPs offer several advantages, which include minimal activity restrictions, few steps for the patient to perform, and few dressing changes (except when used to maintain continuous infusions or intermittent infusion devices). Implanted devices are easier to maintain than external devices. For instance, they require heparinization only once after each use (or periodically if not in use). They also pose less risk of infection because they have no exit site to serve as an entry for microorganisms.

Because VAPs create only a slight protrusion under the skin, many patients find them easier to accept than external infusion devices. Because the device is implanted, however, it may be harder for the patient to manage, particularly if he'll be administering medication or fluids daily or frequently. And because accessing the device requires inserting a needle through subcutaneous tissue, patients who fear or dislike needle punctures may be uncomfortable using a VAP and may require a local anesthetic. In addition, implantation and removal of the device require surgery and hospitalization.

Implanted VAPs are contraindicated in patients who have been unable to tolerate other implanted devices and in those who may develop an allergic reaction.

Equipment

Implanting a VAP

Noncoring needles of appropriate type and gauge (a noncoring needle has a deflected point, which slices the port's septum) ♦ VAP ♦ sterile gloves ♦ mask ♦ 2% chlorhexidine swabs ♦ extension set tubing, if needed ♦ local anesthetic (lidocaine without epinephrine) ♦ ice pack ♦ 10- and 20-ml syringes ♦ normal saline and heparin flush solutions ♦ I.V. solution ♦ sterile dressings ♦ luer-lock injection cap ♦ clamp ♦ adhesive skin closures ♦ suture removal set

Administering a bolus injection

Extension set ♦ 10-ml syringe filled with normal saline solution ♦ clamp ♦ syringe containing the prescribed medication ♦ optional: sterile syringe filled with heparin flush solution

Administering a continuous infusion

Prescribed I.V. solution or drugs ♦ I.V. administration set ♦ filter, if ordered ♦ extension set ♦ clamp ♦ 10-ml syringe filled with normal saline solution ♦ adhesive tape ♦ sterile 2″ × 2″ gauze pad ♦ sterile tape ♦ transparent semipermeable dressing

Some health care facilities use an implantable port access kit.

Preparation

- Confirm the size and type of the device and the insertion site with the physician.
- Attach the tubing to the solution container, prime the tubing with fluid, fill the syringes with saline or heparin flush solution, and prime the noncoring needle and extension set.
- All priming must be done using strict sterile technique, and all tubing must be free from air.
- After you've primed the tubing, recheck all connections for tightness. Make sure that all open ends are covered with sealed caps.

Key steps

- Wash your hands to prevent the spread of microorganisms.

Assisting with implantation of a VAP

- Reinforce to the patient the practitioner's explanation of the procedure, its benefit to the patient, and what's expected of him during and after implantation.
- Although the physician is responsible for obtaining consent for the procedure, make sure that the written document is signed, witnessed, and in the chart.
- Allay the patient's fears and answer questions about movement restrictions, cosmetic concerns, and management regimens.
- Check the patient's history for hypersensitivity to local anesthetics or iodine.
- The surgeon will surgically implant the VAP, probably using a local anesthetic (similar to insertion of a central venous [CV] catheter). Occasionally, a patient may receive a general anesthetic for VAP implantation.
- First, the surgeon makes a small incision and introduces the catheter, typically into the superior vena cava through the subclavian, jugular, or cephalic vein. After fluoroscopy verifies correct placement of the catheter tip, the physician creates a subcutaneous pocket over a bony prominence in the chest wall. Then he tunnels the catheter to the pocket. Next, he connects the catheter to the reservoir, places the reservoir in the pocket, and flushes it with heparin solution. Finally, he sutures the reservoir to the underlying fascia and closes the incision.

Understanding VAPs

Typically, a vascular access port (VAP) is used to deliver intermittent infusions of medication, chemotherapy, and blood products. Because the device is completely covered by the patient's skin, the risk of extrinsic contamination is reduced. Patients may prefer this type of central line because it doesn't alter the body image and requires less routine catheter care.

The VAP consists of a catheter connected to a small reservoir. A septum designed to withstand multiple punctures seals the reservoir.

To access the port, a special noncoring needle is inserted perpendicular to the reservoir.

Top-entry VAP

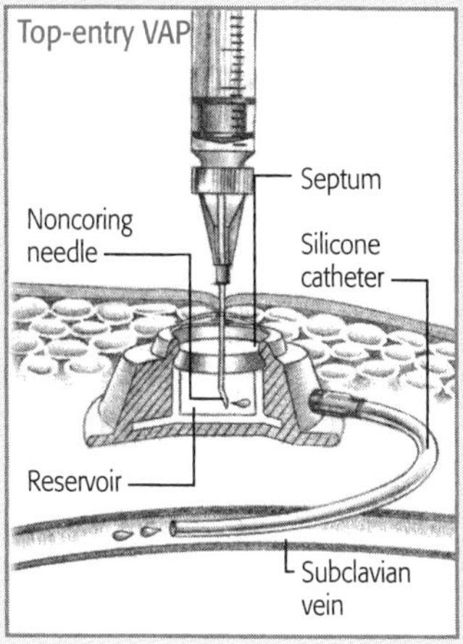

Preparing to access the port

- The VAP can be used immediately after placement, although some edema and tenderness may persist for about 72 hours. This makes the device initially difficult to palpate and slightly uncomfortable for the patient.

- Confirm the patient's identity using two patient identifiers according to facility policy.
- Prepare to access the port, following the specific steps for top-entry ports.
- Using sterile technique, inspect the area around the port for signs of infection or skin breakdown.
- Place an ice pack over the area for several minutes to alleviate possible discomfort from the needle puncture. Alternatively, administer a local anesthetic after cleaning the area.
- Wash your hands thoroughly. Put on sterile gloves and a mask and wear them throughout the procedure.
- Clean the area with an alcohol pad, starting at the center of the port and working outward with a firm, circular motion over a 4″ to 5″ (10 to 12.5 cm) diameter. Repeat this procedure twice. Allow the site to dry, then clean the area with 2% chlorhexidine swabs in the same manner. Repeat this procedure twice.
- If facility policy calls for a local anesthetic, check the patient's record for possible allergies. As indicated, anesthetize the insertion site by injecting 0.1 ml of lidocaine (without epinephrine).
- Palpate the area over the port to find its septum.
- Anchor the port with your nondominant hand. Then, using your dominant hand, aim the needle at the center of the device.
- Insert the needle perpendicular to the port septum. Push the needle through the skin and septum until you reach the bottom of the reservoir.
- Check needle placement by aspirating for blood return.
- If you can't obtain blood, remove the needle and repeat the procedure. Inability to obtain blood may indicate sludge buildup (from medications) in the port reservoir. If so, you may need to use a fibrinolytic agent to free the occlusion. Ask the patient to raise his arms and perform Valsalva's maneuver. If you still don't get a blood return, notify the practitioner; a fibrin sleeve on the distal end of the catheter may be occluding the opening. (See *Managing VAP problems*.)
- Flush the device with normal saline solution. If you detect swelling or if the patient reports pain at the site, remove the needle and notify the practitioner.

Administering a bolus injection

- Attach the 10-ml syringe filled with saline solution to the end of the extension set and remove all the air. Now attach the extension set to the noncoring needle. Check for blood return. Then flush the port with normal saline solution, according to facility policy.
- Clamp the extension set and remove the saline syringe.
- Connect the medication syringe to the extension set. Open the clamp and inject the drug, as ordered.
- Examine the skin surrounding the needle for signs of infiltration, such as swelling or tenderness. If you note these signs, stop the injection and intervene appropriately.
- When the injection is complete, clamp the extension set and remove the medication syringe.
- Open the clamp and flush with 5 ml of normal saline solution after each drug injection to minimize drug incompatibility reactions.
- Flush with heparin solution according to facility policy.

Administering a continuous infusion

- Remove all air from the extension set by priming it with an attached syringe of normal saline solution. Now attach the extension set to the noncoring needle.
- Flush the port system with normal saline solution. Clamp the extension set and remove the syringe.
- Connect the administration set, and secure the connections with sterile tape if necessary.
- Unclamp the extension set and begin the infusion.
- Affix the needle to the skin. Then apply a transparent semipermeable dressing. (See *Continuous infusion: Securing the needle*, page 594.)
- Examine the site carefully for infiltration. If the patient complains of stinging, burn-

Managing VAP problems

This chart outlines common problems with vascular access ports (VAPs) along with possible causes and nursing interventions.

Problems and possible causes	Nursing interventions
Inability to flush the device or draw blood	
Catheter lodged against vessel wall	▪ Reposition patient. ▪ Teach patient to change his position to free catheter from vessel wall. ▪ Raise the arm that's on same side as catheter. ▪ Roll patient to his opposite side. ▪ Have patient cough, sit up, or take a deep breath. ▪ Infuse 10 ml of normal saline solution into catheter. ▪ Regain access to catheter or VAP using a new needle.
Clot formation	▪ Assess patency by trying to flush VAP while patient changes position. ▪ Notify practitioner; obtain an order for fibrinolytic agent instillation. ▪ Teach patient to recognize clot formation, to notify practitioner if it occurs, and to avoid forcibly flushing VAP.
Incorrect needle placement or needle not advanced through septum	▪ Regain access to device. ▪ Teach home care patient to push down firmly on noncoring needle device in septum and to verify needle placement by aspirating for blood return.
Kinked catheter, catheter migration, or port rotation	▪ Notify practitioner immediately. ▪ Tell patient to notify practitioner if he has trouble using VAP.
Kinked tubing or closed clamp	▪ Check tubing or clamp.
Inability to palpate the device	
Deeply implanted port	▪ Note portal chamber scar. ▪ Use deep-palpation technique. ▪ Ask another nurse to try locating VAP. ▪ Use a 1½" or 2" noncoring needle to access VAP.

ing, or pain at the site, discontinue the infusion and intervene appropriately.

▪ When the solution container is empty, obtain a new I.V. solution container, as ordered.

▪ Flush with normal saline solution followed by heparin solution according to facility policy.

Special considerations

▪ After implantation, monitor the site for signs of hematoma and bleeding. Edema and tenderness may persist for up to 72 hours. The incision site requires routine postoperative care for 7 to 10 days. You'll also need to assess the implantation site for signs of infection, device rotation, or skin

Continuous infusion: Securing the needle

When starting a continuous infusion, you must secure the right-angle, noncoring needle to the skin. If the needle hub isn't flush with the skin, place a folded sterile dressing under the hub, as shown. Then apply adhesive skin closures across it.

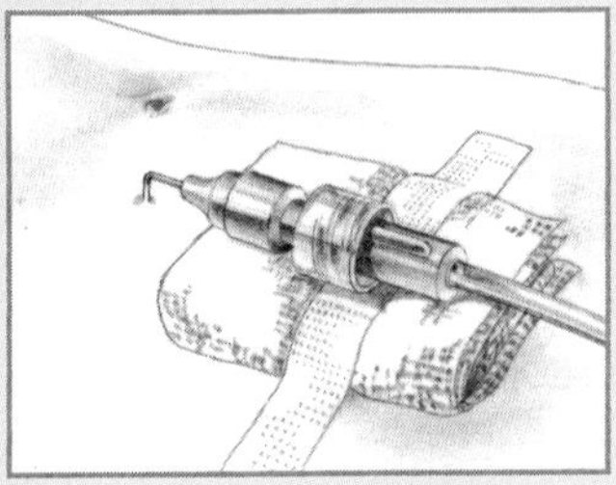

Secure the needle and tubing, using the chevron-taping technique.

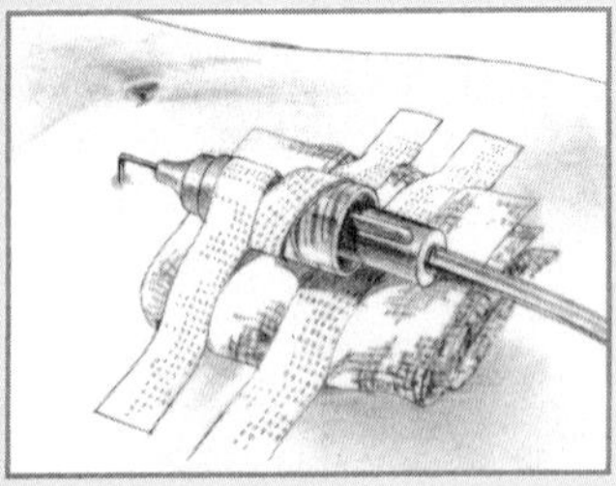

Apply a transparent semipermeable dressing over the entire site.

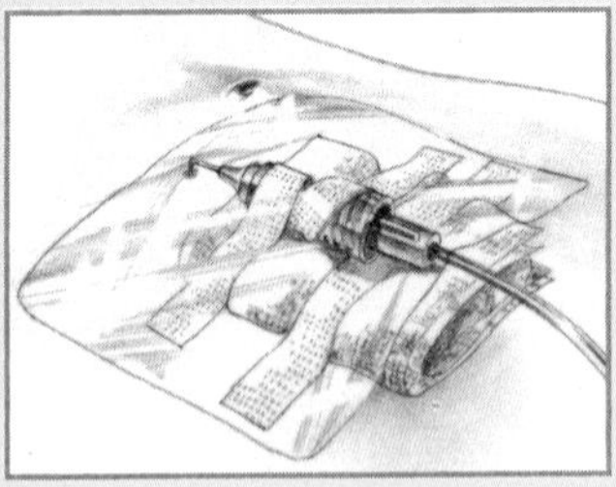

erosion. You don't need to apply a dressing to the wound site except during infusions or to maintain an intermittent infusion device.

- While the patient is hospitalized, a luer-lock injection cap may be attached to the end of the extension set to provide ready access for intermittent infusions. Besides saving nursing time, a luer-lock cap reduces the discomfort of accessing the port and prolongs the life of the port septum by decreasing the number of needle punctures.
- If the patient is receiving a continuous or prolonged infusion, change the dressing and needle every 7 days. You'll also need to change the tubing and solution, as you would for a long-term CV infusion. If the patient is receiving an intermittent infusion, flush the port periodically with heparin solution. When the VAP isn't being used, flush it every 4 weeks. During the course of therapy, you may have to clear a clotted VAP, as ordered.
- If clotting threatens to occlude the VAP, the practitioner may order a fibrinolytic agent to clear the catheter. Because such agents increase the risk of bleeding, fibrinolytic agents may be contraindicated in patients who have had surgery within the past 10 days; in those who have active internal bleeding such as GI bleeding; and in those who have experienced central nervous system damage, such as infarction, hemorrhage, traumatic injury, surgery, or primary or metastatic disease, within the past 2 months.
- Besides performing routine care measures, you must be prepared to handle several common problems that may arise during an infusion with a VAP. These common problems include an inability to flush the VAP, withdraw blood from it, or palpate it.

Complications

- Similar risks to those associated with CV catheters: infection, thrombus formation, and occlusion (see *Risks of VAP therapy*)

Patient teaching

- If the patient will be accessing the port himself, explain that the most uncomfortable part of the procedure is the actual insertion of the needle into the skin.
- Stress the importance of pushing the needle into the port until the patient feels the needle bevel touch the back of the port. Many patients tend to stop short of

Risks of VAP therapy

This chart shows possible complications of vascular access port (VAP) therapy and outlines signs and symptoms, possible causes, and nursing interventions.

Complication	Signs and symptoms	Possible causes	Nursing interventions
Extravasation	▪ Burning sensation or swelling in subcutaneous tissue	▪ Needle dislodged into subcutaneous tissue ▪ Needle incorrectly placed in VAP ▪ Needle position notconfirmed; needle pulled out of septum ▪ Rupture of catheter along tunnel route	▪ Stop infusion, but don't remove needle. ▪ Notify practitioner; prepare to administer an antidote, if ordered. **Prevention** ▪ Teach patient how to gain access to device, verify its placement, and secure needle before initiating an infusion.
Fibrin sheath formation	▪ Blocked port and catheter lumen ▪ Inability to flush port or administer infusion ▪ Possible swelling, tenderness, and erythema in neck, chest, and shoulder	▪ Adherence of platelets to catheter	▪ Notify practitioner; prepare to administer a thrombolytic agent. **Prevention** ▪ Use port only to infuse fluids and medications; don't use it to obtain blood samples. ▪ Administer only compatible substances through port.
Site infection or skin breakdown	▪ Erythema and warmth at port site ▪ Oozing or purulent drainage at VAP site or pocket ▪ Fever	▪ Infected incision or VAP pocket ▪ Poor postoperative healing	▪ Assess site daily for redness; note drainage. ▪ Notify practitioner. ▪ Administer antibiotics, as prescribed. ▪ Apply warm soaks for 20 minutes four times per day. **Prevention** ▪ Teach patient to inspect for and report redness, swelling, drainage, or skin breakdown at port site.
Thrombosis	▪ Inability to flush port or administer infusion	▪ Frequent blood sampling ▪ Infusion of packed red blood cells (RBCs)	▪ Notify practitioner; obtain an order to administer a fibrinolytic agent. **Prevention** ▪ Flush VAP thoroughly right after obtaining a blood sample. ▪ Administer packed RBCs as a piggyback with normal saline solution and use an infusion pump; flush with normal saline solution between units.

the back of the port, leaving the needle bevel in the rubber septum.

- Stress the importance of monthly flushes when no more infusions are scheduled. If possible, instruct a family member in all aspects of care.

Documentation

Record your assessment findings and interventions according to facility policy. Include the type, amount, rate, and duration of the infusion; appearance of the site; and adverse reactions and nursing interventions.

Also keep a record of all needle and dressing changes for continuous infusions; blood samples obtained, including the type and amount; and patient teaching topics covered. Finally, document the removal of the infusion needle, the status of the site, the use of the heparin flush, and any problems you found and resolved.

Venipuncture

Venipuncture is the primary method for acquiring blood samples for laboratory testing and involves inserting a hollow-bore needle into the lumen of a large vein to obtain a sample.

Typically, venipuncture is performed at the antecubital fossa. If necessary, however, it can be performed on a vein in the wrist, the dorsum of the hand or foot, or another accessible location. Although laboratory personnel usually perform this procedure in the hospital setting, nurses may also perform it.

Before attempting venipuncture, the nurse should inform the patient of the need for venipuncture and its possible risks and assess the patient's understanding of the procedure. This will reduce the patient's anxiety and promote cooperation during venipuncture.

Every upper-extremity venipuncture carries the risk of inadvertently puncturing or nicking a nerve. To avoid this complication, the Infusion Nurses Society recommends limiting the number of attempts of venipuncture on a patient. After two unsuccessful tries, the nurse should either ask another colleague to try or consult the I.V. team, nurse-anesthetist, or anesthesiologist.

For most adults, the hand is the common site for I.V. access. Using the patient's hand—preferably the nondominant one—leaves more proximal sites available for subsequent venipunctures. The nurse should avoid using the hands with elderly patients, who have lost subcutaneous tissue surrounding the veins; they're at increased risk for hematoma.

The nurse should also determine if special conditions exist before venipuncture. It's important that the patient be assessed for possible risks of venipuncture, such as anticoagulant therapy, low platelet count, bleeding disorders, and other abnormalities that increase the risk of bleeding and hematoma formation.

When selecting a catheter, the nurse should consider the patient's condition and the type of solution to be infused over the next 48 to 72 hours. Using the smallest-gauge catheter in the largest vein possible diminishes chemical and mechanical irritation to the vein wall.

Equipment

Tourniquet ♦ gloves ♦ syringe or evacuated tubes and needle holder ♦ alcohol or chlorhexidine pads ♦ 20G or 21G needle for the forearm or 25G needle for the wrist, hand, and ankle and for children ♦ color-coded collection tubes containing appropriate additives ♦ labels ♦ laboratory request form ♦ 2″ × 2″ gauze pads ♦ adhesive bandage (see *Guide to color-top collection tubes*)

Preparation

- If you're using evacuated tubes, open the needle packet, attach the needle to its holder, and select the appropriate tubes. If you're using a syringe, attach the appropriate needle to it. Be sure to choose a syringe large enough to hold all the blood required for the test.
- Label all collection tubes clearly with the patient's name and room number, the practitioner's name, and the date and time of collection.

Guide to color-top collection tubes

Tube color	Draw volume	Additive	Purpose
Red	2 to 20 ml	None	Serum studies
Lavender	2 to 10 ml	EDTA	Whole-blood studies
Green	2 to 15 ml	Heparin (sodium, lithium, or ammonium)	Plasma studies
Blue	2.7 or 4.5 ml	Sodium citrate and citric acid	Coagulation studies on plasma
Black	2.7 or 4.5 ml	Sodium oxalate	Coagulation studies on plasma
Gray	3 to 10 ml	Glycolytic inhibitor, such as sodium fluoride, powdered oxalate, or glycolytic-microbial inhibitor	Glucose determinations on serum or plasma
Yellow	12 ml	Acid-citrate-dextrose	Whole-blood studies

Key steps

- Wash your hands thoroughly and put on gloves.
- Confirm the patient's identity using two patient identifiers according to facility policy.
- Tell the patient that you're about to take a blood sample, and explain the procedure to ease his anxiety and ensure his cooperation. Ask him if he has ever felt faint, sweaty, or nauseated when having blood drawn. If the patient is a child, try using distraction with a toy or game to reduce anxiety.
- If the patient is on bed rest, ask him to lie supine, with his head slightly elevated and his arms at his sides. Ask the ambulatory patient to sit in a chair and support his arm securely on an armrest or table.
- Assess the patient's veins to determine the best puncture site. (See *Common venipuncture sites*, page 598.)
- Observe the patient's skin for the vein's blue color, or palpate the vein for a firm rebound sensation.
- Tie a tourniquet 2″ (5 cm) proximal to the area chosen. By impeding venous return to the heart while still allowing arterial flow, a tourniquet produces venous dilation. If arterial perfusion remains adequate, you'll be able to feel the radial pulse. (If the tourniquet fails to dilate the vein, have the patient open and close his fist repeatedly. Then ask him to close his fist as you insert the needle and to open it again when the needle is in place.)
- Clean the venipuncture site with an alcohol or chlorhexidine pad. Wipe in a circular motion, spiraling outward from the site to avoid introducing potentially infectious skin flora into the vessel during the procedure. If you use alcohol, apply it with friction for 30 seconds, or until the final pad comes away clean. Allow the skin to dry before performing venipuncture.
- Immobilize the vein by pressing just below the venipuncture site with your thumb and drawing the skin taut.
- Position the needle holder or syringe with the needle bevel up and the shaft parallel to the path of the vein and at a 30-degree angle to the arm. Insert the needle into the vein. If you're using a syringe, venous blood will appear in the hub; with-

Common venipuncture sites

These illustrations show the anatomic locations of veins commonly used for venipuncture. The most commonly used sites are on the forearm, followed by those on the hand.

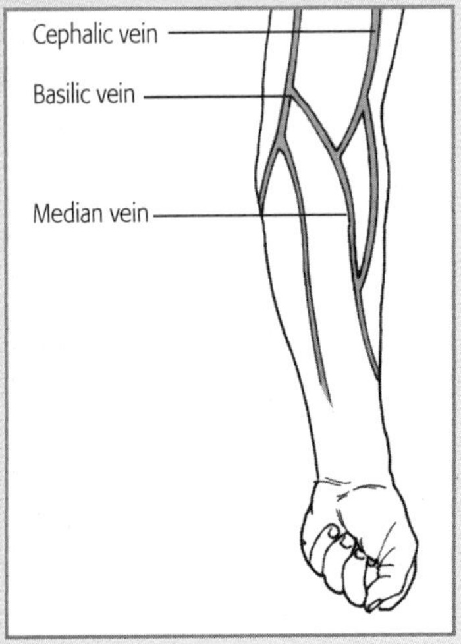

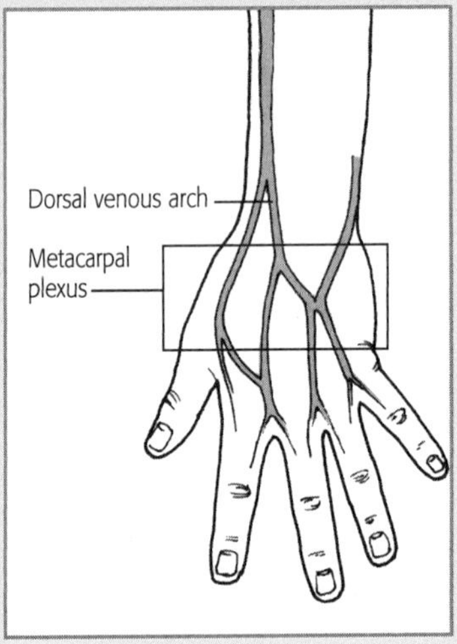

draw the blood slowly, pulling the plunger of the syringe gently to create steady suction until you obtain the required sample. Pulling the plunger too forcibly may collapse the vein. If you're using a needle holder and an evacuated tube, grasp the holder securely to stabilize it in the vein, and push down on the collection tube until the needle punctures the rubber stopper. Blood will flow into the tube automatically.

- Remove the tourniquet as soon as blood flows adequately to prevent stasis and hemoconcentration, which can impair test results. If the flow is sluggish, leave the tourniquet in place longer, but always remove it before withdrawing the needle.
- Continue to fill the required tubes, removing one and inserting another. Gently rotate each tube as you remove it to help mix the additive with the sample.
- After you've drawn the sample, place a gauze pad over the puncture site, and slowly and gently remove the needle from the vein. When using an evacuated tube, remove it from the needle holder to release the vacuum before withdrawing the needle from the vein.
- Apply gentle pressure to the puncture site for 2 or 3 minutes or until bleeding stops. This prevents extravasation into the surrounding tissue, which can cause a hematoma.
- After bleeding stops, apply an adhesive bandage.
- If you've used a syringe, transfer the sample to a collection tube. Detach the needle from the syringe, open the collection tube, and gently empty the sample into the tube, being careful to avoid foaming, which can cause hemolysis.
- Finally, check the venipuncture site to see if a hematoma has developed. If it has, apply pressure to the site.
- Discard syringes, needles, and used gloves in the appropriate containers.

Special considerations

- Never draw a venous sample from an arm or leg that's already being used for I.V. therapy or blood administration because this may affect test results; I.V. fluids may dilute blood.

- Don't collect a venous sample from an infection site because this may introduce pathogens into the vascular system. Similarly, avoid drawing blood from edematous areas or sites of previous hematoma or vascular injury because the vessel wall may be damaged.

DO'S & DON'TS

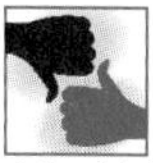

Don't use an arm on the side of a mastectomy because reduced lymphatic drainage increases the risk of infection at the site.

- Never use an arm with an arteriovenous fistula because of the increased risk of clotting and bleeding.
- If the patient has large, distended, highly visible veins, perform venipuncture without a tourniquet to minimize the risk of hematoma formation. If the patient has a clotting disorder or is receiving anticoagulant therapy, maintain firm pressure on the venipuncture site for at least 5 minutes after withdrawing the needle to prevent hematoma formation.
- Avoid using veins in the patient's legs for venipuncture, if possible, because this increases the risk of thrombophlebitis.
- If a large-bore catheter is necessary, consider using a topical or subcutaneous anesthetic agent to reduce pain.

Complications

- Hematoma at the needle insertion
- Infection resulting from poor technique

Documentation

Record the date, time, and site of venipuncture; name of the test; the time the sample was sent to the laboratory; the amount of blood collected; the patient's temperature; and any adverse reactions to the procedure.

Ventricular assist device

A temporary life-sustaining treatment for a failing heart, the ventricular assist device (VAD) diverts systemic blood flow from a diseased ventricle into a centrifugal pump. It temporarily reduces ventricular work, allowing the myocardium to rest and contractility to improve. Although used most commonly to assist the left ventricle, this device may also assist the right ventricle or both ventricles. (See *VAD: Help for the failing heart,* page 600.)

Candidates for VAD include patients with massive myocardial infarction, irreversible cardiomyopathy, acute myocarditis, an inability to be weaned from cardiopulmonary bypass, valvular disease, or bacterial endocarditis, and those who have experienced a heart transplant rejection. The device may also be used in those awaiting a heart transplant.

Equipment

The VAD is inserted in the operating room.

Key steps

- Before surgery, explain to the patient that food and fluid intake must be restricted and that you will continuously monitor his cardiac function (using an electrocardiogram, a pulmonary artery catheter, and an arterial line). Offer the patient reassurance. Before sending him to the operating room, make sure he has signed a consent form.
- If time permits, scrub the patient's chest with an antiseptic solution.
- When the patient returns from surgery, administer analgesics as ordered.
- Frequently monitor vital signs and intake and output.
- Keep VAD exit sites immobile. The patient should be encourage to rehabilitate as soon as clinically stable.
- Monitor pulmonary artery pressures. If you've been prepared to adjust the pump, maintain cardiac output at 5 to 8 L/minute, central venous pressure at 8 to 16 mm Hg, pulmonary capillary wedge pressure at 10 to 20 mm Hg, mean arterial pressure at more than 60 mm Hg, and left atrial pressure between 4 and 12 mm Hg.
- Assess the patient who has a left VAD for signs and symptoms of right-sided heart failure.
- Monitor the patient for signs and symptoms of poor perfusion and ineffective pumping, including arrhythmias, hypotension, slow capillary refill, cool skin, olig-

VAD: Help for the failing heart

The ventricular assist device (VAD) functions somewhat like an artificial heart. The major difference is that the VAD assists the heart, whereas the artificial heart replaces it. The VAD is designed to aid one or both ventricles. The pumping chambers themselves may be implanted in the patient or may be external, depending on the VAD system.

A VAD with an implanted pump receives power through the skin either through a percutaneous lead or through a belt of electrical transformer coils (worn externally as a portable battery pack). It can also operate off an implanted, rechargeable battery for up to 1 hour at a time, depending on the VAD system.

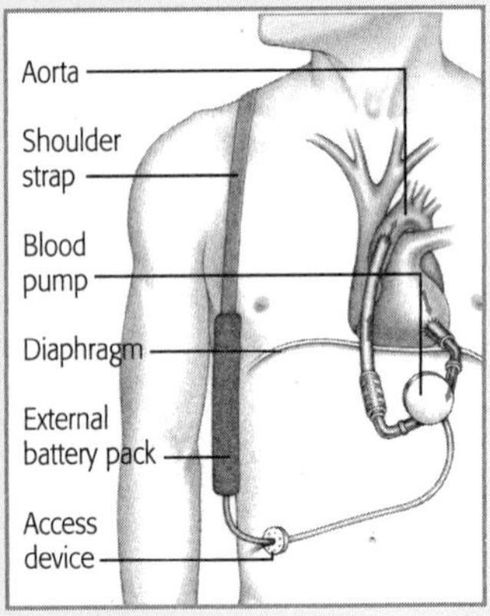

uria or anuria, confusion, anxiety, and restlessness.

- Administer heparin, as ordered, to prevent clotting in the pump head and thrombus formation. Check for bleeding, especially at the operative sites. Monitor laboratory studies, as ordered, especially complete blood count and coagulation studies.
- Assess the patient's incisions and the cannula insertion sites for signs of infection. Monitor the white blood cell count and differential daily, and take rectal or core temperature every 4 hours. Maintain stability of all device exit sites to promote tissue healing and decrease the risk of infection.
- Change the dressing over the cannula sites daily or according to facility policy.
- Provide supportive care, including range-of-motion exercises and mouth and skin care.
- If VAD support is to be maintained for a prolonged period, follow your facility's protocol for assessments, dressing, and patient mobility as the patient's condition progresses.

Special considerations

- If ventricular function fails to improve within a few days, the patient may need a transplant. If so, provide psychological support for the patient and his family. You may also be asked to initiate the transplant process by contacting the appropriate agency.
- The left ventricular assist device has also been approved as a permanent therapy for patients with end-stage heart failure who are ineligible for heart transplantation. This device helps prolong the life of select patients.
- The psychological effects of the VAD can produce stress in the patient, his family, and his close friends. If appropriate, refer them to other support personnel.

Complications

- Damaged blood cells thereby increasing the likelihood of thrombus formation and subsequent pulmonary embolism or stroke
- Infection and device failure

Documentation

Note the patient's condition following insertion of the VAD. Document any pump adjustments as well as any complications and interventions.

Violent and assaultive patient management

To manage violent and assaultive behavior in patients, the nursing staff must use the least amount of force possible to bring the situation under control. The key to managing this type of situation is encouraging the patient to talk about his feelings rather than acting them out. It's important to treat the patient with respect and dignity during this stressful situation.

Equipment

No specific equipment needed

Key steps

- Talk with the patient to ascertain what's upsetting him. Assess his behavioral controls and ability to cooperate. Speak in a calm, reassuring—but firm—manner.
- Encourage the patient to vent his hostility verbally. Divert his attention or help him to redirect his energy to appropriate activities or exercise.
- Provide a private, nonstimulating environment in which the patient can relax or talk.
- Be honest with the patient, answer his questions truthfully, and don't provide false promises.
- Define his limits in a firm but nonthreatening manner.
- Allow the patient to lie down in a quiet room. You may remain with the patient or observe him frequently.
- Assess the need for medication or chemical restraint and notify the physician. The physician is responsible for ensuring that an acutely disturbed patient receives appropriate medication and amounts to prevent as much violent behavior as possible.
- Give the medication as needed before using seclusion or physical restraints. Oral liquid medication is preferred over tablets, capsules, or the I.M. route.
- If all efforts fail to assist the patient in regaining or maintaining self-control, use seclusion or physical restraints.
- Obtain a practitioner's order for seclusion or restraints and plan the strategy for approach and application away from the patient. It's challenging to the patient, not reassuring, if he perceives that there will be a struggle to control his behavior.
- Make sure you have enough staff available to help but have them remain on the periphery and assist only as directed in a show of force. Tell the patient quietly and calmly what you're going to do and keep repeating it as you approach him.
- Use firm but humane physical holds to place the patient in seclusion or restraints.
- If the patient responds inappropriately to seclusion by becoming harmful to himself, remove him from seclusion and place him in restraints and a private room. When a patient is in physical restraints, give a chemical restraint to reduce the amount of time spent in physical restraints.
- Obtain a practitioner's order within 1 hour of initiation of restraint or seclusion. Verbal orders must be cosigned within 8 hours of initiation. Each order must state a time limit and can't exceed 4 hours for an adult. A registered nurse may continue this order for two 4-hour periods, according to the practitioner's order, if reassessment by the registered nurse indicates continued need. After a maximum of 12 hours, the practitioner must conduct a face-to-face-assessment of the patient and write a new order and progress note.
- Review the incident with the patient after control is achieved.
- If the problem can't be solved using the actions described, contact your local police department.

Special considerations

- Make every effort to calm the patient using the following techniques before the use of restraint or seclusion:
  - –Treat the patient with dignity and respect.
  - –Convey a willingness to understand the patient and show concern for his welfare.
  - –Keep communications simple, concise, and clear.
  - –Strive to establish trust. Don't threaten the patient.
  - –Avoid power struggles. Don't argue with the patient.
  - –Convey the expectation that if he doesn't maintain self-control, you'll take measures to prevent him from harming himself or others.
  - –Allow the patient time to express his feelings and deal with his frustrations.
  - –Define clear limits with the patient.

- Quietly clear the area of other patients and any objects that could be used to inflict harm.
- Continue to assess the patient's level of behavioral controls and his ability to cooperate.

Complications
- None known

Documentation
Document as soon as possible and be specific. Document all interventions and the patient's response to these interventions.

Volume-control set
A volume-control set—an I.V. line with a graduated chamber—delivers precise amounts of fluid and shuts off when the fluid is exhausted, preventing air from entering the I.V. line. It may be used as a secondary line in adults for intermittent infusion of medication.

A volume-control set is used as a primary line in children for continuous infusion of fluids or medication.

Equipment
Volume-control set ♦ I.V. pole (for setting up a primary I.V. line) ♦ I.V. solution ♦ 20G to 22G 1" needle or needle-free adapter ♦ alcohol pads ♦ medication in labeled syringe ♦ tape ♦ label

Although various models of volume-control sets are available, each one consists of a graduated fluid chamber (120 to 250 ml) with a spike and a filtered air line on top and administration tubing underneath. Floating-valve sets have a valve at the bottom that closes when the chamber empties; membrane-filter sets have a rigid filter at the bottom that, when wet, prevents the passage of air.

Preparation
- Ensure the sterility of all equipment and inspect it carefully to ensure the absence of flaws.
- Take the equipment to the patient's bedside.

Key steps
- Wash your hands, and explain the procedure to the patient. If an I.V. line is already in place, observe its insertion site for signs of infiltration and infection.
- Remove the volume-control set from its box, and close all the clamps.
- Remove the protective cap from the volume-control set spike, insert the spike into the I.V. solution container, and hang the container on the I.V. pole.
- Open the air vent clamp and close the upper slide clamp. Then open the lower clamp on the I.V. tubing, slide it upward until it's slightly below the drip chamber, and close the clamp (as shown below).

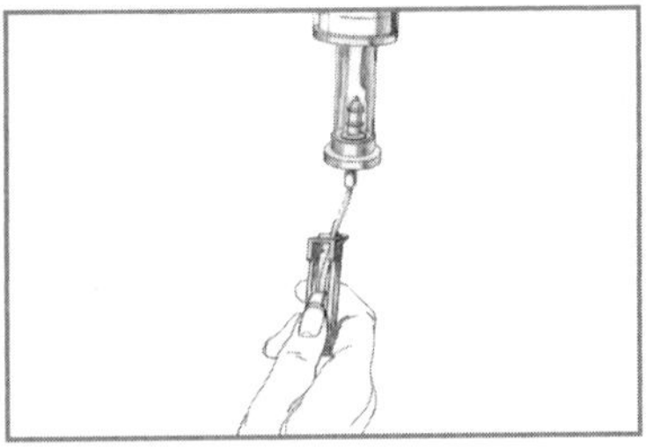

- If you're using a valve set, open the upper clamp until the fluid chamber fills with about 30 ml of solution. Then close the clamp and carefully squeeze the drip chamber until it's half full.
- If you're using a volume-control set with a membrane filter, open the upper clamp until the fluid chamber fills with about 30 ml of solution, and then close the clamp.
- Open the lower clamp and squeeze the drip chamber flat with two fingers of your opposite hand (as shown below). If you squeeze the drip chamber with the lower clamp closed, you'll damage the membrane filter.

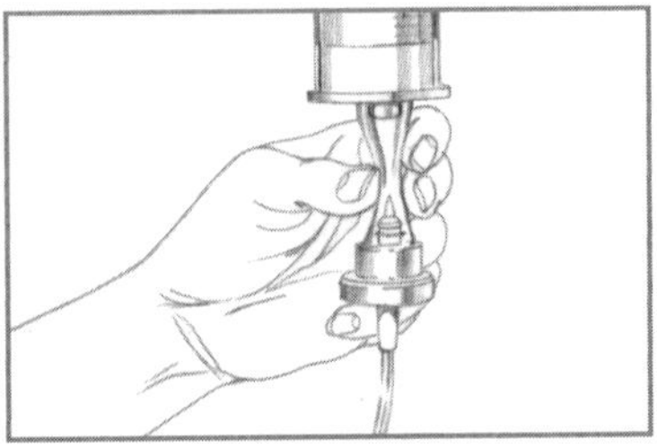

- Keeping the drip chamber flat, close the lower clamp. Now release the drip chamber so that it fills halfway.
- Open the lower clamp, prime the tubing, and close the clamp. To use the set as a primary line, insert the distal end of the tubing into the catheter or needle hub. To use the set as a secondary line, attach a needle to the adapter on the volume-control set. Wipe the Y-port of the primary tubing with an alcohol pad, and insert the needle. Then tape the connection.
- If you're using a needle-free system, attach the distal end of the tubing to the Y-port of the primary tubing, following the manufacturer's instructions.
- To add medication, wipe the injection port on the volume-control set with an alcohol pad, and inject the medication. Place a label on the chamber, indicating the drug, dose, and date. Don't write directly on the chamber because the plastic absorbs ink.

ALERT

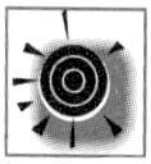

Inadequate drug mixing can result in adverse effects. To avoid complications, never add medications to a hanging I.V. solution.

- Open the upper clamp, fill the fluid chamber with the prescribed amount of solution, and close the clamp. Gently rotate the chamber (as shown below) to mix the medication.

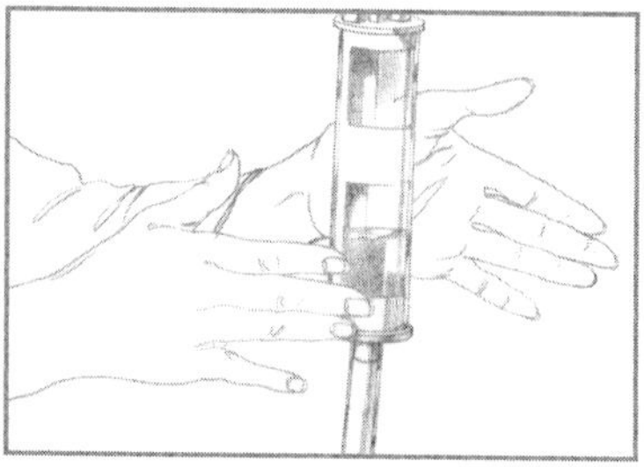

- Turn off the primary solution (if present) or lower the drip rate to maintain an open line.
- Open the lower clamp on the volume-control set, and adjust the drip rate as ordered. After completion of the infusion, open the upper clamp and let 10 ml of I.V. solution flow into the chamber and through the tubing to flush them.
- If you're using the volume-control set as a secondary I.V. line, close the lower clamp and reset the flow rate of the primary line. If you're using the set as a primary I.V. line, close the lower clamp, refill the chamber to the prescribed amount, and begin the infusion again.

Special considerations

- Always check compatibility of the medication and the I.V. solution. If you're using a membrane-filter set, avoid administering suspensions, lipid emulsions, blood, or blood components through it.
- If you're using a floating-valve set, the diaphragm may stick after repeated use. If it does, close the air vent and upper clamp, invert the drip chamber, and squeeze it. If the diaphragm opens, reopen the clamp and continue to use the set.
- If the drip chamber of a floating-valve diaphragm set overfills, immediately close the upper clamp and air vent, invert the chamber, and squeeze the excess fluid from the drip chamber back into the graduated fluid chamber.

Complications

- None known

Documentation

If you add a drug to the volume-control set, record the amount and type of medication, amount of fluid used to dilute it, and date and time of infusion.

W
XY

Walker use

Walkers are used for patients who don't have sufficient strength and balance to use crutches or a cane. A walker provides the maximum support for the patient; however, use of a walker requires a slow gait.

A walker consists of a metal frame with handgrips and four legs that buttresses the patient on three sides. Attachments for standard walkers and modified walkers help meet special needs. For example, a walker may have a platform added to support an injured arm.

Before a patient starts using a walker, the correct height must be determined. To check for the correct height, have the patient stand inside the walker frame with arms at his sides. The walker handles should be at wrist level so that the patient's elbows are flexed 15 to 30 degrees when holding the walker. (See *Teaching safe use of a walker*.)

Equipment

Walker ♦ platform or wheel attachments, as necessary

Various types of walkers are available. The standard walker is used by the patient with unilateral or bilateral weakness or an inability to bear weight on one leg. It requires arm strength and balance. Platform attachments may be added to a standard walker for the patient with arthritic arms or a casted arm, who can't bear weight directly on his hand, wrist, or forearm. With the practitioner's approval, wheels may be placed on the front legs of the standard walker to allow the extremely weak or poorly coordinated patient to roll the device forward, instead of lifting it. However, wheels are applied infrequently because they may be a safety hazard. Four-wheeled walkers are used by patients who require a larger base of support but don't rely on it to bear weight. They are used for patients who walk long distances and are at higher functioning.

The stair walker—used by the patient who must negotiate stairs without bilateral handrails—requires good arm strength and balance. Its extra set of handles extends toward the patient on the open side. The rolling walker—used by the patient with very weak legs—has four wheels and a seat. The reciprocal walker—used by the patient with very weak arms—allows one side to be advanced ahead of the other.

Preparation

- Obtain the appropriate walker with the advice of a physical therapist, and adjust it to the patient's height: His elbows should be flexed at a 15- to 30-degree angle when standing comfortably within the walker with his hands on the grips.
- To adjust the walker, turn it upside down, and change the leg length by pushing in the button on each shaft and releasing it when the leg is in the correct position.
- Make sure that the walker is level before the patient attempts to use it.

Key steps

- Confirm the patient's identity using two patient identifiers according to facility policy.

Teaching safe use of a walker

Sitting down

- First, tell the patient to stand with the back of his stronger leg against the front of the chair, his weaker leg slightly off the floor, and the walker directly in front.
- Tell him to grasp the armrests on the chair one arm at a time while supporting most of his weight on the stronger leg. (In the illustrations below, the patient has left leg weakness.)
- Tell the patient to lower himself into the chair and slide backward. After he's seated, he should place the walker beside the chair.

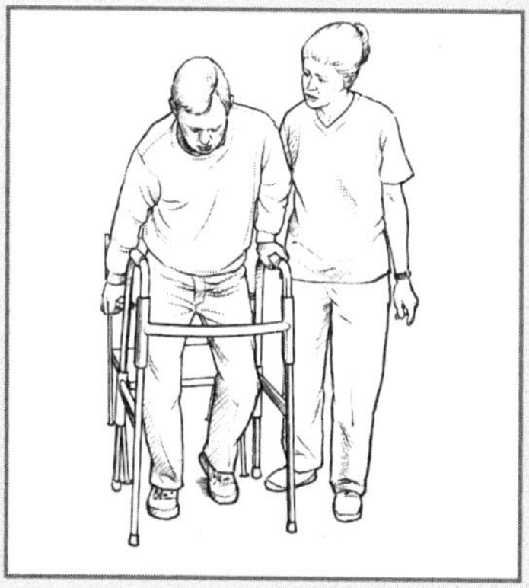

Getting up

- After bringing the walker to the front of his chair, tell the patient to slide forward in the chair. Placing the back of his stronger leg against the seat, he should then advance the weaker leg.
- Next, with both hands on the armrests, the patient can push himself to a standing position. Supporting himself with the stronger leg and the opposite hand, the patient should grasp the walker's handgrip with his free hand.
- Then have the patient grasp the free handgrip with his other hand.

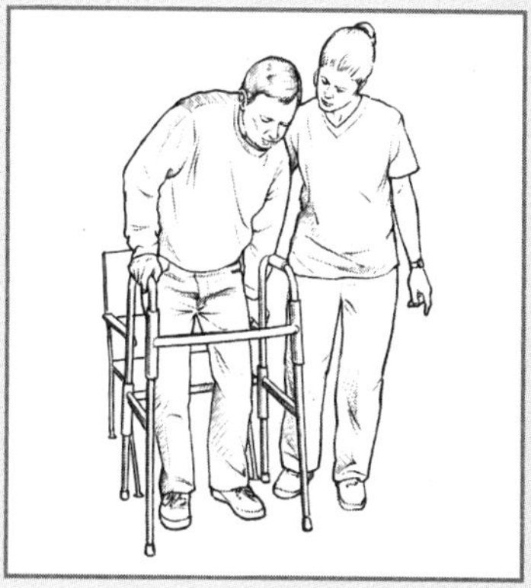

- Help the patient stand within the walker, and instruct him to hold the handgrips firmly and equally. Stand behind him, closer to the involved leg.
- If the patient has one-sided leg weakness, tell him to advance the walker 6″ to 8″ (15 to 20 cm) and to step forward with the involved leg and follow with the uninvolved leg, supporting himself on his arms. Encourage him to take equal strides. If he has equal strength in both legs, instruct him to advance the walker 6″ to 8″ and to step forward with either leg. If he can't use one leg, tell him to advance the walker 6″ to 8″ and to swing onto it, supporting his weight on his arms.
- If the patient is using a wheeled or stair walker, reinforce the physical therapist's instructions. Stress the need for caution when using a stair walker.

Special considerations

- If the patient starts to fall, support his hips and shoulders to help maintain an upright position if possible.

Complications

- None known

Patient teaching

- If the patient is using a reciprocal walker, teach him the two-point gait. Instruct the patient to stand with his weight evenly distributed between his legs and the walker. Stand behind him, slightly to one side. Tell him to simultaneously advance the walker's right side and his left foot. Have the patient advance the walker's left side and his right foot.

- If the patient is using a reciprocal walker, you may also teach him the four-point gait. Instruct the patient to evenly distribute his weight between his legs and the walker. Stand behind him and slightly to one side. Have him move the right side of the walker forward. Have the patient move his left foot forward. Next, instruct him to move the left side of the walker forward. Have him move his right foot forward.
- Teach the patient how to lower himself into a chair safely.

Documentation

Record the type of walker and attachments used, patient teaching, the degree of guarding required, the distance walked, and the patient's tolerance of ambulation.

Wound dehiscence and evisceration

Surgical wounds usually heal well; however, edges of a wound may fail to join or may separate even after they seem to be healing normally. This separation may lead to more serious complications of evisceration, in which a portion of the viscera (usually a bowel loop) protrudes through the incision. Evisceration can lead to peritonitis and septic shock.

Dehiscence and evisceration are most likely to occur 6 or 7 days after surgery, when sutures may have been removed and the patient can cough easily and breathe deeply—which strain the incision. (See *Recognizing dehiscence and evisceration*.)

Conditions are caused by:

- poor nutrition (from inadequate intake or condition such as diabetes mellitus)
- chronic pulmonary or cardiac disease and metastatic cancer because the injured tissue doesn't get needed nutrients and oxygen
- localized wound infection may limit closure, delay healing, and weaken the incision
- stress on the incision from coughing or vomiting may cause abdominal distention or severe stretching. (A midline abdominal incision, for instance, poses a high risk of wound dehiscence.)

Equipment

Two sterile towels ♦ 1 L of sterile normal saline solution ♦ sterile irrigation set, including a basin, a solution container, and a 50-ml catheter-tip syringe ♦ several large abdominal dressings ♦ sterile, waterproof drape ♦ linen-saver pads ♦ sterile gloves

Returning to the operating room

All previous equipment ♦ I.V. administration set and I.V. fluids ♦ equipment for nasogastric (NG) intubation ♦ sedative, as ordered ♦ suction apparatus

Key steps

- Provide reassurance and support to ease the patient's anxiety.
- Tell him to stay in bed. If possible, stay with him while someone else notifies the practitioner and collects necessary equipment.
- Place a linen-saver pad under him to keep sheets dry when you moisten the exposed viscera.
- Using sterile technique, unfold a sterile towel to create a sterile field.
- Open the package containing the irrigation set, and place the basin, solution container, and 50-ml syringe on the sterile field.
- Open the bottle of normal saline solution and pour about 400 ml into the solution container. Also pour about 200 ml into the sterile basin.
- Open several large abdominal dressings and place them on the sterile field.
- Put on the sterile gloves and place one or two of the large abdominal dressings into the basin to saturate them with normal saline solution.
- Place the moistened dressings over the exposed viscera; place a sterile, waterproof drape over the dressings to prevent the sheets from getting wet.
- Moisten the dressings every hour by drawing normal saline solution into a syringe and squirting solution on the dressings.

Recognizing dehiscence and evisceration

In wound dehiscence, the layers of the surgical wound separate. With evisceration, the viscera (in this case, a bowel loop) protrude through the surgical incision.

Wound dehiscence

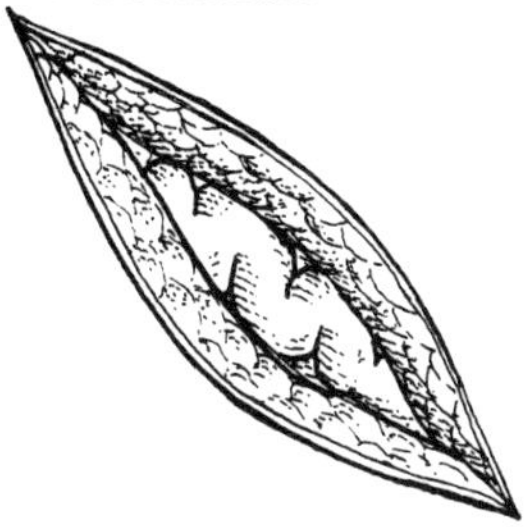

Evisceration of bowel loop

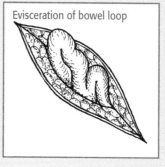

■ When you moisten the dressings, inspect the color of the viscera.

ACTION STAT!

If the viscera appears dusky or black, notify the practitioner immediately. With its blood supply interrupted, a protruding organ may become ischemic and necrotic.

■ Keep the patient on absolute bed rest in low Fowler's position (no more than 20 degrees' elevation) with his knees flexed to prevent injury and reduce stress on an abdominal incision.

DO'S & DON'TS

Don't allow the patient to eat or drink anything by mouth, to decrease the risk of aspiration during surgery.

■ Monitor the patient's pulse, respirations, blood pressure, and temperature every 15 minutes to detect shock.
■ If necessary, prepare him to return to the operating room. After gathering the appropriate equipment, start an I.V. infusion, as ordered.
■ Insert an NG tube and connect it to continuous or intermittent low suction, as ordered.
■ Give preoperative drugs to the patient as ordered.
■ Depending on circumstances, some of these procedures may not be done at the bedside.
■ NG intubation may make the patient gag or vomit, causing further evisceration; the practitioner may choose to have the NG tube inserted in the operating room with the patient under anesthesia.
■ Continue to reassure the patient while you prepare him for surgery.
■ Make sure the patient signed a consent form and the operating room staff has been informed about the procedure.

Special considerations

■ If you're caring for a postoperative patient who's at risk for poor healing, make sure he gets an adequate supply of protein, vitamins, and calories. Monitor his dietary deficiencies; discuss problems with the practitioner and dietitian.
■ When changing wound dressings, always use sterile technique.
■ Inspect the incision with each dressing change; if you recognize early signs of infection start treatment before dehiscence or evisceration can occur.
■ If local infection develops, clean the wound, as necessary, to eliminate a buildup of purulent drainage.
■ Make sure bandages aren't so tight that they limit blood supply to the wound.

Complications

■ Infection

- Peritonitis
- Septic shock
- Necrosis

Documentation

Note when the problem occurred. Record the patient's activity preceding the problem. Document the patient's condition and the time the practitioner was notified. Describe the appearance of the wound or eviscerated organ; the amount, color, consistency, and odor of drainage; and nursing actions taken. Record vital signs, the patient's response to the incident, and the practitioner's actions. Change the care plan to reflect nursing actions needed to promote proper healing.

Wound irrigation

Irrigation cleans tissues and flushes cell debris and drainage from an open wound. Irrigation with a commercial wound cleaner helps the wound heal properly from the inside tissue layers outward to the skin surface; it also helps prevent premature surface healing over an abscess pocket or infected tract. Performed properly, wound irrigation requires strict sterile technique. After irrigation, open wounds usually are packed to absorb additional drainage. Always follow the standard precaution guidelines of the Centers for Disease Control and Prevention (CDC).

Equipment

Waterproof trash bag ♦ linen-saver pad ♦ emesis basin ♦ clean gloves ♦ sterile gloves ♦ goggles ♦ gown, if indicated ♦ prescribed irrigant such as sterile normal saline solution ♦ sterile water or normal saline solution ♦ soft rubber or plastic catheter ♦ sterile container ♦ materials as needed for wound care ♦ sterile irrigation and dressing set ♦ commercial wound cleaner ♦ 30-ml piston syringe with 19G needle or catheter ♦ skin protectant wipe

Preparation

- Assemble all equipment in the patient's room. Check the expiration date on each sterile package and inspect for tears. Check the sterilization date and the date that each bottle of irrigating solution was opened; don't use any solution that's been open longer than 24 hours.
- Using aseptic technique, dilute the prescribed irrigant to the correct proportions with sterile water or normal saline solution, if necessary. Let the solution stand until it reaches room temperature, or warm it to 90° to 95° F (32.2° to 35° C).
- Open the waterproof trash bag, and place it near the patient's bed. Position the bag to avoid reaching across the sterile field or the wound when disposing of soiled articles. Form a cuff by turning down the top of the trash bag to provide a wide opening, which will keep instruments or gloves from touching the bag's edge, thus preventing contamination.

Key steps

- Check the practitioner's order, and assess the patient's condition. Identify the patient's allergies, especially to povidone-iodine or other topical solutions or medications.
- Explain the procedure to the patient, provide privacy, and position the patient correctly for the procedure. Place the linen-saver pad under the patient to catch any spills and avoid linen changes. Place the emesis basin below the wound so that the irrigating solution flows from the wound into the basin.
- Wash your hands thoroughly. If necessary, put on a gown to protect your clothing from wound drainage and contamination. Put on clean gloves.
- Remove the soiled dressing; then discard the dressing and gloves in the trash bag.
- Establish a sterile field with all the equipment and supplies you'll need for irrigation and wound care. Pour the prescribed amount of irrigating solution into a sterile container so you won't contaminate your sterile gloves later by picking up unsterile containers. Put on sterile gloves, gown, and goggles, if indicated.
- Fill the syringe with the irrigating solution; then connect the catheter to the syringe. Gently instill a slow, steady stream of irrigating solution into the wound until the syringe empties. (See *Irrigating a deep wound.*) Make sure the solution flows from

the clean to the dirty area of the wound to prevent contamination of clean tissue by exudate. Also make sure the solution reaches all areas of the wound.

- Refill the syringe, reconnect it to the catheter, and repeat the irrigation.
- Continue to irrigate the wound until the solution returns clear. Note the amount of solution administered. Then remove and discard the catheter and syringe in the waterproof trash bag.
- Keep the patient positioned to allow further wound drainage into the basin.
- Clean the area around the wound with normal saline solution; wipe intact skin with a skin protectant wipe and allow it to dry well to help prevent skin breakdown and infection.
- Pack the wound, if ordered, and apply a sterile dressing. Remove and discard your gloves and gown.
- Make sure the patient is comfortable.
- Properly dispose of drainage, solutions, and trash bag, and clean or dispose of soiled equipment and supplies according to facility policy and CDC guidelines. To prevent contamination of other equipment, don't return unopened sterile supplies to the sterile supply cabinet.

Special considerations

- Try to coordinate wound irrigation with the practitioner's visit so that he can inspect the wound.
- Use only the irrigant specified by the practitioner because others may be erosive or otherwise harmful.
- Remember to follow your facility's policy and CDC guidelines concerning wound and skin precautions.
- Irrigate with a bulb syringe if the wound is small or not particularly deep or if a piston syringe is unavailable. However, use a bulb syringe cautiously because this type of syringe doesn't deliver enough pressure to adequately clean the wound.

Complications

- Increased risk of pain and excoriation from wound irrigation
- Trauma to the wound due to pressure over 15 psi that directs bacteria back into the tissue

Irrigating a deep wound

When preparing to irrigate a wound, attach a 19G needle or catheter to a 30-ml piston syringe. This setup delivers an irrigation pressure of 8 psi, which is effective in cleaning the wound and reducing the risk of trauma and wound infection. To prevent tissue damage or, in an abdominal wound, intestinal perforation, avoid forcing the needle or catheter into the wound.

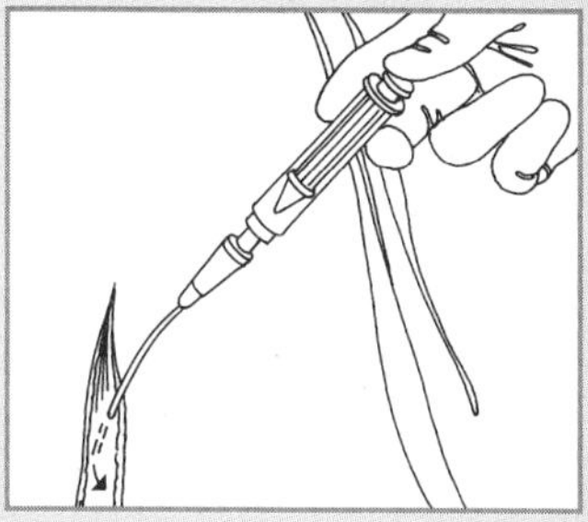

Irrigate the wound with gentle pressure until the solution returns clean. Then position the emesis basin under the wound to collect any remaining drainage.

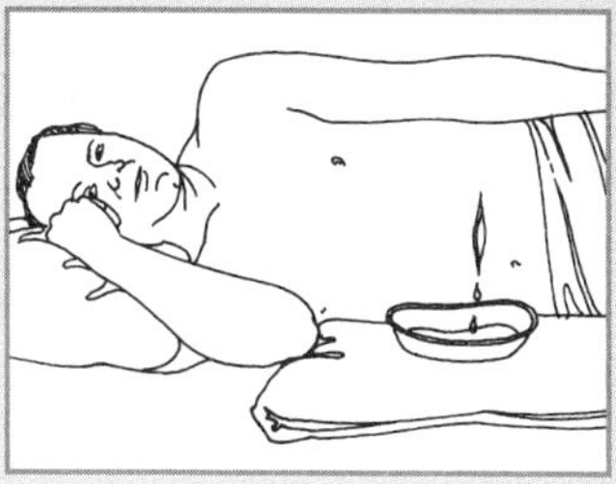

Patient teaching

- If the wound must be irrigated at home, teach the patient or a family member how to perform this procedure using strict aseptic technique. Ask for a return demonstration of the proper technique. Provide written instructions.
- Arrange for home health supplies and nursing visits, as appropriate.

Choosing a dressing

Wounds aren't static entities; their needs change as they progress or deteriorate. Ongoing assessment of the wound is critical for successful management. Use a general performance-based approach to choose a wound dressing, following these guidelines:

- Examine the wound and the periwound skin to determine exactly what the wound needs.
- Review product literature and examine the comparative clinical studies to determine what the product does and how well it performs.
- Assess the patient's medical and psychosocial status to determine what the patient needs.
- Evaluate what's available in your facility, what's covered by the patient's insurance, and what's practical, focusing on the goal of treatment.

Adapted with permission from Ovington, L.G., and Schaum, K.D. "Wound Care Products: How to Choose," *Home Healthcare Nurse* 19(4):224-32, 240, April 2001.

- Urge the patient to call the practitioner if he detects signs of infection.

Documentation

Record the date and time of irrigation, amount and type of irrigant, appearance of the wound, sloughing tissue or exudate, amount of solution returned, skin care performed around the wound, dressings applied, and the patient's tolerance of the treatment.

Wound management, surgical

The primary goal of surgical wound management is the promotion of healing and the prevention of infection. The two primary methods used to manage a draining surgical wound are dressing and pouching. Dressing is preferred unless caustic or excessive drainage is compromising your patient's skin integrity. Usually, lightly seeping wounds with drains and wounds with minimal purulent drainage can be managed with packing and gauze dressings. Some wounds, such as those that become chronic, may require an occlusive dressing.

A wound with copious, excoriating drainage calls for pouching to protect the surrounding skin. If your patient has a surgical wound, you must monitor him and choose the appropriate dressing.

Dressing a wound calls for sterile technique and sterile supplies to prevent contamination. To choose a dressing, use a performance-based approach focusing primarily on what the wound needs. (See *Choosing a dressing.*)

Be sure to change the dressing often enough to keep the skin dry. Always follow standard precautions set forth by the Centers for Disease Control and Prevention (CDC).

Equipment

Waterproof trash bag ♦ clean gloves ♦ sterile gloves ♦ gown and face shield or goggles, if indicated ♦ sterile 4″ × 4″ gauze pads ♦ large absorbent dressings, if indicated ♦ sterile cotton-tipped applicators ♦ sterile dressing set ♦ povidone-iodine swabs ♦ topical medication, if ordered ♦ adhesive or other tape ♦ soap and water ♦ optional: skin protectant, nonadherent pads, collodion spray or acetone-free adhesive remover, sterile normal saline solution, graduated container, Montgomery straps, a fishnet tube elasticized dressing support, or a T-binder

Wound with a drain

Sterile scissors ♦ sterile 4″ × 4″ gauze pads without cotton lining ♦ sump drain ♦ ostomy pouch or another collection bag ♦ sterile precut tracheostomy pads or drain dressings ♦ adhesive tape (paper or silk tape if the patient is hypersensitive) ♦ surgical mask

Pouching a wound
Collection pouch with drainage port ♦ sterile gloves ♦ skin protectant ♦ sterile gauze pads

Preparation
- Ask the patient about allergies to tapes and dressings.
- Assemble all equipment in the patient's room.
- Check the expiration date on each sterile package, and inspect for tears.
- Open the waterproof trash bag, and place it near the patient's bed. Position the bag to avoid reaching across the sterile field or the wound when disposing of soiled articles.
- Form a cuff by turning down the top of the trash bag to provide a wide opening and to prevent contamination of instruments or gloves by touching the bag's edge.

Key steps
- Premedicate the patient for pain if indicated, 20 minutes before dressing change.
- Explain the procedure to the patient to allay his fears and ensure his cooperation.

Removing the old dressing
- Check the practitioner's order for specific wound care and medication instructions. Be sure to note the location of surgical drains to avoid dislodging them during the procedure.
- Assess the patient's condition.
- Identify the patient's allergies, especially to adhesive tape, povidone-iodine or other topical solutions, or medications.
- Provide the patient with privacy, and position him as necessary. To avoid chilling him, expose only the wound site.
- Wash your hands thoroughly. Put on a gown and face shield, if necessary. Put on clean gloves.
- Loosen the soiled dressing by holding the patient's skin and pulling the tape or dressing toward the wound. This protects the newly formed tissue and prevents stress on the incision. Moisten the tape with acetone-free adhesive remover, if necessary, to make the tape removal less painful (particularly if the skin is hairy). Don't apply solvents to the incision because they could contaminate the wound.
- Slowly remove the soiled dressing. If the gauze adheres to the wound, loosen the gauze by moistening it with sterile normal saline solution.
- Observe the dressing for the amount, type, color, and odor of drainage.
- Discard the dressing and gloves in the waterproof trash bag.

Caring for the wound
- Wash your hands. Establish a sterile field with all the equipment and supplies you'll need for suture-line care and the dressing change, including a sterile dressing set and povidone-iodine swabs. If the practitioner has ordered ointment, squeeze the needed amount onto the sterile field. If you're using an antiseptic from a nonsterile bottle, pour the antiseptic cleaning agent into a sterile container so you won't contaminate your gloves. Put on sterile gloves. (See *How to put on sterile gloves,* page 612.)
- Saturate the sterile gauze pads with the prescribed cleaning agent. Avoid using cotton balls because they may shed fibers in the wound, causing irritation, infection, or adhesion.
- If ordered, obtain a wound culture, and then proceed to clean the wound.
- Pick up the moistened gauze pad or swab, and squeeze out the excess solution.
- Working from the top of the incision, wipe once to the bottom, and then discard the gauze pad. With a second moistened pad, wipe from top to bottom in a vertical path next to the incision (as shown below).

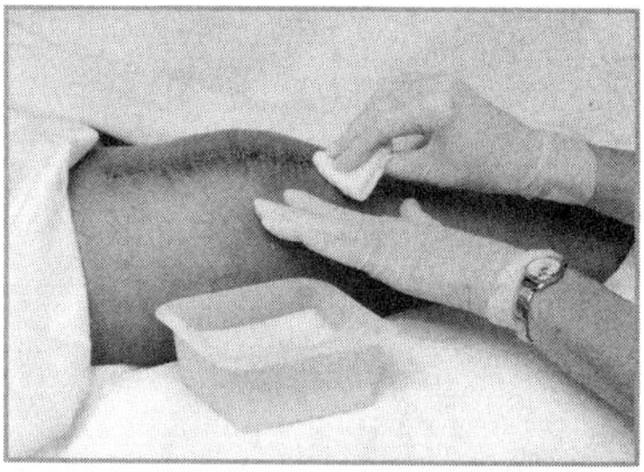

How to put on sterile gloves

1. Using your nondominant hand, pick up the opposite glove by grasping the exposed inside of the cuff.

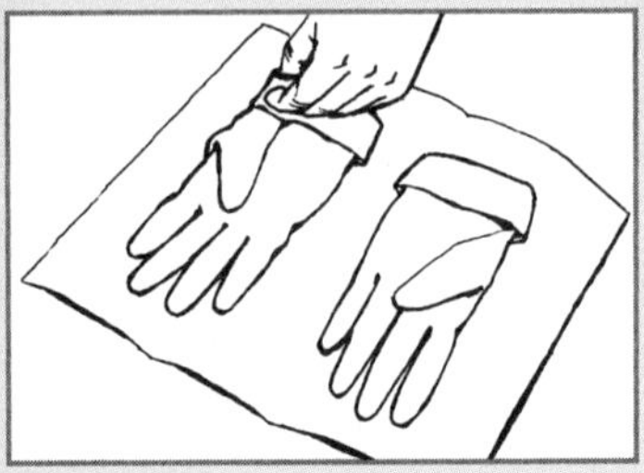

2. Pull the glove onto your dominant hand. Be sure to keep your thumb folded inward to avoid touching the sterile part of the glove. Allow the glove to come uncuffed as you finish inserting your hand, but don't touch the outside of the glove.

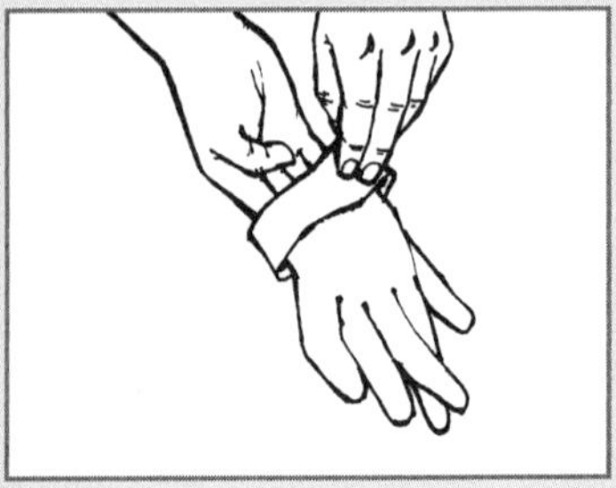

3. Slip the gloved fingers of your dominant hand under the cuff of the loose glove to pick it up.

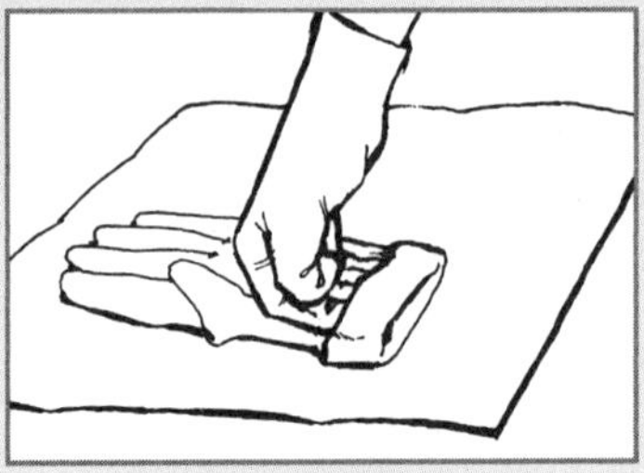

4. Slide your nondominant hand into the glove, holding your dominant thumb as far away as possible to avoid brushing against your arm. Allow the glove to come uncuffed as you finish putting it on, but don't touch the skin side of the cuff with your other gloved hand.

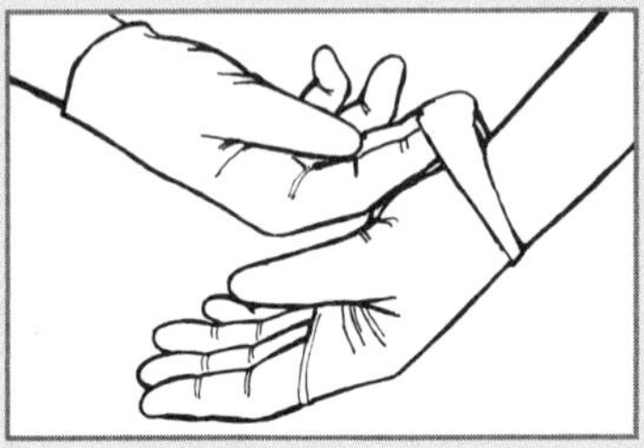

- Continue to work outward from the incision in lines running parallel to it. Always wipe from the clean area toward the less clean area (usually from top to bottom). Use each gauze pad or swab for only one stroke to avoid tracking wound exudate and normal body flora from surrounding skin to the clean areas. Remember that the suture line is cleaner than the adjacent skin and the top of the suture line is usually cleaner than the bottom because more drainage collects at the bottom of the wound.
- Use sterile cotton-tipped applicators for efficient cleaning of tight-fitting wire sutures, deep and narrow wounds, or wounds with pockets. Because the cotton on the swab is tightly wrapped, it's less likely than a cotton ball to leave fibers in the wound. Remember to wipe only once with each applicator.
- If the patient has a surgical drain, clean the drain's surface last. Because moist drainage promotes bacterial growth, the drain is considered the most contaminated area. Clean the skin around the drain by wiping in half or full circles from the drain site outward.
- Clean all areas of the wound to wash away debris, pus, blood, and necrotic material. Try not to disturb sutures or irritate the incision. Clean to at least 1″ (2.5 cm) beyond the end of the new dressing. If you

aren't applying a new dressing, clean to at least 2″ (5 cm) beyond the incision.

- Check to make sure the edges of the incision are lined up properly, and check for signs of infection (heat, redness, swelling, induration, and odor), dehiscence, or evisceration. If you observe such signs or if the patient reports pain at the wound site, notify the practitioner.
- Irrigate the wound, as ordered.
- Wash skin surrounding the wound with soap and water, and pat dry using a sterile 4″ × 4″ gauze pad. Avoid oil-based soap because it may interfere with pouch adherence. Apply any prescribed topical medication.
- Apply a skin protectant, if needed.
- If ordered, pack the wound with gauze pads or strips folded to fit, using sterile forceps. Pack the wound using the wet-to-damp method. Soaking the packing material in solution and wringing it out so it's slightly moist provides a moist wound environment that absorbs debris and drainage. But removing the packing won't disrupt new tissue.

DO'S & DON'TS

Don't pack the wound tightly; doing so will exert pressure and may damage the wound.

Applying a fresh gauze dressing

- Gently place sterile 4″ × 4″ gauze pads at the center of the wound, and move progressively outward to the edges of the wound site. Extend the gauze at least 1″ beyond the incision in each direction, and cover the wound evenly with enough sterile dressings (usually two or three layers) to absorb all drainage until the next dressing change. Use large absorbent dressings to form outer layers, if needed, to provide greater absorbency.
- Secure the dressing's edges to the patient's skin with strips of tape to maintain the sterility of the wound site (as shown top of next column). Or secure the dressing with a T-binder or Montgomery straps to prevent skin excoriation, which may occur with repeated tape removal necessitated by frequent dressing changes. (See *How to make Montgomery straps,* page 614.) If the wound is on a limb, secure the dressing with a fishnet tube elasticized dressing support.

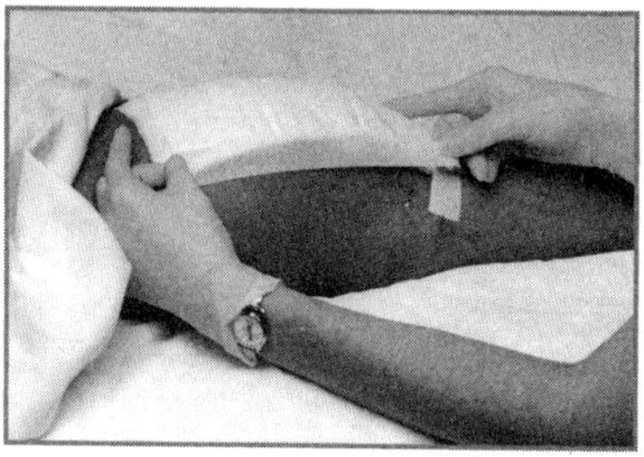

- Make sure the patient is comfortable.
- Properly dispose of the solutions and trash bag, and clean or discard soiled equipment and supplies according to facility policy. If your patient's wound has purulent drainage, don't return unopened sterile supplies to the sterile supply cabinet because this could cause cross-contamination of other equipment.

Dressing a wound with a drain

- Prepare a drain dressing by using sterile scissors to cut a slit in a sterile 4″ × 4″ gauze pad. Fold the pad in half; then cut inward from the center of the folded edge. Don't use a cotton-lined gauze pad because cutting the gauze opens the lining and releases cotton fibers into the wound. Prepare a second pad the same way, or use commercially precut gauze.
- Gently press one folded pad close to the skin around the drain so that the tubing fits into the slit. Press the second folded pad around the drain from the opposite direction so that the two pads encircle the tubing.
- Layer as many uncut sterile 4″ × 4″ gauze pads or large absorbent dressings around the tubing as needed to absorb expected drainage. Tape the dressing in place, or use a T-binder or Montgomery straps.

Pouching a wound

- If your patient's wound is draining heavily or if drainage may damage surrounding skin, you'll need to apply a pouch.

How to make Montgomery straps

An abdominal dressing requiring frequent changes can be secured with Montgomery straps to promote the patient's comfort. If ready-made straps aren't available, follow these steps to make your own:

- Cut four to six strips of 2" to 3" wide hypoallergenic tape of sufficient length, allowing the tape to extend about 6" (15 cm) beyond the wound on each side. (The length of the tape varies, depending on the patient's size and the type and amount of dressing.)
- Fold one of each strip 2" to 3" back on itself (sticky sides together) to form a nonadhesive tab. Cut a small hole in the folded tab's center, close to its top edge. Make as many pairs of straps as you'll need to snugly secure the dressing.
- Clean the patient's skin to prevent irritation. After the skin dries, apply a skin protectant. Apply the sticky side of each tape to a skin barrier sheet composed of opaque hydrocolloidal or nonhydrocolloidal materials, and apply the sheet directly to the skin near the dressing. Next, thread a separate piece of gauze tie, umbilical tape, or twill tape (about 12" [30.5 cm]) through each pair of holes in the straps, and fasten each tie as you would a shoelace. Don't stress the surrounding skin by securing the ties too tightly.
- Repeat this procedure according to the number of Montgomery straps needed.
- Replace Montgomery straps whenever they become soiled (every 2 to 3 days). If skin maceration occurs, place new tapes about 1" (2.5 cm) away from any irritation.

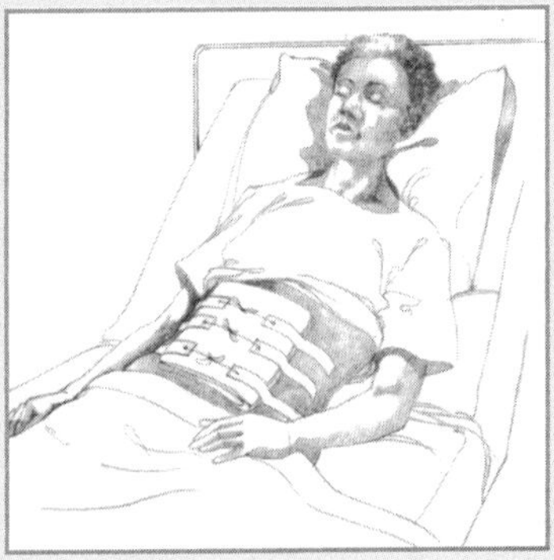

- Measure the wound. Cut an opening ⅜" (1 cm) larger than the wound in the facing of the collection pouch (as shown below).

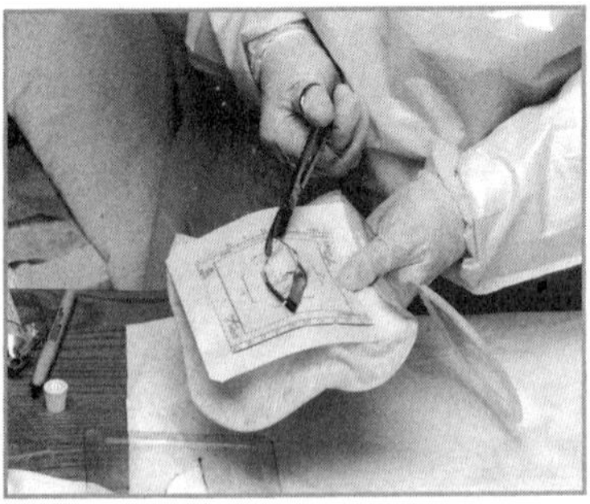

- Apply a skin protectant as needed. (Some protectants are incorporated within the collection pouch and also provide adhesion.)
- Before you apply the pouch, keep in mind the patient's usual position. Plan to position the pouch's drainage port so that gravity facilitates drainage.
- Make sure the drainage port at the bottom of the pouch is closed firmly to prevent leaks. Gently press the contoured pouch opening around the wound, starting at its lower edge, to catch drainage (as shown below).

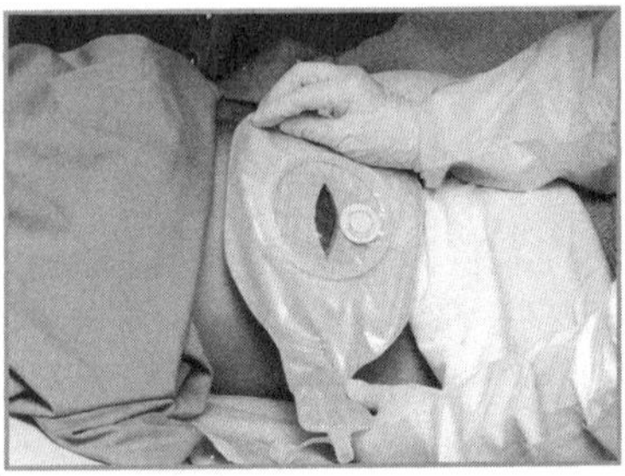

▪ To empty the pouch, put on gloves and a face shield or mask and goggles to avoid splashing. Insert the pouch's bottom half into a graduated biohazard container, and open the drainage port (as shown below). Note the color, consistency, odor, and amount of fluid. If ordered, obtain a culture specimen and send it to the laboratory immediately. Remember to follow the CDC's standard precautions when handling infectious drainage.

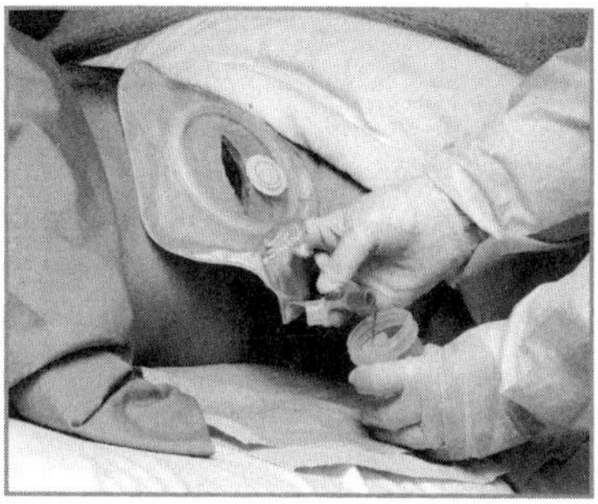

▪ Wipe the bottom of the pouch and the drainage port with a gauze pad to remove drainage that could irritate the patient's skin or cause an odor. Reseal the port. Change the pouch only if it leaks or fails to adhere. More frequent changes are unnecessary and only irritate the patient's skin.

Special considerations

▪ If the patient has two wounds in the same area, cover each wound separately with layers of sterile 4″ × 4″ gauze pads. Cover each site with a large absorbent dressing secured to the patient's skin with tape. Don't use a single large absorbent dressing to cover both sites because drainage quickly saturates a pad, promoting cross-contamination.

▪ When packing a wound, don't pack it too tightly because this compresses adjacent capillaries and may prevent the wound edges from contracting. Avoid overlapping damp packing onto surrounding skin because it macerates the intact tissue.

▪ To save time when dressing a wound with a drain, use precut tracheostomy pads or drain dressings instead of custom-cutting gauze pads to fit around the drain. If your patient is sensitive to adhesive tape, use paper or silk tape because it's less likely to cause a skin reaction and will peel off more easily than adhesive tape. Use a surgical mask to cradle a chin or jawline dressing; this provides a secure dressing and avoids the need to shave the patient's hair.

▪ If ordered, use a collodion spray or similar topical protectant instead of a gauze dressing. Moisture- and contaminant-proof, this covering dries in a clear, impermeable film that leaves the wound visible for observation and avoids the friction caused by a dressing.

▪ If a sump drain isn't adequately collecting wound secretions, reinforce it with an ostomy pouch or another collection bag. Use waterproof tape to strengthen a spot on the front of the pouch near the adhesive opening; then cut a small "X" in the tape. Feed the drain catheter into the pouch through the "X" cut. Seal the cut around the tubing with more waterproof tape, and then connect the tubing to the suction pump. This method frees the drainage port at the bottom of the pouch so you don't have to remove the tubing to empty the pouch. If you use more than one collection pouch for a wound or wounds, record drainage volume separately for each pouch. Avoid using waterproof material over the dressing because it reduces air circulation and promotes infection from accumulated heat and moisture.

▪ Because many practitioners prefer to change the first postoperative dressing themselves to check the incision, don't change the first dressing unless you have specific instructions. If you have no such order and drainage comes through the dressings, reinforce the dressing with fresh sterile gauze. Request an order to change the dressing, or ask the practitioner to change it as soon as possible. A reinforced dressing shouldn't remain in place longer than 24 hours because it's an excellent medium for bacterial growth.

▪ For the recent postoperative patient or a patient with complications, check the dressing every 15 to 30 minutes or as ordered. For the patient with a properly

Documenting surgical incision care

Besides documenting vital signs and the level of consciousness when the patient returns from surgery, pay particular attention to maintaining records pertaining to the surgical incision and drains and the care you provide. Read the records that travel with the patient from the postanesthesia care unit. Look for a physician's order to determine whether you or the physician will perform the first dressing change. Be sure to document:

- date, time, and type of wound management procedure
- amount of soiled dressing and packing removed
- wound appearance (including size, condition of margins, and presence of necrotic tissue) and odor (if present)
- type, color, consistency, and amount of drainage (for each wound); the presence and location of drains
- additional procedures, such as irrigation, packing, or application of a topical medication
- type and amount of new dressing or pouch applied
- patient's tolerance of the procedure.

healing wound, check the dressing at least once every 8 hours.

- If the dressing becomes wet from the outside (for example, from spilled drinking water), replace it as soon as possible to prevent wound contamination.

Complications

- Allergic reaction to an antiseptic cleaning agent, a prescribed topical medication, or adhesive tape leading to skin redness, a rash, excoriation, or infection
- Wound dehiscence and evisceration or infection

Patient teaching

- If your patient will need wound care after discharge, provide appropriate teaching.
- If he'll be caring for the wound himself, stress the importance of using aseptic technique, and teach him how to examine the wound for signs of infection and other complications. Show him how to change dressings, and give him written instructions for all procedures to be performed at home.

Documentation

Document special or detailed wound care instructions and pain management steps and the patient's response on the care plan. Record the color and amount of drainage on the intake and output sheet. (See *Documenting surgical incision care.*)

Wound management, traumatic

Traumatic wounds include abrasions, lacerations, puncture wounds, and amputations. In an abrasion, the skin is scraped, with partial loss of the skin surface. In a laceration, the skin is torn, causing jagged, irregular edges; the severity of a laceration depends on its size, depth, and location. A puncture wound occurs when a pointed object, such as a knife or glass fragment, penetrates the skin. Traumatic amputation refers to the removal of part of the body, a limb, or part of a limb.

When caring for a patient with a traumatic wound, first assess his ABCs—airway, breathing, and circulation. It may seem natural to focus on a gruesome injury, but a patent airway and pumping heart take first priority. Once the patient's ABCs are stabilized, you can turn your attention to the traumatic wound. Initial management concentrates on controlling bleeding, usually by applying firm, direct pressure and elevating the extremity. If bleeding continues, you may need to compress a pressure point. Assess the condition of the wound. Management and cleaning technique usually depend on the specific type of wound and degree of contamination.

Equipment

Sterile basin ♦ normal saline solution ♦ sterile 4″ × 4″ gauze pads ♦ sterile gloves ♦ clean gloves ♦ sterile cotton-tipped applicators ♦ dry sterile dressing, nonadherent pad, or petroleum gauze ♦ linen-saver pad ♦ optional: scissors, towel, goggles, mask, gown, 30-ml catheter-tip syringe, surgical scrub brush, antibacterial ointment, porous tape, sterile forceps, sutures and suture set, hydrogen peroxide

Preparation

- Place a linen-saver pad under the area to be cleaned. Remove any clothing covering the wound. If necessary, cut hair around the wound with scissors to promote cleaning and treatment.
- Assemble needed equipment at the patient's bedside.
- Fill a sterile basin with normal saline solution.
- Make sure the treatment area has enough light to allow close observation of the wound.
- Depending on the nature and location of the wound, wear sterile or clean gloves to avoid spreading infection.

Key steps

- Check the patient's medical history for previous tetanus immunization and, if needed and ordered, arrange for immunization.
- Administer pain medication, if ordered.
- Wash your hands.
- Use appropriate protective equipment, such as a gown, a mask, and goggles, if spraying or splashing of body fluids is possible.

Abrasion

- Flush the scraped skin with normal saline solution.
- Remove dirt or gravel with a sterile 4″ × 4″ gauze pad moistened with normal saline solution. Rub in the opposite direction from which the dirt or gravel became embedded.
- If the wound is extremely dirty, you may use a surgical brush to scrub it.
- With a small wound, allow it to dry and form a scab. With a larger wound, you may need to cover it with a nonadherent pad or petroleum gauze and a light dressing. Apply antibacterial ointment if ordered.

Laceration

- Moisten a sterile 4″ × 4″ gauze pad with normal saline solution. Clean the wound gently, working outward from its center to about 2″ (5 cm) beyond its edges. Discard the soiled gauze pad and use a fresh one as necessary. Continue until the wound appears clean.
- If the wound is dirty, you may irrigate it with a 30-ml catheter-tip syringe and normal saline solution.
- Assist the practitioner in suturing the wound edges using the suture kit, or apply sterile strips of porous tape.
- Apply the prescribed antibacterial ointment to help prevent infection.
- Apply a dry sterile dressing over the wound to absorb drainage and help prevent bacterial contamination.

Puncture wound

- If the wound is minor, allow it to bleed for a few minutes before cleaning it.
- For a larger puncture wound, you may need to irrigate it before applying a dry dressing.
- Stabilize any embedded foreign object until the physician can remove it. After he removes the object and bleeding is stabilized, clean the wound as you'd clean a laceration or deep puncture wound.

Amputation

- Apply a gauze pad moistened with normal saline solution to the amputation site. Elevate the affected part, and immobilize it for surgery.
- Recover the amputated part, and prepare it for transport to a facility where microvascular surgery is performed.

Special considerations

- When irrigating a traumatic wound, avoid using more than 8 psi of pressure. High-pressure irrigation can seriously interfere with healing, kill cells, and allow bacteria to infiltrate the tissue.
- To clean the wound, you may use normal saline or hydrogen peroxide (its foaming action facilitates debris removal). However, peroxide should never be instilled into a deep wound because of the risk of embolism from the evolving gases. Be sure to rinse your hands well after using hydrogen peroxide.
- Avoid cleaning a traumatic wound with alcohol because alcohol causes pain and tissue dehydration. Also, avoid using antiseptics for wound cleaning because they can impede healing. In addition, never use a cotton ball or cotton-filled gauze pad to clean a wound because cotton fibers left in the wound can cause contamination.
- After a wound has been cleaned, the physician may want to debride it to remove dead tissue and reduce the risk of infection and scarring. If this is necessary, pack the wound with gauze pads soaked in normal saline solution until debridement.
- Observe for signs and symptoms of infection, such as warm red skin at the site or purulent discharge. Be aware that infection of a traumatic wound can delay healing, increase scar formation, and trigger systemic infection, such as septicemia.
- Observe all dressings. If edema is present, adjust the dressing to avoid impairing circulation to the area.

Complications

- Temporary increase in patient's pain due to cleaning and care of traumatic wounds
- Further disruption of tissue integrity resulting from excessive, vigorous cleaning

Documentation

Document the date and time of the procedure, wound size and condition, medication administration, specific wound care measures, and patient teaching.

Z

Z-track injection

The Z-track method of I.M. injection prevents leakage, or tracking, into the subcutaneous tissue. It's typically used to administer drugs that irritate and discolor subcutaneous tissue, primarily iron preparations such as iron dextran. It may also be used in elderly patients who have decreased muscle mass. Lateral displacement of the skin during the injection helps to seal the drug in the muscle.

This procedure requires careful attention to technique because leakage into the subcutaneous tissue can cause patient discomfort and may permanently stain some tissues.

Equipment

Patient's medication record and chart ♦ two 20G 1¼″ to 2″ needles ♦ prescribed medication ♦ gloves ♦ 3- or 5-ml syringe ♦ two alcohol pads

Preparation

- Verify the order on the patient's medication record by checking it against the prescriber's order.
- Wash your hands.
- Make sure the needle you're using is long enough to reach the muscle. As a rule of thumb, a 200-lb (90.7-kg) patient requires a 2″ needle; a 100-lb (45-kg) patient, a 1¼″ to 1½″ needle.
- Attach one needle to the syringe, and draw up the prescribed medication. Then draw 0.2 to 0.5 cc of air (depending on facility policy) into the syringe.
- Remove the first needle and attach the second to prevent tracking the medication through the subcutaneous tissue as the needle is inserted.

Key steps

- Confirm the patient's identity using two patient identifiers according to facility policy. Explain the procedure, and provide privacy.
- If your facility uses a bar code scanning system, be sure to scan your ID badge, the patient's ID bracelet, and the medication's bar code.
- Place the patient in the lateral position, exposing the gluteal muscle to be used as the injection site. The patient may also be placed in the prone position.
- Clean an area on the upper outer quadrant of the patient's buttock with an alcohol pad.
- Put on gloves. Then displace the skin laterally by pulling it away from the injection site. (See *Displacing the skin for Z-track injection*, page 620.)
- Insert the needle into the muscle at a 90-degree angle.
- Aspirate for blood return; if none appears, inject the drug slowly, followed by the air. Injecting air after the drug helps clear the needle and prevents tracking the medication through subcutaneous tissues as the needle is withdrawn.
- Wait 10 seconds before withdrawing the needle to ensure dispersion of the medication.
- Withdraw the needle slowly. Then release the displaced skin and subcutaneous tissue to seal the needle track. Don't mas-

Displacing the skin for Z-track injection

By blocking the needle pathway after an injection, the Z-track technique allows I.M. injection while minimizing the risk of subcutaneous irritation and staining from such drugs as iron dextran. The illustrations here show how to perform a Z-track injection.

Before the procedure begins, the skin, subcutaneous fat, and muscle lie in their normal positions.

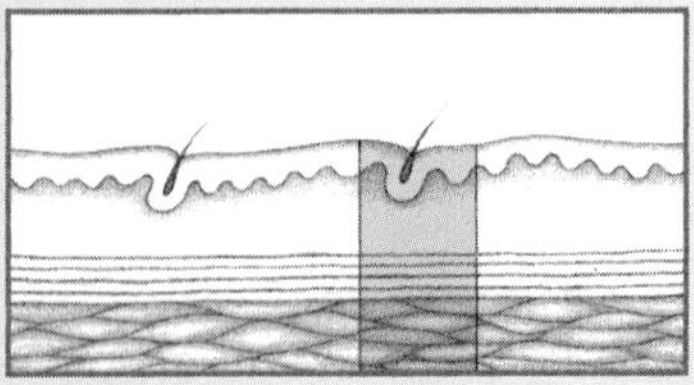

To begin, place your finger on the skin surface, and pull the skin and subcutaneous layers out of alignment with the underlying muscle. You should move the skin about ½" (1.3 cm).

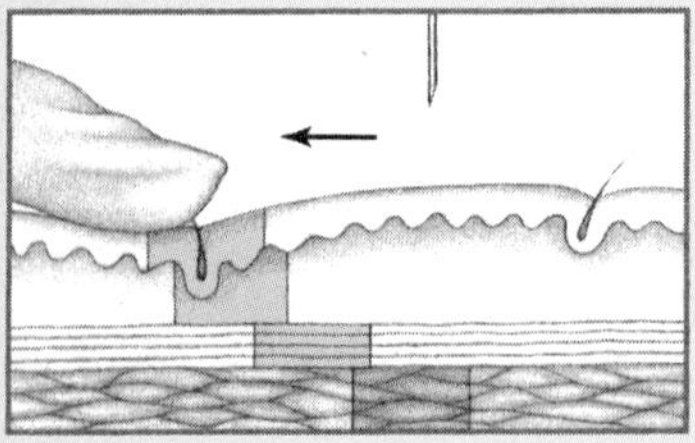

Insert the needle at a 90-degree angle at the site where you initially placed your finger. Inject the drug and withdraw the needle.

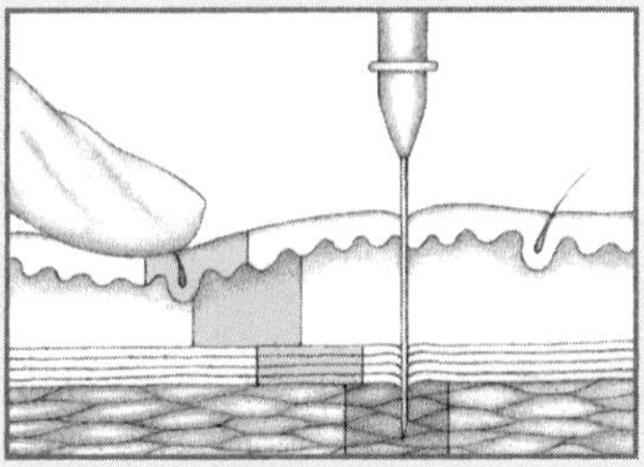

Finally, remove your finger from the skin surface, allowing the layers to return to their normal positions. The needle track (shown by the dotted line) is now broken at the junction of each tissue layer, trapping the drug in the muscle.

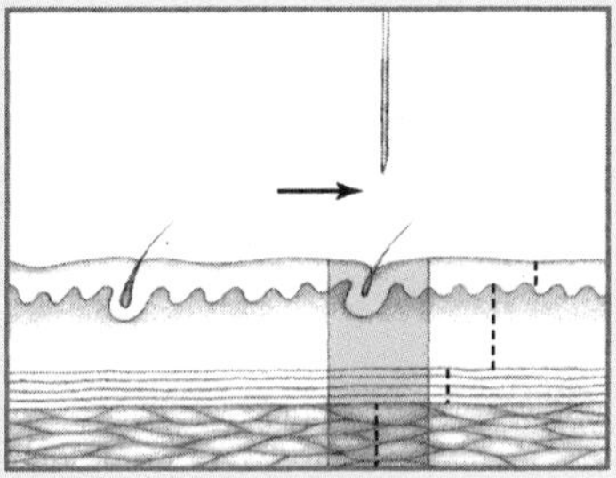

sage the injection site or allow the patient to wear a tight-fitting garment over the site because it could force the medication into subcutaneous tissue.
- Encourage the patient to walk or move about in bed to facilitate absorption of the drug from the injection site.
- Discard the needles and syringe in an appropriate sharps container. Don't recap needles to avoid needle-stick injuries.
- Remove and discard your gloves.

Special considerations
- Never inject more than 5 ml of solution into a single site using the Z-track method. Alternate gluteal sites for repeat injections.
- Always encourage the patient to relax the muscle you'll be injecting because injections into tense muscle are more painful and may bleed more readily.
- If the patient is on bed rest, encourage active range-of-motion (ROM) exercises or perform passive ROM exercises to facilitate absorption from the injection site.
- I.M. injections can damage local muscle cells, causing elevated serum enzyme levels (for example, of creatine kinase) that can be confused with the elevated enzyme levels resulting from damage to cardiac muscle, as in myocardial infarction. If measuring enzyme levels is important, suggest that the physician switch to I.V.

administration and adjust dosages accordingly.

Complications

- Discomfort and tissue irritation resulting from drug leakage into subcutaneous tissue
- Interference with medication absorption due to failure to rotate sites in patients who require repeated injections causing unabsorbed medications to build up in deposits; such deposits reducing the desired pharmacologic effect and leading to abscess formation or tissue fibrosis

Documentation

Record the medication, dosage, date, time, and site of injection on the patient's medication record. Include the patient's response to the injected drug.

Selected references

"2005 International Consensus on Cardiopulmonary Resuscitation and Emergency Cardiovascular Care," *Circulation* 112(suppl IV), 2005.

American Association for Respiratory Care. "AARC Clinical Guideline: Blood Gas Analysis and Hemoximetry. 2001 Revision and Update," *Respiratory Care* 46(5):498-505, May 2001.

American Association for Respiratory Care. "AARC Clinical Practice Guideline: Nasotracheal Suctioning," *Respiratory Care* 49(9):1080-84, September 2004.

American Association of Neuroscience Nurses. *Core Curriculum for Neuroscience Nursing,* 4th ed. Philadelphia: W.B. Saunders Co., 2004.

American Heart Association. "Practice Standards for Electrocardiographic Monitoring in Hospital Settings," *Circulation* 110:2721-46, 2004.

American Society of Anesthesiologists. "Practice Guidelines for Pulmonary Artery Catheterization: An Updated Report by the American Society of Anesthesiologist Task Force," *Anesthesiology* 99(4):988-1014, October 2003.

Baranoski, S., and Ayello, E. *Wound Care Essentials: Practice and Principles.* Philadelphia: Lippincott Williams & Wilkins, 2004.

Bickely, L., and Szilagyi, P. *Bates' Guide to Physical Examination and Health History Taking,* 9th ed. Philadelphia: Lippincott Williams & Wilkins, 2007.

The Brain Trauma Foundation. The American Association of Neurological Surgeons. The Joint Section on Neurotrauma and Critical Care. "Indications for Intracranial Pressure Monitoring," *Journal of Neurotrauma* 17(6-7):479-91. June-July 2000.

Bridges, E.J. "Monitoring Pulmonary Artery Pressures: Just the Facts," *Critical Care Nurse* 20(6):59-80, December 2000.

Canale, S. "Wrong-Site Surgery: A Preventable Complication," *Clinical Orthopaedics & Related Research* (433):26-29, April 2005.

Centers for Disease Control and Prevention. "Guidelines for Prevention of Intravascular Catheter-Related Infections," *Morbidity and Mortality Monthly Report* 51(rr-10):1-29, August 2002.

Centers for Disease Control and Prevention. National Institute for Occupational Safety and Health. "Latex Allergy: A Prevention Guide," Department of Health and Human Services (NIOSH) Publication No. 98-113. *www.cdc.gov/niosh/98-113.html*

Craven, R.F., and Hirnle, C.J. *Fundamentals of Nursing Human Health and Function,* 5th ed. Philadelphia: Lippincott Williams & Wilkins, 2006.

Garner, J.S. "Hospital Infection Control Practices Advisory Committee Guidelines for Isolation Precautions in Hospitals," *Infection Control and Hospital Epidemiology* 17(1):53-80, January 1996. *www.cdc.gov/ncidod/hip/isolat/isopart2.htm*

Geerts, W.H., et al. Seventh AACP Conference on Antithrombotic and Thrombolytic Therapy. "Prevention of Venous Thromboembolism," *Chest* 126(3 Suppl): 338S-400S, September 2004.

Gould, P.A., et al. "Biventricular Pacing in Heart Failure: A Review," *Expert Review of Cardiovascular Therapy* 4(1):97-109, January 2006.

Guenter, P., and Silkroski, M. *Tube Feeding: Practical Guidelines and Nursing Protocols.* Gaithersburg, Md.: Aspen Pubs., Inc., 2001.

Holmes, S.B., and Brown, S.J. "Skeletal Pin Site Care: NAON Guidelines for Orthopaedic Nursing," *Orthopaedic Nursing* 24(2):99-107, March-April 2005.

"Infusion Nursing Standard of Practice," *Journal of Intravenous Nursing* 29(1S), January-February 2006.

Joint Commission on Accreditation of Healthcare Organizations, "Patient Safety Goals 2006." *www.jcaho.org*

Kübler-Ross, E. *Questions and Answers on Death and Dying*. New York: Simon & Schuster, 1997.

Lynn-McHale Wiegand, D.J., and Carlson, K.K. *AACN Procedure Manual for Critical Care*, 5th ed. Philadelphia: W.B. Saunders Co., 2005.

Macklin, D. "How to Manage PICCs," *AJN* 97(9):26-33, September 1997.

Manno, M. "Preventing Adverse Drug Events," *Nursing* 36(3):56-61, March 2006.

McCalister, F., and Straus, S. "Evidenced-Based Treatment of Hypertension. Measurement of Blood Pressure: An Evidenced-Based Review," *British Medical Journal* 322(7291): 908-11, April 2001.

Mendez-Eastman, S. "Burn Injuries," *Plastic Surgical Nursing* 25(3):133-39, July-September 2005.

O'Hare, A., and Fenlon, H. "Virtual Colonoscopy in the Detection of Colonic Polyps and Neoplasms," Best Practice Research. *Clinical Gastroenterology* 20(1):79-92, February 2006.

Owen, B. "Preventing Injuries Using an Ergonomic Approach," *AORN Journal* 72(6): 1031-36, December 2000.

Perry, A., and Potter, P. *Clinical Nursing Skills and Techniques*, 6th ed. St Louis: Mosby–Year Book, Inc., 2005.

Phillips, L.D. *Manual of I.V. Therapeutics*, 3rd ed. Philadelphia: F.A. Davis Co., 2001.

Pruitt, B., and Jacobs, M., "Best-practice interventions: How can you prevent ventilator-associated pneumonia?" *Nursing* 36(2):36-41, February 2006.

Rebmann, T. "Management of Patient Infected with Airborne-Spread Diseases: An Algorithm for Infection Control Professionals," *American Journal of Infection Control* 33(10):571-79, December 2005.

Sluka, K.A. "The Basic Science Mechanisms of TENS and Clinical Implications," *APS Bulletin* 11(2), March- April 2001.

Task Force of the American College of Critical Care Medicaine, Society of Critical Medicine. "Practice Parameters for Hemodynamic Support of Sepsis in Adult Patients: 2004 Update," *Critical Care Medicine* 32(9):1928-48, September 2004.

Thomas, J., and Feliciano, C. "Measuring BP with a Doppler Device," *Nursing2003* 33(7):52-53, July 2003.

Tracy, S., et al., "Translating Best Practices in Nondrug Postoperative Pain Management.," *Nursing Research* 55(2) Supplement 1:S57-S67, March/April 2006.

Vengelen-Tyler, V., ed. *Technical Manual*, 13th ed. Bethesda, Md.: American Association of Blood Banks 1999.

Webb, J.G. "Percutaneous Aortic Valve Implantation Retrograde from the Femoral Artery," *Circulation* 113(6):842-50, February 2006.

Wipke-Tevis, D., and Sae-Sia, W. "Management of Vascular Leg Ulcers," *Advances in Skin & Wound Care* 18(8):446-47, October 2005.

Wojcik, J. "Central Venous Catheters," *Advance for Nurses* 7(23):25-28, October 2005.

Index

A

B

i refers to an illustration; t refers to a table.

C

i refers to an illustration; t refers to a table.

i refers to an illustration; t refers to a table.

F

G

i refers to an illustration; t refers to a table.

i refers to an illustration; t refers to a table.

J

K

L

M

i refers to an illustration; t refers to a table.

N

O

P

i refers to an illustration; t refers to a table.

i refers to an illustration; t refers to a table.

i refers to an illustration; t refers to a table.

i refers to an illustration; t refers to a table.

U

V

W

XY

Z

i refers to an illustration; t refers to a table.